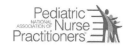

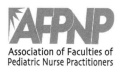

Association of Faculties of
Pediatric Nurse Practitioners

D1561156

CORE REVIEW FOR PRIMARY CARE PEDIATRIC NURSE PRACTITIONERS

Volume Editor

Victoria P. Niederhauser DrPH, APRN, BC, PNP
Associate Professor and Graduate Chair
Director, Nurse Practitioner Program
University of Hawaii
School of Nursing & Dental Hygiene
Honolulu, Hawaii

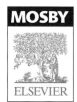

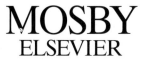

MOSBY
ELSEVIER

11830 Westline Industrial Drive
St. Louis, Missouri 63146

CORE REVIEW FOR PRIMARY CARE
PEDIATRIC NURSE PRACTITIONERS

ISBN-13: 978-0-323-02757-1
ISBN-10: 0-323-02757-1

Notice

Knowledge and best practice in this field are constantly changing. As new research and experience broaden our knowledge, changes in practice, treatment and drug therapy may become necessary or appropriate. Readers are advised to check the most current information provided (i) on procedures featured or (ii) by the manufacturer of each product to be administered, to verify the recommended dose or formula, the method and duration of administration, and contraindications. It is the responsibility of the practitioner, relying on their own experience and knowledge of the patient, to make diagnoses, to determine dosages and the best treatment for each individual patient, and to take all appropriate safety precautions. To the fullest extent of the law, neither the Publisher nor the Editor assumes any liability for any injury and/or damage to persons or property arising out or related to any use of the material contained in this book.

The Publisher

Library of Congress Cataloging-in-Publication Data
Library of Congress Control Number: 2006940734

Acquisitions Editor: Sandra Clark Brown
Senior Developmental Editor: Cindi Anderson
Publishing Services Manager: Gayle May
Project Manager: Tracey Schriefer
Design Direction: Amy Buxton

Working together to grow
libraries in developing countries

www.elsevier.com | www.bookaid.org | www.sabre.org

ELSEVIER   BOOK AID International   Sabre Foundation

Printed in the United States of America
Last digit is the print number: 9   8   7   6   5   4   3   2   1

Acknowledgements

This book would not be possible without the guidance, support and encouragement of many people. First, I would like to acknowledge the many authors, who through their daily work make a difference in the health and well being of children and families. In addition to demanding jobs and personal commitments, they found time to make significant contributions to this book. Secondly, I offer a big thanks to Karen Kelly-Thomas, the executive director of NAPNAP, for all her guidance and support throughout this endeavor. Thirdly, I would like to acknowledge the tremendous support of Dr. Shirley Menard, who reviewed all the chapters in this book. Finally, "Mahalo Nui Loa" to my husband, Glen, and three great children, Travis, Matt and Emily, who provide me love, laughter and wisdom on a daily basis.

The multiple choice questions and rationales in this book were created by nursing faculty and practicing clinicians. They have been reviewed by members of the Association of Faculties of Pediatric Nurse Practitioners; however the questions have not undergone in-depth psychometric testing. I welcome your feedback on the text, questions and rationales.

Victoria P. Niederhauser

Contributors

Patricia Jackson Allen, RN, MS, PNP, FAAN
Professor, Director of Pediatric Nurse
Practitioner Specialty
Yale University School of Nursing
New Haven, Connecticut
Chapter 27. Common Illness of the Head, Eyes, Ears, Nose, and Throat; Chapter 28. Common Illness of the Pulmonary System

Shirley A. Alvaro, APRN, CPNP, MPH, MS
Faculty/Clinical Instructor
Community Health Nursing & Nurse
Practitioner Programs
University of Hawaii School of Nursing &
Dental Hygiene
Honolulu, Hawaii
Chapter 19. Newborns and Infants

Richelle T. Magday Asselstine, MS, RN, CMC
RN Care Coordinator
Shriners Hospital for Children
Honolulu, Hawaii
Chapter 48. Juvenile Rheumatoid Arthritis

Cheri Barber, MSN, CRNP
Coordinator, Pediatric Nurse Practitioner
Program
Thomas Jefferson University
Jefferson College of Health Professions
Jefferson School of Nursing
Philadelphia, Pennsylvania
Chapter 10. Assessment of the Integumentary System

Lisa Marie Bernardo, PhD, MPH, RN, HFI
Associate Professor
University of Pittsburgh School of Nursing
Pittsburgh, Pennsylvania
Chapter 52. Readiness for Handling Pediatric Emergencies in the Primary Care Office

Linda S. Blasen, MS, APRN, BC, ACNP, FNP
Instructor
USF Health College of Nursing
University of South Florida
Tampa, Florida
Associate Lecturer
Fitzgerald Health Education Associates, Inc.
North Andover, Massachusetts
Chapter 57. Nonpharmacologic Treatments and Pediatric Procedures

Stephanie Bonney, MS, RN, CPNP
Pediatric Nurse Practitioner
St. Mary's Hospital for Children
Bayside, New York
Chapter 44. Diabetes Types 1 and 2

Mirella Vasquez Brooks, APRN, MSN, PhD, FNP
Assistant Professor
School of Nursing & Dental Hygiene
University of Hawaii
Honolulu, Hawaii
Chapter 47. Hemoglobinopathies

Terry A. Buford, RN, CPNP, PhD
Clinical Associate Professor
University of Missouri-Kansas City
School of Nursing
Kansas City, Missouri
Chapter 36. Asthma

Janet M. Camacho, APRN, MSN, MPH, CPNP
Certified Pediatric Nurse Practitioner
Kaiser Permanente
Honolulu, Hawaii
Chapter 15. Immunizations

Maria S. Chico, RN, MS, CCRN, CPNP
Pediatric Nurse Practitioner
Comprehensive Epilepsy Program
Medical College of Wisconsin
Children's Hospital of Wisconsin
Milwaukee, Wisconsin
Chapter 46. Epilepsy

Kari Crawford, MS, APRN, BC, CPNP-AC
Pediatric Nurse Practitioner
Brenner Children's Hospital
Winston-Salem, North Carolina
*Chapter 42. Congenital Heart Disease; Chapter
58. Evolving Roles for Pediatric Nurse
Practitioners*

**Sharron L. Docherty, PhD, CPNP-AC
(AC/PC)**
Assistant Professor
Director, Pediatric Acute/Chronic Care
Advanced Practice Specialty
Duke University School of Nursing
Pediatric Nurse Practitioner
Valvano Day Hospital
Duke University Medical Center
Durham, North Carolina
Chapter 38. Childhood Cancer

Karen Duderstadt, MS, RN, CPNP
Associate Clinical Professor
Department of Family Health Care Nursing
School of Nursing
University of California San Francisco
San Francisco, California
*Chapter 13. Assessment of the Neurologic
System*

Amy K. Foy, MSN, CPNP
Pediatric Nurse Practitioner
Tuckahoe Orthopaedics
Richmond, Virginia
*Chapter 24. Sports Participation: Evaluation
and Monitoring; Chapter 55. Pain Management
in Children*

**Mary Margaret Gottesman, PhD, RN,
CPNP, FAAN**
Associate Professor, Clinical
Pediatric Nurse Practitioner Specialty
Program Director
College of Nursing
The Ohio State University
Columbus, Ohio
*Chapter 17. Preconceptional and Prenatal Role of
the Pediatric Nurse Practitioner*

**Mary Enzman Hagedorn, RN, PhD, CNS,
CPNP, AHN-BC**
Professor
Beth-El College of Nursing and Health
Sciences
University of Colorado
Colorado Springs, Colorado
Chapter 20. Preterm Infant Follow-up Care

**Mary Blaszko Helming, PhD, APRN, BC,
FNP, AHN-BC**
Assistant Professor of Nursing
Family Nurse Practitioner Track Coordinator
Quinnipiac University
Hamden, Connecticut
*Chapter 11. Assessment of the Hematologic and
Lymphatic Systems*

Gail Hornor, RNC, MS, CPNP
Pediatric Nurse Practitioner
Center for Child and Family Advocacy
Children's Hospital
Columbus, Ohio
*Chapter 9. Assessment of the Reproductive and
Urologic Systems*

Amy J. Howells RN, CPNP
Pediatric Nurse Practitioner
Texas Children's Hospital
Baylor College of Medicine
Houston, Texas
*Chapter 53. Diagnostic Tests for Pediatric
Clinical Decision Making*

Dana K. Ing, MSN, APRN, NNP
Certified Neonatal Clinician
Kaiser Permanente
Honolulu, Hawaii
*Chapter 18. Care of the Newborn Before Hospital
Discharge*

Jean B. Ivey, DSN, PNP
Associate Professor
Coordinator Pediatric Graduate Options
University of Alabama School of Nursing
University of Alabama at Birmingham
Birmingham, Alabama
Chapter 26. Sexuality and Birth Control

Ritamarie John, CPNP, DrNP
Assistant Professor of Clinical Nursing
Columbia University
New York, New York
Chapter 35. Common Illness of the Neurologic System

Melanie S. Klein, MSN, CNP
Nurse Practitioner
University Hospitals of Cleveland
Rainbow Babies and Children's Hospital
Cleveland, Ohio
Chapter 50. Renal Failure

Joyce M. Knestrick, PhD, FNP, ARNP-BC
Associate Professor of Nursing
Wheeling Jesuit University
Wheeling, West Virginia
Family Nurse Practitioner
Primary Care Center of Mt. Morris
Mt. Morris, Pennsylvania
Chapter 29. Common Illness of the Cardiovascular System

Patricia Biller Krauskopf , PhD, RN, APRN, BC, FNP
Coordinator, Family Nurse Practitioner Program
Assistant Professor
Shenandoah University
Winchester, Virginia
Chapter 14. Core Concepts in Genetics; Chapter 16. Nutrition

Irma Lara, RN, MSN, FNP, BC
Assistant Professor
Texas A&M International University
Laredo, Texas
Chapter 2. Essential Elements of the Advanced Practice Role for Pediatric Nurse Practitioners; Chapter 40. Common Genetic Conditions in Children; Chapter 54. Pharmacodynamic Considerations Unique to Neonates, Infants, Children, and Adolescents

Lori Lei Lundberg, RN, MNE, CMC
RN Care Coordinator
Shriners Hospital for Children
Honolulu, Hawaii
Chapter 37. Cerebral Palsy

Margaret Anne McNulty, DrPH, APRN, FNP-C, PNP-C
Assistant Professor
Department of Nursing
University of Hawaii at Manoa
Honolulu, Hawaii
Chapter 31. Common Illness of the Reproductive and Urologic Systems

MaryAnne C. Murray, MSN, EdD, APRN-BC, FNP
Family Nurse Practitioner
Oakland Bay Pediatrics
Shelton, Washington
Chapter 21. Child Abuse and Neglect

Victoria P. Niederhauser DrPH, APRN, BC, PNP
Associate Professor and Graduate Chair
Director, Nurse Practitioner Program
University of Hawaii
School of Nursing & Dental Hygiene
Honolulu, Hawaii
Chapter 7. Assessment of the Cardiovascular System; Chapter 39. Cleft Lip and Palate

Lois Pancratz, ARNP
Coordinator, Family Nurse Practitioner Program
Clarke College
Dubuque, Iowa
Chapter 43. Cystic Fibrosis

Ruey Jane Ryburn, DrPH, RN, AHN-BC
Professor Emeritus
School of Nursing
University of Hawaii
Director
Sacred Path Healing, LLC
Honolulu, Hawaii
Chapter 56. Complementary and Alternative Therapy

Rose A. Saldivar, MSN, FNP, BC
Assistant Professor
Canseco School of Nursing
Texas A & M International University
Laredo, Texas
Chapter 2. Essential Elements of the Advanced Practice Role for Pediatric Nurse Practitioners; Chapter 40. Common Genetic Conditions in Children; Chapter 54. Pharmacodynamic Considerations Unique to Neonates, Infants, Children, and Adolescents

Barbara Hoyer Schaffner, PhD, CPNP
Chair, Professor of Nursing
Otterbein College
Westerville, Ohio
Chapter 34. Common Illness of the Musculoskeletal System

Naomi A. Schapiro, RN, MS, CPNP
Associate Clinical Professor
Department of Family Health Care Nursing
University of California San Francisco
School of Nursing
San Francisco, California
Chapter 25. Early Adolescents, Late Adolescents, and College-age Young Adults

Vicki W. Sharrer, MS, RN, CPNP
Professor, Department of Nursing
Ohio University-Zanesville
Zanesville, Ohio
Chapter 32. Common Illness of the Integumentary System

Deborah Shelton, PhD, RN, BC
Associate Dean for Research
Associate Professor
School of Nursing
University of Connecticut
Storrs, Connecticut
Chapter 23. Mental Health Promotion and Mental Health Screening for Children and Adolescents; Chapter 41. Common Mental Health Disorders in Children and Adolescents; Chapter 49. Learning Disorders and Attention Deficit Hyperactivity Disorder

Leigh Small, PhD, RN, CPNP
Assistant Professor & Coordinator
Pediatric Nurse Practitioner Graduate Program
College of Nursing and Health Care Innovation
Arizona State University
Phoenix, Arizona
Chapter 8. Assessment of the Gastrointestinal System; Chapter 30. Common Illness of the Gastrointestinal System

Mary Sobralske, PhD, MSN, APRN
Nurse Practitioner
Pediatric Orthopedics
Shriners Hospital for Children
Honolulu, Hawaii
Chapter 12. Assessment of the Musculoskeletal System

Mariailiana J. Stark DrPH, APRN, CPNP
Assistant Professor
Department of Nursing
University of Hawaii at Manoa
Child Developmental Specialist
Kaiser Permanente
Honolulu, Hawaii
Chapter 4. Measures of Child Growth and Development; Chapter 22. Toddlers, Preschoolers, and School-agers; Chapter 31. Common Illness of the Reproductive and Urologic Systems

Stacey Teicher, MS, RN-CS, CNS, CPNP
Pediatric Nurse Practitioner
Pediatric Nurse Practitioner
Oakland Children's Hospital
Oakland, California
Chapter 58. Evolving Roles for Pediatric Nurse Practitioners

Michele A. Tholcken, RN, MSN, CPNP, CRRN, RN-BSN
Assistant Professor
Director RN-BSN Program
School of Nursing
University of Texas Medical Branch
Undergraduate Program
Galveston, Texas
Chapter 51. Spina Bifida and Other Myelodysplasias

Paula Grace Dunn Tropello, BS, MN, EdD, FNP
Associate Professor
Evelyn L. Spiro School of Nursing
Wagner College
Staten Island, New York
Chapter 1. Evolution of the Pediatric Nurse Practitioner Role

Julee Waldrop, MS, FNP, PNP
Clinical Associate Professor
School of Nursing and School of Medicine
The University of North Carolina
Chapel Hill, North Carolina
Chapter 5. Assessment of the Head, Eyes, Ears, Nose, and Throat; Chapter 6. Assessment of the Pulmonary System

Kiersten Wells, CPNP
Certified Pediatric Nurse Practitioner
Department of Pediatric Cardiology
Lucille Packard Children's Hospital
Palo Alto, California
Chapter 45. Eating Disorders

Diane M. Wink, EdD, FNP, ARNP
Professor
University of Central Florida School of Nursing
Orlando, Florida
Chapter 3. Clinical Reasoning and Clinical Decision-Making

Adele E. Young
Assistant Professor
College of Health & Human Services
George Mason University
Fairfax, Virginia
Chapter 33. Common Illness of the Hematologic and Lymphatic Systems

Reviewers

Linda S. Gilman, MSN, EdD
Associate Professor
Department of Family Health
Indiana University School of Nursing
Indianapolis, Indiana

Jean B. Ivey, DSN, CRNP
Associate Professor and Coordinator,
Pediatric Graduate Options
The University of Alabama at Birmingham
Birmingham, Alabama

Jean T. Martin, DNSc, RN, CPNP
Associate Professor
Kirkhof College of Nursing
Director of Graduate Programs
Grand Valley State University
Grand Rapids, Michigan

Shirley Menard, PhD, RN, CPNP, FAAN
Retired Professor
University of Texas Health Science Center
San Antonio, Texas

Beth Richardson DNS, RN, CPNP
Associate Professor
Coordinator of the Pediatric Nurse
Practitioner Program
Indiana University School of Nursing
Indianapolis, Indiana

Contents

Preface

AFPNP and NAPNAP are pleased to present the review questions that accompany the 2006 Core Curriculum for Primary Care Pediatric Nurse Practitioners edited by Nancy Ryan-Wenger and contributed to by more than 50 NAPNAP members and other nurse practitioners. These review questions correspond to each chapter in the 2006 Core Curriculum for Primary Care Pediatric Nurse Practitioners.

Preparing for a new role, a new job, and even certification is an anxious time. We sincerely hope that these review questions will stimulate your thinking and help you in your review of knowledge needed to take care of children you see in your primary care practice.

Readers will find these self assessment questions useful primarily in testing knowledge acquired as a result of reading and reviewing the Core Curriculum. These questions have not been tested over time for reliability and validity. We welcome all feedback about specific questions and overall questions related to each chapter. We hope to continuously improve this review exercise as a means to help nurse practitioners caring for children assess knowledge acquired as a result of reading the core curriculum.

Best wishes in your new role.

Pat Clinton, PhD, RN, CPNP, FAANP
President, NAPNAP

Patricia Jackson, MS, PNP, FAAN
President, AFPNP

ROLE OF THE NURSE PRACTITIONER

1 Evolution of the Pediatric Nurse Practitioner Role

PAULA GRACE DUNN TROPELLO

Select the best answer for each of the following questions:

1. The original nurse practitioner program was a joint project between Dr. Loretta Ford and Dr. Henry Silver at which of the following medical university complexes?
   A. University of Kansas.
   B. University of Colorado.
   C. University of Virginia.
   D. Boston University.

2. The original nurse practitioner program was institutionalized as a(n):
   A. Geriatric program.
   B. Adult program.
   C. Pediatric program.
   D. Women's health program.

3. The two chief disciplines involved in establishing the role expansion were:
   A. Sociology and nursing.
   B. Sociology and medicine.
   C. Psychology and nursing.
   D. Nursing and medicine.

4. The initial rationales for the creation of the expanded nursing role included all of the following EXCEPT that:
   A. An increased need existed for child health services.
   B. Nurses could assume a role in extending child health services.
   C. Nurses could be taught to do physical exams and counsel.
   D. Nurses could work in inpatient settings providing acute care management.

5. Titles early on included which of the following?
   A. Pediatric nurse clinicians.
   B. Pediatric nurse practitioners.
   C. Pediatric nurse associates.
   D. All of the above.

6. Degrees required were not initially standardized and included certification beyond:
   A. Master's degree.
   B. Bachelor's degree.
   C. Associate's degree or diploma.
   D. All of the above.

7. The first recognized formal nurse practitioner demonstration project began in:
   A. 1952.
   B. 1970.
   C. 1965.
   D. 1980.

8. The very first nurse practitioner membership organization to form was:
   A. NAPNAP.
   B. AANP.
   C. AAWH.
   D. AACCN.

9. By 2005, there were at least how many programs for pediatric nurse practitioners?
   A. More than 100.
   B. Just over 50.
   C. Fewer than 50.
   D. None of the above.

10. The first meeting of NAPNAP took place with what group in 1973?
   A. AMA

B. ACOG
C. AAP
D. ANCC

11. Goals of NAPNAP continue to be relevant and include all of the following EXCEPT:
A. Standards development for pediatric nurse practitioner education and practice.
B. Provision of continuing education relevant to pediatrics.
C. Support of legislation to improve child health.
D. Donate money to important child heath organizations.

12. Which of the following was NOT a part of the 2000 strategic planning model?
A. Education and research.
B. Health policy leadership.
C. Practice collaboration.
D. Disciplinary issues.

13. The rationale for forming a separate certification board from NAPNAP in 1975 was:
A. To ensure a high quality standard of certification.
B. To incorporate practice and educational excellence in evaluation.
C. To satisfy state boards as more nurse practitioners began training and concerns about competencies emerged.
D. All of the above.

14. To sit for certification by the National Certification Board of Pediatric Nurse Practitioners, the nurse must hold a minimum of a:
A. Bachelor's degree.
B. Post-master's degree.
C. Master's degree.
D. Associate's degree.

15. Which of the following are examples of marketing to increase pediatric nurse practitioner recognition?
A. *The PNP Advantage.*
B. *Why a PNP Is Right for Your Child.*
C. Both of the above.
D. Neither "a" nor "b."

16. The legislative listserv was created for all of the following purposes EXCEPT to:
A. Inform about legislative issues.
B. Alert pediatric nurse practitioners on issues in the legislature affecting their practice.
C. Allow rapid dissemination of legislative information.
D. Allow for members of Congress to get in touch with their constituents.

17. One of the most effective campaigns to slow infant deaths caused by SIDS is:
A. ASTRA campaign.
B. KySS campaign.
C. Baby Steps campaign.
D. Back to Sleep campaign.

18. The SIDS campaign that is presently effective in the U.S. caused NAPNAP to do which of the following in order to show its support?
A. Put the SIDS initials on the NAPNAP logo.
B. Add a logo of a baby in the prone position.
C. Eliminate its logo of a sleeping baby in the prone position.
D. Donate money to the campaign.

19. What is the title of NAPNAP's official journal now?
A. *Pediatric Nursing.*
B. *Maternal and Child Health Nursing.*
C. *Journal of Pediatric Health Care.*
D. *Baby Steps.*

20. NAPNAP hired a lobbyist to work in Washington, D.C. to assist with legislative issues. The lobbyist visited several members of Congress to discuss the negative effects of passing a bill to ban thimerisol-containing vaccinations. This would be an example of:
A. Removing barriers to pediatric nurse practitioner practice.
B. Representing pediatric nurse practitioners' health-related concerns.
C. Advocating for children's programs.
D. Negotiating areas of reimbursement in managed care.

21. Two levels of ANCC credentialing and their acronyms are:
   A. Board Certified (BC) and Certified (RN,C).
   B. Certified (CPNP) and Board Certified (BC, PNP).
   C. Board Certified (C, PNP) and Certified (RN,C).
   D. Certified (NC) and Board Certified (NCB).

22. Pediatric nurse practitioners who are certified through the PNCB use the credential:
   A. PNP.
   B. PNPC.
   C. CPNP.
   D. PNCB.

23. Presently, in the majority of states, a pediatric nurse practitioner may do all the following EXCEPT:
   A. Receive third-party reimbursement.
   B. Prescribe medications.
   C. Receive Medicaid and Medicare reimbursement.
   D. Work completely independently.

NOTES

ANSWERS

1. *Answer:* B
   Rationale: The first nurse practitioner program was established at the University of Colorado.

2. *Answer:* C
   Rationale: The program was institutionalized as a pediatric nurse practitioner program.

3. *Answer:* D
   Rationale: The two disciplines involved in program startup were nursing and medicine, Dr. Ford and Dr. Silver.

4. *Answer:* D
   Rationale: The rationale for the expanded role included the extension of child health services, teaching nurses to conduct physical examinations, diagnose and manage illness, and counseling. The acute care role was not part of the initial rationale for the expanded role for nurses.

5. *Answer:* D
   Rationale: All of the titles of pediatric nurse associates, nurse clinicians, and pediatric nurse practitioners were utilized initially.

6. *Answer:* D
   Rationale: Degrees were not standardized at first, but included all who went through the certificate program.

7. *Answer:* C
   Rationale: The first nurse practitioner program began in 1965.

8. *Answer:* A
   Rationale: The very first ever membership organization for nurse practitioners was NAPNAP.

9. *Answer:* A
   Rationale: There were over 100 pediatric nurse practitioner programs in 2005.

10. *Answer:* C
    Rationale: The first meeting of the NAPNAP took place with the AAP.

11. *Answer:* D
    Rationale: The goals of NAPNAP still include setting standards, continuing education, and support of legislation to improve child health. Donating money is not a goal of NAPNAP.

12. *Answer:* D
    Rationale: Discipline was not part of the NAPNAP 2000 strategic planning model.

13. *Answer:* D
    Rationale: A separate board was formed apart from NAPNAP for certification purposes.

14. *Answer:* C
    Rationale: To become certified by this organization, a nurse must hold a minimum of a master's degree now.

15. *Answer:* C
    Rationale: Marketing pediatric nurse practitioner role was the goal of *The PNP Advantage* and *Why a PNP Is Right for Your Child*.

16. *Answer:* D
    Rationale: The listserv is useful for information dissemination and to alert pediatric nurse practitioners about important legislative issues. The listserv does not allow individual Congress members to contact their constituents.

17. *Answer:* D
    Rationale: The Back to Sleep Campaign is effective against SIDS.

18. *Answer:* C
    Rationale: NAPNAP eliminated its prone sleeping logo to support the Back to Sleep Campaign.

19. *Answer:* C
    Rationale: The official journal title today for NAPNAP is the *Journal of Pediatric Health Care*.

20. *Answer:* B
    Rationale: Lobbyists are hired for Washington to advocate for children, remove prac-

tice barriers, and negotiate the health care system. This is an example of how the lobbyist can address pediatric health-related concerns of NAPNAP members.

21. *Answer:* A
Rationale: The two levels of ANCC credentialing are Board Certified and Certified and the acronyms are BC and RN,C, respectively.

22. *Answer:* C
Rationale: The correct credential to utilize in writing for a certified pediatric nurse practitioner through the PNCB is CPNP.

23. *Answer:* D
Rationale: Pediatric nurse practitioners can receive third-party reimbursement, prescribe, and receive Medicare and Medicaid payments. To date, 14 states permit nurse practitioners to practice independently, 23 states require some type of collaborative agreement as a condition for practice, and 13 states still use supervisory language in their practice act.

BIBLIOGRAPHY

American Nurses Credentialing Center (ANCC). (2005). ANCC certification for professional nurses—certifying excellence in nursing practice. Retrieved on March 7, 2006 from http://nursingworld.org/ancc/inside.html.

Clinton, P., Novak, J.C. (2001). NAPNAP and NCBPNP: A history intertwined. *PNP Newsletter, 12*(6), 1-2.

Ford, L.C. (1994). Nurse practitioners: Myths and misconceptions. An article excerpted from "Myths and misconceptions regarding the nurse practitioner" in "Critical issues in American nursing in the twentieth century," (1994), published by the Foundation of the New York State Nurses Association, Inc. *Pulse, 32*(4), 9-10.

Ford, L.C. (1997). A voice from the past: 30 fascinating years as a nurse practitioner. *Clin Ex Nurse Pract, 1*(1), 3-6.

Ford, L.C. (1999). NP 2000. Thoughts for the 21st century. *Nurse Pract: Am J Prim Health Care, 24*(5), 17.

HEAT (2006). "Healthy eating and activity together" initiative. Retrieved on March 8, 2006 from http://www.napnap.org/index.cfm?page=198&sec=220.

Hobbie, C. (1998). NAPNAP: The first 25 years. *J Pediatr Health Care, 28*(5), part 2, S3-S8.

KySS (2006). "Keep your children/yourself safe and secure" program. Retrieved on March 8, 2006 from http://www.napnap.org/index.cfm?page=198&sec=221.

National Association of Pediatric Nurse Practitioners Annual Reports 1973–74 to 2002-2003.

National Association of Pediatric Nurse Practitioners. (2004). *Scope and standards of practice.* Cherry Hill, NJ: NAPNAP.

National Association of Pediatric Nurse Practitioners. (2006a). About NAPNAP. Retrieved on March 8, 2006 from www.napnap.org/index.cfm?page=9.

National Association of Pediatric Nurse Practitioners. (2006b). Position statements. Retrieved on March 8, 2006 from http://www.napnap.org/index.cfm?page=10&sec=54.

Pediatric Nurses Certification Board (PNCB). (2005). Personal communication with executive director Jan Wyatt on June 29, 2005. See also www.pncb.org/ptistore/control/index.

Pulcini, J., Wagner, M. (2002). Nurse practitioner education in the United States: A success story. *Clin Ex Nurse Pract, 6*(2), 51-56.

2

Essential Elements of the Advanced Practice Role for Pediatric Nurse Practitioners

ROSE A. SALDIVAR AND IRMA LARA

Select the best answer for each of the following questions:

1. As part of a health fair activity, a pediatric nurse practitioner provides immunization screening and health education to a community group. What ethical principle most likely underlies the decision to offer this activity?
   A. Autonomy
   B. Justice
   C. Beneficence
   D. Fidelity

2. Seatbelt laws, bicycle safety helmet laws, and child safety restraint laws present a conflict between which ethical principles?
   A. Veracity and beneficence.
   B. Autonomy and fidelity.
   C. Justice and veracity.
   D. Nonmaleficence and autonomy.

3. While conducting a community assessment of an inner-city housing development, through data collection from high crime rate statistics, a nurse practitioner has identified safety issues as a community need. Community residents were surveyed to collect further data. A high-priority need which they identified was recreation activities or playground areas for their children. The pediatric nurse practitioner's decision to address the community residents' recreational needs is an example of which ethical principle?
   A. Autonomy.
   B. Respect for others.
   C. Justice.
   D. Veracity.

4. Agencies like the Joint Commission on Accreditation of Healthcare Organizations (JCAHO) have an established process for assessing quality of care or services in which an organization demonstrates that it meets a set of minimum standards. What is this process called?
   A. Certification.
   B. Licensure.
   C. Accreditation.
   D. Quality assurance/quality improvement.

5. Which ethical principle supports the public health system of the United States?
   A. Beneficence
   B. Justice
   C. Fidelity
   D. Veracity

6. The process performed by a health care institution which grants the nurse practitioner specific authority to perform designated clinical activities in their facility is termed:
   A. Credentialing.
   B. Accrediting.
   C. Privileging.
   D. Certification.

7. Mrs. Garcia is new to your clinic. She comments to you that she recently took her 1-month-old son to a *curandero* (spiritual healer) for fever. As a culturally competent nurse practitioner, the most appropriate initial response to Mrs. Garcia's comment would be:
   A. Advising Mrs. Garcia not to return to the *curandero*.
   B. Advising Mrs. Garcia to continue to see the *curandero*.

C. Asking Mrs. Garcia what occurred during the visit to the *curandero.*

D. Informing Mrs. Garcia that folk medicine interferes with western medicine.

8. Levels of prescriptive authority for a pediatric nurse practitioner vary from state to state. Which of the following statements is correct?

A. Prescription authority (including controlled substances) for a pediatric nurse practitioner is independent of physician involvement in approximately half of the states.

B. Prescription authority (including controlled substances) for a pediatric nurse practitioner has some degree of physician involvement or delegation of prescription writing in more that half of the states.

C. Prescription authority (excluding controlled substances) for a pediatric nurse practitioner is independent of physician involvement in approximately half of the states.

D. Prescription authority (excluding controlled substances) for a pediatric nurse practitioner is not independent of physician involvement in all of the states.

9. Mrs. Rodriques is a first-time mom of a 1-year-old baby girl. She brings her child to the clinic with complaints of fever, abdominal pain, and emesis. Ms. Rodriques states that she feels this to be a punishment from God (*castigo*) for not breastfeeding her child. As the pediatric nurse practitioner, your best response is to:

A. Inform Mrs. Rodriques that her belief is not the best approach to use.

B. Disregard Mrs. Rodriques' beliefs and discuss medical conditions that can cause stomach pain.

C. Accept Mrs. Rodriques' belief, but explain that the child may need further examination and treatment.

D. Encourage Mrs. Rodriques to seek her culture's folk healer (*curandero*) to manage the pain.

10. Long-term planning of health care in the United States should include data on trends in the ethnicity of the country. It has been estimated that by the early twenty-first century, over 50% of the population will be minority, with the largest group being:

A. African American.

B. Asian American.

C. Hispanic American.

D. Native American.

11. The American Medical Association (AMA) publishes current procedural terminology (CPT) codes yearly. Guidelines for evaluation and management (E/M) services use descriptors for these services. These descriptors recognize seven components. These are history, examination, medical decision making, counseling, coordination of care, nature of presenting problem, and time. Key components identified by AMA for use when selecting a level of E/M service are:

A. Counseling, coordination of care, and nature of presenting problem.

B. Examination, medical decision making, and counseling.

C. Medical decision making, coordination of care, and time.

D. History, examination, and medical decision making.

12. The American Medical Association (AMA) publishes current procedural terminology (CPT) codes yearly. Guidelines for evaluation and management (E/M) services use descriptors for these services. These descriptors recognize seven components. These are history, examination, medical decision making, counseling, coordination of care, nature of presenting problem, and time. Contributory factors identified by the AMA important to E/M services but are NOT required to be provided in every patient encounter are:

A. Counseling, coordination of care, and nature of presenting problem.

B. Examination, medical decision making, and counseling.

C. Medical decision making, coordination of care, and time.

D. History, examination, and medical decision making.

13. Under which authority can a pediatric nurse practitioner receive and/or dispense medication samples?
    A. Scope of Practice.
    B. Board of Medical Examiners.
    C. Pharmacy Practice Act.
    D. Health Care Financing Agency.

14. In order for a pediatric nurse practitioner to prescribe controlled substances, he or she must apply for and receive a:
    A. Medicaid number.
    B. Drug Enforcement Agency (DEA) number.
    C. Food and Drug Agency (FDA) number.
    D. Medicare number.

15. Amy, a pediatric nurse practitioner, is asking about national certification examinations. Which of the following organizations provide certification for pediatric nurse practitioners?
    A. American Academy of Pediatrics (AAP).
    B. Pediatric Nurse Certification Board (PNCB).
    C. American Academy of Nurse Practitioners (AANP).
    D. Society for Pediatric Nurses (SPN).

16. Which governing agency grants pediatric nurse practitioners a Medicare personal identification number (PIN)?
    A. Health Care Financing Administration.
    B. State Department of Health.
    C. Joint Commission Accreditation of Health Care Organization.
    D. National Association of Pediatric Nurse Practitioners.

17. A new graduate pediatric nurse practitioner working at the local clinic believes that current procedural terminology (CPT) coding for services is the function and responsibility of the billing department. Who is responsible for utilizing this coding?
    A. Insurance provider.
    B. Health care provider at time of service.
    C. Clinic billing department.

    D. Contractual department.

18. What is the best definition for a collaborative practice agreement, otherwise known as an *employment contract*?
    A. Verbal legally binding agreement between the employer and prospective employee.
    B. Written legally binding agreement between the employer and prospective employee.
    C. Written legally binding agreement between the government and prospective employee.
    D. Verbal legally binding agreement between the government and prospective employee.

19. Andy, a 2-month-old Hispanic infant, is brought in for a well baby check. The mother tells you that the infant's grandmother wants her to place a charm on a string that the baby wears as a necklace to fight of the evil spirit (*mal de ojo*). A culturally sensitive response would be to:
    A. Ignore the comment and go on with your well baby check.
    B. Inform the mother that the charm is ineffective and serves no purpose.
    C. Inform the mother that the grandmother's suggestion is inaccurate and she should not listen to her.
    D. Inform the mother to keep the charm on the string and to place this around the baby's wrist to avoid a choking incident.

20. Andy's grandmother becomes offended because you have suggested that they ignore her request to apply a charm necklace to ward off the evil spirits (*mal de ojo*). To be culturally sensitive means:
    A. Familiarizing yourself with the Hispanic culture and understanding that the patient's family would not object to your request to remove the charm.
    B. Looking after the child's safety and best interest and not worrying about what the patient's family thinks.
    C. Understanding that you insulted the patient's family and placed the nurse-patient relationship at risk.

D. Acknowledging the grandmother's offense and continue with your exam.

21. A pediatric nurse practitioner is offered a position in the pediatric outpatient clinic at a health maintenance organization. The human resources manager asks where she went to nurse practitioner school and what organization granted her national certification. The pediatric nurse practitioner asks why she needs this information. The HRM replies, "We need this information for:
   A. Credentialing.
   B. Privileging.
   C. Security validation.
   D. Licensure.

22. What is the Advanced Practice Registered Nurse Compact (APRN)?
   A. An agreement between selected states for mutual recognition of RN and APRN licenses to practice.
   B. An agreement between the government for mutual recognition of RN and APRN licenses to practice.
   C. An agreement between the local governing agencies to keep RN and APRN licenses in practice.
   D. An agreement between schools of nursing for mutual recognition of RN and APRN licenses to practice.

23. Medicare will reimburse pediatric nurse practitioners at what fee for services?
   A. 100%
   B. 75%
   C. 85%
   D. 90%

24. Which of the following is the specialty organization for pediatric nurse practitioners?
   A. Advance Pediatric Nurse Practitioners Association (APNPA).
   B. National Pediatric Nurse Practitioners Association (NPNPA).
   C. National Association of Pediatric Nurses and Practitioners (NAPNAP).
   D. National Advance Pediatric Nurse Association (NAPNA).

25. Which of the following theories used by pediatric nurse practitioners proceeds from the simple to the complex?
   A. Structural functional theory.
   B. Communication theory.
   C. General systems theory.
   D. Developmental theory.

ANSWERS

1. **Answer:** C
   Rationale: Beneficence is the desire to act in the best interest of others. It is perhaps the strongest guiding ethical principle of health professionals.

2. **Answer:** D
   Rationale: Autonomy is the right of an individual to self-determination, where an individual freely governs his or her own actions. Nonmaleficence is to do no harm. The act of nonmaleficence is violated by omission and putting others at risk. An individual can decide not to use a child safety restraint and thus place the child at risk for harm.

3. **Answer:** B
   Rationale: Respect for others is the capacity to appreciate and recognize other people's judgments or beliefs. Selecting to work with community residents on their perceived needs versus those perceived by others is an example of respect for others.

4. **Answer:** C
   Rationale: Accreditation is process for assessing quality of care or quality of services. An organization must demonstrate that it meets a set of minimum standards in order to receive accreditation.

5. **Answer:** B
   Rationale: Justice is the fair distribution of rights and resources. Allocation of resources is fair and of greatest good to the most people.

6. **Answer:** C
   Rationale: Privileging is the correct response. Credentialing is performed by the employing institution to validate a pediatric nurse practitioner's licensure, educational preparation, and certification in a clinical practice area. National organizations, such as ANCC, use predetermined standards in certification to validate a nurse's knowledge, skills, and ability in a clinical area.

7. **Answer:** C

Rationale: A culturally competent provider accepts the rights of others to participate with their health care provider. Options (a) and (c) are not sensitive to a person's health care beliefs. Option (b) does not expand on the visit to the spiritual healer so that a complementary approach could be considered.

8. **Answer:** B
   Rationale: Prescriptive authority for the pediatric nurse practitioner, which includes controlled substances, has some degree of physician involvement or delegation of prescription writing with written documentation in 39 states, and without written documentation in one state.

9. **Answer:** C
   Rationale: A culturally competent provider recognizes cultural issues and interacts with patients in culturally sensitive ways. Options (a) and (b) are not sensitive to a person's health care belief. Option (d) does not expand on the visit to the spiritual healer so that a complementary approach could be considered.

10. **Answer:** C
    Rationale: The Census Bureau projects that by 2040, there will be 87.5 million Hispanic individuals, comprising 22.3% of the population.

11. **Answer:** D
    Rationale: Evaluation and management services guidelines identify history, examination, and medical decision making as the key components in selecting a level of E/M services. These components must be present in every patient encounter.

12. **Answer:** A
    Rationale: The American Medical Association publishes CPT codes yearly. Evaluation and management service guidelines identify counseling, coordination of care, and nature of presenting problem as the contributory components in selecting a level of E/M service. Counseling and coordination of care are important E/M services but are not

required to be provided in every patient encounter.

13. *Answer:* A
    Rationale: Nurse practitioners are required to follow their practicing state's standards and guidelines when dispensing drug samples. Nurse practitioners may acquire, store, dispense, and dispose of medications in accordance with state and federal legislation.

14. *Answer:* B
    Rationale: Nurse practitioners with full authorization to practice and valid prescription authorization are eligible to prescribe certain categories of controlled substances. After the controlled substances permit has been issued, the nurse practitioners may apply for a Drug Enforcement Agency registration number.

15. *Answer:* B
    Rationale: The PNCB certifies pediatric nurse practitioners. Certification is valid for 7 years and requires annual documentation.

16. *Answer:* A
    Rationale: Nurse practitioners can bill directly for their services or reassign payments to an employer with Medicare personal identification number (PIN). Health Care Financing Administration (HCFA) is a federal agency of the U.S. Department of Health and Human Services. HCFA administers the Medicare and Medicaid programs.

17. *Answer:* B
    Rationale: American Medical Association publishes the CPT manual. All CPT coding is the responsibility of the health care provider at the time the service is provided.

18. *Answer:* B
    Rationale: A contract is an agreement between two or more parties, especially if it is written and enforceable by law.

19. *Answer:* D
    Rationale: Mal de ojo, or evil eye, is a Hispanic belief that results when a person with "strong eyes" looks at a child. To be cultur-

ally sensitive requires an awareness of or acceptance of *mal de ojo* which would have allowed one to recognize that the charm was placed there to protect the infant.

20. *Answer:* C
    Rationale: Showing respect for the dignity of all human beings, acceptance of families' rights to choose care providers and type of care, acknowledging your own personal beliefs and biases, recognizing cultural issues, and acting in a culturally sensitive manner are all ways the pediatric nurse practitioner can provide culturally sensitive care. In this case, the pediatric nurse practitioner recognizes that she has placed her relationship with the patient in jeopardy because she was not sensitive to this cultural practice.

21. *Answer:* A
    Rationale: Credentialing occurs once the pediatric nurse practitioner is hired by an institution. Credentialing collects, assesses, and validates professional licensure, clinical experiences, educational preparation, certification, references, and professional activity. Privileging is the process that an employer conducts to grant authority to perform designated clinical activities.

22. *Answer:* A
    Rationale: Currently 18 states participate in the Nurse Licensure Compact Agreement. This agreement allows nurses to practice in participating member states without relicensure. Nurses may be licensed in more than one state either by examination or by the endorsement of a license issued by another state.

23. *Answer:* C
    Rationale: Medicare will compensate pediatric nurse practitioners 85% of the physician fee schedule.

24. *Answer:* C
    Rationale: The National Association of Pediatric Nurses and Practitioners is the specialty organization for pediatric nurse practitioners.

25. *Answer:* D

Rationale: Developmental theory explains human growth and development. This model outlines the eight consecutive stages in the family life cycle that offer a predictive overview of the activities that occur in families over time.

BIBLIOGRAPHY

Abood, S., & Keepnews, D. (2000a). *Understanding payment for advanced practice nursing services, volume 1: Medicare reimbursement.* Washington DC: American Nurses Publishing.

Abood, S., & Keepnews, D. (2000b). *Understanding payment for advanced practice nursing services, volume 2: Fraud and abuse.* Washington DC: American Nurses Publishing.

Agency for Health Care Research and Quality. (2006a). Clinical practice guidelines, 1992–1996. Retrieved March 10, 2006, from www.ahrq.gov/clinic/cpgsix.htm.

Agency for Healthcare Research and Quality. (2006b). Evidence-based practice centers. Retrieved March 10, 2006, from www.ahrq.gov/clinic/epc.

Agency for Healthcare Research and Quality. (2006c). Evidence report topics and technical reviews. Retrieved March 10, 2006, from www.ahrq.gov/clinic/epcix.htm.

Agency for Healthcare Research and Quality. (2006d). State and local policy makers. Retrieved March 10, 2006, from www.ahrq.gov/news/ulpix.htm.

American Academy of Pediatrics. (2006a). Clinical practice guidelines. Retrieved March 10, 2006, from http://aappolicy.aappublications.org./practice_guidelines/index.dtl.

American Academy of Pediatrics. (2006b). Policy statements. Retrieved March 10, 2006, from http://aappolicy.aappublications.org/policy_statement/index.dtl.

American Association of Colleges of Nursing (1996). *The essentials of master's education for advanced practice nursing.* Washington D.C.: American Association of Colleges of Nursing Publishing.

American Association of Colleges of Nursing. (2006). Position statement on nursing research. Retrieved April 20, 2006, from www.aacn.nche.edu/Publications/positions/rscposst.htm.

American Medical Association. (2006). *Current procedural terminology: CPT 2006: Professional edition.* Chicago: American Medical Association.

American Nurses Association. (1996). *Scope and standards of advanced practice registered nursing.* Washington DC: American Nurses Publishing.

American Nurses Association. (2002). *Code of ethics for nurses, with interpretive statements.* Washington DC: American Nurses Publishing.

American Nurses Association. (2006). Position statements. Retrieved March 10, 2006, from www.nursingworld.org/readroom/position.

American Nurses Credentialing Center. (2006). Homepage. Retrieved March 10, 2006, from www.nursingworld.org/ancc.

Annie E. Casey Foundation. (2006). Kids count. Retrieved March 10, 2006, from www.aecf.org/kidscount.

Association of Faculties of Pediatric Nurse Practitioner Programs (AFPNP). (1996). *Philosophy, conceptual model, terminal competencies for the education of pediatric nurse practitioners.* Cherry Hill, NJ: AFPNP/NAPNAP.

Bandolier Journal. (2006). Home page. Retrieved March 10, 2006, from www.jr2.ox.ac.uk/bandolier/aboutus.html.

Boyd, M.D. (1998). *Health teaching in nursing practice: A professional model* (3rd ed.). Stamford, CT: Appleton Lange.

Boynton, R.W., Dunn, E.S, Stephens, G.R., & Pulcini, J. (2003). *Manual of ambulatory pediatrics* (5th ed.) Philadelphia: Lippincott Williams & Wilkins.

Burns, C.E., Brady, M.A., Dunn, A.M., et al. (2004). *Pediatric primary care: A handbook for nurse practitioners* (3rd ed.). Philadelphia: Elsevier Science.

Centers for Disease Control and Prevention. (2006). Office of Minority Health. *Reports and publications.* Retrieved March 10, 2006, from www.cdc.gov/omh/reportspubs.htm.

Centers for Medicare and Medicaid Services. (January 24, 2003). Clinical laboratory improvement program. Retrieved March 10, 2006, from www.cms.hhs.gov/clia.

Centers for Medicare and Medicaid Services. (2006). State Children's Health Insurance Programs. Retrieved on March 10, 2006, from www.cms.hhs.gov/schip.

Children's Defense Fund. (2006). Mission of the Children's Defense Fund. Retrieved on March 10, 2006, from www.childrensdefense.org.

Clinical Laboratory Improvement Amendments. (2006). Home page. Retrieved on March 10, 2006 at http://www.phppo.cdc.gov/clia/default.aspx.

[The] Cochrane Collaboration (2006). Cochrane reviews: abstracts and full-text access. Retrieved November 8, 2006, from www.cochrane.org/reviews/index.htm.

Department of Health and Human Services Office for Civil Rights. (2006). HIPAA medical privacy—National standards to protect the privacy of personal health information. Retrieved on March 10, 2006, from www.hhs.gov/ocr/hipaa.

Drug Enforcement Agency. (2006a). *Drug registration applications.* Retrieved on March 10, 2006, from www.deadiversion.usdoj.gov/drugreg/index.html.

Drug Enforcement Agency. (2006b). Midlevel practitioners authorization by state. Retrieved on March 10, 2006, from www.deadiversion.usdoj.gov/drugreg/practioners/index.html.

Fadiman, A. (1997). *The spirit catches you and then you fall down.* New York: Farrar, Straus & Giroux.

Fleischman, A.R., Collogan, L.K. (2004). Addressing ethical issues in everyday practice. *Pediatr Ann, 33*(11), 740-745.

Green-Hernandez, C., Quinn, A.A., Denman-Vitale, S., et al. (2004). Making primary care culturally competent. *Nurse Pract, 29*(6), 49-55.

Guido, G.W. (2006). *Legal and ethical issues in nursing.* (4th ed.). Upper Saddle River, NJ: Prentice Hall.

Joint Commission on Accreditation of Healthcare Organizations. (2006). How to become accredited. Retrieved on March 10, 2006, from www.jcaho.org/htba/index.htm.

Jones, D. (2002). Reimbursement, privileging and credentialing for pediatric nurse practitioners. Paper presented at the National Association of Pediatric Nurse Associates and Practitioners 23rd Annual Nursing Conference for Pediatric Primary Care, April 10–13, 2002, Reno, Nevada. Retrieved October 15, 2004, from www.medscape.com/viewarticle/433372.

Kaplan, L., & Brown, M.A. (2004). Prescriptive authority and barriers to practice. *Nurse Pract, 29*(3), 28-35.

Leininger, M.M. (2001). *Cultural care diversity and universality: A theory of nursing.* Sudbury, MA: Jones and Bartlett.

National Association of Pediatric Nurse Practitioners. (2000). *Continuing education.* Retrieved January 6, 2006, from http://www.napnap.org/index.cfm?page=10&sec=54&ssec=61.

National Association of Pediatric Nurse Practitioners. (2001a). *Access to care.* Retrieved January 6, 2006, from http://www.napnap.org/index.cfm?page=10&sec=54&ssec=55.

National Association of Pediatric Nurse Practitioners. (2001b). *Certification.* Retrieved January 6, 2006, from http://www.napnap.org/index.cfm?page=10&sec=54&ssec=58.

National Association of Pediatric Nurse Practitioners. (2002a). *Age parameters for pediatric nurse practitioner practice.* Retrieved January 6, 2006, from http://www.napnap.org/index.cfm?page=10&sec=54&ssec=170.

National Association of Pediatric Nurse Practitioners. (2002b). *Pediatric health care home.* Retrieved January 6, 2006, from http://www.napnap.org/index.cfm?page=10&sec=54&ssec=68.

National Association of Pediatric Nurse Practitioners. (2003a). *Credentialing and privileging for pediatric nurse practitioners.* Retrieved January 6, 2006, from http://www.napnap.org/index.cfm?page=10&sec=54&ssec=63.

National Association of Pediatric Nurse Practitioners. (2003b). *PNP prescriptive privilege.* Retrieved January 6, 2006, from http://www.napnap.org/Docs/pos_prescriptive.pdf.

National Association of Pediatric Nurse Practitioners. (2004a). *Protection of children involved in research studies.* Retrieved January 6, 2006, from http://www.napnap.org/Docs/pos-child-esearch.pdf.

National Association of Pediatric Nurse Practitioners. (2004b). *Reimbursement for nurse practitioner services.* Retrieved January 6, 2006, from http://www.napnap.org/Docs/ps-eimbursement.pdf.

National Association of Pediatric Nurse Practitioners. (2004c). *Scope and standards of practice: Pediatric nurse practitioner (PNP).* Retrieved January 6, 2006, from http://www.napnap.org/Docs/Final-Scope2–25.pdf.

National Association of Pediatric Nurse Practitioners. (2004d). *School-based and school-linked centers.* Retrieved January 6, 2006, from http://www.napnap.org/index.cfm?page=10&sec=54&ssec=74.

National Association of Pediatric Nurse Practitioners. (2005). *Nurse practitioner career resource guide.* Retrieved on January 6, 2006, from http://www.napnap.org/index.cfm?page=10&sec=463.

National Association of Pediatric Nurse Practitioners. (2006a). Home page. Retrieved January 8, 2006, from http://www.napnap.org.

National Association of Pediatric Nurse Practitioners. (2006b). *Position statements.* Retrieved January 8, 2006, from http://www.napnap.org/practice/positions/.

National Association of Pediatric Nurse Practitioners (2006c). *Practice issues: Frequently asked questions.* Retrieved January 6, 2006, from http://www.napnap.org/index.cfm?page=10&sec=390.

National Center for Health Statistics. (2005). *International classification of diseases, 9th revision, clinical modification (ICD-9-CM)* (6th ed.). Retrieved March 10, 2006, from www.cdc.gov/nchs/about/otheract/icd9/abticd9.htm.

National Committee for Quality Assurance. (2006). *NCQA programs.* Retrieved March 10, 2006, from www.ncqa.org. index.htm.

National Council of State Boards of Nursing. (2006). *Nurse licensure compact: Advanced practice model legislative language.* Retrieved on March 10, 2006, from www.ncsbn.org/nlc/aprncompact.asp.

National Organization of Nurse Practitioner Faculties (NONPF). (2000). *Cultural guidelines.* Washington, DC: NONPF.

National Organization of Nurse Practitioner Faculties (NONPF). (2006). *Sample collaborative agreement.* Retrieved March 10, 2006, from www.nonpf.com/fpcollabagreesample.htm.

Occupational Safety and Health Administration (OSHA). (2006). *Bloodborne pathogens and needlestick prevention.* Retrieved March 10, 2006, from www.osha.gov/SLTC/bloodbornepathogens/index.html.

Pearson, L.J. (2006a). A national overview of nurse practitioner legislation and healthcare issues. *Amer J Nurse Pract, 10*(1), 15-84.

Pearson, L.J. (2006b). A national overview of nurse practitioner legislation and healthcare issues. *Amer J Nurse Pract, 10*(2), 13-84.

Pediatric Nursing Certification Board (PNCB). (2006). Retrieved March 10, 2006, from www.pncb.org/ptistore/control/index.

Phillips, S.J. (2006). Eighteenth annual legislative update. *Nurse Pract, 31*(1), 6-38.

Sackett, D.L., Rosenberg, W.M.C., Muir, J.A., et al. (1996). Evidence based medicine: What it is and what it isn't. *BMJ, 312,* 71-72.

United States Department of Health and Human Services (HHS). 2006. *Insure kids now! Linking the nation's children to health insurance.* Retrieved March 10, 2006, from www.insurekidsnow.gov.

NOTES

3 Clinical Reasoning and Clinical Decision Making

DIANE M. WINK

Select the best answer for each of the following questions:

1. A 19-year-old mother brings her 2½-month-old boy to your clinic with a concern that the baby has become less interested in his feedings over the past 2 or 3 days, taking in only about half the normal amount of formula before becoming tired and falling asleep. His birth history is normal and he has normal development and weight gain. His temperature is 100.2° F (axillary) now. He has no respiratory symptoms and your physical examination reveals no identifiable source of fever. Which of the following questions/observations would be MOST helpful in establishing a diagnosis?
   A. "Is anyone else at home ill at this time?"
   B. "How sick do you think he is?"
   C. "Has he ever had a temperature before?"
   D. "Did you have any infection or rash when you were pregnant?"

2. When evaluating a child for a sick visit, the pediatric nurse practitioner should start the visit with:
   A. As little information from the chart as possible so as not to bias her questions.
   B. A small set of broad questions based on the reported reason for the visit.
   C. A large number of differentials which will be ruled out as the assessment of the child progresses.
   D. A narrow focused question.

3. Clinical reasoning is generally optimal in the pediatric nurse practitioner who:
   A. Relies on content presented in his initial RN and pediatric nurse practitioner education.
   B. Consults with his physician colleagues on almost every case.
   C. Follows evidence-based recommendations very strictly.
   D. Reads extensively in his practice area.

4. Which of the following pediatric nurse practitioners is best demonstrating critical thinking?
   A. Mary, who uses the approaches her collaborating physician uses in all practice situations.
   B. Joanne, who collaborates with peers in difficult situations to determine the best approach to care.
   C. Susan, who always uses drug and protocol books on her PDA to determine needed care.
   D. Terry, who bases care on the most common approaches which work in his practice.

5. Clinical reasoning is similar to the nursing process, in that both require identification of:
   A. Nursing diagnoses.
   B. Nursing care plans.
   C. Essential assessment data.
   D. Care based on assessment of the child rather than the child, family, and community.

6. The pediatric nurse practitioner seeking to increase critical thinking skills should:

A. Identify his or her personal stereotypes and biases.
B. Keep visits on time to maximize use of clinical practice time.
C. Conduct a full developmental assessment at every visit.
D. Involve all members of the practice's staff in the care of the children.

7. An aim of evidence-based practice is to:
A. Limit the scope of pediatric nurse practitioners' decision making.
B. Use research to support clinical practice decisions.
C. Eliminate individualization of care.
D. Decrease time needed for visits.

8. A pediatric nurse practitioner is seeing a child with an unusual problem she has rarely treated. The parents bring in written material they keep to help educate their daughter's health care providers. When reviewing the material, the pediatric nurse practitioner should:
A. Be polite with the parents, but not use the material since it was gathered by a nonprofessional.
B. Consider the author and source of the materials to determine its usefulness in this situation.
C. Use only material copied from print resources and discard materials obtained from the Internet.
D. Explain to the parents that providers have access to similar information and they needn't trouble themselves getting this material.

9. The study of rare diseases by the pediatric nurse practitioner:
A. Is of little importance because they can always refer children with complex or rare problems to other providers.
B. Is a waste of time, because pediatric nurse practitioners need to focus on common problems.
C. Can help the pediatric nurse practitioner recognize and treat both common and complex problems.
D. Allows pediatric nurse practitioners to prove their value to the practice.

10. Of the following, the best example of evaluation data that indicate an alternative diagnosis should be considered is:
A. Response to treatment is not as expected.
B. Parent is unhappy with the diagnosis.
C. Child does not like the treatment.
D. Plan of care has not been used in the practice before.

11. Clinical reasoning and decision-making skills are difficult to develop because:
A. Everyday problems are messy and ill-defined.
B. Pediatrics is such an old specialization.
C. Patients change over time.
D. Books become outdated quickly.

12. During the clinical decision-making process, it is important to:
A. Have a rationale for accepting and rejecting diagnoses.
B. Include parents throughout the process.
C. Come to diagnostic conclusions quickly.
D. Focus on physical assessment findings rather than history.

13. A concept map may help a pediatric nurse practitioner develop clinical reasoning skills. The concept map uses symbols, lines, and arrows to:
A. Verbally present pathology.
B. Illustrate nursing theory.
C. Show a timeline of care since birth.
D. Relate pathology to health assessment findings and treatment.

14. Which of the following activities would be most effective to help a pediatric nurse practitioner identify errors in her clinical reasoning process?
A. Reading of case studies.
B. Development of a personal portfolio.
C. Use of simulated patient encounters.
D. Completion of web-based learning modules.

15. Of the following, the best way an interdisciplinary care team can promote clinical

reasoning among team members is through the use of:
- A. Grand rounds.
- B. Practice-based quality assurance initiatives.
- C. Having team members do online case studies.
- D. Paying costs for continuing education programs.

16. The learning of the diagnostic process and clinical decision making is best supported by the:
- A. Study of algorithms.
- B. Engaging in debate.
- C. Reading case studies.
- D. Keeping a personal journal with reflections on practice.

17. When reevaluating a child with a respiratory illness, which of the following is the most useful data to support clinical decision making?
- A. The child complains of nausea after eating.
- B. The child's respiratory rate has dropped from 36 to 28 breaths per minute.
- C. The child likes taking his liquid medication.
- D. The child's weight is higher than at the last visit.

18. Which of the following is a standard for nursing ethics?
- A. ANA Standards for Nursing Practice.
- B. The Nurse Practice Act.
- C. The Nightingale Pledge.
- D. ANA Code for Nurses.

19. A pediatric nurse practitioner is considering using one of four web sites as a resource. Which of these is best?
- A. A site maintained by a professional organization.
- B. A site with a hit counter showing 100 hits a day and many postings from practicing nurse practitioners but no information on who runs the site.
- C. A site with weekly dated updates by a person supporting expansion of pediatric nurse practitioner practice.

- D. A site maintained by the manufacturer of a widely used infant care product.

20. Assessment data should be organized:
- A. In the manner the parent(s) presented it.
- B. From least to most important.
- C. So related findings are grouped together.
- D. In the order the data are collected.

21. A verified laboratory result obtained during a routine screening of an apparently healthy 1-year-old is just below the upper limit of normal. The pediatric nurse practitioner demonstrating clinical decision making will:
- A. Repeat the test at least one more time.
- B. Implement routine care, since the value is within the normal range.
- C. Consider reasons for why the finding could be close to an abnormal value.
- D. Initiate a quality assurance study related to this finding for other children in the practice.

22. Which of the following pediatric nurse practitioners is most likely to identify an unusual presentation of a particular disease? The pediatric nurse practitioner who:
- A. Has a full schedule of visits each day, often needing to stay late to finish paperwork.
- B. Has blocks of time in his week to review difficult case presentations.
- C. Feels he knows almost all there is to know and rarely consults with a peer.
- D. Goes to a lot of drug company dinner presentations.

23. A pediatric nurse practitioner is precepting a pediatric nurse practitioner student. Which of the following approaches will best help the student develop clinical reasoning skills?
- A. Asking the student to explain why he or she chose an intervention.
- B. Focusing on the details of the PE skill set to ensure all skills are perfected.
- C. Having the student see as many children in a day as possible.

D. Telling the student the best drugs to choose after both preceptor and student assess the child.

24. When assessing a child with an acute illness, the diagnostic conclusion of the pediatric nurse practitioner will be best supported if:
   A. The diagnosis is frequently seen in that community.
   B. Assessment data are congruent with that expected for this problem.
   C. Immunizations which could have prevented the problem are identified.
   D. The collaborating physician agrees.

25. A pediatric nurse practitioner is precepting a pediatric nurse practitioner student. Which of the following approaches will best help the student develop clinical reasoning skills?
   A. Using as few resources as possible.
   B. Encouraging the student to follow approaches taken at that practice.
   C. Exploring alternative explanations for assessment and diagnostic test findings.
   D. Having the student observe staff members rather than provide care so she can see how different providers work.

NOTES

ANSWERS

1. *Answer:* A
   Rationale: This question will give you data essential to the visit today. While the mother's opinion about how sick the child is will help you appraise her view of this illness, it will not help with the diagnostic process. Items C and D elicit data not related to the problem today.

2. *Answer:* B
   Rationale: Starting with a few broad questions rather than a single narrow focused question will increase the likelihood the major concerns which caused the parent to bring the child in for the visit will be elicited. It is essential to review the child's record at the start of the visit. While it is good to have a few differentials in mind to help structure the start of the assessment, having too large a number will make it difficult to proceed efficiently.

3. *Answer:* D
   Rationale: The more the pediatric nurse practitioner reads about topics related to practice (from child development to family dynamics to assessment and treatment of acute and chronic as well as common and rare problems), the better his or her knowledge foundation for clinical reasoning and decision making will be. Knowledge gained in prior formal education programs quickly becomes incomplete or outdated. Consultation, while of value, is not needed or necessary on a regular basis except for the pediatric nurse practitioner new to practice. While evidence-based recommendations are very important, they must be used in light of the individual child.

4. *Answer:* B
   Rationale: Collaboration with peers when a case is difficult or complex will help the pediatric nurse practitioner validate findings and decision making. Collaboration also helps the pediatric nurse practitioner avail him- or herself of the knowledge and insights of peers. Protocols are useful, but basing care totally on protocols can result in care that does not meet the needs of an individual child or fails to consider an unusual presentation or treatment approach.

5. *Answer:* C
   Rationale: Both the nursing process and clinical reasoning require that the pediatric nurse practitioner gather essential assessment data which will be the foundation for clinical decisions. Nursing diagnoses and plans of care are drawn from clinical decisions, as will be the medical diagnoses made by the pediatric nurse practitioner. Both the nursing process and clinical reasoning are based on an assessment of the child, family, and their community.

6. *Answer:* A
   Rationale: Identification of personal stereotypes and biases is an essential step in the refinement of critical thinking skills, since both can result in the incorrect gathering and/or interpretation of data as well as development of inappropriate or ineffective plans of care. Maximizing use of time per visit, completion of full developmental assessments, and working collaboratively with staff can all have value, but they are not as closely linked to development of critical thinking skills.

7. *Answer:* B
   Rationale: Research findings form the foundation on which clinical reasoning, decision making, and practice are built. While evidence-based practice may seem to limit choices, its actual effect is wider use of effective rather than ineffective plans of care where there is clear evidence that one approach is superior to another. Individualization of care and time of visit can remain the same.

8. *Answer:* B
   Rationale: Material brought in by a parent can be very helpful. As with all newly obtained data, the pediatric nurse practitioner should verify that the source of the material is of good quality. Good quality resources may be from a reputable and accurate web site as well as from lay and professional publications and books.

9. *Answer:* C
Rationale: While a pediatric nurse practitioner may never see a rare disease or unusual presentation of a common problem, learning about them will increase overall knowledge, the foundation of effective critical thinking and clinical reasoning. In addition, it will improve the pediatric nurse practitioner's ability to recognize such problems if they do occur. Referral and consultation may still be needed, but increased knowledge will make this a more thoughtful process.

10. *Answer:* A
Rationale: A key clue that more assessment or an alternate plan of care is needed is that the response to treatment is not as expected. The parent and/or child's response to care or the treatment regimen must be respected and considered, but these can result from factors other than the correctness of the plan of care. A practice's usual approach to care should be known by all providers but when data indicate that approach is not having the intended outcome, more data and possibly a change in care are needed.

11. *Answer:* A
Rationale: While some texts and other resources present content (e.g., pathophysiology, relevant assessments, and recommended care) becomes outdated, the real world of the child and his or her family makes the assessment, planning, implementation, and evaluation of care more difficult because each child is different and certain situations are unique.

12. *Answer:* A
Rationale: As the diagnostic process evolves, it is necessary to have a reason to either accept or reject each differential. The speed with which diagnostic conclusions are reached, specific physical examination findings, and the parents' participation are important, because they provide needed data for keeping or discarding a diagnosis.

13. *Answer:* D
Rationale: A concept map is a depiction of the relationship among assessment findings, pathology, diagnostic testing results, treatment, and other aspects of the child and

his or her care. This may reflect a theory, but does not usually show a timeline (e.g., since birth) or only present pathology.

14. *Answer:* C
Rationale: A simulated patient encounter is an excellent methodology to help a student, as well as more experienced nurse practitioner, develop clinical reasoning skills. By practicing care in a setting where they can get feedback about therapeutic communication, questioning skills, and physical examination techniques as well as their therapeutic conclusions and plan of care, the pediatric nurse practitioner can refine a wide arrange of abilities. A professional portfolio helps document accomplishments. Reading case studies and web-based learning modules can also help increase knowledge, but they do not provide the high-quality feedback of a simulation.

15. *Answer:* A
Rationale: Grand rounds provide an opportunity for professionals from a wide range of disciplines to review and discuss care. Quality assurance activities promote evaluation of care, although there may be some learning about clinical decision making from reading the documentation of others and having your own care reviewed. Online case studies and continuing education programs are good learning activities but are not interdisciplinary.

16. *Answer:* A
Rationale: Algorithms guide the clinician through the steps of the decision-making process for a particular problem. Engaging in debate, reading case studies, and keeping a personal journal are all ways to promote knowledge, but they do not directly teach or refine clinical reasoning.

17. *Answer:* B
Rationale: When collecting data as part of the decision-making process, the more precise the data, the more useful they are. In this case, the specific respiratory rates are the most precise.

18. *Answer:* D

Rationale: The ANA code for nurses is the ethical code for the nursing profession.

19. *Answer:* A

Rationale: When evaluating the quality of a web site, the authority of the group or individual that maintains the site is an important consideration. A site maintained by a professional organization is backed up by the organization and is more likely to have internal review to ensure accuracy and lack of bias. Sites maintained by a single pediatric nurse practitioner or posted by someone who supports pediatric nurse practitioners can be of high quality but often lack the quality and accuracy review of professional organizations' sites. Sites by manufacturers can have a great deal of useful and accurate information, but their internal bias must always be considered.

20. *Answer:* C

Rationale: Grouping of data so you can see how they relate is an important part of the clinical decision-making process. There are a variety of ways of grouping data and often data can be placed in different groups. However, simple grouping from least to most important, in the order collected or in the manner the parent presented the data, are not useful grouping mechanisms.

21. *Answer:* C

Rationale: Any unusual or unexpected lab value should be further explored to verify there is no action needed in that child's case and that routine care is appropriate. While another repeat of the test may be appropriate in a limited number of situations, one repeat with the same outcome should be enough. A pattern of marginally normal results may be a reason to do a study of children in the practice (e.g., to identify a new pattern of a problem in the community), but only one almost abnormal is not usually a strong reason for this.

22. *Answer:* B

Rationale: Having time to think about care and reflect on what was, was not, and could be done, supports the clinical reasoning process.

23. *Answer:* A

Rationale: Questioning a student about his or her decision-making process helps the student refine clinical reasoning as well as take on responsibility for those decisions. While questioning the "why" of the PE develops critical reasoning, simply focusing on PE skills is more useful for development of the psychomotor skill itself. Seeing many patients in a day and the provision of answers by the preceptors do not promote development of critical thinking skills.

24. *Answer:* B

Rationale: Evaluating if data obtained is congruent with that expected is an essential component of clinical reasoning. The pediatric nurse practitioner must learn to recognize both what is there and what is not.

25. *Answer:* C

Rationale: Activities which encourage and support students in going beyond first impressions and obvious answers will help them increase depth and scope of their clinical decision making. Students must use resources both to learn and also to validate their conclusions. While the "usual approaches" taken in a practice may be firmly based in good practice, a student needs to learn the "whys" of that care, not just to do it because that is what is done. Pure observation has a role in the education of the advanced practice nurse but it should not replace actual provision of care.

BIBLIOGRAPHY

Abegglen, J., & Conger, C.O. (1997). Critical thinking in nursing: Classroom tactics that work. *J Nurs Educ, 36*(10), 452-458.

Alfaro-LeFevre, R. (2004). *Critical thinking and clinical judgment: A practical approach* (3rd ed.). St. Louis: Saunders.

Barnsteiner, J., Deatrick, J., Grey, M., et al. (1993). Future of pediatric advanced nursing practice. *Pediatr Nurs, 19*(2), 196-197.

Benner, P. (1984). *From novice to expert*. Menlo Park, CA: Addison-Wesley. (Reprinted in 2001).

Benner, P. (1994). The role of articulation in understanding practice and experience as sources of knowledge in clinical nursing. In J. Tully, & D. M. Weinstock, Eds., *Philosophy in an age of plu-*

ralism: *The philosophy of Charles Taylor in question*. Cambridge, NY: Cambridge University Press.

Bickley, L.S., & Szilagyi, P.G. (Eds.) (2003). *Bates' guide to physical assessment and history taking* (8th ed.). Philadelphia: J.B. Lippincott.

Bonnel, W.B. (2000). Adding the detail for clinical decision making: Web-based modules as classroom adjunct. In M.K. Crabtree (Ed.). *Teaching clinical decision making in advanced practice nursing* (pp. 75-81). Washington, DC: NONPF.

Burman, M.E., Stepans, M.B., Jansa, N., & Steiner, S. (2002). How do NPs make clinical decisions? *Nurse Pract, 27*(5), 59-64.

Cabana, M.D., Medzihradsky, O.F., Rubin, H.R., & Freed, G.L. (2001). Applying clinical guidelines to pediatric practice. *Pediatr Ann, 30*(5), 274-282.

Candela, L., Michael, S.R., & Mitchell, S. (2003). Ethical debates: Enhancing critical thinking in nursing students. *Nurse Educ, 28*(1), 37-39.

DeToma, H.R. (2000). Clinical decision making: A student perspective on problem-based learning. In M.K. Crabtree (Ed.). *Teaching clinical decision making in advanced practice nursing* (pp. 91-96). Washington, DC: NONPF.

Dexter, P., Applegate, M., Backer, J., et al. (1997). A proposed framework for teaching and evaluating critical thinking in nursing. *J Prof Nurs, 13*(3), 160-167.

Dumas, M.A. (2000). Problem based learning: Using case studies and elaboration to teach clinical decision making. In M.K. Crabtree (Ed.). *Teaching clinical decision making in advanced practice nursing* (pp. 97-119). Washington, DC: NONPF.

Flagler, S. (2000). Recognizing the thinking processes behind clinical decision making. In M.K. Crabtree (Ed.). *Teaching clinical decision making in advanced practice nursing*. Washington, DC: NONPF.

Gray, M.T. (2003). Beyond content: Generating critical thinking in the classroom. *Nurse Educ, 28*(3), 136-140.

King, M., & Shell, R. (2002). Critical thinking strategies: Teaching and evaluating critical thinking with concept maps. *Nurse Educ, 27*(5), 214-216.

Lee, J.E., & Ryan-Wenger, N. (2000). Standard methods of teaching clinical decision making: Strengths, limitations, and enhancements. In M.K. Crabtree (Ed.). *Teaching clinical decision making in advanced practice nursing*. Washington, DC: NONPF.

Lipman, T.H., & Deatrick, J.A. (1997). Preparing advanced practice nurses for clinical decision making in specialty practice. *Nurse Educ, 22*(2), 47-50.

Logan, S. & Gilbert, R. (2000). Framing questions. In V.A. Moyer, E.J. Elliott, R.L. Logsdon, M.C., & Merkt, J.T. (2000). Reflection: An aid to clinical decision making. In M.K. Crabtree (Ed.). *Teaching clinical decision making in advanced practice nursing*. Washington, DC: NONPF.

Melnyk, B.M., & Fineout-Overholt, E. (2004). Evidence-based practice in nursing and healthcare. Philadelphia: Lippincott, Williams & Wilkins.

McKusick, K.A. (1967). Foreword. In W.B. Bean, *Rare diseases and lesions: Their contributions to clinical medicine*. Springfield, IL: Thomas.

Myrick, F., & Yonge, O. (2002). Preceptor behaviors integral to the promotion of student critical thinking. *J Nurs Staff Dev, 18*(3), 127-135.

Rosner, A.M. (2002). Teaching tools: "Puzzle patients" and critical thinking. *Nurse Educ, 27*(4), 155-156.

Steiner, S.H., & Burman, M.E. (2000). Integrating clinical decision making and advanced assessment. In M.K. Crabtree (Ed.). *Teaching clinical decision making in advanced practice nursing*. Washington, DC: NONPF.

Thompson, J.E., Kershbaumer, R.M., & Krisman-Scott, M.A. (2001). *Educating advanced practice nurses and midwives: From practice to teaching*. New York: Springer.

Webber, P.B. (2000). Clinical decision making: Components, processes, and outcomes. In M.K. Crabtree (Ed.). *Teaching clinical decision making in advanced practice nursing*. Washington, DC: NONPF.

HEALTH ASSESSMENT AND PHYSICAL EXAMINATION

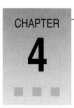

Measures of Child Growth and Development

MARIAILIANA J. STARK

Select the best answer for each of the following questions:

1. Which of the following is NOT used in the selection of an appropriate growth chart:
   A. Gender.
   B. Age.
   C. Ethnicity.
   D. Copyright year.

2. From which of the following resources can the most up-to-date standardized growth charts be obtained?
   A. They can be downloaded at www.cdc.gov/growthcharts.
   B. Each health care institution has developed their own unique growth charts for their health care providers.
   C. The formula companies are responsible for distribution of the growth charts.
   D. Regional departments of health have a limited supply of growth charts for their community health centers.

·3. Which of the following factors in serial measurements is NOT appropriate to include to establish growth patterns or to evaluate growth patterns?
   A. Gestational age.
   B. Formula brand.
   C. Birth weight.
   D. Genetic influence and genetic disorder.

4. When do infants typically gain more weight?
   A. Between 9 months to 12 months.
   B. After solids have been introduced.

C. The first week of life.
D. Between birth and 7 months.

5. Which one of the following statements is NOT true regarding the updated CDC growth charts?
   A. BMI-for-age charts are currently used for all age groups.
   B. The 85th percentile to identify children at risk for becoming overweight was added to the BMI-for-age and weight-for-stature charts.
   C. The 3rd and 97th percentiles were added to the growth charts.
   D. The lower limits of length and height were extended.

6. The anthropometric index that considers a child's weight, height, and age is:
   A. Weight-for-stature.
   B. Weight-for-length.
   C. BMI-for-age.
   D. Weight-for-age.

7. Select one of the following. Ideally, weighing an infant should be performed:
   A. Only in the evening after all the major feedings.
   B. Without any clothing including the diaper.
   C. Using an upright/platform scale.
   D. With clothing on to prevent hypothermia.

8. Kawika is a 13-month-old male child who presents at the clinic today for his well child exam. On the standardized growth charts, Kawika's weight has steadily increased from the 75th percentile to above the

97th percentile on serial measurements. His length has remained steady between the 30th and 50th percentile. His weight-for-length is over the 97th percentile. His physical examination and development are within normal limits. The correct response to Kawika's parent is which of the following?

    A. Overweight children usually lose the weight as they become adolescents and adults.

    B. "Baby fat" is normal at this age; once Kawika starts school, he will lose the weight.

    C. I am concerned about Kawika's weight; the prevalence of overweight children and adolescents in the United States has increased.

    D. Oral intake is the only known cause for overweight children and adolescents.

9.   Malia's weight is 16.6 kg and her height is 99.1 cm. What is Malia's BMI?

    A. 15.2

    B. 16.9

    C. 17.1

    D. 18.2

10. Jose is a 3-year-old male child. His height is 39.7 inches, his weight is 41 lbs., and his BMI is 18.3. You plot his weight on the BMI-for-age chart and he falls above the 95th percentile. Which of the following best describes Jose's weight?

    A. Underweight.

    B. Normal.

    C. At risk of overweight.

    D. Overweight.

11. Kealii is a 17-year-old adolescent male and his height falls at the 3rd percentile. Which of the following should NOT be included in the differential diagnosis for his short stature?

    A. Genetic conditions.

    B. Inhaled steroids used once for his asthma management.

    C. Constitutional delay.

    D. Endocrine condition.

12. Mandy is concerned about her weight. She asks you how to tell if she is overweight.

What is the BEST method to determine Mandy's weight status?

    A. Body mass index.

    B. Tricep skin-fold measurement.

    C. Weight-for-height ratio.

    D. Percent of ideal body weight.

13. Nia is a 15-month-old female child seen today for her well child exam. At her last visit at 12 months, her weight-for-stature ratio was at the 10th percentile. Today, her weight-for-stature has dropped to less than the 3rd percentile. Which of the following actions would NOT be appropriate?

    A. Assessment of developmental milestones.

    B. Hospitalization for observation and assessment of feeding pattern.

    C. Assessment of Nia's nutritional status including the growth parameters.

    D. Complete health history and complete physical exam.

14. Bright Futures gives health care providers guidelines for health supervision of infants, children, and adolescents. One of the major tasks of these guidelines is:

    A. Cutting the time of the health care visit.

    B. Building effective partnerships.

    C. Using directive questions.

    D. Reducing the cost to the health care provider.

15. In each section of the Bright Futures Guidelines an overview is given for each age group focusing on which of the following areas?

    A. Anthropometric measurements.

    B. Psychological testing.

    C. Physical, cognitive, social-emotional, and health behaviors.

    D. Regulatory laws on the environment.

16. Angela is a 3½-year-old female in your clinic for her well child health care visit. You administer the Denver II. To pass the item "name one color," Angela must:

    A. Point to one color correctly when examiner names it.

    B. Name one color correctly when examiner points to it.

C. Point to one color correctly when parent names it.
D. Must be 4 years of age to administer this item.

17. Before administering the Denver II to Angela, the pediatric nurse practitioner should explain the Denver II is:
   A. Administered to determine the child's current developmental status.
   B. An IQ test.
   C. Made up of 125 items and the child is expected to pass all the items administered.
   D. Completed by parent interview.

18. Jacob comes into the clinic for his 9-month well baby exam. Jacob's parents want to know if there is an alternate developmental screening test that can be given to him. He is asleep at the time of his well child exam. Your best response is:
   A. He will be documented as being asleep during the screening.
   B. Jacob will be referred for further diagnostic testing because it is unusual that a 9-month-old child would be sleepy during the daytime.
   C. Have parents keep him awake.
   D. The parents can complete the Ages and Stages Questionnaire and mail it into the clinic.

19. Carissa's parents report that she is a fussy child and is a very picky eater. You note on the growth chart she is at the less than 3rd percentile for weight and stature for a 10-month-old child. Which of the following assessment tools would be the most appropriate to use to assess the caregiver-infant interaction?
   A. Denver II.
   B. Clinical Linguistic and Auditory Milestone Scale (CLAMS).
   C. Nursing Child Assessment Satellite Training (NCAST).
   D. Mullen Scales.

20. Having a child draw figures (shapes) or a person evaluates which of the following skill(s)?
   A. Visual-perceptual and cognitive.

B. Language.
C. Adaptive behavior.
D. Gross motor.

21. At the 18-month well child exam, the mother tells you that her child says "mama" and "dada," points and gestures if he wants something and follows simple one-step commands. Your best response is:
   A. Your child's language development is at the appropriate age level.
   B. Usually boys are delayed in their speech compared to girls.
   C. A hearing and language evaluation should be completed.
   D. Evaluate the child again at 2 years of age.

22. Which of the following is NOT a test for infants and toddlers for speech and language evaluation?
   A. ELM (Early Language Milestone scale).
   B. Fluharty-2.
   C. Clinical Linguistic and Auditory Milestone test (CLAMS/CAT).
   D. REEL (Receptive and Expressive Emergent Language).

23. Kainoa is a 2-year-old with a history of eight episodes of otitis media, no meaningful language, loves playing in water, and variable eye contact. Which of the following is NOT included in your differential diagnosis?
   A. Hearing impaired.
   B. Conduct disorder.
   C. Autism spectrum disorder
   D. Fragile X syndrome.

24. Natalie was born at 27 weeks gestation. Her mother wants to know if her long-term development will be affected. Your best response is:
   A. For the most part, premature infants develop at the same rate as term infants.
   B. Premature infants are always slower than term infants and there is no catching up.

C. There are no developmental tests available to evaluate children who are premature.

D. Once a child reaches 40 weeks adjusted age, age correction factors are unnecessary.

25. Which of the following is not a common cause of gross motor delay?
    A. Normal variation.
    B. Mental retardation.
    C. Autism spectrum disorder.
    D. Cerebral palsy.

NOTES

ANSWERS

1. *Answer:* C
    Rationale: A limitation of the 1977 growth charts was the nonrepresentative sample of primarily formula-fed, white, middle-class infants that did not accurately reflect the national population. The most current growth charts include BMI percentiles for children from 2 to 18 years.

2. *Answer:* A
    Rationale: The CDC Growth Charts consist of revised versions of the growth charts developed by the National Center for Health Statistics in 1977 and the addition of BMI-for-age charts.

3. *Answer:* B
    Rationale: Serial measurements are needed to establish growth patterns and are affected by such factors as gestational age, birth weight, genetic influence and genetic disorders, environmental influences, and biological influences.

4. *Answer:* D
    Rationale: Infants gain more weight between birth and 7 months than between 7 and 12 months. A single measurement between birth and 7 months may falsely indicate unusual weight gain. Infants typically lose 5% to 10% of their birth weight immediately after birth.

5. *Answer:* A
    Rationale: The BMI-for-age charts are for children and adolescents aged 2 to 20, not for infants and children younger than 2 years of age.

6. *Answer:* C
    Rationale: Body mass index (BMI) is an anthropometric index of weight and height combined with age. BMI-for-age is used to identify children and adolescents as underweight, overweight, or at risk of overweight.

7. *Answer:* B
    Rationale: Infants should be weighed without clothing or with a clean diaper if the weight of the clean diaper is taken into account.

8. *Answer:* C
    Rationale: Based on data from 1999-2000 NHANES, 21% of 2- to 5-year-olds, 30% of 6- to 11-year-olds, and 30% of all teens in the United States are now overweight or at risk of overweight. Overweight results when energy intake exceeds energy needs for growth, maintenance, and activity.

9. *Answer:* B
    Rationale: Using the metric system formula of weight (kg)/height (cm)^2 × 10,000 (16.6 kg/99.1 cm/99.1 cm) × 10,000 = 16.9; or using the English system formula of weight (lbs)/height (in)^2 × 703 (36.5 lbs/39 in/39 in) × 703 = 16.9. Using this calculation, Malia's BMI is 16.9.

10. *Answer:* D
    Rationale: BMI screening criteria CDC 2006: Overweight greater than or equal to 95th percentile; at risk of overweight, 85th to less than 95th percentile; normal weight 5th to less than 85th percentile; underweight less than 5th percentile.

11. *Answer:* B
    Rationale: The major categories of cause for short stature include genetic, constitutional delay; chronic disease; and chromosomal, endocrine, psychosocial, and intrauterine problems .

12. *Answer:* A
    Rationale: Early recognition of increases in weight to linear growth can be assessed by calculating and plotting BMI routinely on standardized growth charts; tracking BMI increases provider, teen, and parent awareness of trends in weight.

13. *Answer:* B
    Rationale: There is no consensus on the definition of failure to thrive. It is a descriptive rather than a diagnostic term. A comprehensive history and meticulous physical examination are necessary. In addition, a nutritional assessment, including feeding patterns and review of growth patterns, needs to be completed.

14. *Answer:* B

Rationale: A clinical partnership is a relationship in which participants join together to ensure health care delivery in a way that recognizes the critical roles and contributions of child, family, health care provider, and community.

15. *Answer:* C
    Rationale: The mission of Bright Futures is to promote and improve the health, social development, and well-being of infants, children, adolescents, families, and communities.

16. *Answer:* B
    Rationale: The Denver II is designed to be used with well children from birth to 6 years of age. The test must be administered in the standardized manner.

17. *Answer:* A
    Rationale: Since the evaluation using the Denver II may cause anxiety for the child's caregiver, it is essential to explain that the Denver II is administered to determine the child's current developmental status. It is not an IQ test, and the child is not expected to pass all of the items administered.

18. *Answer:* D
    Rationale: The Ages and Stages Questionnaire (ASQ) is a parent report covering ages 4 months through 60 months. It includes six questions in each of the five domains: communication, gross motor, fine motor, problem solving, and personal-social, and the parents note whether the child can perform the skill identified.

19. *Answer:* C
    Rationale: The Nursing Child Assessment Satellite Training (NCAST) is an assessment technique that provides observable behaviors that describe the parent-child interaction, infant behavior, and parental behavior. The provider must complete a training course before using this tool.

20. *Answer:* A
    Rationale: The child is given a sheet of paper and instructed to draw a person or asked to make a shape. The child is given one point for each detail present on the drawing of the person or an age equivalent for the shape completed. The scores are compared to norms for age. The ability to execute these figures requires visual-perceptual, fine motor, and cognitive abilities.

21. *Answer:* C
    Rationale: An evaluation of hearing is mandatory in any setting of significant speech/language delay. Language screening is divided into expressive, visual, and receptive language skills. Because language and cognitive skills are intricately interwoven, any delays noted should alert the provider to proceed with diagnostic follow-up and early intervention services.

22. *Answer:* B
    Rationale: Fluharty-2 tests articulation and language performance in children 3 to 6 years of age.

23. *Answer:* B
    Rationale: Failure to acquire speech developmental milestones should prompt the provider to explore the etiology and make a referral for early intervention services.

24. *Answer:* A
    Rationale: In ongoing developmental assessments, premature infants for the most part catch up to their chronological peers. Early in life, the extent of prematurity must be taken into account during assessments.

25. *Answer:* C
    Rationale: Normal variation is the most common cause of motor delay, followed by mental retardation and then cerebral palsy. The three essential features of autism are: impaired social interaction, absent or abnormal speech/language development, a narrow range of interest, and stereotyped or repetitive response to objects.

BIBLIOGRAPHY

Accardo, P. & Capute, A. (2005). *The Capute Scales: Cognitive Adaptive Test and Clinical Linguistic and Auditory Milestone Scale (CAT/CLAMS).* Baltimore: Brookes.

AGS Publishing. (2004). Fluharty-2: Fluharty preschool speech and language screening test. Retrieved March 11, 2006 from www.agsnet.com/Group.asp?nMarketInfoID=42&nCategoryInfoID=2668&nGroupInfoID=a11390.

American Academy of Pediatrics, Committee on Nutrition. (2004). *Pediatric nutrition handbook* (5th ed.). Elk Grove Village, IL: American Academy of Pediatrics.

Bricker, D. & Squires, J. (1999). *Ages and Stages Questionnaires: A parent-completed, child-monitoring system (2nd ed.).* Baltimore: Brookes.

Centers for Disease Control and Prevention. (2002). National health and nutrition examination survey: Overweight among U.S. children and adolescents. Retrieved March 11, 2006, from www.cdc.gov/nchs/data/nhanes/databriefs/overwght.pdf.

Centers for Disease Control and Prevention. (2006a). Accurately weighing and measuring. Module 1: Equipment; Module 2: Technique. Retrieved March 11, 2006, from http://depts.washington.edu/growth.

Centers for Disease Control and Prevention. (2006b). CDC table for calculated body mass index values for selected heights and weights for ages 2 to 20 years. Retrieved March 11, 2006, from www.cdc.gov/nccdphp/dnpa/bmi/00binaries/bmi-tables.pdf.

Centers for Disease Control and Prevention. (2006c). Growth chart training. Retrieved March 11, 2006, from http://depts.washington.edu/growth.

Centers for Disease Control and Prevention. (2006d). Overview of the CDC growth charts. Retrieved March 11, 2006 from www.cdc.gov/nccdphp/dnpa/growthcharts/training/modules/module2/text/page1a.htm.

Centers for Disease Control and Prevention. (2006e). The CDC growth charts for children with special health care needs. Retrieved March 11, 2006, from http://depts.washington.edu/growth/cshcn/text/page1a.htm.

Denver Developmental Materials, Inc. (1999). Denver II. Retrieved March 11, 2006, from www.denverii.com/DenverII.html.

Denver Developmental Materials, Inc. (1973). Denver Articulation Screening Exam (DASE). Retrieved March 11, 2006, from www.denverii.com/DASE.html.

Goldbloom, R. (2003). Assessment of physical growth. In R. Goldbloom (Ed.). *Pediatric clinical skills* (3rd ed., pp. 23-48). New York: Churchill Livingstone.

Green, M. & Palfrey, J.S. (Eds.). (2002). *Bright futures: Guidelines for health supervision of infants, children, and adolescents.* (3rd ed.). Arlington, VA: National Center for Education in Maternal and Child Health.

Koppitz, E. (1984). *Psychological evaluation of human figure drawings by middle school pupils.* Orlando, FL: Grune & Stratton, Inc.

Koppitz, E. (1968). *Psychological evaluation of children's human figure drawings.* New York: Grune & Stratton.

Kube, D., Wilson, W., Peterssen, M., & Palmer, F. (2000). CAT/CLAMS: Its use in detecting early childhood cognitive impairment. *Pediatr Neurol, 23*(3), 208–215.

Maternal and Child Health Bureau. (2006). Identifying poor growth in infants and toddlers. Retrieved March 11, 2006, from http://depts.washington.edu/growth/poorgrowth/text/intro.htm.

Morrison, J., Barton, B. Obarzanek, E. et al. (2001). Racial differences in the sums of skinfolds and percentage of body fat estimated from impedance in black and white girls, 9 to 19 years of age: The National Heart, Lung, and Blood Institute Growth and Health Study. *Obesity Res, 9*(5), 97.

National Health and Nutrition Examination Survey. (2002). *Anthropometry procedures manual.* Retrieved March 11, 2006 from www.cdc.gov/nchs/data/nhanes/nhanes_01_02/body_measures_year_3.pdf.

National Health and Nutrition Examination Survey (2000). *Body composition procedures manual.* Retrieved March 11, 2006 from www.cdc.gov/nchs/data/nhanes/bc.pdf.

NCAST AVENUW. (2004). *NCAST Programs, University of Washington.* Retrieved March 11, 2006, from www.ncast.org.

Roberts, S. & Dallal, G. (2001). The new childhood growth charts. *Nutr Rev, 59*(2), 31.

Robinson, T., Kiernan, M., Matheson, D.M., & Haydelet, K.F. (2001). Is parental control over children's eating associated with childhood obesity? Results from a population-based sample of third graders. *Obesity Res, 9*(5), 306.

Ryan-Wenger, N. (2001). Use of children's drawings for measurement of developmental level and emotional status. *J Child Fam Nurs, 4*, 139.

Skybo, T., & Ryan-Wenger, N. (2003). Measures of overweight status in school-age children. *J Sch Nurs, 19*(3), 172.

Strauss, R., & Pollack, H. (2001). Epidemic increase in childhood overweight: 1986–1998. *JAMA, 286*(22), 2845.

Sumner, G., & Spietz, G. (1994). *NCAST caregiver/parent-child interaction feeding manual.* Seattle: NCAST Publications, University of Washington, School of Nursing.

Talbot, L., & Lister, Z. (1995). Assessing body composition: The skinfold method. *AAOHN J, 43*(12), 605.

Tanita. (2003). Tanita: FatCheck. Retrieved March 11, 2006, from www.fatcheck.com/home.html.

U.S. Department of Health and Human Services. (2003a). *Criteria for determining disability in infants and children: Short stature.* (AHRQ Publication No. 03-E025). Rockville, MD: Author. Retrieved March 13, 2006, from www.ahrq.gov/clinic/epcsums/shorts.htm.

U.S. Department of Health and Human Services. (2003b). *Criteria for determining disability in infants and children: Failure to thrive.* (AHRQ Pub-lication No. 03-E019). Rockville, MD: Author. Retrieved March 13, 2006, from www.ahrq.gov/clinic/epcsums/fthrivesum.htm.

Utter, A., Scott, J., Oppliger, R., et al. (2001). A comparison of leg-to-leg bioelectrical impedance and skinfolds in assessing body fat in collegiate wrestlers. *J Strength Cond Res, 15*(2), 157.

Zemel, B., Riley, E., & Stallings, V. (1997). Evaluation of methodology for nutritional assessment in children: Anthropometry, body composition, and energy expenditure. *Annu Rev Nutr, 17,* 211.

NOTES

5

Assessment of the Head, Eyes, Ears, Nose, and Throat

JULEE WALDROP

Select the best answer for each of the following questions:

1. If a child is born with a cleft palate, the problem occurred during which period of gestation?
   A. Less than 4 weeks.
   B. 6 to 12 weeks.
   C. 13 to 24 weeks.
   D. More than 24 weeks.

2. When taking the prenatal history of a baby with a cleft palate, it would be important to ask about:
   A. Medications or substance use during pregnancy.
   B. Gestational hypertension.
   C. Weight gain during pregnancy.
   D. Problems during labor and delivery.

3. Robert is a new patient to your practice. He is here for a 9-month checkup. His head circumference measurement is plotted at greater than the 98th percentile. The most helpful history question at this point would be:
   A. Does Robert have a shunt?
   B. Which parent has the big head?
   C. When Robert's head has been measured in the past, has it always been large for his age?
   D. Has Robert had a head ultrasound before?

4. The average size for a newborn anterior fontanelle is:
   A. 0.5 cm.
   B. 1.0 cm.
   C. 1.5 cm.
   D. 2.1 cm.

5. Kara is 7 years old. Her visual acuity was screened using the Snellen alphabet chart. She scored 20/50 with her right eye and 20/20 with her left eye. Based on these results you will:
   A. Advise her to come back in 6 months and get rescreened.
   B. Tell her that her vision is within normal limits for her age.
   C. Refer her to an ophthalmologist.
   D. Keep testing her; she will get better with practice.

6. Anna is a 4-year-old. Which of the following screening tests for visual acuity would be good to use with her?
   A. HOTV matching chart.
   B. Snellen alphabet.
   C. Newsprint.
   D. Letter recognition.

7. Which of the following is used for hearing assessment in children aged 4 years and older?
   A. Brainstem auditory evoked response (BAER).
   B. Moro reflex.
   C. Whisper test.
   D. Audiometry.

8. Kevin's mom wants to know when he will stop "going cross-eyed." He is 3 months old. You tell her that it is:
   A. Not normal to be cross-eyed and he needs to be referred to an ophthalmologist.

B. Normal at his age and should resolve by 6 months.
C. Normal at his age and should resolve by 9 months.
D. Normal at his age and should resolve by 12 months.

9. Kevin is now 9 months old and he missed his 6-month checkup. His mom is concerned that his left eye still looks crossed sometimes. You perform the cover-uncover test on Kevin. A normal response, once you uncover the right eye is:
   A. No movement in the right eye.
   B. Dilation in the right eye.
   C. Right eye deviates inward.
   D. Left eye deviates outward.

10. Another test that can be used to screen for strabismus is:
    A. The Bruckner test or red reflex.
    B. Fundoscopy.
    C. Corneal light reflex.
    D. Cardinal fields of gaze.

11. The Bruckner or red reflex is done in the newborn period to rule out:
    A. Congenital cataracts.
    B. Decreased visual acuity.
    C. Strabismus.
    D. Corneal abrasions.

12. David is 6 months old and was brought to the emergency department because his mom found her boyfriend shaking him when the baby wouldn't stop crying. You do a fundoscopic exam to rule out:
    A. Corneal abrasion.
    B. Retinal hemorrhage.
    C. Retinoblastoma.
    D. Intracranial hemorrhage.

13. When examining a newborn, you assess for ear placement. The superior tip of the ear should be located:
    A. Below an imaginary line that extends from the outer canthus of the eye.
    B. At an imaginary line that extends from the outer canthus of the eye.
    C. In front of an imaginary line that extends from the junction of the coronal and sagittal sutures of the skull.

D. Behind an imaginary line that extends from the junction of the coronal and sagittal sutures of the skull.

14. Grace's mother brings her to the office. She says that her left ear is draining. On exam you see that the external canal has an orange-colored runny substance in it but the tympanic membrane appears normal. The ear canal is not inflamed. This is consistent with:
    A. Otitis externa.
    B. Otitis media.
    C. Otitis media with effusion.
    D. Excessive cerumen.

15. On examining Oliver, you visualize a slight crease across his nose where the nasal bone ends. This may be a sign of:
    A. Allergic rhinitis.
    B. Sinusitis.
    C. An upper respiratory infection.
    D. Asthma.

16. Kathryn is 6 years old. She is in the office complaining of a sore throat. On exam her tonsils are touching each other. You record this finding as tonsils:
    A. 1+.
    B. 2+.
    C. 3+.
    D. 4+.

17. In a child with chronic allergic rhinitis you might also observe:
    A. The epiglottis for exudate.
    B. Cobblestoning of the posterior pharynx.
    C. Petechiae of the palate.
    D. Bifid uvula.

18. Which of the following glands are involved in mumps?
    A. Submandibular
    B. Tonsilar
    C. Parotid
    D. Sublingual

19. Primary dentition erupts between:
    A. 6 and 24 months.
    B. 1 and 5 years.
    C. 6 months and 3 years.

D. 6 and 11 years.

20. One way to assess for increased intra-cranial pressure is palpation of the fontanelle in infants. The best position for the infant during this assessment is:
A. The supine position.
B. The prone position.
C. In a sitting position.
D. While crying in a sitting position.

21. At what age should the anterior fontanelle no longer be palpable?
A. 26 months.
B. 2 months.
C. 18 months.
D. 6 months.

22. At 10 months of age, you can assess receptive language ability by asking the:
A. Parent if the child says "mama" or "dada."
B. Child to perform one action with a verbal command.

C. Child to point to objects according to their use.
D. Parent if the child can speak at least 20 words.

23. Jeannine's mom is worried about 24-month-old Jeannine because her older daughter was talking in sentences by the same age. What do you expect Jeannine should be able to do with verbal expression?
A. Speak three-word sentences.
B. Use plurals.
C. Use gestures to seek help.
D. Name all body parts.

24. A flat philtrum and a thin upper lip are signs of:
A. Down syndrome.
B. Trisomy 13.
C. Fetal alcohol syndrome.
D. Russell Silver syndrome.

NOTES

ANSWERS

1. *Answer:* B
   Rationale: The palate and other midline structures develop during the second half of the first trimester, weeks 6 through 12. The fetus' major organ systems and cellular differentiation occur from 4 through 12 weeks gestation.

2. *Answer:* A
   Rationale: Medications or exposure to drugs or toxins may interfere with the developing fetus and be associated with birth defects like cleft palate. Gestational hypertension, weight gain, and problems during labor and delivery all occur after the first trimester when the fetus is most at risk for developmental insults.

3. *Answer:* C
   Rationale: It is most important to know if this is normal for Robert or is something new before further questions are asked. A head circumference of greater than the 98th percentile can still be benign. It does not automatically indicate hydrocephalus and the practitioner should not jump to conclusions or raise alarm unnecessarily.

4. *Answer:* D
   Rationale: Although the range of size of the newborn fontanelle is wide, the mean newborn anterior fontanelle size is 2.1 cm. The posterior fontanelle size is 0.5 to 0.7 cm.

5. *Answer:* C
   Rationale: At 7 years of age, Kara should have developed optimal visual acuity and rechecking will only delay her receiving the appropriate prescriptive help. She should also not need to practice the test; at 7 years of age she should be developmentally able to perform the test. Kara has more than a two-line difference between her eyes. This necessitates a referral to an ophthalmologist, as she may be suffering from strabismus and early treatment can prevent amblyopia.

6. *Answer:* A
   Rationale: At 4 years of age, Anna may not yet know her alphabet, so the Snellen chart, letter recognition, and newsprint would not be appropriate. The HOTV matching chart has two advantages for use in preschoolers: It does not require letter recognition and also does not require talking, just pointing.

7. *Answer:* D
   Rationale: Audiometry can be used in children starting at the age of 4 for assessment of the ability to hear frequencies (Hertz) and loudness (decibels). The BAER only tests nerve conduction and is used in infant hearing screening. The whisper test is a gross test of hearing and the Moro reflex is not a hearing test.

8. *Answer:* B
   Rationale: Binocular vision is not established until 6 months of age.

9. *Answer:* A
   Rationale: Cover-uncover test is used to detect strabismus. In a normal result, the covered eye will not deviate when uncovered.

10. *Answer:* C
    Rationale: The corneal light reflex demonstrates binocular fixation. If the corneal light reflex occurs equally, then strabismus is unlikely. The red reflex test demonstrates the absence of retinoblastoma or congenital cataracts. Fundoscopic exam evaluates the fundus, which is not related to visual fixation. Cardinal fields of gaze demonstrate extraocular movement.

11. *Answer:* A
    Rationale: The red reflex rules out congenital cataracts and retinoblastoma. You cannot detect strabismus or visual acuity in the newborn period. A corneal abrasion would not be visible while doing the Bruckner test.

12. *Answer:* B
    Rationale: The fundoscopic exam allows you to visualize structures at the back of the eye, such as the retinal vessels. Retinal hemorrhage, a common sequel when a baby is shaken, can be visualized with a fundoscopic exam. Often flourescein staining is required

to see a corneal abrasion. Although a retinoblastoma can be seen during fundoscopic exam, it is not caused by shaking. Intracranial hemorrhage is not visible on fundoscopic exam.

13. *Answer:* B

Rationale: Having low-set ears below the outer canthus is a red flag for many congenital syndromes such as Down syndrome.

14. *Answer:* D

Rationale: Cerumen can be copious and orange to yellow color is common. A normal tympanic membrane and no inflammation of the external canal rules out the other diagnoses.

15. *Answer:* A

Rationale: The nasal crease is often caused by the child repeatedly wiping the nose with the palm of the hand in an upward manner as with chronic allergic rhinitis (known as the *allergic salute*). On visual inspection there are usually no visible signs of sinusitis, upper respiratory infection, or asthma.

16. *Answer:* D

Rationale: Tonsils can be large in children. An objective evaluation on a scale helps to communicate accurately the size of the tonsils.

17. *Answer:* B

Rationale: Chronic exposure to postnasal exudates causes an inflammatory response with a bumpy or "cobblestone" appearance in the posterior pharynx.

18. *Answer:* C

Rationale: The mumps virus causes significant swelling of the parotid gland. Other glands are often part of the generalized lymph adenopathy that occurs in viral infections of the upper respiratory tract.

19. *Answer:* A

Rationale: By 24 months, most children will have all of the 20 teeth of the primary dentition.

20. *Answer:* C

Rationale: The sitting position decreases the effect of gravity or crying and gives the most accurate assessment. Crying will cause increased tone in the fontanelle.

21. *Answer:* A

Rationale: The anterior fontanelle closes by 24 to 26 months. The posterior fontanelle is usually closed by 2 months.

22. *Answer:* B

Rationale: At 10 months, a child should be able to understand (receive) language enough to comply with a one-action command like "wave bye-bye." Speech is considered part of expressive language. Identifying objects and their function is a more complex skill, developed in the second year of life.

23. *Answer:* A

Rationale: By 2 years of age, Jeannine should be able to put two words together frequently and use three-word sentences. Using only gestures to seek help at this age would indicate a delay. Naming body parts is also a skill usually learned before sentence construction, but using plurals is a more developed skill.

24. *Answer:* C

Rationale: A flat philtrum and thin upper lip are classic signs of fetal alcohol syndrome. This is not a facial characteristic associated with the trisomies. (Low-set ears and epicanthal folds are more common.) Facial features associated with Russell Silver syndrome are more subtle at birth.

BIBLIOGRAPHY

American Academy of Pediatrics. (2003). Oral health risk assessment timing and establishment of the dental home. *Pediatrics*, *111*(5), 1113-1116.

American Academy of Pediatrics, Committee on Practice and Ambulatory Medicine and Section on Ophthalmology. (2002). Use of photoscreening for children's vision screening. *Pediatrics*, *109*(3), 524-525.

American Academy of Pediatrics. (2003). Hearing assessment in infants and children: Recommendations beyond neonatal screening. *Pediatrics, 111*(2), 436-440.

Colyar, M.R. (2003). *Well-child assessment for primary care providers*. Philadelphia: F.A. Davis.

Cunningham, M., Cox, E.O. (2003). American Academy of Pediatrics Committee on Practice and Ambulatory Medicine and the Section on Otolaryngology and Bronchoesophagology. Hearing assessment in infants and children: Recommendations beyond neonatal screening. *Pediatrics, 111*(2), 436-440.

Curnyn, K.M., & Kaufman, L.M. (2003). The eye examination in the pediatrician's office, *Pediatr Clin North Am, 50*(1), 25-40.

Goldbloom, R.B. (2003). *Pediatric clinical skills* (3rd ed.). Philadelphia: Saunders.

Larsen, W.J. (2001). *Human embryology*. New York: Churchill Livingstone.

Moore, K.L., & Persaud, T.V.N. (2003). *The developing human: Clinically oriented embryology*. Philadelphia: Saunders.

Moses, S. (2005). Fontanelle. Family practice notebook. Retrieved on August 8, 2005, from www. fpnotebook.com/NIC25.htm.

Seidel, H.M., Ball, J.W., Dains, J.E., & Benedict, G.W. (2003). *Mosby's guide to physical examination* (5th ed.). St. Louis: Mosby.

U.S. Preventive Services Task Force. (2004). *Screening for visual impairment in children younger than age 5 years: Recommendation statement*. May 2004. Rockville, MD: Agency for Healthcare Research and Quality. Retrieved August 8, 2005, from www.ahrq.gov/clinic/3rduspstf/visionscr/vischrs.htm.

NOTES

Assessment of the Pulmonary System

JULEE WALDROP

Select the best answer for each of the following questions:

1. Which cells present in the alveoli produce surfactant?
   A. Type I cells.
   B. Type II cells.
   C. Goblet cells.
   D. Epithelial cells.

2. When taking the neonatal history of a 6-month-old patient new to your office, which of the following factors will have an effect on current lung function?
   A. Low gestational age at birth.
   B. Low Apgar scores.
   C. IUGR.
   D. SGA.

3. In taking a past medical history with a new teenage patient, he reports all of the following. Which one represents continued respiratory risk?
   A. Asthma.
   B. Pneumonia.
   C. Foreign body aspiration.
   D. Respiratory syncitial virus.

4. Gregory is 12 months old and his mom brings him in today because he has coughing fits and can't catch his breath. It is scaring her. You review his chart and quickly notice he has not been in for a well child visit since his 2-month-old checkup. His mother denies going anywhere else for care. Based on the chief complaint, you are concerned about Gregory's incomplete vaccination series with:
   A. IPV.
   B. HIB.
   C. DTaP.
   D. PCV7.

5. Which of the following respiratory conditions can be detected with prenatal testing?
   A. Asthma.
   B. Allergies.
   C. Bronchopulmonary dysplasia.
   D. Cystic fibrosis.

6. All children's respiratory health is significantly compromised by which of the following environmental factors?
   A. Crowded living conditions.
   B. Exposure to second-hand smoke.
   C. Pets.
   D. Dust.

7. In which age group is it normal to have an A:P chest diameter of 1:1?
   A. Infant.
   B. Toddler.
   C. School-age.
   D. Adolescent.

8. A respiratory rate of 50 would be normal in what age group?
   A. Infant.
   B. Toddler.
   C. School-age.
   D. Adolescent.

9. On physical examination of a newborn, you notice that one side of the chest wall is more prominent than the other. This could indicate:

A. Delayed opening of the bronchioles and alveoli on the less prominent side.
B. Pectus excavatum.
C. Pectus carinatum.
D. Spontaneous pneumothorax.

10. Peak flow meter measurements are based on the child's:
A. Age.
B. Height.
C. Weight.
D. BMI.

11. Airway compromise can be evaluated using a peak flow meter in patients with asthma. At what age can you reliably begin to use this tool for assessment?
A. Infant.
B. Toddler.
C. Preschool.
D. School-age.

12. Ms. Jones is in the office for her baby's newborn checkup. She is concerned because "sometimes Adrienne's breathing is really fast and sometimes she hardly seems to be breathing." What do you tell her?
A. Infants have irregular breathing rates and rhythm.
B. Because infants' breathing rate is so fast, it is difficult to see all the breaths they take.
C. Infants breathe so shallowly you can miss some breaths.
D. Infants' respiratory rate should be regular and she is right to be concerned.

13. Auscultation is important in the evaluation of the respiratory system; however, what other assessment can give you a lot of information about how well the respiratory system is functioning?
A. Heart rate.
B. Skin color.
C. Bowel sounds.
D. Reflexes.

14. Francisco is 3 years old. His mom brings him in because she ran out of his asthma medicine last week and he is getting worse without it. On auscultation you expect to find:

A. Stridor.
B. Wheezing.
C. Crackles.
D. Clear lung fields.

15. Another sign of increased work of breathing that you might find on Francisco's exam is:
A. Grunting.
B. Tracheal deviation.
C. Crepitus.
D. Tactile fremitus.

16. Percussion of the lung fields is helpful in determining:
A. Gas exchange.
B. Expiratory volume.
C. Areas of consolidation.
D. Tidal volume.

17. Lynne is a 15-year-old female who arrives at the urgent care center where you work at 8 PM complaining of chest pain. You suspect she has had a spontaneous pneumothorax because on percussion of her right chest, you detect:
A. Resonance.
B. Dullness.
C. Hyperresonance.
D. Tympany.

18. When auscultating a child's lung fields over the posterior chest, you expect to hear:
A. Tracheal lung sounds.
B. Bronchial lung sounds.
C. Vesicular lung sounds.
D. Bronchovesicular lungs sounds.

19. Audrey is 8 years old. Her father brings her in because she has been saying that "it hurts to breathe deep." On auscultation, you hear a harsh grating sound with respirations. This is indicative of a:
A. Friction rub.
B. Crackles.
C. Wheezing.
D. Stridor.

20. Elizabeth's father rushes her to the emergency department in the middle of the night because she developed this terrible "barking" cough. On auscultation you expect to hear:

A. Wheezing.
B. Stridor.
C. Crackles.
D. Friction rub.

21. Dylan presents with a complaint of abrupt onset of fever and cough for 24 hours. On exam, you find decreased breath sounds in the right lower lobe. With percussion, you believe you hear dullness. The last test you could do to confirm your suspicion of pneumonia is whispered pectoriloquy. You expect to find:
   A. Increased quality of loudness of whispered sounds.
   B. Decreased quality of loudness of whispered sounds.
   C. Abnormal voice sounds.
   D. Normal voice sounds.

22. The primary immune system cells involved in protection from infection contracted via the airways are:
   A. Epithelial cells.
   B. Macrophages.
   C. T cells.
   D. Clara cells.

23. Steven is 4 months old and his mom brings him to the office because he has had a cold for a few days but over the last 24 hours he has not been nursing well. She says he just takes a few sucks then stops and breathes. You tell the mother that:

   A. Difficulty nursing as described above can be related to respiratory system compromise.
   B. All babies suck in a start and stop manner. This does not sound so unusual.
   C. It is normal for babies with a cold to not be able to feed well. Don't worry.
   D. She needs to come back the next time Jackson needs to nurse so you can observe the feeding.

24. Lillian's parents are waiting until she is 12 months old to receive any vaccinations. She has had two episodes of otitis media in the last 2 months. Which of the following vaccines may have prevented these episodes?
   A. DTaP
   B. IPV
   C. Hep B
   D. PCV7

25. Madeleine is 4 days old and at the office for a newborn checkup. Her parents are worried because she looks like she is always cold. Her hands and feet often have a bluish tinge. You explain that this is:
   A. A sign of poor oxygenation and must be further evaluated.
   B. A sign of cardiovascular compromise and must be further evaluated.
   C. A sign that she is too cold and they need to keep mittens and socks on her at all times.
   D. Normal in new babies and will resolve on its own in a week or so.

ANSWERS

1. *Answer:* B
   Rationale: There is one type II for every seven type I cells in the alveoli. Type II cells produce surfactant for keeping the alveoli open even at low pressures. Goblet cells produce mucus and epithelial cells line the upper airways.

2. *Answer:* A
   Rationale: Prematurity is the greatest risk factor for chronic lung disease, which can continue to cause problems in a 6-month-old. A low Apgar only indicates the status of the infant at 1 and 5 minutes after birth. IUGR or SGA are related to weight or size of the infant and not lung maturity.

3. *Answer:* A
   Rationale: Asthma is the only chronic problem in this list. The others are acute problems which should resolve without sequelae.

4. *Answer:* C
   Rationale: Paroxysmal coughing is a hallmark sign of pertussis. Gregory's incomplete vaccine series for DTaP puts him at risk for contracting pertussis.

5. *Answer:* D
   Rationale: Cystic fibrosis is the only genetic disease that can be detected prenatally. Asthma and allergies have not had a specific gene associated with them. Bronchopulmonary dysplasia or chronic lung disease is a consequence of prematurity not a genetic disease.

6. *Answer:* B
   Rationale: All children are harmed by second-hand smoke, whereas only children with allergies are affected by exposure to pet dander or dust. Crowded living conditions are not necessarily harmful to respiratory health.

7. *Answer:* A
   Rationale: Infants normally have a barrel-shaped chest. In all other age groups, this would be a sign of chronic lung compro-

mise such as that seen in chronic lung disease or cystic fibrosis.

8. *Answer:* A
   Rationale: Normal respiratory rate for infants is 30 to 80. Respiratory rate decreases with age.

9. *Answer:* D
   Rationale: Asymmetry of the chest wall shape is most likely due to a pathological cause such as pneumothorax. Pectus excavatum and pectus carinatum are deformities of the middle chest. Delayed opening of bronchioles and alveoli is not detected on visual inspection.

10. *Answer:* B
    Rationale: Height is most closely correlated with lung volume.

11. *Answer:* D
    Rationale: Children must be able to mechanically perform the exercise as well as follow directions. This reliably occurs by school-age, although there may be exceptions.

12. *Answer:* A
    Rationale: Infants may take shallow, rapid breaths and have irregular respiratory rates and rhythms. This is normal and not a cause for concern.

13. *Answer:* B
    Rationale: Any change in skin color toward blue or gray, whether circumoral or generalized, is a sign of poor gas exchange and respiratory or cardiorespiratory compromise. Heart rate may increase after peripheral vessels have constricted. The GI tract and nervous system will not manifest changes initially.

14. *Answer:* B
    Rationale: Wheezing is a hallmark finding in asthma. Stridor is a sign of croup and crackles can indicate consolidation.

15. *Answer:* A
    Rationale: Grunting is another sign of increased effort to expel air from the small airways. Crepitus is a sign of air in the sub-

cutaneous tissues. Tactile fremitus will be increased in areas of consolidation and tracheal deviation is a sign of pneumothorax.

16. *Answer:* C
    Rationale: Percussion is useful to determine air-filled, fluid-filled, or solid structures underlying the chest wall. Gas exchange, expiratory volume, and tidal volume are all assessments of lung function that are not part of the physical exam.

17. *Answer:* C
    Rationale: Hyperresonance on percussion is evidence of underlying air-filled area. The other sounds indicate increasing levels of solidity from resonance to tympany to dullness.

18. *Answer:* D
    Rationale: Bronchiovesicular lung sounds are softer than bronchial sounds of the larger airways and are fairly equal on inspiration and expiration. Tracheal sounds can only be heard over the trachea. Bronchial and vesicular lungs sounds are best heard anteriorly.

19. *Answer:* A
    Rationale: Friction rubs are present when there is inflammation and two surfaces are moving across each other. Crackles are caused by consolidation or fluid accumulation. Wheezes and stridor are caused by airway narrowing.

20. *Answer:* B
    Rationale: Stridor is a hallmark sign of viral croup infection, also characterized by a "barking cough." Wheezing is heard primarily on inhalation and associated with asthma or bronchiolitis. Crackles are heard over consolidation as in pneumonia and a friction rub usually causes pain, not a "barking cough."

21. *Answer:* A
    Rationale: When there is consolidation of a lung field, whispered sounds will be clearer and louder but not normal over the area on auscultation. Decreased quality of loudness and abnormal voice sounds are normal find-ings and should be present in the unaffected lung.

22. *Answer:* B
    Rationale: Macrophages perform the job of engulfing foreign materials when they come in contact with the epithelium. T cells are present in the serum and lymph and clara cells produce surfactant.

23. *Answer:* A
    Rationale: When a baby must stop nursing to breathe, this is a concern and he is at risk for dehydration. Babies breathe through their noses during feeding and the baby's airway is compromised. Although babies do nurse in a start and stop manner, they do not unlatch to breathe through their mouths.

24. *Answer:* D
    Rationale: The PCV7 (Prevnar) protects against *Streptococcus pneumoniae* which is one of the most common causes of bacterial meningitis and otitis media. Diphtheria and pertussis affect the lower respiratory tract. Hepatitis B affects the liver and polio attacks the neuromuscular system.

25. *Answer:* D
    Rationale: This is called *acrocyanosis* and is normal in newborns and presumed to be related to an immature vascular system. It does not reflect oxygenation status or core temperature. Central cyanosis is indicative of cardiorespiratory compromise.

BIBLIOGRAPHY

Asthma and Allergy Information and Research. (3/24/2003). Asthma: What should my child's peak flow be? Retrieved August 8, 2005, from www.users.globalnet.co.uk/~aair/asthma_PEFCH.htm.

CATS—*Computer assisted teaching system*. University of Vermont College of Medicine. Retrieved August 8, 2005, from http://cats.med.uvm.edu.

Colyar, M.R. (2003). *Well-child assessment for primary care providers*. Philadelphia: F.A. Davis.

Dorland's Illustrated Medical Dictionary. (2002). Philadelphia: Saunders. Retrieved August 8, 2005, from www.Mercksource.com.

Goldbloom, R.B. (2003). *Pediatric clinical skills* (3rd ed.). Philadelphia: Saunders.

Larsen, W.J. (2001). *Human embryology*. New York: Churchill Livingstone.

Moore, K.L., & Persaud, T.V.N. (2003). *The developing human: Clinically oriented embryology*. Philadelphia: Saunders.

RNCeus. (2004). Normal breath sounds. Retrieved August 8, 2005, from www.rnceus.com/resp/respnorm.html.

Seidel, H.M., Ball, J.W., Dains, J.E., & Benedict, G.W. (2003). *Mosby's guide to physical examination* (5th ed.). St. Louis: Mosby.

NOTES

7 Assessment of the Cicardiovascular System

VICTORIA P. NIEDERHAUSER

Select the best answer for each of the following questions:

1. All of the following syndromes are associated with congenital heart conditions EXCEPT:
   A. Turner's syndrome.
   B. Fetal alcohol syndrome.
   C. Noonan's syndrome.
   D. Marfan syndrome.

2. The fetal heart has four chambers by:
   A. 2 weeks.
   B. 8 weeks.
   C. 16 weeks.
   D. 24 weeks.

3. Maternal rubella infection during the first trimester has been associated with:
   A. Venous hum.
   B. Patent ductus arteriosus.
   C. Mitral stenosis.
   D. Tetralogy of Fallot.

4. What is the normal capillary refill time in a child?
   A. 1 to 2 seconds.
   B. 3 to 5 seconds.
   C. 5 to 7 seconds.
   D. 10 to 12 seconds.

5. Vickie, a pediatric nurse practitioner, is doing a cardiac assessment on an 18-month-old. Where would she expect to find the point of maximal impulse (PMI)?
   A. Second intercostal space at the mid-clavicular line.
   B. Second intercostal space at the right sternal border.
   C. Fourth intercostal space at the mid-clavicular line.
   D. Fourth intercostal space at the right sternal border.

6. Vickie notes the PMI is difficult to find, thready, and easy to obliterate. What is the correct way to document this impulse quality?
   A. 0
   B. +1
   C. +2
   D. +3

7. What is the correct way to assess for thrills?
   A. Listen carefully over the carotid arteries.
   B. Check bilateral femoral pulses.
   C. Observe the lips for cyanosis.
   D. Feel the chest with the base of the fingers.

8. Penny, a pediatric nurse practitioner, is conducting a well baby exam on Samantha, a 6-month-old. What is the best way for Penny to assess Samantha's femoral pulses?
   A. One at a time, using the bell of the stethoscope.
   B. Using the first and second digits of her dominant hand.
   C. One at a time, using the diaphragm of the stethoscope.
   D. Simultaneously while conducting the Ortolani's maneuver.

9. Penny listens for the first heart sound (S₁). She knows that this sound:
   A. Is created when the mitral and tricuspid valves close.
   B. Marks the beginning of diastole.
   C. Is very soft in children with mitral stenosis.
   D. Is created when the pulmonary and aortic valves close.

10. Which of the following characteristics of a heart murmur in a child would cause the GREATEST concern?
   A. Changes with position.
   B. Vibratory in nature.
   C. Grade II/VI.
   D. Occurs during diastole.

11. Trisha, a 3-year-old, has a Still's murmur. What would you expect to find when you auscultate her heart?
   A. Split S₂ and S₃.
   B. Musical quality and is louder when she is supine.
   C. Grade IV or higher.
   D. High pitch and radiates to the right chest.

12. The pediatric nurse practitioner notes a grade III venous hum murmur during a 4-year-old boy's physical examination. What is the BEST action?
   A. Reassure the parents and child that this is an innocent murmur.
   B. Order an EKG immediately.
   C. Refer to the pediatric cardiologist.
   D. Order an echocardiogram.

13. At what age should all well children get a blood pressure screening?
   A. 12 months.
   B. 18 months.
   C. 24 months.
   D. 36 months.

14. The clinic medical assistant obtained a blood pressure on a 4-year-old using an automated machine. The pediatric nurse practitioner noted the measurement was less than the 90th percentile. What would be the BEST initial action to take?
   A. Repeat the test using the other automated machine at the clinic.
   B. Refer to the pediatric cardiologist.
   C. Repeat the test using the manual auscultation method.
   D. Schedule a repeat test in 24 to 48 hours.

15. Observation of the chest is an important component in cardiac assessment. Chest movement that is described as "forceful outward movements" is called:
   A. Heaves.
   B. Bruits.
   C. Thrills.
   D. Splits.

16. While making newborn rounds on a 12-hour-old newborn, which finding would NOT be considered normal?
   A. Soft, grade III systolic murmur.
   B. Blood pressure reading of 70/40.
   C. Apical heart rate of 62.
   D. Capillary refill rate of 2 seconds.

17. What is the BEST way to measure blood pressure in a 5-year-old child?
   A. Standing straight against the wall.
   B. Lying supine on the examination table.
   C. Sitting with back supported and arm supported at heart level.
   D. Carried in a parent's arms.

18. Jana is a 16-year-old who comes into the clinic for a sports physical examination. Her blood pressure, measured twice, is 130/88 and 128/90, respectively. Based on her blood pressure readings, she is considered:
   A. Antihypertensive.
   B. Normotensive.
   C. Prehypertensive.
   D. Hypertensive.

19. Blood pressure percentages are based on:
    A. Age, gender, and percentage of height.
    B. Age, gender, and percentage of weight.
    C. Age, height, and weight.
    D. Age and weight.

20. A parent of a child diagnosed with an innocent heart murmur asks you to explain what causes this sound. The BEST response is:
    A. There is an obstruction as the blood flows through the child's heart valves.
    B. The structures of your child's heart are different from a normal heart.
    C. The sound is caused by turbulent blood flow in the heart.
    D. The pressure in the heart is high in children.

NOTES

ANSWERS

1. ***Answer:*** A
    Rationale: Several syndromes, including Down syndrome, fetal alcohol syndrome, Marfan syndrome, and Noonan's syndrome are associated with congenital heart disease.

2. ***Answer:*** B
    Rationale: During fetal development of the cardiovascular system, by 8 weeks there are four chambers in the heart.

3. ***Answer:*** B
    Rationale: Maternal rubella infections during the first trimester can cause congenital heart defects such as patent ductus arteriosus and pulmonary artery stenosis. A venous hum is an innocent heart murmur.

4. ***Answer:*** A
    Rationale: The normal capillary refill is 1 to 2 seconds. Longer capillary refill times indicate poor perfusion.

5. ***Answer:*** C
    Rationale: The PMI in infants and children under 4 years of age is located at the mid-clavicular line, fourth intercostal space.

6. ***Answer:*** B
    Rationale: Impulse quality is recorded on a 0 to 4 scale. 0 indicates the impulse is not palpable; +1 indicates a thready and difficult-to-find impulse; +2 is difficult to find and pressure may obliterate; +3 is normal, easy to find, difficult to obliterate; and +4 is strong, bounding, and cannot be obliterated.

7. ***Answer:*** D
    Rationale: Thrills are coarse, low-frequency vibrations that are felt with your hands.

8. ***Answer:*** B
    Rationale: The best way to assess femoral pulses is to use the finger pads of the dominant hand. Femoral pulses cannot be assessed while conducting the Ortolani's test or using a stethoscope.

9. ***Answer:*** A

Rationale: The S_1 heart sound is produced when the mitral and tricuspid valves close. The S_2 heart sound is produced when the aortic and pulmonary valves close, which marks the onset of diastole.

10. ***Answer:*** D
    Rationale: Murmurs that occur during diastole are never innocent murmurs; therefore, this finding should raise concern and indicate further investigation. Murmurs that change with position, are not loud (grade I-II), and are vibratory in nature are characteristic of innocent murmurs.

11. ***Answer:*** B
    Rationale: A Still's murmur is an innocent heart murmur with a musical, vibratory quality. They are common in children 2 to 6 years old and are loudest when the child is lying supine.

12. ***Answer:*** A
    Rationale: A venous hum is an innocent murmur, common in children ages 2 to 8 years. They are best heard when a child sits and changes when he or she is lying down and when he or she turns the head to the side.

13. ***Answer:*** D
    Rationale: Routine screening of blood pressure in healthy children should begin at 3 years of age.

14. ***Answer:*** C
    Rationale: National guidelines recommend that blood pressure readings of less than the 90th percentile be confirmed using the manual auscultation method.

15. ***Answer:*** A
    Rationale: Heaves are detected during the observation stage of the cardiac examination and are forceful outward movements in the chest wall. Split refers to the heart sounds; thrills are felt with palpation and are a vibratory sensation produced by turbulent blood flow that is usually secondary to valvular abnormalities. Carotid bruits are heard over the carotid arteries and are sounds created by turbulent flow within the blood vessel.

16. *Answer:* C

Rationale: The normal apical heart rate in a newborn is 80 to 180 beats per minute. A soft, grade III/IV systolic murmur found in the first 24 hours after birth is normal because the ductus arteriosus may not be closed. A normal newborn systolic blood pressure is between 65 and 95 mm Hg and the normal diastolic blood pressure is between 30 and 60 mm Hg. Capillary refill of 1 to 2 seconds is a normal finding.

17. *Answer:* C

Rationale: To get the most accurate reading, the best position to measure the blood pressure in this 5-year-old child is sitting, with his back against the chair and arm extended at the level of the heart.

18. *Answer:* C

Rationale: Any adolescent with a blood pressure of greater than or equal to 120/80 mm Hg is considered prehypertensive. Elevated blood pressure readings should be repeated twice during a clinic visit and the two systolic readings and two diastolic reading should be averaged.

19. *Answer:* A

Rationale: The most recent tables for blood pressure percentiles are based on the child's gender, age, and height percentiles on standardized growth charts.

20. *Answer:* C

Rationale: Innocent heart murmurs are common in children and are caused by the turbulent blood flow at the origin of the great vessels.

BIBLIOGRAPHY

Allen, H., Phillips, J., & Chan, D. (2001). History and physical examination. In H. Allen, H. Gutgesell, E. Clark, & D. Driscoll (Eds.). *Moss and Adams' heart disease in infants, children, and adolescents, volume 1* (6th ed.). Philadelphia: Lippincott Williams & Wilkins.

Arafat, M., & Mattoo, T. (1999). Measurement of blood pressure in children: Recommendations and perceptions on cuff selection. *Pediatrics, 104*(3), e30-34.

Barkauskas, V., Baumann, L., & Darling-Fisher, C. (2002). *Health and physical assessment* (3rd ed.). Philadelphia: Elsevier.

Bernstein, D. (2004). Evaluation of the cardiovascular system. In R. Behrman, R. Kliegman, & H. Jenson (Eds.). *Nelson textbook of pediatrics* (17th ed.). Philadelphia: Saunders.

Bickley, L., & Szilagyi. P. (2004). *Bates' guide to physical examination & history taking* (8th ed.). Philadelphia: Lippincott.

Engel, J. (2002). *Pocket guide to pediatric assessment.* St. Louis: Mosby.

Hoffman, J. (2003). The circulatory system. In A.M. Rudolph & C.D. Rudolph (Eds.). *Rudolph's pediatrics* (21st ed.). New York: McGraw-Hill.

Johnson, W., & Moller, J. (2001). *Pediatric cardiology.* Philadelphia: Lippincott Williams & Wilkins.

Larsen, W.J. (2001). *Human embryology.* New York: Churchill Livingstone.

Moore, K.L., & Persaud, T.V.N. (2003). *The developing human: Clinically oriented embryology.* Philadelphia: Saunders.

National High Blood Pressure Education Program (NHBPEP) working group on high blood pressure in children and adolescents (2004). Fourth report on the diagnosis, evaluation and treatment of high blood pressure in children and adolescents. *Pediatrics, 114*(2), 555-576.

Pelech, A.N. (1999). Evaluation of the pediatric patient with a cardiac murmur. *Pediatr Clin North Am, 46*(2), 167-188.

Roy, D. (2003). Cardiovascular assessment of infants and children. In R. Goldbloom (Ed.). *Pediatric clinical skills* (3rd ed.). Philadelphia: Saunders.

Seidel, H., Ball, J., Dains, J., & Benedict, G. (2003). *Mosby's guide to physical examination* (5th ed.). St. Louis: Mosby.

8 Assessment of the Gastrointestinal System

LEIGH SMALL

Select the best answer for each of the following questions:

1. Fecal material that is tarry, black, and foul-smelling is called:
   A. Hematochezia.
   B. Guiac.
   C. Melena.
   D. Hemocult.

2. If brown or black spots are noted on the lips of a 6-year-old child it would be important to ask if others in the family have which of the following disorders?
   A. Celiac disease.
   B. Marfan syndrome.
   C. Inflammatory bowel disease.
   D. Peutz-Jeghers syndrome.

3. Where is a child's stomach located?
   A. Right upper quadrant.
   B. Left upper quadrant.
   C. Right lower quadrant.
   D. Left lower quadrant.

4. Umbilical hernias are often found in infants and premature infants because:
   A. The abdominal pressure from birth causes the muscles to separate.
   B. The diastasis recti muscles entrap the umbilical cord during embryological development.
   C. The small intestines herniate into the umbilicus during embryological development.
   D. Infants perform a Valsalva's maneuver in response to birth, increasing abdominal pressure that creates a hernia.

5. Can the absolute measure of body mass index (BMI) be accurately used to describe a child's adiposity or degree of overweight?
   A. Yes, because this measure of body composition is arithmetically derived from a child's height and weight.
   B. Yes, because BMI correlates with doubly labeled water studies, which is the "gold standard" measure.
   C. No, because absolute BMI does not take into account the rate of growth based on a child's age and gender.
   D. No, because BMI has been determined to not take into account body mass that is muscle versus body mass that is adipose tissue.

6. A child is classified as being overweight if his or her BMI percentile is greater than the:
   A. 85th percentile.
   B. 90th percentile.
   C. 95th percentile.
   D. 99th percentile.

7. A 6-month-old infant whose head circumference and height measurements have been accelerating consistently at the 20th percentiles and the weight measurement has been decelerating and is now at the 3rd percentile can be characterized as:
   A. Small for gestational age.
   B. Underweight.
   C. Constitutional growth delay.
   D. Failure to thrive.

8. Upon physical examination, a specific area of tenderness may be found midway be-

tween the right iliac crest and the umbilicus. This should be documented as:

A. Point tenderness at McBurney's point.
B. A positive Phren's sign.
C. Psoas sign.
D. Rebound rigidity.

9. What is the normal liver size in a 3-year-old?

A. 2 cm.
B. 4 cm.
C. 6 cm.
D. 8 cm.

10. All of the following should be included in a physical assessment when determining a child's level of hydration EXCEPT:

A. Capillary refill.
B. Mucous membranes.
C. Elasticity of the skin.
D. Esophageal pH levels.

11. The presence of rectal fistulas and skin tags suggest that the examiner may want to ask which of the following questions?

A. Does anyone in your immediate family have a history of peptic ulcer disease?
B. Does anyone in your family have a history of inflammatory bowel disease?
C. Does anyone in your family have a history of having duodenal polyps?
D. Does anyone in you family have a history of gastroesophageal reflux?

12. Melissa is a 4-year-old child who has been brought to see you today for a 6-month history of constipation and intermittent rectal bleeding. Given this presentation, a thorough exam including a digital rectal exam is performed. What findings would NOT be considered normal on the digital rectal examination?

A. Stool in the rectal vault.
B. Sphincter tone intact.
C. Lubricated gloved finger easily inserted.
D. Fecal occult blood test negative.

13. While conducting a newborn examination, you note that the edge of a 3-day-old infant's liver can be felt 2 centimeters below the right costal margin. This newborn is the product of a 40-week gestation and normal vaginal delivery with Apgar scores of 9 and 10. His newborn course has been uneventful and the nurses have noted him to be otherwise well, voiding and stooling normally, and breastfeeding well. He has exhibited a 4% weight loss to date and no signs of jaundice. His mother is recovering well without any history of health problems. What is your assessment of the liver?

A. This would be a normal finding given the age of the infant.
B. This would be a normal finding given the gender of the infant.
C. This would be an abnormal finding and needs to be followed up immediately.
D. This would be an abnormal finding and the infant should be evaluated frequently for the next 6 months.

14. While conducting a 2-week newborn well child checkup, you determine from the maternal report that the infant didn't have a stool for 48 hours after birth, the stool looked odd and the nurse called it a "meconium plug." The infant appears to be healthy, breastfeeding well, and stooling normally; although the infant is at birth weight today. What might be the best next question you would want to ask this mother?

A. Is there a history of chronic constipation in any immediate family members?
B. Do any family members have a history of irritable bowel syndrome?
C. Are there any family members who have been diagnosed with cystic fibrosis?
D. Do you consume many milk products or other constipating foods?

15. The contour of the abdomen in toddlers is usually:

A. Flat.
B. Scaphoid.
C. Protuberant.
D. Obese.

16. When lightly palpating the abdomen of a 14-year-old female, you note that

she responds with tensing of her abdominal muscles. This persists when you distract her and when you hold her hand, techniques that can be used to reduce the patient's sensitivity during abdominal palpation. The technical term for her response to your palpation is:

A. Rigidity.
B. Preparing.
C. Guarding.
D. Abdominal tension.

17. A complete physical examination should include checking for an anal wink. This is done to check:

A. That cranial nerve X is intact and properly functioning.
B. If the superficial reflexes are intact.
C. If the patient has suffered from sexual abuse.
D. If the patient has normal sensory neurological function.

18. One method used to auscultate the liver and approximate its size is the scratch test. This is performed by:

A. Scratching the liver and listening with a stethoscope to the resultant bowels sounds.
B. Placing the stethoscope over the liver and then scratching on the lower abdomen. Noise created while scratching on the abdomen is heard best over the liver.
C. Listening with a stethoscope to the noise created when scratching in a counterclockwise pattern beginning over the gastric bubble.
D. Scratching the skin overlying the liver and listening with a stethoscope to the loud sounds that change to quieter sounds when the scratching goes beyond the edge of the liver.

19. A 17-year-old male comes to see you today for a complaint of fatigue and abdominal pain. Upon physical examination, you determine that his spleen is 2 cm below the lower left costal border. Which of the following would be the BEST comment that you could make following this examination finding of his spleen?

A. Some people have larger spleens than other people. Your spleen is larger than many people your age and given your symptoms we should do more testing.
B. Your spleen is in a slightly different location than most teenagers' spleens and I will note this in your chart.
C. Your spleen is normal in size and is unlikely to be the cause of your symptoms.
D. Do you play football or other contact sports?

20. During a routine history and physical of a teen who has come to be seen for recurrent abdominal pain, you identify a family history of migraines (on the maternal side). Which of the following is the BEST response?

A. This is important information, because maternal migraine headaches increase the risk of migraine headaches in their offspring more so than do paternal migraines.
B. Migraines can be a familial disorder, but have little bearing on your symptom of recurrent abdominal pain.
C. A family history of chronic pain syndromes can result in children who develop chronic functional pain syndromes.
D. A family history of migraine headaches is related to the occurrence of abdominal migraines.

ANSWERS

1. *Answer:* C
Rationale: Melena refers to blood lost from the upper portion of the gastrointestinal system, such as the stomach or small intestines, which is visible in fecal material. The blood is denatured in the lower intestines resulting in changes in color, consistency, and odor.

2. *Answer:* D
Rationale: Peutz-Jeghers syndrome is an autosomal dominant hereditary disorder characterized by small brown or black spots on the lips and/or in the mouth. There is an increased risk for cancer of the gut, breasts, or ovaries in people with this condition.

3. *Answer:* B
Rationale: The stomach, spleen, left lobe of the liver, body of the pancreas left kidney and part of the transverse and decending colon are located in the left upper quadrant.

4. *Answer:* C
Rationale: At the end of the fifth week of embryological development, the liver and the spleen are large. This decreases the intraabdominal space available for the small intestines. If the organs don't decrease in size by week 10, the intestine cannot return to the mid-gut, resulting in an umbilical hernia.

5. *Answer:* C
Rationale: BMI has been found to closely correspond with adipose measures in adults and has been accepted as a universal measure of body mass and adiposity; however, in children, BMI changes with the normal and expected growth that occurs in childhood. The rate of growth depends on the child's age and gender; therefore, BMI percentile is the most accurate accepted measure of childhood adiposity.

6. *Answer:* C
Rationale: According to the Centers for Disease Control and Prevention and the American Academy of Pediatrics, children whose BMI is at or greater than the 95th percentile are overweight. Children at greater than 85th percentile and less than 95th percentile are at risk for overweight.

7. *Answer:* D
Rationale: A child whose weight is failing to accelerate as the height and head circumference are normally accelerating is "failing to thrive" and the cause of this must be investigated.

8. *Answer:* A
Rationale: McBurney's point is located halfway between the right iliac crest and the umbilicus. If a specific area is tender this should be identified as point tenderness; however, if the examiner were to elicit exquisite pain by pushing down and then quickly releasing, this would be rebound tenderness that may be characteristic of inflammation of the appendix.

9. *Answer:* B
Rationale: The normal liver size in a 6-month-old is 2 cm, in a 3-year-old is 4 cm, in a 10-year-old is 6 cm, and in an adult is 8 cm.

10. *Answer:* D
Rationale: A child's level of dehydration can be assessed by examining the moistness of the mucous membranes, skin turgor, capillary refill, level of alertness/irritability, and urinary output and specific gravity; however, esophageal pH levels are measured to assess for gastric reflux.

11. *Answer:* B
Rationale: The presence of rectal or anal skin tags or fistulas is suggestive that this patient may have inflammatory bowel disease, which often has a familial history.

12. *Answer:* A
Rationale: While a 6-month history of rectal bleeding is very concerning, realizing that this occurred with constipation is less worrisome. Physical examination finding of a full rectal vault is not normal and may indicate that this child suffered from chronic constipation and withholding. This will likely need a long course of treatment to resolve. This is a common diagnosis in children during toilet-training years; however, it requires

a full examination, a laboratory evaluation, and then a treatment trial. The other differential diagnosis to consider is Hirschprung's disease; however, this condition is much less common.

13. *Answer:* A
    Rationale: It is common and thus normal to feel the soft smooth edge of the liver 1 to 2 cm below the costal margin in an infant. This finding alone should not result in further testing and evaluation.

14. *Answer:* C
    Rationale: Meconium plug syndrome may be the result of immaturity of the colon and most often is a functional problem rather than the sign of a pathologic process. Other processes that may result in a delayed first stool would include Hirschprung's disease, cystic fibrosis, ileus, necrotizing enterocolitis (NEC), volvulus, and/or intussusception. From the history of normal defecation and breastfeeding, the pediatric nurse practitioner can rule out the pathologic processes of Hirschprung's disease, NEC, volvulus, and intussusception. In this case it is important to determine if there is a family history of cystic fibrosis because this inherited genetic disease causes mucus to be thick and sticky, resulting in a wide variety of gastrointestinal and respiratory disturbances.

15. *Answer:* C
    Rationale: The contour the toddler's abdomen is usually protuberant, or pot-belly–like.

16. *Answer:* C
    Rationale: If a patient tenses the abdominal muscles despite methods of distraction and reducing sensitivity the examiner should suspect that the patient's is reflexively tensing the muscles to protect the lower abdominal structures; this is known as *guarding*.

17. *Answer:* B
    Rationale: The anal wink is a reflex that occurs in response to slight stimulation of the anus (i.e., stroking, light touch) during which the external anal sphincter tenses or puckers. Testing the anal wink is an important compo-

nent of superficial reflex testing and evaluation of the intact functioning of the neurological system originating from the lowest sacral segments of the spinal cord

18. *Answer:* D
    Rationale: When scratching the surface of the skin that overlies solid organs, such as the liver in the abdominal cavity, the sound waves will be more readily conducted and thus will be louder than scratching the skin overlying the hollow structures or structures not in direct contact with the overlying skin.

19. *Answer:* A
    Rationale: Only 3% of adolescents have palpable spleens. These findings warrant further investigation.

20. *Answer:* D
    Rationale: Family history of migraine headaches is associated with abdominal migraines. Abdominal migraines, a type of migraine seen most frequently in children ages 5 to 9 years, consists primarily of abdominal pain, nausea, and vomiting.

BIBLIOGRAPHY

Bickley, L.S., & Szilagyi, P.G. (2003). *Bates' guide to physical examination and history taking* (8th ed.). New York: Lippincott Williams & Wilkins.

Boynton, R.W., Dunn, E.S., Stephens, G.R., & Pulcini, J. (2003). *Manual of ambulatory pediatrics* (5th ed.). New York: Lippincott Williams & Wilkins.

Burns, C.E., Brady, M.A., Blosser, C., et al. (2004). *Pediatric primary care: A handbook for nurse practitioners* (3rd ed.). New York: Saunders.

Colyar, M.R. (2003). *Well-child assessment for primary care providers.* Philadelphia: F.A. Davis.

Fox, J.A. (2003). *Primary health care of infants, children, & adolescents* (2nd ed.). St. Louis: Mosby.

Goldbloom, R.B. (2003). *Pediatric clinical skills* (3rd ed.). Philadelphia: Saunders.

Larsen, W.J. (2001). *Human embryology.* New York: Churchill Livingstone.

Moore, K.L., & Persaud, T.V.N. (2003). *The developing human: Clinically oriented embryology.* Philadelphia: Saunders.

Schwartz, M.W. (2003). *Clinical handbook of pediatrics* (3rd ed.). New York: Lippincott Williams & Wilkins.

9 Assessment of the Reproductive and Urologic Systems

GAIL HORNOR

Select the best answer for each of the following questions:

1. Melissa, a healthy 3-year-old, comes into the clinic for a well child check. You have a discussion with mother regarding sexual behaviors and she expresses concerns regarding the following: Melissa touches her own genitals, and while playing with a 4-year-old boy, both children were seen touching each other's genitals. What is the most appropriate intervention for this child/family?
   A. Inform the mother that it is likely her child has been sexually abused and refer to the sexual abuse treatment center.
   B. Refer Melissa to play therapy as this behavior is very abnormal and unusual.
   C. Notify child protective services of this event.
   D. Reassure mother that this is normal, age-appropriate behavior and discuss approaches to deal with this behavior.

2. David comes into the clinic for a well child check. He is 5 years old and in kindergarten. During the well child exam, you discuss sexual behaviors with mother and she expresses concern regarding the following incident. David and Ben, a 10-year-old neighbor, were playing together last week and when David's mother walked into the room, both boys had their clothes off and David's penis was in Ben's mouth. During the exam, you talk with David about his body parts and David shares that he and Ben have engaged in reciprocal oral-genital contact on multiple occasions. David's ano-genital exam is nor-

mal today in clinic. The most appropriate initial intervention would be to:
   A. Reassure his mother that this is normal sexual play.
   B. Report this information to child protective services.
   C. Refer David to the urologist.
   D. Discuss homosexuality with David's mother.

3. When is it most appropriate to complete a physical exam of the genitourinary system?
   A. At every well child physical exam and whenever specific genitourinary complaints arise.
   B. At every well child and ill child visit regardless of presenting problem.
   C. During the first 12 months of life.
   D. Only during sports participation examinations.

4. Anne, a healthy 4-year-old, comes into the clinic for her well child check. Mother reports no medical, behavioral, or social concerns. What are appropriate question(s) to ask Anne to screen for sexual abuse?
   A. Did your Daddy hurt your pee-pee (vagina)?
   B. It is not appropriate for a primary care provider to ask questions regarding sexual abuse, especially if the parent has not identified a concern of sexual abuse.
   C. Do you have parts of your body that no one is supposed to look at, touch, kiss, or tickle? Has anyone ever touched, tickled, kissed, or hurt those body parts?

D. Anne is too young to be questioned about potential sexual abuse experiences.

5. Sally, age 16 years, comes to the clinic for her well child checkup. Sally began menses at age 10 and her last menstrual period was 2 weeks ago. At an appropriate time during the examination, you ask mother to leave the exam room so that you and Sally can speak privately. What is the most appropriate initial question to ask Sally regarding sexuality?
   A. It is not appropriate to ask questions about sexuality to a teenager without a parent present.
   B. What is your definition of sex?
   C. Have you ever had sex?
   D. Have you ever had nonconsensual sexual experiences?

6. A hydrocele is best described as:
   A. Eversion of posterior wall of the bladder.
   B. Urethral opening located on the ventral surface of the penis.
   C. Peritoneal fluid between the parietal and visceral layers of the tunica vaginalis, anterior to the testicle.
   D. Downward concave curvature of penis.

7. What is the name for a cultural practice observed in 26 African countries, in the Middle East, and Muslim populations of Indonesia and Malaysia which involves removal of part or all of the clitoris and labia minora; labia majora are reapproximated to cover the urethra and introitus, leaving a small opening for the passage of urine and menstrual blood?
   A. Female circumcision.
   B. Female dissection.
   C. Female circumvent.
   D. Female chastity.

8. Potential health benefits of male circumcision include:
   A. Improves sexual prowess.
   B. Decreases the risk of prostate cancer.
   C. Prevents the transmission of sexually transmitted diseases.

D. Decreases the risk for penile cancer.

9. Ashley, a 10-year-old female, comes to clinic for her well child exam. After explaining the genital exam, Ashley's mother states she does not want you looking at Ashley's genitals as this will embarrass Ashley. The most appropriate response would be:
   A. Allow mother and Ashley to have control of the situation and simply do not examine Ashley's genitalia.
   B. State to mother that Ashley's embarrassment over the exam is abnormal and leads you to be concerned that she has been sexually abused.
   C. Quickly examine Ashley's genitals before she realizes what is happening.
   D. Utilizing a calm, matter-of-fact attitude, again explain the genital exam to Ashley and mother and the reasons why it is important to examine all the parts of Ashley's body.

10. Adam, a healthy 6-month-old, comes to the clinic for a well child exam. It is the first time you have seen Adam. Upon physical exam, you note that his urethral opening is on the dorsum of his penis. The most appropriate intervention would be:
   A. Explain to his mother that Adam has a congenital anomaly known as *epispadias* and he needs to be seen by a urologist.
   B. Explain to his mother that this is a normal variation and provide reassurance that no intervention is necessary.
   C. Explain to his mother that Adam has a congenital anomaly known as a *hydrocele* and should be seen by a surgeon.
   D. Explain to his mother that Adam has a congenital anomaly known as *chordee* and should be seen by a urologist.

11. Chris, an 11-year-old healthy male, comes to the clinic for a well child exam. Upon examination, you note that he is uncircumcised. You attempt to retract the foreskin and are unable to do so. The most appropriate intervention would be:
   A. Attempt to forcefully retract the foreskin. If unable to do so, refer to urology.

B. No intervention is needed as this is a normal finding, typically the foreskin cannot be retracted until puberty.

C. Explain that the condition is called *phimosis*. Discuss genital hygiene and foreskin care. Refer to urology for evaluation.

D. Instruct Chris to use 1% hydrocortisone cream twice a day to assist with the release of the foreskin.

12. John, a healthy 13-year-old male, presents to the clinic for a sports physical. When determining sexual maturation, you note enlargement of scrotum and testes without enlargement of penis. Scrotum is reddened in color. You also note a few, long, light straight hairs at the base of the penis. What Tanner stage of development is Chris?
   A. Tanner I.
   B. Tanner II.
   C. Tanner III.
   D. Tanner IV.

13. Megan, a healthy 16-year-old female, comes to the clinic for her well child exam. When determining sexual maturation, you note the following: pubic hair of adult color and texture but covering the pubis area with no spread to the medial thighs. What Tanner stage of development is Megan?
   A. Tanner I.
   B. Tanner II.
   C. Tanner III.
   D. Tanner IV.

14. To conduct an examination of the hymen on 10-year-old Debbie, you apply traction to visualize the opening. You are unable to visualize the hymenal opening so you release traction, then reapply traction, attempt to float opening with normal saline, and place Debbie in knee-chest position. Despite these maneuvers, the hymen opening is not visible. This exam is consistent with:
   A. Imperforate hymen.
   B. Crescentic hymen.
   C. Cribriform hymen.
   D. Perforate hymen.

15. A pubertal hymen can best be described as:

A. Smooth and delicate hymenal edge.
B. Typically very sensitive to touch.
C. Thickened, redundant, moist, and pale.
D. Thickened, redundant, and very sensitive to touch.

16. Hymenal variants that require referral to gynecology are:
   A. Cribriform, imperforate, and crescentic.
   B. Imperforate, cribriform, microperforate, and septate.
   C. Septate, imperforate, and annular.
   D. Imperforate, cribriform, microperforate, and annular.

17. Gina, a healthy 3-year-old, presents to the clinic for her well child exam. Appropriate techniques to utilize to facilitate visualization of the hymenal opening are:
   A. Examine in supine/frog-leg position and change to knee-chest if needed; apply gentle traction pulling labia toward the examiner; palpate hymen with a cotton applicator.
   B. Apply gentle traction pulling labia toward the examiner; flush area with a small amount of water or saline; gently palpate hymen with cotton applicator.
   C. Apply traction on labia pulling toward the examiner; flush area with a small amount of water or saline using a syringe; place child in knee-chest position or switch to supine frog-leg position.
   D. Examine only in supine frog-leg position; avoid knee-chest position as it does not facilitate hymenal visualization; flush area with a small amount of water or normal saline.

18. Which statement is true regarding techniques for palpating the testicles?
   A. Place index finger and thumb over the lower part of the scrotal sac along the penile shaft and palpate upward.
   B. Place index finger and thumb over the upper part of the scrotal sac along the inguinal canal.

C. Place pinky finger and thumb over the upper part of the scrotal sac along the urethral meatus.
D. Always palpate testicles with thumb high in the inguinal canal.

19. The cremasteric reflex can be stimulated by:
A. Warmth, touch, excitement, or exercise.
B. Warmth, touch, sleep, or exercise.
C. Cold, touch, sleep, or exercise.
D. Cold, touch, excitement, or exercise.

20. All of following are indications for pelvic examinations in adolescents EXCEPT:
A. Irregular vaginal bleeding.
B. Severe dysmenorrhea.
C. Sexually inactive teen with vaginal discharge.
D. Sexually active teen with vaginal discharge.

21. Choose the BEST statement regarding speculum examinations.
A. Reassure the patient that the exam will not be uncomfortable even if the patient has not had sexual intercourse.
B. Speculum examinations are not always necessary; always perform the least invasive examination that will answer the clinical question.
C. Contraindications include amenorrhea and sexually active adolescent with vaginal discharge.
D. Never conduct a speculum examination in patients with irregular vaginal bleeding or unexplained abdominal or pelvic pain.

22. An essential fact for practitioners to understand regarding sexual abuse is:

A. From 70% to 95% of children who give history of sexual abuse involving penile penetration of the vagina will have an abnormal genital exam.
B. A normal genital exam negates the possibility of sexual abuse.
C. A normal genital exam does not negate the possibility of sexual abuse.
D. From 70% to 95% of children who give history of sexual abuse will have a sexually transmitted infection.

23. Sadie, a healthy 6-year-old female, presents to the clinic for her well child exam. Upon genitourinary examination, you note a green-yellow vaginal discharge which you culture for Chlamydia/GC/wet prep. You address the issue of sexual abuse with Sadie and her mother separately and both deny any concerns of sexual abuse. Three days later you are notified by the lab that the vaginal GC culture is positive. The most appropriate intervention, in addition to treating the infection with the most appropriate antibiotic, is:
A. Discuss the importance of good hygiene with Sadie and her parents.
B. Discuss with her parents that a positive GC culture is diagnostic of sexual abuse and you must report this to child protective services.
C. Tell Sadie's parents to contact the school regarding Sadie's diagnosis so they can test other children for this infection.
D. Interview Sadie at length regarding the sexual abuse concern and report to child protective services only if Sadie gives history of sexual abuse.

ANSWERS

1. *Answer:* D
   Rationale: Touching own genitals and sex play involving touching and looking at genitals of age-mates are common, normal sexual behaviors in prepubertal children. The pediatric nurse practitioner can suggest that mother direct Melissa to touch her genitals only when in an appropriate private setting, such as her room, and provide closer supervision when Melissa is playing with her friend.

2. *Answer:* B
   Rationale: Oral-genital contact between children, even age-mates, is a behavior that raises a concern of possible sexual abuse and should be referred to child protective services. David's and Ben's scenario is even more concerning because of the greater than 4-year age difference.

3. *Answer:* A
   Rationale: Routine genitourinary exams increase diagnostic skills, provide a baseline for compliance with the exam, and may reveal previously undiscovered anomalies or trauma.

4. *Answer:* C
   Rationale: It is vital for the practitioner to screen their patients for sexual abuse at all routine well child examinations. This provides the child with education regarding sexual abuse and provides an opportunity for the disclosure of sexual abuse.

5. *Answer:* B
   Rationale: Adolescent sexuality must be explored by the practitioner to ensure that the adolescent's health care needs are met. Once the definition of sex is identified, then ask Sally if she has ever had sex. If the answer is yes, inquire about the age of sexual partners, the number of sexual partners, the gender of partners, and use of "safe sex" practices and birth control. Explore with Sally any nonconsensual sexual experiences (rape or sexual abuse).

6. *Answer:* C

Rationale: A hydrocele is defined as peritoneal fluid between the parietal and visceral layers of the tunica vaginalis, anterior to the testicle. If the hydrocele is the communicating form, the amount of fluid fluctuates. Refer to a physician for surgical repair if no spontaneous resolution by 1 year.

7. *Answer:* A
   Rationale: Female circumcision or female genital mutilation affects approximately 80 to 110 million females; it is usually performed between 4 and 10 years of age without anesthesia; legs of the girl are bound from ankle to hip for up to 40 days to allow scar tissue to heal.

8. *Answer:* D
   Rationale: Potential health benefits to circumcision include prevention of penile cancer, local infection, phimosis, and urinary tract infection in the first year of life. Also decreases the risk for HIV infections and other sexually transmitted diseases such as chancroid and syphilis.

9. *Answer:* D
   Rationale: The pediatric nurse practitioner should understand that preadolescents and adolescents may be embarrassed and apprehensive with the exam.

10. *Answer:* A
    Rationale: Epispadias is a congenital anomaly where the anterior urethra terminates on the dorsum of the penis; refer to urology.

11. *Answer:* C
    Rationale: At approximately 6 years of age, the foreskin is retracted during the physical exam. Gently retract uncircumcised foreskin if child is more than 6 years old. Phimosis is the tightening of the foreskin that prevents its retraction over the glans penis. If severe, it may require circumcision.

12. *Answer:* B
    Rationale: Typically in male sexual maturation, testicles and scrotum begin growing, then pubic hair develops, and finally the pe-

nis enlarges. Tanner Stage II notes the beginning of sexual maturation when the scrotum and testes enlarge, a few immature pubic hairs exist, and penile enlargement has not yet occurred.

13. *Answer:* D
    Rationale: Typically in female sexual maturation, pubic hair becomes progressively coarser, darker, and curlier and spreads to mons pubis and then to the medial thighs as sexual maturation progresses. Tanner Stage IV notes nearly complete sexual maturation where pubic hair is adult-like but covering a smaller area with no spread to thighs.

14. *Answer:* A
    Rationale: An inability to visualize a hymenal opening after using various techniques to provide visualization of the opening may indicate an imperforate hymen. An imperforate hymen is defined as no hymenal opening. An imperforate hymen requires a referral to gynecology and a hymenotomy may be needed. Crescentic hymen is a normal anatomical variant and no referral is needed.

15. *Answer:* C
    Rationale: Due to the release of estrogen, the pubertal hymen becomes thickened, redundant, moist, and pale in color. The pubertal hymen is no longer sensitive to touch.

16. *Answer:* B
    Rationale: A simple hymenotomy is required at the time of diagnosis for imperforate hymen. A hymenotomy may be required before tampon use or sexual intercourse with the diagnosis of microperforate, cribriform, and septate hymen. In these cases, referral to a specialist is warranted.

17. *Answer:* C
    Rationale: When inspecting the external female genitalia, it may be difficult to view the hymenal orifice. Gently apply traction on the labia pulling toward the examiner. Flush area with a small amount of water or saline using a syringe or angiocath attached to a syringe. Place child in knee-chest position for

the best view of the hymen; can place in a frog-leg position if child is unable to cooperate with knee-chest position. Prepubertal hymen is very sensitive to touch; avoid touching with an applicator.

18. *Answer:* B
    Rationale: Warm your hands; retraction of testes can be stimulated by cold. A proper palpation technique involves placing index finger and thumb over the upper part of the scrotal sac along the inguinal canal. Testicles are normally smooth and equal in size. If the testicle is not palpated in the scrotum, it is proper technique to palpate the inguinal canal for a soft mass and attempt to move the testicle to the scrotum.

19. *Answer:* D
    Rationale: The cremasteric reflex, retraction of the testes into the abdomen, can be stimulated by cold, touch, excitement, or exercise.

20. *Answer:* C
    Rationale: Indications for an adolescent pelvic exam include irregular vaginal bleeding, complaints of unexplained abdominal or pelvic pain, severe dysmenorrhea, amenorrhea, consensual sexual intercourse with a vaginal discharge, and sexual abuse/assault with unexplained vaginal bleeding. In a sexually inactive teenager with vaginal discharge, cultures can be obtained without using a speculum by touching the vagina with a cotton-tipped applicator.

21. *Answer:* B
    Rationale: It is important for the medical provider to always perform the least invasive examination that will answer the clinical question. An adolescent who is denying sexual activity and has a vaginal discharge should have cultures obtained by touching vagina with an applicator. For adolescents with primary amenorrhea, a cotton-tipped applicator can be used to determine vaginal length, followed by one-finger vaginal-abdominal exam.

22. *Answer:* C

Rationale: It is essential for the practitioner to remember that a normal ano-genital exam does not negate the possibility of sexual abuse. From 70% to 95% of children who give history of sexual abuse, including penile penetration of the vagina and/or anus, will have a normal genital exam.

23. *Answer:* B

Rationale: If a prepubertal child or a nonconsensually sexually active adolescent has a positive culture for GC, a report to child protective services is mandatory.

BIBLIOGRAPHY

Adams, J.A. (1996). Genital findings in adolescent girls referred for suspected sexual abuse. *Arch Pediatr Adolesc Med, 150*(8), 850-856.

Alanis, M.C., & Lucidi, R.S. (2004). Neonatal circumcision: A review of the world's oldest and most controversial operation. *Obstet Gynecol Surv, 59*(5), 379-395.

Berkowitz, C.D. (2000) *Pediatrics: A primary care approach.* Philadelphia: Saunders.

Elford, K.J., & Spence, J.E.H. (2002). The forgotten female: Pediatric and adolescent gynecological concerns and their reproductive consequences. *J Pediatr Adolesc Gynecol, 15*(2), 65-77.

Heger, A.H., Ticson, L., Guerra, L., et al. (2002). Appearance of the genitalia in girls selected for nonabuse: Review of hymenal morphology and nonspecific findings. *J Pediatr Adolesc Gnecol, 15*(1), 27-35.

Hornor, G. (2002). Child sexual abuse: Psychological risk factors. *J Pediatr Health Care, 16*(4), 187-192.

Hornor, G., & Ryan-Wenger, N. (1999). Aberrant genital care practices: An unrecognized form of child sexual abuse. *J Pediatr Health Care, 13*(1), 12-17.

Hymel, K.P., & Jenny, C. (1996). Child sexual abuse. *Pediatr Rev, 17*(7), 236-249.

Johnson, C.F. (2002). Child maltreatment 2002: Recognition, reporting and risk. *Pediatr Int, 44*(5), 554-560.

Kolon, T.F. (2006). Cryptorchidism. Retrieved on March 13, 2006 from http://www.emedicine.com/med/topic2707.htm.

Miller, G.P. (2002). Circumcision: Cultural-legal analysis. *Virginia J Soc Policy & Law, 9*, 497-985.

Schoen, E., Wiswell, T., & Moses, S. (2000). New policy on circumcision: Cause for concern. *Pediatrics, 105*(3 Pt 1), 620-623.

10 Assessment of the Integumentary System

CHERI BARBER

Select the best answer for each of the following questions:

1. Which of the following is found in the epidermal layer?
   A. Melanocytes.
   B. Nerves.
   C. Sebaceous glands.
   D. Sweat glands.

2. What type of hair is darkly pigmented and found primarily on the scalp and face of males?
   A. Vellus
   B. Terminal
   C. Lanugo
   D. Bulb

3. A 2-month-old baby girl arrives for her well baby checkup. You notice she has a congenital nevus. Which of the following questions could be included in a focused history?
   A. What is the ethnicity of this child?
   B. Has there been any change in the size, color, or shape of the nevus?
   C. What type of skin moisturizer is used?
   D. How much sun exposure has this baby had?

4. A 5-year-old girl arrives for her yearly well child exam. As you examine her perineal area, you notice that the labial area is quite erythematous. Which of the following would you find most helpful to include in your history taking?
   A. Dietary intake.
   B. Type of soap used to bathe the child.

   C. Allergies to chocolate.
   D. Exposure to a child with varicella.

5. A 3-year-old boy was brought into clinic because his mother noticed a very distinct erythematous area with a defined border on his waistline. The area was slightly indurated but intact. Which factor would be key in your assessment?
   A. Food allergies.
   B. Recent injury.
   C. Recent illness.
   D. Use of a belt.

6. A 10-year-old boy returned from an outside camping trip with a red macular, confluent rash on his arms and legs. The most pertinent factor in your assessment is:
   A. Health status of family members.
   B. Contact with vegetation or exposure to animals.
   C. Exposure to sun.
   D. Temperature.

7. A 2-year-old with a history of asthma and nasal allergies arrives for her 2-year well child visit and upon examination, you notice a dry scaly patch on the inner aspect of her elbows. Which of the following conditions would you suspect?
   A. Eczema.
   B. Bacterial infection.
   C. Viral infection.
   D. Fungal infection.

8. Which of the following would be most helpful to include when assessing a child's perineal area?
   A. How long the infant sleeps.

B. The foods recently consumed by the infant.

C. Type of diaper and barrier creams used.

D. The amount of liquid normally ingested.

9. You are examining a teenager who has come in because of a rash that he noticed along his hairline. Which factor would be most important to include in your history taking?

A. Foods consumed in the last 24 hours.

B. Use of illicit drugs.

C. Use of hair gels or hair-coloring products.

D. History of allergies.

10. Which of the following would be used in the preparation of a specimen for KOH smear?

A. Scissors.

B. Wood's lamp.

C. A catheter.

D. Wool's lamp.

11. When assessing hair, which of the following is most important?

A. Hair loss or bald spots.

B. Last haircut.

C. Hair line and length.

D. Color.

12. What is the normal nail angle?

A. 90 degrees.

B. 180 degrees.

C. 160 degrees.

D. 140 degrees.

13. Capillary refill should occur within how many seconds?

A. One

B. Two

C. Three

D. Four

14. Which term refers to a configuration of a skin lesion that is arc-shaped?

A. Arculate

B. Grouped

C. Confluent

D. Arctoid

15. What are the dimensions of a nodule?

A. Less than 1 cm.

B. Greater than l cm but less than 2 cm.

C. Less than or equal to 2 cm.

D. Greater than 2 cm.

16. Which matches the definition: Linear crack from epidermis into dermis.

A. Erosion

B. Fissure

C. Atrophy

D. Ulcer

17. Characteristics of vesicles are:

A. Raised, fluid-filled lesions less than 1 cm such as blisters or herpes simplex.

B. Flat, elevated, superficial papules.

C. Plugged openings of sebaceous glands.

D. Superficial area of cutaneous edema such as hives or insect bites.

18. Which ethnicity has a bluish tinge of the lips?

A. Mediterranean

B. Asian

C. Black

D. Hispanic

19. How often does the strateum corneum or horny cell layer shed and have a complete turnover in cells?

A. Every 1 to 2 weeks.

B. Every 2 to 3 weeks.

C. Every 3 to 4 weeks.

D. Every 4 to 5 weeks.

20. At what age is the average onset of acne?

A. 10 years old.

B. 12 years old.

C. 14 years old.

D. 16 years old.

21. At what age should a health care provider begin to discuss sun exposure with parents?

A. Birth.

B. 6 months.

C. 12 months.

D. 2 years.

22. A parent of a 6-year-old comes in for a sick visit with a complaint of circular patches with raised borders and bald spots on the head. The diagnosis is probably:
   A. Lice.
   B. Scabies.
   C. Tinea capitis.
   D. Herald patches.

23. Johnny comes into the office with an allergic reaction to an insect bite on his left arm. He presents with:
   A. An erythematous circular hive around the bite.
   B. A bruise 3 cm below the bite.
   C. A hypopigmented area below the bite.
   D. A keratotic lesion.

NOTES

ANSWERS

1. *Answer:* A
   Rationale: The epidermis is the thin outer layer which is comprised of five layers of stratified squamous epithelium. The sebaceous glands, nerves, and sweat glands are located in the dermis (the middle layer of the skin).

2. *Answer:* B
   Rationale: Types of hair are lanugo (thin, short hair shed before term), vellus hair (short, soft, distributed over the body, unpigmented), terminal hair (long, coarse, found on the scalp, beard, eyebrows, eyelashes, and axillary and pubic hair). Bulb matrix is new hair cells.

3. *Answer:* B
   Rationale: The physical examination should include: Skin type; recent or long-term changes in size, shape, or color of the nevus. Skin care products, ethnicity, and exposure to sun are important questions to ask for a general skin history and assessment; however, those questions are not directly related to the nevus.

4. *Answer:* B
   Rationale: In general, mild soaps such as Dove, Neutrogena, Aveeno, or Purpose are less damaging to the skin. Bubble baths are especially irritating and should be avoided.

5. *Answer:* D
   Rationale: Contact dermatitis is an acute or chronic inflammation of the skin. A common type of contact dermatitis is nickel dermatitis caused by jewelry, belts, snaps, or eyeglasses.

6. *Answer:* B
   Rationale: Contact dermatitis is an acute or chronic inflammation of the skin. A common type of contact dermatitis is plant oleoresis such as poison ivy, oak, or sumac.

7. *Answer:* A
   Rationale: Eczema (sometimes used interchangeably with the term *atopic dermatitis*) has clinical findings of dry, scaly patches ap-

pearing on the hands, popliteal and antecubital fossae, creases, and flexural areas.

8. *Answer:* C
   Rationale: Factors that contribute to diaper dermatitis include improper hygiene and cleansing method, and chemical irritation caused by prolonged contact with skin products, urine, or feces.

9. *Answer:* C
   Rationale: Clinical findings of contact dermatitis are repeated exposure to any substances or items, contact with new or unusual substances, generally localized to one area.

10. *Answer:* B
    Rationale: KOH preparation provides a rapid and reliable method for evaluating fungal elements; once added to the specimen, it is heated over an alcohol lamp. This is called a *Wood's lamp.*

11. *Answer:* A
    Rationale: The physical examination of the hair includes thickness, loss, and texture.

12. *Answer:* C
    Rationale: The normal nail angle is 160 degrees. This angle changes in conditions such as clubbing.

13. *Answer:* B
    Rationale: Normal capillary refill should occur within 2 seconds; however, environmental temperature may cause peripheral vasoconstriction.

14. *Answer:* A
    Rationale: Configurations of skin lesions are: arcuate (arc-shaped lesions), grouped (lesions appearing in the same body location in clusters), and confluent (lesions that run together). Arctoid is not a valid term.

15. *Answer:* C
    Rationale: A *nodule* is defined as a raised, firm, movable lesion with indistinct borders of 2 cm or smaller.

16. *Answer:* B

Rationale: A *fissure* is defined as a linear crack from the epidermis into the dermis.

17. *Answer:* A

Rationale: Vesicles are less than 1 cm in size and appear as serous-filled lesions.

18. *Answer:* A

Rationale: Inspection of the skin includes overall appearance, including color and skin tone. Note any racial or ethnic differences: Black people will have a bluish tinge on their gums, tongue, and nail borders; whereas people of Mediterranean descent have a bluish tinge on their lips.

19. *Answer:* C

Rationale: The stratum corneum or horny cell layer begins to develop at the 21st week and sheds with a complete turnover in cells every 3 to 4 weeks.

20. *Answer:* B

Rationale: Acne occurs in 80% to 85% of all people 12 to 24 years of age, with the average onset at 12 years of age.

21. *Answer:* A

Rationale: At the newborn and 2-month visit, it is important to include in your anticipatory guidance that risk factors for skin cancer include sunburn, and that sunscreen is not to be used before to 6 months of age. Infants should be out of the sun completely, kept in the shade, and wearing a wide-brimmed hat and protective clothing.

22. *Answer:* C

Rationale: Tinea capitis appears clinically as diffuse scaling with discrete hair loss and raised borders.

23. *Answer:* A

Rationale: Mild reactions to insect bites appear as local redness, pruritus, pain, edema, or possibly generalized urticaria.

BIBLIOGRAPHY

Alaiti, S. (2005). Hair growth. Retrieved on March 13, 2006, from http://www.emedicine.com/ent/topic16.htm.

American Heart Association. (2002). *Pediatric advanced life support provider manual*. Dallas: American Heart Association.

Bickley, L.S., & Szilagyi, P.G. (2004). *Bates guide to physical examination and history taking* (8th ed.) Philadelphia: Lippincott Williams & Wilkins.

Engel, J. (2002). *Mosby's pocket guide series: Pediatric assessment* (4th ed.). St. Louis: Mosby.

Furdon, S.A., & Clark, D.A. (2003). Scalp hair characteristics in the newborn infant. *Advances in Neonatal Care, 3*(6), 286-296.

Jarvis, C. (2004). *Physical examination and health assessment* (4th ed.). Philadelphia: Elsevier.

McCance, K.L., & Heuther, S.C. (2002). Structure, function, and disorders of the integument. In K.L. McCance, & S.C. Heuther, *Pathophysiology: The biologic basis for disease in adults and children* (4th ed.). St. Louis: Mosby.

Moore, K.L., & Persaud, T.V.N. (2003). *The developing human: Clinically oriented embryology* (7th ed.). Philadelphia: Saunders.

Sibert, J. (2004). Bruising, coagulation disorder, and physical child abuse. *Blood coagulation and fibrinolysis: An international journal in haemostasis and thrombosis, 15*(Suppl. 1), S33-S39.

Swartz, M.H. (2004). *Textbook of physical diagnosis, history and examination* (4th ed.). Philadelphia: Elsevier.

11 Assessment of the Hematologic and Lymphatic Systems

MARY BLASZKO HELMING

Select the best answer for each of the following questions:

1. Which of the following statements is correct?
   A. Hemoglobin F is adult-type hemoglobin formed in the spleen.
   B. Hemoglobin F is fetal hemoglobin with a higher affinity for oxygen than hemoglobin A.
   C. At 6 months of age, hemoglobin F is approximately 60% of hemoglobin.
   D. Hemoglobin A remains unchanged throughout the gestational period.

2. The formation of erythrocytes is determined by:
   A. Erythropoietin, which is produced by the renal system in response to tissue hypoxia.
   B. The amount of iron and iron-binding capacity.
   C. The amount of bilirubin that is excreted by the liver.
   D. The number of circulating reticulocytes in the serum.

3. Which of the following blood types contains no agglutinins on the erythrocyte, although it contains agglutinins in plasma?
   A. Type A.
   B. Type B.
   C. Type AB.
   D. Type O.

4. The three types of granulocytes that act in phagocytosis are:
   A. Macrophages, monocytes, and lymphocytes.
   B. Bands, polys, and monocytes.
   C. Neutrophils, eosinophils, and basophils.
   D. Thrombocytes, monocytes, and lymphocytes.

5. The type of leukocytes that are active in parasitic infections and allergic reactions are the:
   A. Basophils.
   B. Mast cells.
   C. Macrophages.
   D. Eosinophils.

6. A type of immature neutrophil that proliferates in infection and inflammation is termed a:
   A. Band.
   B. Seg.
   C. Mast cell.
   D. Reticulocyte.

7. Which of the following statements is FALSE regarding the extrinsic coagulation cascade?
   A. Tissue injury promotes this response.
   B. The cascade is evaluated by the partial thromboplastin time (PTT).
   C. Tissue factor is released by exposure of collagen to a vessel surface.
   D. Factors II, VII, and X are required.

8. Which of the following clusters contain the body's bone marrow reserve?
   A. Femur, cranium, spleen, and myeloid tissue.
   B. Liver, spleen, hip, and spine.
   C. Pelvis, skull, sternum, and long bones.

D. Lymphatic tissue, myeloid tissue, pelvis, and sternum.

9. All of the following medications may possibly prolong bleeding EXCEPT:
A. Oral contraceptives.
B. Sulfonamides.
C. Penicillins.
D. Anticonvulsants.

10. High altitude, chronic hypoxia, and congenital heart disease are among the issues that can cause:
A. Iron deficiency anemia.
B. Polycythemia.
C. Leukocytosis.
D. Leukopenia.

11. A subtle measure for iron deficiency anemia includes which of the following tests?
A. WBC differential.
B. Partial thromboplastin time (PTT).
C. Hemoglobin electrophoresis.
D. Red cell distribution width (RDW).

12. The definition of a *left shift* is:
A. Abnormal morphology of platelets.
B. Rise in reticulocyte count.
C. Increase in percentage of band WBCs.
D. Decrease in total neutrophil count.

13. The type of lymphocyte that makes IgM antibodies and eventually IgG, IgA, and IgE antibodies on reexposure to the antigen is:
A. B lymphocyte.
B. T lymphocyte.
C. Natural killer (NK) lymphocyte.
D. Cytokines.

14. A pediatric nurse practitioner is examining a 15-year-old male with severe pharyngitis. She notes that one tonsil is more edematous and erythematous than the other and the uvula is deviating toward that tonsil. The teen is having difficulty swallowing. What is the MOST important action the pediatric nurse practitioner must take?
A. Send the teen home on amoxicillin 500 mg three times a day for 10 days.

B. Send a confirmatory group A beta hemolytic strep test to the lab for full culture.
C. Refer the teen to an ENT physician immediately for emergency evaluation of peritonsillar abscess.
D. Send the teen home on Zithromax Z-pack for 5 days with one refill.

15. The pediatric nurse practitioner finds a fixed, nontender, rubbery 1.5 cm anterior cervical lymph node in a 12-year-old girl. What is the MOST important action the pediatric nurse practitioner must take?
A. Administer a group A beta hemolytic strep test.
B. Send the child home on amoxicillin 250 mg three times a day for 10 days.
C. Refer the child immediately to a pediatric oncologist.
D. Order a heterophile test.

16. The pediatric nurse practitioner is aware that patients presenting with enlarged supraclavicular lymph nodes are at risk for:
A. Mediastinal lymphadenopathy.
B. Tuberculosis.
C. Pneumonia.
D. Infectious mononucleosis.

17. A 5-year-old male presents with tonsillar erythema, edema, white exudate, a temperature of 101° Fahrenheit, and a fetid odor. The pediatric nurse practitioner administers a throat culture. The most likely diagnosis is:
A. Bacterial infection.
B. Viral pharyngitis.
C. Infectious mononucleosis.
D. Herpangina.

18. A worried parent brings her 8-year-old well child to see the pediatric nurse practitioner, due to feeling anterior cervical adenopathy. This child has a history of recurrent tonsillitis. the pediatric nurse practitioner notes that the nodes are soft, minimally tender, mobile, less than 0.5 cm, and multiple. After determining the child has a mild upper respiratory infection, the pediatric nurse practitioner tells the mother that the:
A. Amount of lymphatic tissue peaks in middle childhood.

B. Lymph nodes she is feeling are potentially malignant.

C. Child will require a complete blood count at this time.

D. Child will require testing for infectious mononucleosis.

19. A pediatric nurse practitioner receives back a lab report on a 3-year-old girl revealing anemia, neutropenia, and blasts. What action must be taken immediately?

A. Repeat the lab test because it cannot be correct.

B. Tell the child's parents to start an iron supplement.

C. Refer the child to a pediatric hematologist-oncologist promptly.

D. Check RBC morphology for MCV, MCH, and MCHC.

20. A 6-year-old female has a low hemoglobin at her routine well child checkup. If the pediatric nurse practitioner decides to do further lab testing, which of the following are the MOST important tests to order?

A. Complete blood count, reticulocyte count, red cell distribution width (RDW).

B. Iron-binding capacity and ferritin levels.

C. PT/PTT.

D. B_{12} and folic acid levels.

21. A 12-year-old male with abdominal pain shows a high total WBC count with elevated neutrophils and the presence of bands. What is the likely etiology in this case?

A. Bacterial infection.

B. Physiological stress response.

C. Leukemia.

D. Viral infection.

22. The pediatric nurse practitioner is examining an infant during a well child exam. She questions whether the spleen is enlarged, but also knows that the:

A. Spleen may extend more than 2 cm in an infant.

B. Spleen is normally 1 to 2 cm below the left costal margin in infants and children.

C. Spleen might feel hard in some infants.

D. Liver edge may extend beyond 2 cm in the right costal margin in infants.

23. Pallor of the skin, petechiae (especially on the gums and soft palate), and diffuse bruising in a child should prompt the pediatric nurse practitioner to FIRST:

A. Consider domestic violence.

B. Check the family history for hemophilia.

C. Order a CBC and platelet count.

D. Order iron and iron-binding tests.

24. A pediatric nurse practitioner is taking care of a pediatric oncology patient. This child is suffering from neutropenia due to the chemotherapy regimen. The pediatric nurse practitioner is aware that:

A. There is no treatment for the neutropenia.

B. The child is at no risk for infection.

C. The patient should have a reticulocyte count drawn.

D. The child can be treated with recombinant growth factors to accelerate hematopoiesis.

25. When there is a family history of a bleeding disorder, which of the following questions is an essential part of the medical history?

A. History of pica.

B. History of hyperbilirubinemia.

C. Frequent episodes of epistaxis.

D. Oligomenorrhea in teenage girls.

ANSWERS

1. *Answer:* B
   Rationale: Hemoglobin F is fetal hemoglobin, while hemoglobin A is adult hemoglobin. Approximately 65% of hemoglobin is comprised of hemoglobin F at 2 weeks of age, while at 6 months of age, hemoglobin F drops to its normal level of 2%. Hemoglobin F maintains a higher affinity for oxygen.

2. *Answer:* A
   Rationale: Erythrocytes are red blood cells (RBCs) whose production is regulated by erythropoietin that the kidney produces when there is tissue hypoxia. Bilirubin is a breakdown product of RBCs which is excreted into the bile. Iron stores are reused to produce new RBCs.

3. *Answer:* D
   Rationale: Blood type is determined by the absence or presence of agglutinins on RBC surfaces and in the plasma. The role of agglutinins is to destroy "foreign" RBCs. Type O blood is the only type which carries no agglutinins on the RBC, although it carries A and B type agglutinins in the plasma.

4. *Answer:* C
   Rationale: Granulocytes are considered phagocytes that fight foreign substances. There are three types of leukocytes, or white blood cells (WBCs); these are granulocytes, monocytes, and lymphocytes. The granulocytes are further divided into neutrophils, basophils, and eosinophils.

5. *Answer:* D
   Rationale: Eosinophils are a type of granulocyte that is active in destroying parasites and fighting anaphylactic hypersensitivity and allergic reactions. Basophils, another type of granulocyte, are also called *mast cells* and they are responsible for histamine release and increasing vascular permeability. Macrophages are a type of monocyte that phagocytizes foreign substances as part of the immune response.

6. *Answer:* A
   Rationale: A type of granulocyte is termed a *neutrophil*, also known as a *poly* or *polymorphonuclear* cell. A mature neutrophil has a segmented nucleus and is termed a *seg*. An immature neutrophil has a band-shaped nucleus and is termed a *band*. Increased bands are associated with significant infection as the body attempts to produce more neutrophils to fight. Reticulocytes are immature RBCs.

7. *Answer:* B
   Rationale: The extrinsic cascade is evaluated by the prothrombin time (PT). The intrinsic cascade is evaluated by the partial thromboplastin time (PTT). All other answers are true for the extrinsic cascade.

8. *Answer:* C
   Rationale: The bone marrow contains the precursors of RBCs. There are numerous hematopoietic (blood-forming) organs, including the lymphatic tissues and the liver and spleen. The pelvis, long bones (as in the extremities), sternum, and skull contain the highest amounts of the bone marrow reserve. Bone marrow biopsies are often done in the pelvic area.

9. *Answer:* A
   Rationale: Sulfonamides, penicillins, and anticonvulsant drugs are among those that can intensify bleeding. Oral contraceptives actually can increase the risk of clotting.

10. *Answer:* B
    Rationale: Polycythemia is a state of elevated RBC count associated with increased venous thrombi risk. It occurs in high altitude, chronic hypoxia, congenital heart disease, and hyperproliferative bone marrow. Leukocytosis is an elevated WBC count, while leukopenia is a decreased WBC count. Iron deficiency anemia may be associated with a lower RBC count, but not consistently.

11. *Answer:* D
    Rationale: The red cell distribution width (RDW) measures the variability among RBC sizes and it may be increased in iron deficiency anemia. The hemoglobin electrophoresis measures hemoglobinopathies, such as sickle

cell anemia and Cooley's anemia. The PTT is a measure of blood coagulability, and the WBC differential measures different types of WBCs.

12. *Answer:* C

Rationale: A *left shift* refers to an increase in bands, which are immature neutrophils proliferating to fight infection or inflammation. The total neutrophil count normally rises in infection. Reticulocytes are immature RBCs more involved with anemias and blood loss. Platelets are involved with coagulability.

13. *Answer:* A

Rationale: B lymphocytes are a type of WBC that matures in the bone marrow and helps to form IgM and other antibodies. T lymphocytes arise from the thymus and destroy virus and tumor cells. Natural killer lymphocytes assist B lymphocytes to destroy foreign substances, while cytokines are hormone-like proteins activated by T cells to modulate inflammation and hematopoiesis.

14. *Answer:* C

Rationale: When one tonsil enlarges significantly more than the other, appears erythematous and edematous, and causes the uvula to tend to deviate toward the more enlarged tonsil, there is great risk for peritonsillar abscess. This is considered an emergency, and normally an ENT physician will drain the abscess then begin the patient on an antibiotic regimen. Antibiotics alone may not cure this disorder. The infection may or may not be caused by group A beta hemolytic strep, which will affect the choice of antibiotic but not the fact that this situation requires emergency consultation with a physician.

15. *Answer:* C

Rationale: Nodes over 1 cm in the cervical area that are excessively large fixed, rubbery, and nontender are suspicious for malignancy. A child with a streptococcal pharyngitis would more likely experience less than 1 cm, tender, mobile, and soft cervical adenopathy. Infectious mononucleosis also causes tender, mobile, and soft cervical

adenopathy, although nodes may approach 1.0 cm or more.

16. *Answer:* A

Rationale: Supraclavicular adenopathy is never normal. It is highly suspicious for malignancy, particularly mediastinal lymphadenopathy-associated malignancy. Tuberculosis and pneumonia may not cause adenopathy, although infectious mononucleosis will usually cause cervical and occipital lymphadenopathy.

17. *Answer:* A

Rationale: Tonsillar erythema, edema, white exudate, significant fever, and a fetid odor are more likely associated with a bacterial infection than a viral pharyngitis. The cause may be streptococcus or other bacteria. Infectious mononucleosis may also cause tonsillar erythema with white exudate, but the fever is not as significant and this disease is more common in adolescents and young adults. Herpangina is caused by the Coxsackie virus and appears as small ulcerations on the palate without exudate.

18. *Answer:* A

Rationale: Soft, minimally tender, shotty (less than 0.5 cm) clusters of lymph nodes are characteristic of upper respiratory infections in children, especially as the amount of lymphatic tissue peaks in middle childhood. Children easily develop cervical lymphadenopathy and tonsillar hypertrophy. Malignant lymph nodes would tend to be nontender, firm or rubbery, fixed, and isolated. Infectious mononucleosis presents with significant cervical adenopathy, severe pharyngitis, fatigue, and frequently hepatosplenomegaly. There is no need to check a CBC because the presentation is suggestive of a viral upper respiratory infection.

19. *Answer:* C

Rationale: Laboratory evidence of anemia, neutropenia (decreased neutrophil count), and blasts (primitive cells) suggests a severe hematologic malignancy. Urgent referral is necessary. It is unlikely this represents iron-deficiency anemia, which further

RBC morphology testing might indicate. Although lab tests can be incorrect, a pattern such as this requires urgent referral.

20. *Answer:* A

Rationale: Since many children are iron-deficient, that would be the most likely cause of this anemia. The RDW test and RBC morphologies on a CBC might indicate iron deficiency. The reticulocyte count is an expression of immature RBCs and indicates bone marrow activity in particular. Iron-binding and ferritin levels are more commonly used for adults and B_{12} and folic acid deficiencies are more commonly seen in adulthood.

21. *Answer:* A

Rationale: A high total WBC count with elevated neutrophils and bands suggests the presence of a significant bacterial infection or tissue necrosis. Given the abdominal pain, one must rule out an acute surgical abdomen in this child. Stress can elevate the WBC count slightly, but bands should not increase. In leukemia and viral infections, the WBC count may actually decrease.

22. *Answer:* B

Rationale: In infants and children, the spleen tip may be palpable 1 to 2 cm below the left costal margin, but anything below 2 cm is considered worrisome. The spleen should feel soft. Although the spleen sometimes enlarges along with the liver (hepatosplenomegaly), this is not always the case, and the liver border should never extend more than 2 cm in infants or children.

23. *Answer:* C

Rationale: Pallor, petechiae, and bruising should make the pediatric nurse practitioner concerned about coagulation disorders first. Bruising alone might alert one to domestic violence. Iron deficiency anemia would only cause pallor. Hemophilia is only one of many coagulation disorders. The best choice is to order a CBC and platelet count to begin the differential diagnosis.

24. *Answer:* D

Rationale: Chemotherapy-induced neutropenia currently can be treated with recom-binant growth factors. Children with neutropenia are considered at risk for infections. The reticulocyte count is more significant for bleeding disorders and anemias.

25. *Answer:* C

Rationale: A family history of bleeding disorders might be discerned with historical questions related to bleeding episodes, such as frequent epistaxis, bleeding gums, prolonged bleeding from minor cuts, and menorrhagia. Pica is associated with severe iron deficiency anemia. Hyperbilirubinemia at birth is not necessarily associated with any other deficits.

BIBLIOGRAPHY

American Association for Clinical Chemistry. (2004). The coagulation cascade. Retrieved April 22, 2006, from www.labtestsonline.org/understanding/analytes/coag_cascade/coagulation_cascade.html.

Bickley, L., & Szilagyi, P.G. (Eds.) (2003). *Bates' guide to physical examination and history taking* (8th ed.). Philadelphia: Lippincott Williams & Wilkins.

Corbett, J.V. (2004). *Laboratory tests and diagnostic procedures with nursing diagnoses* (6th ed.). Upper Saddle River, NJ: Pearson/Prentice Hall.

Engel, J. (2002). *Mosby's pocket guide series: Pediatric assessment* (4th ed.). St. Louis: Mosby.

Grethlein, S., & Perez Jr., J.A. (2005). Mucosa associated lymphoid tissue (MALT). Retrieved April 22, 2006, from www.emedicine.com/med/topic3204.htm (updated March 24, 2005).

King, M.W. (2005). Medical biochemistry: Blood coagulation. Retrieved April 22, 2006, from http://web.indstate.edu/thcme/mwking/blood-coagulation.html.

McCance, K.L., & Heuther, S.C. (2002). *Pathophysiology: The biologic basis for disease in adults and children* (4th ed.). St. Louis: Mosby.

Moore, K.L., & Persaud, T.V.N. (2003). *The developing human: Clinically oriented embryology* (7th ed.). Philadelphia: Saunders.

Nathan, D.G., Orkin, S.H., Look, A.T., & Ginsburg, D. (2003). *Nathan and Oski's hematology of infancy and childhood* (6th ed.). Philadelphia: Saunders.

Wong, D.L., Hockenberry-Eaton, M., Wilson, D., et al. (2001). *Wong's essentials of pediatric nursing.* St. Louis: Mosby.

12 Assessment of the Musculoskeletal System

MARY SOBRALSKE

Select the best answer for each of the following questions:

1. The principles of the musculoskeletal assessment include:
   A. Most joints consist of ball and socket.
   B. There are many joints that normally have a 90-degree arc of motion.
   C. Bones normally are asymmetric and have irregular contours and abrupt shapes.
   D. The musculoskeletal system functions to support the body and provide movement.

2. Factors that MOST influence bone growth are:
   A. Ethnicity and gender.
   B. Nutrition and hormones.
   C. Sun exposure and the environment.
   D. Geographic factors such as altitude and latitude.

3. It is important to compare the bones and muscles side to side because:
   A. Children normally have symmetric muscle development, range of joint motion, length, and function.
   B. All children have some asymmetry from side to side.
   C. The muscles of the dominant hand will always be more developed than those of the nondominant hand.
   D. Children do not grow in even amounts side to side.

4. In a newborn assessment, what special tests are especially important in screening for musculoskeletal problems?

A. Galeazzi tests, symmetry of gluteal and thigh folds, and Ortolani's maneuver.
B. McMurray test for subluxation, Ober test for ilial-tibial band tightness, and Patrick test for flexion contractures.
C. Lachman test for ligamentous instability and Apley's distraction test.
D. Upright test for toe walking, tight heel cords, clasped thumbs.

5. Han is a 2-month-old infant with a positive bilateral Babinski reflex, a poor Moro reflex, frog-leg posture when supine, limp ventral suspension, and floppy extremities with poor tone. He has been experiencing respiratory problems. A referral to the pediatric specialist is made. Based on the above findings, you suspect a diagnosis of:
   A. Generalized spasticity with possible cerebral palsy.
   B. Developmental delay with possible genetic syndrome.
   C. Generalized hypotonia with possible spinal muscular atrophy.
   D. General extremity weakness with possible muscular dystrophy.

6. The pediatric specialist agrees with your presumptive diagnosis. You want to prepare Han's parents for the consultation with some likely causes for these findings. Han's prognosis is:
   A. Poor. This is a progressive problem.
   B. Fair. However, he will be mentally retarded.
   C. Good. He will improve as he gets older.

D. Excellent. The pediatric neurologist will find the cause and Han will have a normal life.

7. Joint crepitus is commonly detected by:
   A. Varus-valgus stressing of the ligaments surrounding the joint.
   B. Palpating the joint and surrounding tissue while putting the joint through full range of motion.
   C. Performing the ballottement test for effusion.
   D. Listening over the joint space with a bedside ultrasonic probe.

8. Kendrick is an 18-month-old Hispanic boy whose father is concerned his son has "cowboy legs" (bowed legs) and he falls a lot. What is the most likely diagnosis for these findings?
   A. Genu valgum.
   B. Physiologic genu varum.
   C. Patellar lateral subluxation.
   D. Bilateral varus thrust when walking.

9. What is one of the most common causes of a limp in a 3-year-old girl?
   A. Developmental dysplasia of the hip.
   B. Legg-Calvé-Perthes disease of the hip(s).
   C. Stress fracture of the foot or ankle.
   D. Slipped capital femoral epiphysis.

10. Eric is a 9-year-old Japanese American boy who likes to play soccer with his friends after school. You evaluate him for intermittent bilateral leg pain that mainly occurs at night. According to his mother, sometimes he wakes up during the night screaming that his legs hurt. When asked to identify the location of his pain, he points to the anterior thigh, posterior knees, and posterior calves. Based on the history, you suspect:
   A. Shin splints.
   B. Growing pains.
   C. Osgood-Schlatter disease.
   D. Pes planus.

11. When treating Eric for his pain, what is the MOST important part of the plan?

A. Reassurance that this problem is not pathologic.
B. He should avoid activities that cause the pain.
C. Eric may have long-term disability because of this problem.
D. He needs physical therapy to relearn his gait pattern.

12. Shanta is a 14-year-old female with a lateral curvature of her spine. One side of her pelvis is higher than the other. When she bends over to touch her toes with her knees straight, you note that her curvature becomes more apparent with a prominence of 14 degrees left of the lumbar spine with a coulometer. What is the most appropriate action?
   A. Inform her family that the curvature is caused by a leg length discrepancy.
   B. Order an x-ray of the entire spine in an upright position, either AP or PA view.
   C. Order an MRI of her spine to rule out spinal cord pathology.
   D. Measure and fit for a scoliosis brace.

13. Observing 10-year-old Sean stepping on and off the scale to be weighed is a simple way to partially screen for the following:
   A. Balance and proprioception.
   B. Biceps muscle strength.
   C. Hip range of motion and pelvic position.
   D. Scoliosis and kyphosis.

14. Tim is a very active 15-year-old male. Tim excitedly walks into the urgent care center bearing weight on both feet but limping. About 40 minutes ago, he was playing basketball and "twisted" his ankle while dribbling down the basketball court. He was able to finish the game and his team won. What diagnosis would you first suspect based on the brief history and the clinical presentation?
   A. Torn meniscus.
   B. Fractured mid-foot.
   C. Fractured distal fibula.
   D. Ligamentous ankle sprain.

15. Tobias is a 14-month-old boy with developmental delays and a marked curvature

of his spine. He was diagnosed with congenital scoliosis with vertebral anomalies. What problems might Tobias have that will need to be investigated?

A. Renal and cardiac anomalies.
B. Skin and liver disease.
C. Genital and urinary tract anomalies.
D. Endocrine and acoustic problems.

16. Leilani is a 2-year-old girl whose father reports that she isn't learning as quickly as her older sister and brother did. She was born premature at 35 weeks gestation after a long labor. She started walking at 21 months and still is "a little wobbly." What gait disturbance would be consistent with this history?

A. She falls down a lot.
B. She has ataxia and disequilibrium.
C. She walks on her toes with a stoppage gait.
D. She walks on the lateral borders and heels of her feet.

17. What are the consequences of inadequate calcium intake in a child?

A. Skeletal dysplasia.
B. Vitamin D deficiency (rickets).
C. Juvenile osteoporosis.
D. Cognitive developmental delay.

18. A thorough musculoskeletal assessment should ALWAYS include:

A. The birth history and attainment of developmental milestones.
B. Radiographs of a newborn's hips to rule out hip dysplasia.
C. Ultrasound of the hips to assess for hip dislocation.
D. CPK and alkaline phosphatase lab values.

19. Three-year-old Jimmy in-toes: Three common etiologies of in-toeing are internal tibial torsion, metatarsus adductus, and:

A. Femoral anteversion.
B. Infantile Blount's disease.
C. Muscle imbalance.
D. Bilateral genu valgum.

20. Jamaal is a 12-year-old African American male who presents with right hip pain for the past 2 weeks. He is well over the 95th percentile for height and weight. He cannot recall that he injured himself. What orthopedic problem should be your number one-concern given his body habitus, age, gender, and ethnicity?

A. An acute femoral neck fracture.
B. Slipped femoral capital epiphysis.
C. Dislocated hip.
D. Legg-Calvé-Perthes disease of his right hip.

21. Amber is a 6-year-old girl who recently moved to your city and is new to your practice. Her parents report that she has a history of brittle bone disease but cannot give you the name(s) of physicians or clinics where she has been diagnosed and treated for osteogenesis imperfecta. They tell you she has had several arm fractures in the last few years but they always heal okay. Dad tells you he had several arm fractures when he was a child, but was never taken to a specialist for the breaks. His father would take him to their town doctor and he would "patch him up like new." Before the family leaves your clinic today, what will be very important to accomplish on this initial visit?

A. Radiographs of all the bones in her extremities to look for new fractures.
B. Recommend and offer to schedule Amber for a consultation with a pediatric orthopedic specialist in the very near future.
C. A referral to Child Protection Services for ongoing child abuse.
D. Have her parents complete a medical release of records for prior medical treatment before their move.

22. What foot fracture is commonly seen in school-age children?

A. Distal fibular fracture due to in-line skating.
B. Jones' fracture of the base of the 5th metatarsal due to playing football.
C. Spondylolysis due to hyperextension of the spine during gymnastics.
D. Pathological calcaneal fracture due to long-distance running.

23. Ten-month-old Jamie is brought in by his mother for the first well baby exam at the

clinic. They just moved to the area and his past medical records are not readily available. Mother states he has been healthy except for the birth defect of his right arm. On exam his right arm is internally rotated and will not abduct fully or flex at the elbow. He cannot reach for a toy over his head and constantly uses his left hand to grab things. His right arm is generally weaker and has less muscle development than the left arm. The most probable diagnosis is:

A. Brachial plexus birth palsy.
B. Child abuse.
C. Hemimelia of the right humerus.
D. Muscular torticollis.

24. Gower sign is seen in children with:
A. Developmental dysplasia of the hip.
B. Scoliosis.
C. Duchenne's muscular dystrophy.
D. Asymmetrical knee height.

NOTES

ANSWERS

1. *Answer:* D
   Rationale: Bones, joints, and muscles support the body and provide movement. Only the hip and shoulder joints consist of ball and socket. Most joints have at least a 120-degree arc of motion. Bones are normally symmetric and have softened contours and gradual flares.

2. *Answer:* B
   Rationale: Nutrition and hormones most influence bone growth. Delay in growth can result if there is malnutrition. Rapid bone growth often occurs when there are hormonal changes such as those that occur in puberty. Body habitus such as height varies by gender and ethnicity, but does not directly affect bone growth. While lack of sun exposure may affect levels of vitamin D, as long as a child is getting adequate vitamin D in enriched food, normal growth of bone should not be a problem. Trauma to the open growth plates can cause abnormal bone growth. There is no evidence that altitude and latitude directly affect bone growth.

3. *Answer:* A
   Rationale: Symmetry is usually the norm. A major principle is to look for symmetry, then assess whether the asymmetry is pathologic or physiologic.

4. *Answer:* A
   Rationale: The only answer that is entirely correct is Galeazzi tests, symmetry of skin folds, and Ortolani's maneuver that all assess for hip dysplasia. McMurray test is performed for meniscus tear which one would not commonly seen in infancy. Ober test may be appropriate in a premature infant who has been in a frog-leg hypotonic position for many weeks or months after birth. Patrick test is positive after a fixed hip contracture. Ligamentous laxity is common in a newborn, but not instability. Toe-walking should not be evident until the infant starts walking. Tight heel cords can be seen in congenital clubfoot. Clamped thumbs may be indicative of an underlying neurologic pathology.

5. *Answer:* C
   Rationale: These findings point to spinal muscular atrophy, especially since the child is experiencing respiratory problems. There is no data to support that he has spasticity or syndromic presentation. While poor tone causes generalized weakness, muscular dystrophy initially presents with proximal muscle weakness. This infant has generalized weakness.

6. *Answer:* A
   Rationale: The prognosis is very poor. Spinal muscular atrophy is a progressive disorder and most children die of respiratory failure at a very young age. Your role will be in supporting his family and coordinating and providing referrals to specialists who can help Han and his family.

7. *Answer:* B
   Rationale: Joint crepitus may be found in disorders that involve the articular cartilage friction, such as patellar femoral crepitus.

8. *Answer:* B
   Rationale: Physiologic genu varum (bow legs) is a common and normal finding in a toddler. Patellar subluxation is rarely seen in a toddler. Varus thrust is indicative of infantile Blount's disease. Genu valgum, or knock knees, is a common finding in a child 3 to 6 years old.

9. *Answer:* A
   Rationale: A young child who has not been treated for developmental dysplasia of the hips may have a length discrepancy. This can cause a limp. Legg-Calvé-Perthes disease is caused by avascular necrosis of the femoral head. This would be seen in 5- to 9-year-old children, more commonly boys. Slipped capital femoral epiphysis would be seen in ages 8 to 15, more common in boys than girls. Stress fracture of the foot or ankle is a problem more commonly seen in adolescent age, usually athletes due to overuse.

10. *Answer:* B
    Rationale: Growing pains are poorly understood. They usually occur at night, worsen after activity, are seen in up to 30% of

children 3 to 12 years old, and are more common in girls than in boys. Pes planus, or flat feet, can sometimes cause foot, ankle, and leg pains. This is thought to be caused by overuse. Osgood-Schlatter disease will present with anterior knee pain at the tibial tuberosity when kneeling. Shin splints, or periostitis of the tibias, result from repetitive running on hard surfaces or forceful excessive use of foot dorsiflexors.

11. *Answer:* A
Rationale: Reassure him and his parents that growing pains are normal in child Eric's age. He will eventually outgrow this problem and his gait will not be affected by them. There are no suggested limitations in activity.

12. *Answer:* B
Rationale: Unequal leg lengths can cause a curvature; however, this would not produce a lumbar spinal prominence. After a thorough examination, a screening radiograph of her spine in an upright position will assess the severity of any curvatures. While an MRI of her spine may be necessary, this would not be done unless other findings pointed to a neurologic basis for the curvature. It is not appropriate to put her in a brace at this point.

13. *Answer:* A
Rationale: Stepping on a clinic scale on demand takes balance and a sense of proprioception. This maneuver requires lower extremity strength. Stepping onto a scale would only assess hip flexion and extension, not rotation. Screening for scoliosis and kyphosis requires focused exam of the spine with clothing removed.

14. *Answer:* D
Rationale: He walks fully bearing weight bilaterally. Tim would probably not be walking and bearing weight, let alone finish playing the game, if his fibula were fractured. Twisting the ankle will probably not cause a torn meniscus in the knee. It is unlikely that he fractured his mid-foot dribbling down a basketball court.

15. *Answer:* A
Rationale: The kidneys and heart develop during the same time as the skeletal system in the early first trimester of gestation. Congenital scoliosis is often associated with anomalies of the kidneys and heart.

16. *Answer:* B
Rationale: All children first learning to walk fall down a lot. Her birth history points to cerebral palsy. Spasticity and muscle weakness will contribute to toe walking and stoppage gait. This gait produces the wobbly appearance. Walking on the lateral borders or heels of the feet is caused by other orthopedic problems such as congenital coalitions of the foot bones.

17. *Answer:* B
Rationale: Vitamin D deficiency (rickets) can result from inadequate calcium intake in children. Older adults who as children did not obtain adequate calcium intake are at greater risk for osteoporosis. Inadequate nutrition in general may cause problems with learning; however, there is no evidence to conclude that inadequate calcium causes cognitive delays. Skeletal dysplasia is congenital, not a result of inadequate nutrition in the child.

18. *Answer:* A
Rationale: Birth history and attainment of developmental milestones is one of the most telling parts of the musculoskeletal assessment in a child. Many neuromusculoskeletal problems seen in children can be attributed to birth trauma. Hip ultrasound and radiographs are only obtained if there is suspicion of hip disorders. There are no lab tests that are commonly done on a musculoskeletal assessment unless there are positive orthopedic or neurologic findings that point to specific problems.

19. *Answer:* A
Rationale: Increased internal rotation (femoral anteversion) of the hips is commonly the etiology of in-toeing in young children. Infantile Blount's is a disease of the proximal tibias. Muscle imbalance would not

be a common reason, and may be indicative of underlying neuromuscular disorder. Genu valgum would not cause in-toeing, but may cause out-toeing.

20. *Answer:* B
    Rationale: Slipped capital femoral epiphysis is mostly commonly seen in overweight children, is more common in black and Polynesian children, and affects boys (60%) more often than girls (40%). The average age at onset is 12 years in girls and 13½ years in boys. There is no history of injury that would cause a femoral neck fracture. A dislocated hip would more commonly be seen in a newborn, not a child at puberty. Legg-Calvé-Perthes more commonly presents at ages 5 to 9 years.

21. *Answer:* B
    Rationale: It is never easy to make clinical decisions in a situation like this. Some parents can be poor historians for many different reasons. Although the history is sketchy, Amber could very well have a history of pathologic fractures due to osteogenesis imperfecta, although you would expect to see bowing and marked angulation of the bones that were fractured. A consultation with a pediatric orthopedic specialist is the best and safest way to proceed. Ultimately acquiring previous medical records is necessary for continuity. You have no proof that Amber is abused; however, you should have a high index of suspicion and surveillance and should monitor her often with frequent clinic visits until you can acquire more information.

22. *Answer:* B
    Rationale: Jones' fracture and calcaneal fracture are the only fractures seen in the foot. A pathological fracture is rarely seen in a child without an underlying disorder that affects the density of the bones.

23. *Answer:* A
    Rationale: Brachial plexus birth palsy is the probable cause of unilateral upper extremity weakness and lack of normal and symmetric range of motion. All prudent pediatric nurse practitioners should consider child abuse as a possible cause for injuries in children, but you should not have high index of suspicion after the clinical presentation and exam. There is no evidence that part of the humerus is missing. Muscular torticollis will affect the neck and sometimes appears that the shoulder is involved because the child will try to compensate for lack of motion in the neck.

24. *Answer:* C
    Rationale: Gower sign is seen in children with Duchenne's muscular dystrophy. It occurs when a child who is attempting to stand from the ground, begins with both hands and feet on the floor and works his way up the legs with his hands until standing because of proximal weakness. Infants with developmental dysplasia of the hip will have a positive Ortolani's sign and Barlow test. A positive Galeazzi or Allis sign are related to knee height asymmetry.

BIBLIOGRAPHY

American Academy of Pediatrics, Committee on Quality Improvement (2000). Clinical practice guideline: Early detection of developmental dysplasia of the hip. *Pediatrics, 105*(4), 896-904.

American Academy of Pediatrics, Committee on Sports Medicine and Fitness (2001). Medical conditions affecting sports participation. *Pediatrics, 107*(5), 1205-1209.

Chin, K.R., Price, J.S., & Zimbler, S. (2001). A guide to early detection of scoliosis. *Contemp Pediatr, 18*(9), 77-103.

Colyar, M.R. (2003). *Well-child assessment for primary care providers.* Philadelphia: F.A. Davis.

Goldbloom, R.B. (2003). *Pediatric clinical skills* (3rd ed.). Philadelphia: Saunders.

Ganel, A., Dudkiewicz, I., & Grogan, D.P. (2003). Pediatric orthopedic physical examination of the infant: A 5–minute assessment. *J Pediatr Health Care, 17*(1), 39-41.

Metzl, J.D. (2001). Preparticipation examination of the adolescent athlete: Part 1. *Pediatr Rev, 22*(6), 199-204.

Metzl, J.D. (2001). Preparticipation examination of the adolescent athlete: Part 2. *Pediatr Rev, 22*(7), 227-239.

Neinstein, L.S. (2002). *Adolescent health care: A practical guide* (4th ed.) Baltimore: Williams & Wilkins.

Patel, D.R., Greydanus, D.E., & Pratt, H.D. (2001). Youth sports: More than sprains and strains. *Contemp Pediatr, 18*(3), 45-72.

Taft, E., & Francis, R. (2003). Evaluation and management of scoliosis. *J Pediatr Health Care, 17*(1), 42-44.

U.S. National Cancer Institute's Surveillance, Epidemiology and End Results (SEER) Program. Bone development and growth. Retrieved April 22, 2006, from http://training.seer.cancer.gov/module_anatomy/unit3_3_bone_growth.html.

NOTES

13 Assessment of the Neurologic System

KAREN DUDERSTADT

Select the best answer for each of the following questions:

1. The neurologic examination includes testing children for sensory function. A young verbal child can be assessed for normal cortical sensation by:
   A. Identifying familiar faces.
   B. Identifying objects by handling them.
   C. Identifying shapes drawn on the palm when eyes are closed.
   D. Evaluating abstract reasoning skills.

2. During the physical examination on a 5-year-old, you palpate two soft, rubbery nodular skin lesions on the arm about 2 to 3 cm in diameter that are nontender and the same color as the child's skin. When asked, mother said she had first noticed them on her son's arm a few months ago. You inspect the skin for other abnormal findings consistent with a diagnosis of:
   A. Axillary freckling.
   B. Neurofibroma.
   C. Cutaneous gliomas.
   D. Benign hemangioma.

3. When assessing a 1-year-old who presents with a history of a fall, what indicator would you use to determine appropriate level of consciousness?
   A. Cries in response to being examined.
   B. Grunts when moved.
   C. Responds to a loud noise.
   D. Incomprehensible words.

4. You are evaluating a 6-year-old who presents to the primary care clinic with his mother. The first grade teacher is concerned that he has a poor attention span and difficulty writing his name. What parts of the neurologic history would be most helpful to you in assessing this child for possible learning problems?
   A. Attainment of developmental milestones.
   B. Birthmarks.
   C. Bowel and bladder problems.
   D. Parental consanguinity.

5. A 13-year-old female presents to the school-based clinic with a history of dizziness when walking up stairs. What parts of the neurologic exam would be most helpful in evaluating this teen?
   A. Testing for balance and coordination.
   B. Testing for the cremasteric reflex.
   C. Testing cranial nerves II and VIII.
   D. Testing for level of attention.

6. A 16-year-old male presents to the urgent care clinic for evaluation of high fever to 103.5° F, headache, and stiff neck. As the patient is lying on the exam table during the physical examination, you flex his leg at both the hip and the knee. As you straighten the legs, he experiences severe pain. What is the name of sign you are eliciting during the physical examination?
   A. Lachman's sign.
   B. Babinski's sign.
   C. Kernig's sign.
   D. Brudzinski's sign.

7. You are completing a physical examination on a newborn infant who is less than 24 hours old. As you are observing the infant, he begins to cry and you notice that his fa-

cial expression is asymmetrical. What cranial nerve may have been affected during the birth process that could contribute to a finding of facial asymmetry?

A. Cranial nerve XI.
B. Cranial nerve V.
C. Cranial nerve VI.
D. Cranial nerve VII.

8. A 7-week-old infant presents in the primary care clinic with her mother for a well child checkup. Mother expresses some concern with the infant's feeding pattern. She is slow at sucking and is difficult to position during feeding. What findings on the neurologic exam would cause concern about this infant?

A. Nonsustained clonus.
B. Gower's sign.
C. Plantar flexion.
D. Absent Moro reflex.

9. A 6-month-old infant with Down syndrome presents for a routine primary care visit and immunizations. Over the past few months, mother has noticed rapid, intermittent movement of his eyes when he was gazing at her. The involuntary rapid eye movement in this 6-month-old infant is called:

A. Opsoclonus.
B. Nystagmus.
C. Abducens movement.
D. Ptosis.

10. The body compensates for loss of sensation due to trauma by a complex overlap of sensory fibers called:

A. Myotomes.
B. Neural folds.
C. Dermatomes.
D. Dendrites.

11. Reflex behavior provides the primary assessment of:

A. Brainstem function.
B. Muscle tension.
C. Impulse control.
D. Peripheral nervous system.

12. Developmental reflexes should be evaluated on all infants until:

A. One month of age.

B. Primitive reflexes disappear.
C. The newborn develops head control.
D. Six months of age.

13. *Myoclonus* is defined as:

A. Slow, twisting, writhing muscle movements.
B. Rapid, alternative movements.
C. Sudden, brief, brisk muscle contractions.
D. Rhythmic oscillation of the body.

14. When testing the nervous system for cerebellar function, you are primarily testing:

A. Coordination and balance.
B. Involuntary muscle movements.
C. Position sense.
D. Cortical sensation.

15. Rhythmic tonic-clonic movements of the foot refers to:

A. Tremors.
B. Stepping reflex.
C. Plantar fasciculations.
D. Clonus.

16. Myotomes are:

A. Named according to the spinal nerve that supplies the sensory fibers.
B. A group of muscles primarily innervated by motor fibers from a single nerve root.
C. Specific muscle groups associated with reflexes.
D. Fibers that innervate the skin.

17. The normal function of cranial nerve VII is responsibility for:

A. Conduction of sound.
B. Lateralization.
C. Frowning.
D. Maxillary pain.

18. A normal reflex arc of the deep tendon reflex is a complex function and requires:

A. A functional synapse in the spinal cord.
B. A diminished response of the musculoskeletal system.
C. Free movement of the toes.
D. Hyperactive sensory neurons.

19. Observing normal activities of a new-born infant such as feeding and crying tests:
   A. Cranial nerves X and XII.
   B. Cranial nerve XI.
   C. Cranial nerves VII and X.
   D. Cranial nerve IX.

20. Contraction of the quadriceps muscle and extension of the leg is elicited by:
   A. Stroking the inner aspect of the calf.
   B. Tapping the tendon just below the patella.
   C. Tapping the tuberosity a few centimeters over the knee.
   D. Tapping your thumb on the antecubital fossa.

21. Neuronal messages are transmitted through the cortex by:
   A. Neurotransmitter chemicals.
   B. Synapses.
   C. Dermatomes.
   D. Cognitive activity.

22. During the neurologic examination, school-aged children can be assessed for balance and coordination using tests that are fun and assist the practitioner in assessing cerebellar function. The tests include:
   A. Romberg's test.
   B. Stereognosis.
   C. Graphesthesia.
   D. Two-point discrimination.

23. Tremors can occur in children:
   A. In the facial muscles.
   B. When the child is at rest or active.
   C. When testing tandem walking.
   D. When eliciting rapid alternative movements of the hands.

24. *Chorea* is defined as:
   A. Sudden, brief arrhythmic and asymmetric movements.
   B. Rhythmic tonic-clonic movements of the foot.
   C. Slow, twisting, writhing muscle movements.
   D. Rhythmic oscillation of the body.

NOTES

ANSWERS

1. *Answer:* C
   Rationale: Graphesthesia is the ability to identify shapes traced on the palm with eyes closed and tests children for normal cortical sensation. Children with spatial and proprioceptive dysfunction will be unable to discriminate shapes.

2. *Answer:* B
   Rationale: Neurofibromas are soft, rubbery, nodular lesions noted on the skin and can be palpated in children and adults with neurofibromatosis. Freckling is not nodular and gliomas are tumors generally found in the brain.

3. *Answer:* A
   Rationale: Normal mental status in a 1-year-old with history of a fall would be indicated by crying in response to the physical exam. Grunting would indicate a decreased level of consciousness.

4. *Answer:* A
   Rationale: The attainment of development milestones within the normal range would be the most helpful information of the choices given. Birthmarks in general do not indicate an abnormal finding. The blood type of the parent is not diagnostic of learning problems nor are bowel and bladder problems. Children who have delayed fine and gross motor milestones are at increased risk for learning problems.

5. *Answer:* A
   Rationale: Testing for balance and coordination would be the most helpful of the choices to evaluate her for dizziness.

6. *Answer:* C
   Rationale: Kernig's sign is elicited with the child lying with knees flexed in the supine position. A positive sign is when the practitioner notes pain and resistance when extending/straightening the legs of the child.

7. *Answer:* D
   Rationale: Cranial nerve VII is the facial nerve. Symmetry of the facial movements and facial expression requires an intact cranial nerve VII in the newborn.

8. *Answer:* D
   Rationale: The Moro reflex persists until 4 to 6 months of age in the normal infant. Infants who are hypotonic often have diminished or absent Moro at birth.

9. *Answer:* B
   Rationale: *Nystagmus* is described as rapid involuntary eye movements when the infant is focusing on an object. Ptosis refers to a droopy eyelid.

10. *Answer:* C
    Rationale: Dermatomes are areas of the skin that are innervated by sensory fibers of a single nerve root. The dermatomes overlap so that loss of sensation due to trauma is minimized.

11. *Answer:* A
    Rationale: Reflex behavior provides the primary assessment of brainstem function. Reflexes help maintain appropriate muscle tension, but the impulse or stimulus transmitted when eliciting a reflex requires an intact brainstem. The peripheral nervous system is the messenger to the brainstem.

12. *Answer:* D
    Rationale: Developmental reflexes persist in the infant until 6 months of age. As the initial primitive reflexes begin to diminish or disappear by 4 months of age, the postural reflexes appear between 5 to 6 months of age.

13. *Answer:* C
    Rationale: *Myoclonus* is defined as the sudden, brief, brisk muscle contractions. Tremor is characterized by a rhythmic oscillation of a body part; and slow, twisting, writhing involuntary muscle movements indicate athetosis.

14. *Answer:* A
    Rationale: When testing for cerebellar function, the practitioner is primarily assessing the balance and coordination of the patient. Position sense is only part of testing the cerebrum. The testing requires voluntary

movements and does not involve testing sensation.

15. *Answer:* D
Rationale: Clonus is defined as a rhythmic, tonic-clonic movement of the foot elicited by a brisk dorsiflexion of the foot. The stepping reflex is elicited in the newborn when holding the infant upright over the exam table and allowing the feet to touch.

16. *Answer:* D
Rationale: Myotomes are a group of muscles innervated by the motor fibers of a single nerve root.

17. *Answer:* C
Rationale: Cranial nerve VII is the facial nerve and innervates the facial movements including frowning. Pain in the maxillary area is transmitted by cranial nerve V, the trigeminal nerve.

18. *Answer:* A
Rationale: The reflex arc of the deep tendon reflex requires a functional synapse in the spinal cord.

19. *Answer:* A
Rationale: Cranial nerve X and cranial nerve XII, the vagus and hypoglossal, can be accurately assessed by observing the infant crying and feeding.

20. *Answer:* B
Rationale: The patellar reflex is elicited by tapping the patellar tendon just below the patella. Observe for contraction of the quadriceps and muscle and extension of the leg. The brachioradialis reflex is elicited by tapping your index finger or thumb on the biceps tendon in the antecubital fossa. The result is contraction of the biceps muscle and flexion of the elbow.

21. *Answer:* A
Rationale: Neurotransmitter chemicals are released at the synapses and carry the neuronal messages to the next synapse. The result is normal cognitive function.

22. *Answer:* A
Rationale: Romberg's test assesses for balance and equilibrium in the young child. The child must be able to stand erect with the eyes closed and hands touching the sides. Observe the balance for several seconds while monitoring the child closely. Lesions in the cerebellum can cause the child to stagger and fall. The other tests evaluate normal cortical function.

23. *Answer:* B
Rationale: Tremors can occur when the body is at rest or active. Tremors can occur in any part of the body and are involuntary, generally not elicited by certain activities.

24. *Answer:* A
Rationale: Chorea is sudden, brief arrhythmic and asymmetric movements of the body occurring most often in the extremities, neck, trunk, and facial muscles. *Athetosis* is defined as slow, twisting, writhing movements.

BIBLIOGRAPHY

Colyar, M.R. (2003). *Well-child assessment for primary care providers*. Philadelphia: F.A. Davis.
Goldbloom, R.B. (2003). *Pediatric clinical skills* (3rd ed.). Philadelphia: Saunders.
Fily, A., Truffert, P., Ego, A., et al. (2003). Neurological assessment at five years of age in infants born preterm. *Acta Paediatr, 92*(12), 1433–1437.
Fuller, G. (2004). *Neurological examination made easy* (3rd ed.). Edinburgh: Churchill Livingstone.
Hobdell, E. (2001). Infant neurological assessment. *J Neurosci Nurs, 33*(4), 190–193.
Jarvis, C. (2003). *Physical examination and health assessment* (4th ed.). St. Louis: Elsevier.
Larsen, W.J. (2001). *Human embryology*. New York: Churchill Livingstone.
Miyan, J. (2003) Embryology and neurulation. University of Manchester Institute of Science and Technology. Retrieved April 22, 2006, from www.bi.umist.ac.uk/users/mjfssjm4/OPT-EU/Embryology.htm.
Moore, K.L., & Persaud, T.V.N. (2003). *The developing human: Clinically oriented embryology*. Philadelphia: Saunders.

SPECIAL TOPICS IN HEALTH PROMOTION AND DISEASE PREVENTION

14 Core Concepts in Genetics

PATRICIA BILLER KRAUSKOPF

Select the best answer for each of the following questions:

1. Which of the following was an international research effort to sequence and map all of the genes of *Homo sapiens*?
   A. Human Genome Project.
   B. *Homosapien* Genetic Program.
   C. Deoxyribonucleic Acid (DNA) Protocol.
   D. Genetic Code Project.

2. Which of the following is NOT identified as a role or function of DNA?
   A. Store information.
   B. Transmit itself to subsequent generations.
   C. Determine the precise nature of gene products, including protein structure.
   D. Exist as one long molecule.

3. Each human cell contains which of the following?
   A. A total of 48 chromosomes.
   B. 22 autosomes and 1 sex chromosome.
   C. 23 pairs of chromosomes.
   D. 22 pairs of chromosomes.

4. Which one of the following statements regarding chromosomes is NOT true?
   A. Composed of chromatin that contains genetic information.
   B. Females have one X and one Y chromosome.
   C. Distinct, physically separate microscopic structures contained in the nucleus of every cell.
   D. Visible only during cell division.

5. The basic unit of heredity is which of the following?
   A. Chromosome.
   B. Autosome.
   C. Germ cell.
   D. Gene.

6. Which of the following statements is NOT true regarding genes?
   A. An ordered sequence of nucleotides.
   B. Arranged in a specific locus in a linear fashion along particular chromosomes.
   C. *Heterozygous* describes when genes in a pair are identical.
   D. Regulatory genes encode enzymes and hormones.

7. While obtaining a family history, the pediatric nurse practitioner creates a pictorial representation or diagram of the family history. This is referred to as which of the following?
   A. Pedigree.
   B. Heredity graph.
   C. Familiarity.
   D. Family pictorial.

8. If a genetic disorder is suspected in a patient, the pediatric nurse practitioner is aware that a visual display of chromosome studies arranged in a standardized way may be ordered. The nomenclature includes the number of chromosomes, the sex chromosomes' contribution, and any abnormalities found. This analysis is referred to as which of the following?

A. Genotype
B. Phenotype
C. Pedigree
D. Karyotype

9. Which of the following statements is NOT true regarding mutation?
   A. Occurs when an incorrect nucleotide base is inserted during DNA synthesis.
   B. May produce either a "gain of function" or a "loss of function."
   C. Usually visually apparent or biochemically detectable.
   D. A permanent change in genetic material.

10. A brown-eyed expectant mother and her blue-eyed husband ask the pediatric nurse practitioner what color eyes their child will have. Knowing that brown eyes are usually dominant and blue eyes are usually recessive, which of the following statements is the best reply?
   A. If the father is heterozygous for the blue eye gene, the child's eyes will be blue.
   B. If the mother is heterozygous for the brown eye gene, the child's eyes could be brown or blue.
   C. If the father is homozygous for the blue eye gene, the child's eyes will be blue.
   D. If the mother is homozygous for the brown eye gene, the child's eyes could be brown or blue.

11. Which of the following statements is NOT true of recessive characteristics or traits?
   A. Expressed when one copy of the gene is present at corresponding loci of homologous chromosomes.
   B. Usually remain undetected for generations.
   C. Estimated that each human carries from five to seven recessive rare deleterious alleles in the heterozygous state.
   D. If a carrier of a recessive allele mates with another individual with the same recessive allele, then they may have a child with a homozygous recessive disease.

12. Which of the following is NOT a structural chromosomal abnormality?
   A. Duplications
   B. Transcriptions
   C. Inversions
   D. Deletions

13. Which of the following inherited conditions is NOT autosomal recessive?
   A. Tay-Sachs disease.
   B. Mucopolysaccharide disorders such as Hurler's syndrome.
   C. Adrenogenital syndrome.
   D. Glucose-6-phospate dehydrogenase deficiency.

14. Jeannie is a 23-year-old female who has a sister with cystic fibrosis. She is engaged to be married and is concerned that her children may have cystic fibrosis. Jeannie does not have the disease but she is a carrier. Her fiancé is also a carrier of the cystic fibrosis gene. Which of the following statements, applicable to each pregnancy, would the pediatric nurse practitioner relay to Jeannie?
   A. There is a 75% chance of having an affected child.
   B. There is a 50% chance of having an affected child.
   C. There is a 25% chance of having an affected child.
   D. There is a 50% chance of having an affected child, but only if the child is male.

15. Which of the following inherited conditions has an autosomal dominant inheritance pattern?
   A. Huntington's disease.
   B. Phenylketonuria.
   C. Albinism.
   D. Spinal muscular atrophy.

16. What is the probability of parents having a child with sickle cell disease if the father is a carrier of the sickle cell gene and the mother is not?

A. 100%
B. 50%
C. 25%
D. 0%

17. When obtaining a history from a pregnant patient, the pediatric nurse practitioner is informed that the patient's father has coagulation factor IX deficiency or hemophilia B, also known as Christmas disease, which is an X-linked disorder. If the patient is carrying a male child, which of the following statements would be appropriate for the pediatric nurse practitioner to tell the patient?
   A. The child is not at risk for this disorder.
   B. The child will have this disorder.
   C. There is a 25% chance that the child will be affected by this disorder.
   D. There is a 50% chance that the child will be affected by this disorder.

18. A child is diagnosed with Leber hereditary optic neuropathy (LHON), which the pediatric nurse practitioner recalls is a mitochondrial DNA disorder. Which of the following statements correctly describes this inheritance pattern?
   A. Mitochondria are inherited solely though the mother via her egg.
   B. Mitochondria are inherited solely through the father via his sperm.
   C. Mitochondria may be inherited equally from both the mother or the father.
   D. Only females will exhibit genetic defects associated with this disorder.

19. Prader-Willi syndrome and Angelman syndrome are examples of which inheritance pattern?
   A. Autosomal dominant.
   B. Mutagenesis.
   C. Uniparental disomy.
   D. Germ line mosaicism.

20. Teratogens are any substance that adversely affects fetal development, but do not alter the genetic material. What is the most common human teratogen?
   A. Maternal rubella during pregnancy.

B. Isotretinoin (Accutane) ingested by the mother during pregnancy.
C. Oral contraceptives ingested by the mother during pregnancy.
D. Alcohol ingested by the mother during pregnancy.

21. A newborn has a cleft lip and palate. The parents ask the pediatric nurse practitioner what caused this deformity to occur. The pediatric nurse practitioner relates that the etiology of cleft lip and palate is attributed to which of the following inheritance patterns?
   A. The etiology is unknown at this time.
   B. Multifactorial.
   C. Mutagenesis.
   D. Germ line mosaicism.

22. Taking a patient history, the pediatric nurse practitioner learns that the patient has polydactyly, as does the patient's mother, grandfather, and two of her children, a son and daughter. The pediatric nurse practitioner can determine that this inheritance pattern is which of the following?
   A. X-linked.
   B. Autosomal recessive.
   C. Autosomal dominant.
   D. Multifactorial.

23. A newborn is diagnosed with Marfan syndrome. The parents want to know more about this condition. To aid in describing this condition to the parents, the pediatric nurse practitioner is aware that which of the following defines a *syndrome*?
   A. An abnormal variation in form or structure without inferring a specific cause.
   B. A condition exhibiting an external feature usually seen in the head, hands, feet, or face which may indicate the presence of more serious problems.
   C. A condition associated with significant disability and serious functional problems.
   D. A condition affecting two or more body systems and having one underlying cause.

24. For which of the following inherited conditions is a chromosome analysis NOT indicated?
   A. Phenylketonuria.
   B. Ambiguous genitalia.
   C. Mental retardation.
   D. Suspicion of a known syndrome.

25. A newborn is suspected of having Fragile X syndrome. Which of the following diagnostic tests is indicated for evaluation of this condition?
   A. Biochemical testing.
   B. Chromosome analysis.
   C. DNA analysis of blood.
   D. There is no genetic testing available for this condition.

NOTES

ANSWERS

1. *Answer:* A
Rationale: The Human Genome Project is an international research effort to sequence and map all of the genes of *Homo sapiens*. It was completed in April 2003.

2. *Answer:* D
Rationale: The role of DNA includes the storing of information, the transmission of itself to subsequent generations, and determining the precise nature of gene products, including protein structure. DNA does not exist as one long molecule but as multiple fragments.

3. *Answer:* C
Rationale: Each somatic cell contains 23 pairs of chromosomes, 22 autosomes, and 2 sex chromosomes, a total of 46 chromosomes (called *diploid number*).

4. *Answer:* B
Rationale: Chromosomes are distinct, physically separate microscopic structures in the nucleus of every cell, composed of chromatin that contains genetic information, and visible only during cell division. Females have two X chromosomes; males have one X and one Y.

5. *Answer:* D
Rationale: A gene is the basic unit of heredity.

6. *Answer:* C
Rationale: Genes are individual segments of DNA, an ordered sequence of nucleotides, and are arranged in a specific locus in a linear fashion along particular chromosomes. Structural genes encode cell components. Regulatory genes encode enzymes and hormones. *Homozygous* identifies when genes in pairs are identical. *Heterozygous* describes when one gene in a pair differs from the other.

7. *Answer:* A
Rationale: Pedigree is a pictorial representation or diagram of the family history.

8. *Answer:* D
Rationale: Karyotype is the designation for a visual display of chromosome studies arranged in a standardized way. The nomenclature includes the number of chromosomes, the sex chromosomes' contribution, and any abnormalities found.

9. *Answer:* C
Rationale: A mutation is a permanent change in genetic material, occurs when an incorrect nucleotide base is inserted during DNA synthesis, and some produce a "gain of function" or a "loss of function." Phenotype is the observable expression of a genetically determined trait that is visibly apparent or biochemically detectable.

10. *Answer:* B
Rationale: Because blue eyes are recessive, the father must be homozygous for the blue eye gene and can only contribute a blue eye gene to the child. The mother has brown eyes, but may be homozygous or heterozygous for the brown eye gene. If the mother is homozygous for the brown eye gene, then she can only contribute a brown eye gene, and the child's eyes would be brown, because brown is dominant over the blue eye gene the father will contribute. However, if the mother is heterozygous then she could contribute either a brown eye gene or a blue eye gene and the child's eye color could be either brown or blue, respectively.

11. *Answer:* A
Rationale: Recessive trait or characteristic is expressed only when two copies of the same gene are present at corresponding loci of homologous chromosomes. Each human is estimated to carry from five to seven recessive rare deleterious alleles in the heterozygous state. These usually remain undetected for generations and become apparent when a carrier mates with another individual with the same recessive allele. Then, they may have a child with a homozygous recessive disease.

12. *Answer:* B
Rationale: Structural chromosomal abnormalities include deletions (portions miss-

ing), duplications (portions added), translocations (exchange of chromosome segments), and inversions (reversal of polarity within a chromosome).

13. *Answer:* D

Rationale: Autosomal recessive diseases include cystic fibrosis, Tay-Sachs disease, sickle cell anemia, adrenogenital syndrome, and the mucopolysaccharide disorders such as Hurler's syndrome. Glucose-6-phospate dehydrogenase deficiency is an X-linked recessive disorder.

14. *Answer:* C

Rationale: Cystic fibrosis is an autosomal recessive disorder. Parents who are carriers of the cystic fibrosis gene have a 25% chance with each pregnancy of having an affected child.

15. *Answer:* A

Rationale: Huntington's disease has an autosomal dominant inheritance pattern. Phenylketonuria (PKU), albinism, and spinal muscular atrophy are autosomal recessive.

16. *Answer:* D

Rationale: Sickle cell disease is autosomal recessive. In order for an offspring to have the disease, a sickle cell gene must be received from both parents. If the mother does not carry the gene, then no children from this union will have sickle cell disease.

17. *Answer:* D

Rationale: Hemophilia is an X-linked disorder. If the mother's father had the disease then his female offspring would be carriers. In females, the abnormal gene on one X chromosome is compensated by the normal gene on the other X chromosome. Males are affected because the abnormal gene on the X chromosome is invariably expressed because the Y chromosome is small and mostly inactive. With a mother who is a carrier, there is a 50% chance that the male offspring will be affected.

18. *Answer:* A

Rationale: Leber optic hereditary neuropathy is maternally inherited. Mitochon-

dria are inherited solely through the mother via her egg. The sudden loss of central vision associated with this disease primarily affects males in the second and third decades of life.

19. *Answer:* C

Rationale: Uniparental disomy occurs when inheritance of both chromosomes in a pair is from the same parent rather than inheriting one from each parent, as normally occurs. There is variable phenotypic expression of an abnormal gene depending on whether the abnormal gene was inherited from the mother or father. An example of this inheritance pattern is with chromosome 15 when a specific deleted gene results in Prader-Willi syndrome if it was inherited from the father, or in Angelman syndrome if inherited from the mother.

20. *Answer:* D

Rationale: The most common human teratogen is alcohol.

21. *Answer:* B

Rationale: Cleft lip and palate occurs due to multifactorial causes (hereditary-environmental interactions). Several factors contribute to the total effect. No one factor is sufficient to produce the particular abnormalities, and it probably occurs from the interaction of several genes with environmental factors.

22. *Answer:* C

Rationale: Polydactyly is an example of an autosomal dominant inheritance pattern which usually appears in every generation with little or no skipping, and is transmitted by an affected person to half of his or her children on average. Usually males and females are affected equally, but not always.

23. *Answer:* D

Rationale: A syndrome is a condition affecting two or more body systems and having one underlying cause. Marfan syndrome affects connective tissue but also may have cardiac, skeletal, and ocular manifestations. A congenital anomaly is an abnormal variation in form or structure without inferring a specific cause. A minor anomaly is an external feature usually seen in the head, hands, feet, or face, of which some may indicate the presence of more serious problems. A major anomaly is associated with significant disability, serious functional problems, and/or requires surgery or other medical treatment.

24. *Answer:* A

Rationale: Chromosome analysis is indicated when there are specific indicators, such as suspicion of a known syndrome, ambiguous genitalia, mental retardation, developmental delay, or low birth weight. Biochemical testing is indicated for questions about inborn errors of metabolism such as phenylketonuria.

25. *Answer:* C

Rationale: DNA analysis of blood is indicated to look for abnormalities related to specific conditions such as Fragile X syndrome. In Fragile X syndrome, the fragile site located on the distal long arm of chromosome X at Xq27.3 may not always be visible in chromosome analysis. Chromosome analysis is indicated when there are specific indicators, such as ambiguous genitalia, multiple anomalies, mental retardation, developmental delay, low birth weight, or suspicion of a known

syndrome such as trisomy 21. Biochemical testing is indicated for questions about inborn errors of metabolism.

BIBLIOGRAPHY

American Academy of Pediatrics Committee on Genetics, Section on Endocrinology, and Section on Urology. (2000). Evaluation of newborn with developmental anomalies of external genitalia. *Policy Statement, 106* (1), 138–142.

Behrman, R.E., Kliegman, R.M., & Jenson, H.B. (Eds.). (2004). *Nelson textbook of pediatrics* (17th ed.). Philadelphia: Saunders.

Centers for Disease Control and Prevention (CDC). An overview of the Human Genome Project. Retrieved March 13, 2006, from www.genome.gov/12011238.

Jones, K.L. (1997). *Smith's recognizable patterns of human malformation* (5th ed.). Philadelphia: Saunders.

National Coalition for Health Professional Education in Genetics (NCHPEG). (2000). *Core competencies in genetics essential for all health-care professionals.* Lutherville, MD: NCHPEG.

Professional Genetics Education & March of Dimes. (2006). *Genetics & Your Practice* CD-ROM, Version 2.0. White Plains, NY: March of Dimes.

Williams, J. (2002). Education for genetics and nursing practice. *AACN Clin Issues, 13*(4), 492–500.

15 Immunizations

JANET M. CAMACHO

Select the best answer for each of the following questions:

1. Which of the following is an example of herd immunity?
   A. Immunizations that contain an infectious agent.
   B. Human or animal antibody is administered to an individual who has been exposed or is about to be exposed to a disease.
   C. Antibodies are passed from mother to child during breastfeeding.
   D. As more individuals in the community become immune to any given disease there are fewer opportunities for those still susceptible to that disease to come in contact with it.

2. What is the most recognized resource for health care providers to access information and recommendations on vaccine administration in the U.S.?
   A. State boards of nursing.
   B. Centers for Disease Control and Prevention.
   C. World Health Organization.
   D. Parenting magazines.

3. Which of the following factors is NOT associated with immunization compliance in the pediatric population?
   A. Immunization schedules are complex.
   B. Provider apprehension and discomfort with multiple injections.
   C. There are no state laws regarding immunizations and school attendance.
   D. Parental anxiety.

4. Which of the following statements is accurate about the relationship between MMR vaccine and autism?
   A. MMR is a cause of increasing rate of autism.
   B. There is no causal relationship between thimerosal-containing vaccines and autism.
   C. Administering the components of MMR as separate single antigen vaccines reduces the risk of autism.
   D. Studies have confirmed that delaying the MMR vaccine until older than 2 years of age reduces the risk of autism.

5. What is the difference between whole cell pertussis and acellular pertussis?
   A. There is no difference.
   B. Whole cell pertussis is a live vaccine and acellular pertussis is a killed vaccine.
   C. Acellular pertussis vaccine contains detoxified pertussis toxin and is associated with a much lower incidence of side effects.
   D. Whole cell pertussis vaccine contains detoxified pertussis toxin.

6. Which of the following is a valid contraindication to vaccine administration?
   A. Minor acute illnesses (runny nose, low grade fever).
   B. Prematurity.
   C. Unstable, progressive neurological conditions (encephalopathy).
   D. History of febrile seizure in childhood.

7. Which of the following is NOT required in the documentation of vaccine administration?
   A. Expiration date.
   B. Signature and title of the person who administered the vaccine.
   C. Vaccine name.
   D. The date the CDC Vaccine Information Statement (VIS) was provided and the VIS publication date.

8. The Vaccine for Children Program (VFC) provides immunizations for which of the following groups?
   A. Eligible for Medicaid or who have no health insurance.
   B. People older than 18 years of age.
   C. U.S. citizens.
   D. People with a documented history of a chronic illness.

9. Choose the correct statement regarding vaccination.
   A. Active immunity can result from exposure to a strain of a virus or bacteria or from administration of a vaccine.
   B. A vaccine series should be restarted if the time that has elapsed between doses exceeds the recommended intervals.
   C. Tdap, licensed for use in 2005, is recommended as the primary series for infants at 2, 4, and 6 months of age.
   D. A precaution is a condition in the infant, child, or adolescent that significantly increases the chance of a serious adverse event.

10. Regarding the *Haemophilus influenzae* type B (Hib) conjugate vaccine, which of the following is NOT true?
   A. Clinical efficaciousness is estimated to be between 95% and 100% against typable, encapsulated Hib, the strain responsible for invasive disease (meningitis, epiglottitis, pneumonia, etc.).
   B. Is administered subcutaneously.
   C. Reduced the incidence of invasive Hib disease by 97% in the first 10 years of use.

D. The four licensed brands of Hib conjugate vaccine are all interchangeable for the primary and booster dose.

11. MMRV is a new vaccine combination of MMR and varicella and is approved for use in which of the following circumstances?
   A. MMR and varicella vaccines from separate vials may be drawn up in the same syringe and administered subcutaneously.
   B. Recommended for children greater or equal to 13 years of age where both MMR and varicella vaccines are due.
   C. This vaccine combination can only be used on certain high-risk populations.
   D. MMRV is recommended for infants and children 12 months through 12 years of age.

12. What is the difference between the pediatric DT and adult Td types of diphtheria and tetanus toxoid vaccines?
   A. DT contains standard dose of diphtheria and tetanus toxoids and should be used to immunize all children who are older than 7 years of age when pertussis immunization is not required or is contraindicated.
   B. Td contains a much smaller dose of diphtheria toxoid compared to DT vaccine and is used to immunize children younger than 7 years of age
   C. DT contains standard dose of diphtheria and tetanus toxoids and should be used to immunize all children who are younger than 7 years of age when pertussis immunization is not required or is contraindicated.
   D. A booster dose of DT is required every 10 years to ensure continuing tetanus and diphtheria immunity in adulthood.

13. Which of the following statements is NOT true regarding the immunization schedule for children and adolescents who have delayed immunizations or who are more than 1 month behind?
   A. The vaccine series does not need to be restarted regardless of the time that has elapsed between doses.

B. The fifth dose of DTaP is not necessary if the fourth dose was given on or after the fourth birthday.

C. For children who received an all-IPV or all-OPV schedule series, the fourth dose is not necessary if the third dose was given on or after the fourth birthday.

D. One dose of *Haemophilus Influenzae* type b (Hib) is recommended for children older than 5 years with no documented Hib vaccine.

14. Of the vaccines included in the CDC Recommended Childhood and Adolescent Immunization Schedule, 2006, which one of the following contains live viruses?
   A. Pneumococcal conjugate vaccine.
   B. Varicella vaccine.
   C. Hepatitis A vaccine.
   D. *Haemophilus Influenzae* type b (Hib).

15. Tino, a healthy 4-year-old, comes into the clinic for a well child check. He has had four DTaPs, three IPVs, one MMR, one varicella, and two hepatitis B vaccines. What would you order today?
   A. PCV7, IPV, varicella, DTaP.
   B. Tdap, MMR, hepatitis B, IPV.
   C. DTaP, IPV, MMR, hepatitis B.
   D. PCV7, DTaP, IPV, MMR.

16. Amy comes to the clinic for her well checkup and immunizations. She is 4 months old and had DTaP, hepatitis B, IPV, Hib, and pneumococcal conjugate immunizations at 2 months. She has a viral upper respiratory infection, but is afebrile today. Her older sister, who has cancer, is receiving chemotherapy. Her physical exam is unremarkable. What immunizations would you give today?
   A. DT , Hib, IPV.
   B. DTaP, hepatitis B, IPV, Hib, pneumococcal conjugate.
   C. DTaP, pneumococcal conjugate, hepatitis A.
   D. None. Immunizations are contraindicated due to the viral upper respiratory infection.

17. Abbey is a healthy 18-month-old whose mother has brought her to the clinic for immunizations. Her record states at her 12-month physical exam visit, she received DTaP (third dose), hepatitis B (second dose), MMR (first dose), IPV (second dose), pneumococcal conjugate (fourth dose), and Hib (fourth dose). What do you need to give her today to get her up to date with her immunizations?
   A. MMR and DTaP.
   B. DT, IPV, varicella, pneumococcal conjugate, and hepatitis B.
   C. Hib, pneumococcal conjugate, and IPV.
   D. DTaP, IPV, varicella, hepatitis A, and hepatitis B.

18. Baby Cole returns for his 2-month physical exam. He is healthy, breastfed every 3 to 4 hours, naps during the day, and has one 7-hour sleep stretch at night. Cole has had no immunizations since his hepatitis B at birth. What immunizations will you give today?
   A. DTaP, IPV, hepatitis B, Hib, and pneumococcal conjugate.
   B. HIB, hepatitis B, and MMR.
   C. DPT, IPV, Hib, hepatitis A, and pneumococcal conjugate.
   D. DPT, Hib, and hepatitis B.

19. Which one of the following immunizations was associated with an increased incidence of intussusception in infants?
   A. Rota Shield.
   B. Rubella.
   C. Rota Teq.
   D. Rabies.

20. The parents of a 6-year-old with a history of moderate, persistent asthma call the clinic for advice about the influenza vaccine. The most appropriate advice regarding the recommendation for inactivated influenza virus vaccine is which of the following?
   A. The inactivated influenza vaccine is recommended for infants under 6 months of age.
   B. Two doses of vaccine are necessary each year.
   C. Adults and children who have chronic disorders of the pulmonary or cardiovascular systems, including asthma,

are at increased risk for complications from influenza virus.

D. Inactivated influenza vaccine is only recommended for people older than 65 years.

21. Lucia is a 6-year-old female from the Marshall Islands in the South Pacific. She is here today for her school physical exam. She is reported to be healthy, with no previous history of significant illness or hospitalization. Lucia's immunization status is unknown and there are no available medical records. According to the current recommendations, which immunizations should Lucia receive?
   A. Td, IPV, MMRV, and hepatitis B.
   B. DTaP, IPV, MMRV, hepatitis B, and PPD skin test.
   C. DT, OPV, MMRV, and hepatitis B.
   D. Tdap, IPV, MMRV, and hepatitis B.

22. A Mantoux test (PPD skin test; tuberculin skin test) in a child with no risk factors is considered positive with a reaction of at least:
   A. 5 mm of induration.
   B. 8 mm of induration.
   C. 20 mm of erythema.
   D. 15 mm of induration.

23. Which of the following is the appropriate site for immunization administration in an infant younger than 12 months?
   A. Vastus lateralis muscle in the antero-lateral aspect of the upper thigh.
   B. Deltoid muscle below the acromion process.
   C. Gluteus maximus, medial into the buttock.
   D. Subcutaneous, fatty area in the outer aspect of the lower arm.

24. Corrine is an active 12-month-old female recently adopted from China. This is her first encounter at your clinic. The adopted parents were given an immunization record from China that has not been translated into English. Which of the following is NOT an appropriate management for Corrine?
   A. Only written documentation should be accepted as evidence of immunization status.
   B. All live vaccine immunizations need to be repeated.
   C. Repeating the immunizations is an acceptable option if status is unknown.
   D. The majority of immunizations used internationally are produced with adequate quality control standards. Have the record translated into English and follow the recommended schedule.

25. Hepatitis A vaccine:
   A. Is currently only recommended for children living in communities with the highest disease rates.
   B. Is a three-dose series.
   C. Must be restarted if the interval between the first and second dose is more than 6 months.
   D. Is routinely recommended for infants and children 12 to 23 months of age.

ANSWERS

1. *Answer:* D

   Rationale: Widespread immunization of any given population also has one unique benefit, herd immunity. As the risk of exposure lessens, the group as a whole becomes more immune to infection and illness.

2. *Answer:* B

   Rationale: The many recent changes in immunization recommendations emphasizes the need for all health care providers to be aware of the most current guidelines and recommendations for immunization of populations. The National Immunization Program (NIP) is a part of the Centers for Disease Control and Prevention. As a disease-prevention program, NIP provides leadership for the planning, coordination, and conduct of immunization activities nationwide.

3. *Answer:* C

   Rationale: By 1980, all 50 states had laws covering students' first entering school and Head Start to grade 12. Some states also have immunization requirements for college entrance.

4. *Answer:* B

   Rationale: The Institute of Medicine (2004) report concluded that neither thimerosal-containing vaccines nor MMR vaccine are associated with autism. There is no compelling evidence that thimerosal causes autism, ADHD, or other neuro-developmental disorders.

5. *Answer:* C

   Rationale: The use of acellular pertussis as a component in DTaP has replaced DTP vaccine since the year 2000. Acellular pertussis vaccine contains detoxified pertussis toxin and has a much safer side-effect profile than vaccines containing whole cell pertussis.

6. *Answer:* C

   Rationale: There are many myths and misperceptions about immunization administration. Among the myths and misperceptions are invalid precautions, invalid contraindications, and questionable adverse events from previous doses that were never documented. Whether to or when to administer DTaP to children with proven or suspected underlying neurologic disorders should be decided on an individual basis.

7. *Answer:* A

   Rationale: Documentation regarding vaccine administration is an integral part of a providers' responsibility. The provider should include what vaccine was given and on what date, vaccine manufacturer name, vaccine lot number, signature and title of the person who administered the vaccine, and the address at which it was given.

8. *Answer:* A

   Rationale: VFC programs provide vaccines at no cost for children 18 years and younger, Medicaid eligible, no health plan or are underinsured for vaccines, Native American or Alaskan Native.

9. *Answer:* A

   Rationale: It is not necessary to restart a vaccine series regardless of the time that has elapsed between doses. The recommended use of Tdap is as a booster dose of tetanus-containing vaccine at 11 to 12 years of age and if time elapsed is at least 5 years after the last dose of tetanus-, diphtheria-, and pertussis-containing vaccine. A precaution is a condition in the infant, child, or adolescent that may increase the likelihood of a serious adverse event or may interfere with the immunization's ability to produce immunity.

10. *Answer:* B

    Rationale: The recommended route of administration of Hib conjugate vaccine is intramuscular (IM).

11. *Answer:* D

    Rationale: In September 2005, the Federal Food and Drug Administration (FDA) licensed a live, attenuated measles, mumps, rubella, and varicella (MMRV) vaccine (Proquad, Merck & Co). The following individuals should receive MMRV: Children aged 12 months to 12 years who need a first dose of measles, mumps, rubella (MMR), and varicella vaccine; Children aged 12 months to 12 years who need a second dose of MMR and either a first or second dose (as indicated) of varicella vaccine.

12. *Answer:* C
Rationale: Pediatric DT contains the standard dose of diphtheria and tetanus toxoids, and is recommended for children under 7 years of age when pertussis immunization is not required or is contraindicated. Td has a much smaller dose of diphtheria toxoid compared to DT vaccine. Td is recommended for children under 7 years of age and adults. A booster dose of Td is recommended every 10 years.

13. *Answer:* D
Rationale: The CDC publishes the Recommended Immunization Schedule for Children and Adolescents who start late or who are more than 1 month behind. The tables give catch-up schedules and minimum intervals between doses for children who have delayed immunizations. There is no need to restart a vaccine series regardless of the time that has elapsed between doses. *Haemophilus influenzae* type b (Hib) is not generally recommended for children younger than 5 years.

14. *Answer:* B
Rationale: Varicella vaccine is a live attenuated virus vaccine that is administered subcutaneously. For children through age 12 years, it is administered subcutaneously as a single 0.5 ml dose. People 13 years of age and older should receive two 0.5 ml doses subcutaneously 4 to 8 weeks apart.

15. *Answer:* C
Rationale: According to the 2006 Recommended Childhood and Adolescent Immunization Schedule, this child would need his fifth DTaP, fourth IPV, second MMR, and third hepatitis B immunization during this visit. The PCV7 immunization is not recommended for healthy children over 23 months of age. The Tdap is recommended for children 11 to 12 years old who have completed their primary series of DTaP/DTP.

16. *Answer:* B

Rationale: This child would get the routine immunizations according to the 2006 Recommended Childhood and Adolescent Immunization Schedule. Mild upper respiratory infection is not a contraindication for immunizations. All of these agents are inactivated; therefore, they would not impact the health of the sister with cancer on chemotherapy. Hepatitis A is recommended at 12 months of age.

17. *Answer:* D
Rationale: This child is up to date with Hib, MMR, and pneumococcal conjugate immunizations. She needs to have her varicella and hepatitis A immunizations. In addition, she needs to receive the fourth dose of DTaP, third dose of IPV, and hepatitis B.

18. *Answer:* A
Rationale: According to the 2006 Recommended Childhood and Adolescent Immunization Schedule, infants at 2 months of age should receive DTaP, IPV, hepatitis B, Hib, and PCV7. Hepatitis A and MMR are recommended for children at 1 year of age.

19. *Answer:* A
Rationale: Rota Shield, an oral immunization given to infants to protect against rotavirus infections, was removed from the market soon after it was licensed for use due to an increase incidence of intussusception. In 2006, Rota Teq (Merck & Co, Inc.) was approved for the protection of infants against rotavirus infection, after no increased incidence of intussusception was found in studying over 70,000 children who received the immunization.

20. *Answer:* C
Rationale: Inactivated influenza vaccine can be used to reduce the risk for influenza virus infection and its complications and is approved for people at or older than 6 months, including those with high-risk conditions. Adults and children who have chronic disorders of the pulmonary or cardiovascular systems, including asthma, are one of the target groups recommended to receive annual influenza vaccination.

21. *Answer:* B

Rationale: Health care providers will encounter children with uncertain immunization status or no documentation. These children should be considered susceptible and appropriate immunizations should be started following the catch-up schedule for children age 4 months through 6 years.

22. *Answer:* D

Rationale: Interpretation of results depends on epidemiologic and clinical factors. More than 15 mm of induration is considered positive in everyone.

23. *Answer:* A

Rationale: The vastus lateralis muscle in the anterolateral aspect of the middle/upper thigh is the recommended site for this age group. The gluteus muscles are incompletely developed in some infants. There is potential for injury to the sciatic nerve or the superior gluteal artery if the injection is misdirected. Some vaccinations may be less effective if they are injected into the fat.

24. *Answer:* B

Rationale: The majority of vaccines used worldwide is produced with adequate quality control standards and are potent. Each case should be individually reviewed for special considerations and potential.

25. *Answer:* D

Rationale: Routine vaccination of children is an effective way to reduce hepatitis A incidence in the United States. In 2006, ACIP recommended universal vaccination of infants greater than 12 months of age against hepatitis A.

BIBLIOGRAPHY

American Academy of Family Physicians. (2006). Clinical care and research: Immunization resources. Retrieved on March 13, 2006, from www.aafp.org/x10615.xml.

American Academy of Pediatrics. (2006). Immunization initiatives. Retrieved on March 13, 2006, from www.cispimmunize.org.

Centers for Disease Control and Prevention (2000a). National immunization program use of human cell cultures in vaccine manufacturing. Retrieved March 13, 2006, from www.cdc.gov/nip/vacsafe/concerns/gen/humancell.htm.

Centers for Disease Control and Prevention. (2000b). Preventing pneumococcal disease among infants and young children. Recommendations of the Advisory Committee on Immunization Practices (ACIP), *49*(RR09), 1–38.

Centers for Disease Control and Prevention. (2001). Febrile seizures after MMR and DTP vaccinations. Retrieved March 13, 2006, from www.cdc.gov/nip/issues/mmr-dtp/mmr-dtp.htm.

Centers for Disease Control and Prevention. (2002). Prevention and control of influenza: Recommendations of the Advisory Committee on Immunization Practices (ACIP), *51*(RR03), 1–31.

Centers for Disease Control and Prevention (2004). Oral polio vaccine and HIV/AIDS: Questions and answers. Retrieved March 13, 2006, from www.cdc.gov/nip/vacsafe/concerns/aids/poliovac-hiv-aids-qa.htm.

Centers for Disease Control and Prevention. (2005a). Contraindications to vaccines chart. Retrieved March 13, 2006, from http://www.cdc.gov/nip/recs/contraindications_vacc.htm.

Centers for Disease Control and Prevention. (2005b). Guillain-Barré syndrome (GBS) and influenza vaccine. Retrieved March 13, 2006, from www.cdc.gov/nip/vacsafe/concerns/gbs/default.htm.

Centers for Disease Control and Prevention (2005c). Licensure of a combined live attenuated measles, mumps, rubella, and varicella vaccine. Retrieved February 28, 2006 from http://www.cdc.gov/mmwr/preview/mmwrhtml/mm5447a4.htm.

Centers for Disease Control and Prevention (2005d). Multiple sclerosis and the hepatitis B vaccine. Retrieved March 13, 2006, from www.cdc.gov/nip/vacsafe/concerns/ms/default.htm.

Centers for Disease Control and Prevention (2005e). National immunization program FAQs about measles vaccine and inflammatory bowel disease (IBD). Retrieved March 13, 2006, from www.cdc.gov/nip/vacsafe/concerns/autism/ibd.htm.

Centers for Disease Control and Prevention. (2005f). VAERS: Vaccine adverse effects reporting system. Retrieved March 13, 2006, from http://www.cdc.gov/nip/vacsafe/VAERS/CME-post-mktg-surv.htm.

Centers for Disease Control and Prevention. (2006a). 2006 childhood and adolescent immunization schedule. Retrieved March 13, 2006, from http://www.cdc.gov/nip/recs/child-schedule.htm.

Centers for Disease Control and Prevention (2006b). 2006 immunization catch-up schedule. Retrieved March 14, 2006, from http://www.cdc.gov/nip/recs/childschedule.htm#catchup.

Centers for Disease Control and Prevention. (2006c). Advisory committee on immunization practices. Retrieved on March 13, 2006, from www.cdc.gov/nip/acip.

Centers for Disease Control and Prevention. (2006d). CDC's Advisory Committee recommends new vaccine to prevent rotavirus. Retrieved on March 13, 2006, from http://www.cdc.gov/nip/pr/pr_rotavirus_feb2006.pdf.

Centers for Disease Control and Prevention. (2006e). VACMAN: Vaccine management system. Retrieved March 13, 2006, from http://www.cdc.gov/nip/vacman/Default.htm.

Fredrickson, D., Davis, T., Arnould C., et al. (2004). Child immunization refusal: Provider and parent perceptions. *Fam Med*, *36*(6), 431-439.

Frenkel, L. (Ed.) (2004). Immunization issues in the 21st century, part II. *Pediatr Ann*, *33*(9), 564-616.

Immunization Action Coalition. (2006). Home page. Retrieved on March 13, 2006, from http://www.immunize.org/index.htm.

Irigoyen, M., Findley, S., Chen, S., et al. (2004). Early continuity of care and immunization coverage. *Ambu Pediatr*, *4*(3), 199-203.

Lieber, M., Colden, F., & Colon, A. (2003). Childhood immunizations: A parent education and incentive program. *J Pediatr Health Care*, *17*(5), 240-244.

National Association of Pediatric Nurse Practitioners. (2004). Adolescent immunizations: Nurses can make a difference. Retrieved on March 13, 2006, from http://www.napnap.org/index.cfm?page=10&sec=54&ssec=465.

National Association of Pediatric Nurse Practitioners. (2005). *Immunizations*. Retrieved March 13, 2006, from http://www.napnap.org/index.cfm?page=10&sec=54&ssec=66.

National Network for Immunization Information (2005). IOM reports. Retrieved on February 28, 2006, from www.immunizationinfo.org/iom_reports.cfm.

Niederhauser, V. & Stark, M. (2005). Narrowing the gap in childhood immunization disparities. *Pediatr Nurs*, *31*(5), 380-386.

Raucci, J., Whitehill, J., & Sandritter, T. (2004). Childhood immunizations (part one). *J Pediatr Health Care*, *18*(2), 95-101.

Whitehill, J., Raucci, J. & Sandritter, T. (2004). Childhood immunizations (part two). *J Pediatr Health Care*, *18*(4), 192-199.

16 Nutrition

PATRICIA BILLER KRAUSKOPF

Select the best answer for each of the following questions:

1. An 8-year-old male will be considered overweight when his body mass index for his age is at or above the:
    A. 95th percentile.
    B. 90th percentile.
    C. 85th percentile.
    D. 75th percentile.

2. John, a 4-year-old male, is at risk of developing obesity in adulthood. Which of the following is the strongest predictor of obesity in adulthood?
    A. John's current weight.
    B. John's current body mass index.
    C. Parental obesity.
    D. Sibling obesity.

3. Which of the following does NOT contribute to the development of overweight in childhood?
    A. Unhealthy foods are readily accessible.
    B. Physical education required by schools has decreased.
    C. Fast-food ads focus on children.
    D. Restrict child's access to screen (Television, computers) time.

4. Jason, a 4-year-old male, is overweight. Being overweight puts Jason at risk to experience health consequences. Which of the following is NOT a health-related issue Jason would expect as he gets older due to his overweight status?
    A. Infertility.
    B. Early sexual maturation.

C. Hepatic steatosis.
D. Sleep apnea.

5. The U.S. Department of Agriculture and U.S. Food and Drug Administration establish guidelines for individual's energy and nutrient needs. Which of the following describes "recommended daily allowance" or RDA?
    A. Median usual intake value that should meet the requirements of half of all apparently healthy individuals.
    B. Amount that is adequate for nearly all healthy individuals.
    C. Highest level of intake that should pose no risk of adverse health effects.
    D. Four nutrient-based reference values based on age and sex.

6. Claire and her family do not eat meat or fish but do consume eggs and dairy products. Which of the following is the best classification for this diet?
    A. Strict vegetarian.
    B. Vegan.
    C. Ovolactovegetarian.
    D. Semivegetarian.

7. Amy, a 5-year-old, presents to your office for a well child exam. Amy's family members are vegans and eat no animal products. The pediatric nurse practitioner should consider supplementation of which of the following essential nutrients because it is at risk to be inadequate in Amy's diet?
    A. Magnesium.
    B. Zinc.
    C. Niacin.
    D. Vitamin B_6.

8. The Carters are a family considering becoming vegans. One of the advantages of this lifestyle change is a decrease in the risk of some diseases or disorders. Which of the following diseases or disorders can the Carters NOT expect to be at less risk of developing if they adhere to a vegan diet?
   A. Gallstones
   B. Hypercholesterolemia
   C. Hypertension
   D. Hepatitis

9. Which of the following accounts for most of the fatal and near-fatal food allergy reactions?
   A. Eggs
   B. Fish
   C. Peanuts
   D. Soy

10. Sarah, a 9-year-old, developed anaphylactic shock 60 minutes after ingesting shrimp. This type of reaction is classified as which of the following?
   A. Immediate.
   B. Delayed.
   C. Food hypersensitivity.
   D. Deferred.

11. Kimberley, a 6-year-old, develops acute nausea and vomiting often after ingesting bananas. The pediatric nurse practitioner has decided to administer a food challenge. Kimberley has avoided bananas for the past 2 weeks. What is the the first step in food challenge assessment?
   A. Observe Kimberley for skin, GI, and respiratory changes.
   B. Obtain intravenous access.
   C. Administer graded doses of either bananas or a placebo (both are disguised or placed in capsules).
   D. Confirm negative challenges with a meal-sized portion of the bananas.

12. Marty, an 18-year-old pregnant female, asks the pediatric nurse practitioner about breastfeeding. Which of the following is NOT an advantage that the pediatric nurse practitioner should discuss with Marty?
   A. Breastfeeding infants during painful procedures provides analgesia.

   B. Breastfeeding encourages mother-infant interaction.
   C. Breastfeeding decreases otitis media and upper respiratory infections.
   D. Breastfed infants are satisfied for at least 4 hours.

13. Jennifer, a first-time mother, recalls the importance of maximizing breastfeeding benefits with the "let-down" conditioning reflex of the milk ducts in the breasts, so that hindmilk is accessed by the infant. Which of the following is NOT a good practice to stimulate this reflex?
   A. Concentrate on how frustrating it is to lose that extra pregnancy weight.
   B. Drink a glass of fluid prior to breastfeeding.
   C. Take a warm shower or use warm compresses to soften breasts.
   D. Gently massage breasts starting where the breast meets the chest and stroke toward the nipple.

14. Gina, the mother of a breastfed 1-month-old female, presents for a clinic visit, stating her breasts are sore and appear compressed after nursing. The infant's examination is normal. Birth weight was 6 lbs., 10 oz. and current weight is 7 lbs. Which of the following is most likely the cause of Gina's sore nipples?
   A. The infant's teeth are misshaping the nipples and causing Gina's discomfort.
   B. Improper positioning of the infant's mouth on the breast.
   C. Early hospital discharge did not allow for adequate instruction in breastfeeding.
   D. The nipple changes and discomfort that Gina is experiencing are normal with breastfeeding.

15. Tammy, the mother of a breastfed 2-week-old, presents to the clinic concerned that her son is not getting enough breast milk. In addition to monitoring the neonate's weight, which of the following findings in the neonate would provide reassurance to Tammy that breast milk intake is adequate?

A. The infant produces four to six wet diapers each day.
B. The infant passes black/green, tarry meconium stools.
C. The infant is satisfied for 4 to 5 hours between feedings.
D. Forceful crying is noted after each feeding.

16. Jacob is a 9-day-old breastfed infant who presents to the clinic with his mother who noticed that he was "yellow" on day 3 and this has persisted. Jacob was delivered at term without complications. Mother's blood type is AB-negative and Jacob's blood type is A-negative. A total serum bilirubin is 15.2 mg/dl with a direct bilirubin of 1.0 mg/dl. The pediatric nurse practitioner evaluates this condition as which of the following?
A. Breast milk jaundice.
B. Hemolytic jaundice.
C. Physiologic jaundice.
D. Kernicterus or bilirubin encephalopathy.

17. Katherine, the mother of a breastfed 3-month-old, is planning to return to work. She plans to pump her breast milk and has questions about safe storage of breast milk. Which of the following is correct regarding freshly expressed breast milk?
A. May be stored at room temperature (<78° F) for up to 12 hours.
B. May be refrigerated (<39° F) for up to 7 days.
C. Will keep for 2 weeks in the freezer located inside refrigerator.
D. Will keep for 4 months in the freezer section of refrigerator with a separate door.

18. Which of the following medications is allowed in recommended doses for the breastfeeding mother to ingest?
A. Lithium
B. Methotrexate
C. Acetaminophen
D. Atenolol

19 Emma is nearing 6 months of age which is the time her pediatric nurse practitioner has suggested that solid foods may be introduced into her diet. Which of the following signs would NOT indicate Emma's readiness for solids?
A. Able to sit unassisted and hold head straight.
B. Increased tongue-thrust reflex.
C. Opens mouth when food approaches.
D. Expresses interest in food when others are eating.

20. Keri, a first-time mother of 6-month-old, states her mother-in-law is recommending that she give her son whole milk and eggs when she begins solids. The pediatric nurse practitioner knows that certain foods are to be avoided in order to minimize the likelihood of developing food allergies. Which of the following guidelines would the pediatric nurse practitioner NOT pass on to Keri?
A. Honey is better for infants than processed sugar.
B. Dairy may be introduced at 1 year.
C. Eggs may be introduced at 2 years.
D. Fish may be introduced at 3 years.

21. Jeremiah, a 10-year-old male, has a BMI above the 95th percentile. Which of the following lab tests is NOT routinely recommended to assess for possible underlying health issues in the overweight school-aged child?
A. Fasting blood glucose.
B. Thyroid stimulating hormone.
C. Total cholesterol.
D. Lipid panel.

22. Jill, a 15-year-old, presents to the pediatric nurse practitioner for a sports physical for cheerleading. Her BMI is at the 85th percentile for age and sex and she is Tanner stage III. Jill wants to lose weight and suggests to the pediatric nurse practitioner that she begin a popular trendy diet. The pediatric nurse practitioner responds with which of the following?
A. "I'd like to review your current diet and activity history."
B. "Tell me about your family history including the incidence of obesity."
C. "Tell me about the diet you are suggesting."

D. "Cheerleading will take care of this issue for you, so don't worry about your weight."

23. Which of the following age groups historically has the highest prevalence of unsatisfactory nutritional status?
    A. Toddlers (1 to 3 years).
    B. Preschoolers (4 to 6 years).
    C. School-aged (7 to 11 years).
    D. Adolescents (12 to 21 years).

24. Emily, a 15-year-old, is competing in both cross-country running and soccer this fall. How many calories should she be eating per day based on her gender, age, and activity level?
    A. 1000
    B. 1800
    C. 2400
    D. 3000

NOTES

ANSWERS

1. *Answer:* A
   Rationale: According to the CDC (2005), children with BMI-for-age at or above the 95th percentile are overweight.

2. *Answer:* C
   Rationale: Younger than 5 years of age, parental obesity is a stronger predictor of obesity in adulthood than child's weight at that age.

3. *Answer:* D
   Rationale: Environmental stimuli contributing to overweight include increased access to unhealthy foods; decreased physical activity by children, including a decrease in required physical education by schools; advertising for sweets, soft drinks, cereals, and fast foods focus on children; and increased popularity of TV, videos, video games, and computers. Greater than 4 hours of screen time per day is a risk factor.

4. *Answer:* B
   Rationale: Consequences for overweight children compared with other children include cardiovascular disease, metabolic syndrome, dyslipidemia, glucose intolerance, type 2 diabetes, hypertension, coronary heart disease, hepatic steatosis, cholelithiasis, some cancers (endometrial, breast, and colon), osteoarthritis, infertility, obesity hypoventilation syndrome, sleep apnea, pseudotumor cerebri, and early sexual maturation of females.

5. *Answer:* B
   Rationale: Dietary reference intake (DRI)—a new set of four nutrient-based reference values based on age and sex. Estimated average requirement (EAR)—median usual intake value that should meet the requirements of half of all apparently healthy individuals. Recommended daily allowance (RDA)—amount that is adequate for nearly all healthy individuals. Upper intake level (UL)—highest level of intake that should pose no risk of adverse health effects.

6. *Answer:* C

Rationale: Vegetarians eat fruits, vegetables, nuts, grains, and legumes. Vegans eat no animal products, including honey, gelatin, rennet, and animal fats. Semivegetarians avoid red meat, and usually consume poultry and fish. Ovolactovegetarians will eat eggs and dairy products.

7. *Answer:* B
   Rationale: In vegetarian diets, supplementation of the following may be necessary to provide the following essential nutrients: B_{12}, folic acid, iron, zinc, vitamin D, and occasionally calcium.

8. *Answer:* D
   Rationale: Vegetarian diets are associated with a decrease in the risk of the following diseases and disorders: obesity, heart disease, hypertension, hypercholesterolemia, and gallstones.

9. *Answer:* C
   Rationale: Foods that may cause allergic reactions include milk (90%), eggs, wheat, soy, nuts, and fish. Peanuts are the leading cause of fatal and near-fatal food allergy reactions in the United States.

10. *Answer:* A
    Rationale: Immediate anaphylactic shock is a reaction which occurs within minutes to 2 hours after ingestion. Delayed reactions occur 2 to 48 hours after ingestion.

11. *Answer:* B
    Rationale: Food challenge can be done in the office with strict medical supervision as follows. Patient avoids the suspected food(s) for at least 2 weeks. After intravenous access is obtained, graded doses of either a challenge food or a placebo food are administered (both are disguised in capsules). Ensure access to emergency medications and CPR equipment. Assess patient frequently for skin, GI, and respiratory changes. Terminate challenge when a reaction becomes apparent. Observe for delayed reactions. Confirm negative challenges with a meal-sized portion of the food.

12. *Answer:* D

Rationale: Benefits of breastfeeding include: Human milk is specifically designed for human infants and cannot be duplicated, encourages mother-infant interaction, provides analgesia during painful procedures, decreases otitis media and upper respiratory infections, decreases gastrointestinal problems including gastroesophageal reflux, decreases allergies, antiinflammatory agents in breast milk help decrease atopy, decreases overweight, and costs less than formula. Breastfed infants should be satisfied for at least 2 hours.

13. *Answer:* A
Rationale: Let-down can be under emotional control. It is best for the breastfeeding mother to take 5 minutes to relax and think peaceful thoughts. To facilitate this reflex, she may also take a warm shower or use warm compresses to soften breasts, gently massage breasts by starting where the breast meets the chest and stroke towards the nipple, drink a glass of fluid, and find a comfortable, quiet, safe place to nurse.

14. *Answer:* B
Rationale: Improper position of infant's mouth on the breast or "latching-on" poorly is the number-one cause of sore nipples. Teeth are not an issue. If proper latching-on is occurring, the mother should observe the following: Infant with rhythmic suck and swallow, gulping noise without clicking, and infant's ears should wiggle.

15. *Answer:* A
Rationale: With adequate intake of breast milk, expect 4 to 6 wet diapers per day by age 5 to 7 days. Infant should be satisfied for at least 2 hours and stools change from the black/green, tarry meconium stools to seedy yellow-green within first few days. Crying can be a sign of hunger.

16. *Answer:* C
Rationale: Physiologic jaundice appears around the third day of life in both bottle- and breastfed infants and clears by 2 weeks. Physiologic jaundice presents with an elevated unconjugated serum or direct bilirubin level which does not typically exceed 2 mg/dl. The peak total bilirubin level may be higher in breastfed babies (15-17 mg/dl) than in babies who are given formula (12 mg/dl). Breast milk jaundice typically occurs later between the first and second weeks of life. Hemolytic jaundice usually occurs when an Rh negative mother who has been Rh-sensitized during a previous pregnancy gives birth to a subsequent Rh positive infant. Kernicterus or bilirubin encephalopathy occurs with very high bilirubin levels (>25 mg/dl) and nervous system toxicity results.

17. *Answer:* C
Rationale: Freshly expressed breast milk may be safely stored at room temperature (<78° F) for 6 to 8 hours, refrigerated (<39° F) for 3 to 5 days, 2 weeks in a freezer inside refrigerator, 3 months in the freezer section of refrigerator with a separate door, and 6 to 12 months in a deep freezer (<0° F).

18. *Answer:* C
Rationale: Acetaminophen is a maternal medication usually compatible with breastfeeding. Many medications are contraindicated with breastfeeding due to crossing over into the breast milk. Contraindicated medications include radioactive compounds for diagnostic procedures, drugs for early tuberculosis, street drugs, cancer chemotherapy, lithium, some antidepressants and antipsychotic agents, and some antibiotics which are not recommended for young children. Before prescribing, the pediatric nurse practitioner should consult the most recent recommendations, such as those published by the American Academy of Pediatrics.

19. *Answer:* B
Rationale: Signs of readiness for complementary foods include being between 4 and 6 months of age, having the ability to hold head up straight when sitting, opening mouth when food approaches, displaying interest in food when others are eating, and a decreased tongue-thrust response.

20. *Answer:* A
Rationale: Honey should be avoided due to the risk for botulism. To minimize the chances for development of food allergies,

avoid introducing foods that have a family history of food allergies until the following ages: Wait until 6 months to start solids, dairy at 1 year, eggs at 2 years, and peanuts/nuts/fish at 3 years.

21. *Answer:* B

Rationale: It is recommended to perform a fasting glucose level, total cholesterol, and/or lipid panel to assess for diabetes mellitus, hyperlipidemia, and metabolic syndrome if the school-age child's BMI is greater than the 95th percentile. Thyroid assessment may be indicated if there is a strong family history of this disease, but is not routinely recommended in this age group.

22. *Answer:* A

Rationale: This adolescent is at risk for becoming overweight and because she has expressed that her weight is a concern, this should be addressed. The best approach for the pediatric nurse practitioner is to determine the adolescent's current dietary intake and activity level in order to provide appropriate guidance.

23. *Answer:* D

Rationale: According to National Health and Nutrition Examination Surveys between 1971 and 1991, the highest prevalence of unsatisfactory nutritional status was in the adolescent age group.

24. *Answer:* C

Rationale: Active female teenagers ages 14 to 18 should take in approximately 2400 calories per day.

BIBLIOGRAPHY

Ahluwalia, I.B., Morrow, B., Hsia, J., Grummer-Strawn, L.M. (2003). Who is breast feeding? Recent trends from the pregnancy risk assessment and monitoring system. *J Pediatr, 142*(5), 486-491.

American Academy of Pediatric Dentistry. (2003). *Clinical guideline on fluoride therapy.* Chicago (IL): American Academy of Pediatric Dentistry.

American Academy of Pediatrics Committee on Drugs. (2001). The transfer of drugs and other chemicals into human milk. *Pediatrics, 108*(3), 776-789.

American Academy of Pediatrics Committee on Nutrition. (2000). Hypoallergenic infant formulas. *Pediatrics, 106*(2 Pt 1), 346-349.

American Academy of Pediatrics Committee on Nutrition. (2004). *Pediatric nutrition handbook* (5th ed.). Elk Grove Village, IL: American Academy of Pediatrics.

Anand, M.K., & Routes, J.M. (2004). Hypersensitivity reactions—immediate. Retrieved on June 6, 2006, from www.emedicine.com/med/topic1101.htm.

Bauchner, H. (2004). Failure to thrive. In R.E. Behrman, R.M. Kliegman, & H.B. Jenson (Eds.), *Nelson textbook of pediatrics* (17th ed.). Philadelphia: Saunders.

Brazelton, T.B. (2002). *Touch points. The essential reference*. Reading, MA: Addison-Wesley.

Butte, N., Cobb, K., Dwyer, J., Graney, L., et al. (2004). The Start Healthy Feeding Guidelines for Infants and Toddlers. *J Am Diet Assoc, 104*(3), 42-54.

Centers for Disease Control and Prevention (2001). Recommendations for using fluoride to prevent and control dental caries in the US. *MMWR Recommendations and Reports, 50*(RR-14), 1-42.

Centers for Disease Control and Prevention. (2006). Overweight and obesity. Retrieved June 6, 2006, from www.cdc.gov/nccdphp/dnpa/obesity/index.htm.

Children Now. (2005). Brief: Interactive advertising and children: Issues and implications. Retrieved March 30, 2006, from http://www.childrennow.org/search.jsp?query=interactive+advertising.

Crespo, C.J., Smit, E., Troiano R.P., et al. (2001). Television watching, energy intake, and obesity in U.S. children: results from the third National Health and Nutrition Examination Survey, 1988-1994. *Arch Pediatr Adolesc Med, 155*(3), 360-365.

Dietz, W.H., & Stern, L. (Eds.). (1999). *Guide to your child's nutrition*. New York: Villard.

Donohoue, P.A. (2004). Obesity. In R.E. Behrman, R.M. Kliegman, & H.B. Jenson (Eds.), *Nelson textbook of pediatrics* (17th ed.). Philadelphia: Saunders.

Garrow, A. (2004). Coping patterns in mothers/caregivers of children with chronic feeding problems. *J Pediatr Health Care, 18*(3), 138-144.

Gartner, L.M., & Greer, F.R. (2003). Prevention of rickets and vitamin D deficiency: New guidelines for vitamin D intake. *Pediatrics, 113*(4 Pt 1), 908-910.

Gartner, L.M., Morton, J., Lawrence, R.A. et al. (2005). Breastfeeding and the use of human milk. *Pediatrics, 115*(2), 496-506.

Gray, L., Miller, L.W., Phillip, B.L., & Blass, E.M. (2002). Breastfeeding is analgesic in healthy newborns. *Pediatrics, 109*(4), 590-593.

Hansen, T.W.R. (2002). Jaundice, neonatal. Retrieved on May 9, 2006, from www.emedicine.com/ped/topic1061.htm.

Heird, W.C. (2004a). Food insecurity, hunger and undernutrition. In R.E. Behrman, R.M. Kliegman, & H.B. Jenson (Eds.), *Nelson textbook of pediatrics* (17th ed.). Philadelphia: Saunders.

Heird, W.C. (2004b). The feeding of infants and children. In R.E. Behrman, R.M. Kliegman, & H.B. Jenson (Eds.), *Nelson textbook of pediatrics* (17th ed.). Philadelphia: Saunders.

Host, A. & Halken, S. (2004). Hypoallergenic formulas—when, to whom and how long: After more than 15 years we know the right indication! *Allergy, 59 Suppl 78,* 45-52.

Kennedy, C., Strzempko, F., Danford, C., & Kools, S. (2002). Children's perceptions of TV and health behavior. *J Nurs Schol, 34*(3), 297-302.

Krebs NF, Jacobson MS; American Academy of Pediatrics Committee on Nutrition. (2003). Prevention of pediatric overweight and obesity. *Pediatrics, 112*(2), 424-430.

Merritt, R.J. & Jenks, B.H. (2004). Safety of soy-based infant formulas containing isoflavones: The clinical evidence. *J Nutr, 134*(5), 1220S-1224S.

Moilanen, B.C. (2004). Vegan diets in infants, children, and adolescents. *Pediatr Rev, 25*(5), 174-176.

Morrow, A.L. (2004). Choosing an infant or pediatric formula. *J Pediatr Health Care, 18*(1), 49-52.

National Association of Pediatric Nurse Practitioners (NAPNAP). (2001). Position statement on breastfeeding. Retrieved on March 30, 2006, from http://www.napnap.org/index.cfm?page=10&sec=54&ssec=57.

National Association of Pediatric Nurse Practitioners (NAPNAP). (2006). Identifying and preventing overweight in childhood: Clinical practice guideline. *J Pediatr Health Care, 20*(2), S1-S63.

National Association of Pediatric Nurse Practitioners (NAPNAP). (2005). *Starting solids: Nutrition guide for infants and children 6 to 18 months of age* (brochure). Cherry Hill, NJ: NAPNAP.

National Center for Health Statistics. (2005). Prevalence of overweight among children and adolescents: United States, 1999-2002. Retrieved on March 30, 2006, from http://www.cdc.gov/nchs/products/pubs/pubd/hestats/overwght99.htm.

Osborn, D.A. & Sinn, J. (2004). Soy formula for prevention of allergy and food intolerance in infants. *Cochrane Database of Systematic Reviews: CD003741.*

Sampson, H.A., & Leung, D.Y.M. (2004). Adverse reactions to foods. In R.E. Behrman, R.M. Kliegman, & H.B. Jenson (Eds.), *Nelson textbook of pediatrics* (17th ed.). Philadelphia: Saunders.

Tuohy, P.G. (2003). Soy infant formula and phytoestrogens. *J Paediatr Child Health, 39*(6), 401-405.

U.S. Department of Health & Human Services (HHS) Public Health Service, Office of Assistant Secretary for Health. (2000). *Healthy People 2010: Conference Edition.* Washington, D.C.: HHS.

U.S. Department of Health and Human Services and U.S. Department of Agriculture. (2005). *Dietary guidelines for Americans, 2005* (6th ed.). Washington, D.C.: U.S. Government Printing Office.

17 Preconceptional and Prenatal Role of the Pediatric Nurse Practitioner

MARY MARGARET GOTTESMAN

Select the best answer for each of the following questions:

1. Jennifer is a healthy-appearing 19-year-old college student seen by the pediatric nurse practitioner. She admits that she is considering becoming sexually active for the first time. She denies binge drinking and drug use. Which of the following actions would be LEAST important point to address?
   A. Selection of a method of birth control to use consistently.
   B. Assessment for coercion into sexual activity.
   C. Identification of the need for use of condoms to protect against sexually transmitted infections.
   D. HIV screening for Jennifer.

2. Which of the following conditions does NOT require an increased daily dose of folate for women prior to becoming pregnant?
   A. Kidney disease.
   B. Crohn's disease.
   C. Asthma.
   D. Hypertension.

3. Which of the following maternal immunizations is LEAST critical to fetal well-being?
   A. Rubella.
   B. Varicella.
   C. MCV4.
   D. Hepatitis B.

4. Women with each of the following disorders should take a minimum of 4 mg of folate each day EXCEPT for those with:
   A. Hyperlipidemia.
   B. Seizure disorder.
   C. Spina bifida.
   D. Mental retardation.

5. Each of the following diseases is associated with significant risk during pregnancy for the mother EXCEPT:
   A. Marfan syndrome.
   B. Hypothyroidism.
   C. Systemic lupus erythematosus.
   D. Severe diabetes mellitus.

6. Janet is the 28-year-old mother of Danielle. During Danielle's 2-year-old visit, Janet mentions that she is thinking of having a second child. Which of the following factors is UNLIKELY to pose a risk for the new pregnancy?
   A. The family has two golden retrievers that love duck hunting with Janet's husband in the fall.
   B. Janet and her family live on a farm where corn and soybeans are grown using nonorganic farming methods.
   C. Janet works 3 days each week in her church's daycare during the winter months.
   D. Janet and her husband frequently enjoy relaxing in the hot tub in the evening.

7. Tuesday evening, the pediatric nurse practitioner met with four couples anticipating the birth of their first child. Which of the following couples would be MOST concerning to the nurse practitioner?

A. Jack, 19, and Jody, 18, are married and excited about the new baby. They volunteer that their parents feel they are too young to have a baby but they have read many books and attended prenatal classes. Jody is enrolled in the WIC program. They have an extensive network of family and friends nearby. They are eager to make a good home for the baby, since Jack was adopted at 3 months of age and feels he understands how important a loving home is for a young child.

B. Ben, 24, and Lisa, 26, are long-time partners, but not married. This was an unplanned pregnancy that both partners are happy to accept. Their parents are upset that the couple has not married and there are strained relationships with both sets of grandparents. They have attended childbirth classes and have read a few pamphlets on early infancy care. They are certain little will change in their lives with the arrival of the baby.

C. Brad, 32, and Jennifer, 25, are excited about the unplanned for, but welcomed, new baby. Both parents relate that they have had to curtail their partying lifestyle because of Jennifer's morning sickness and fatigue. They have been so busy working they have been unable to get to prenatal classes yet. They were hoping the nurse practitioner could resolve their ongoing conflict over how strict they need to be as parents.

D. Joe, 30, and Pam, 27, are married and excited about the new baby. All four grandparents accompanied the couple. They have attended childbirth classes and read extensively. Their major concern is how to juggle their graduate studies with the demands of the new baby.

8. Family risk factors suggesting the need for referral for counseling and support before and after delivery of the baby include each of the following EXCEPT:

A. Growing up in a home where there was spousal abuse.
B. Growing up in foster care periodically.
C. Being adopted as a young infant.
D. Experience of neglectful parenting as a child.

9. Which of the following is a protective factor for families?

A. An unplanned pregnancy.
B. Experience in caring for young children.
C. Eligibility for TANF and WIC.
D. Counseling with a geneticist.

ANSWERS

1. *Answer:* D
   Rationale: Jennifer is not sexually active currently and she denies drug use, the major factors that would place her at risk for HIV infection. Practitioners should ensure that women not only protect against pregnancy with birth control but also need to teach about the use of condoms to protect against STIs. Coercion into sexual activity and partner abuse are common among teenage and young adult women. Practitioners should consistently assess for this and advise young women how to handle these threats.

2. *Answer:* C
   Rationale: There is no increased folate requirement associated with asthma. Women with kidney disease, Crohn's disease, or hypertension require a daily intake of at least 1 mg of folate daily compared to the usual recommendation of 400 micrograms per day.

3. *Answer:* C
   Rationale: Rubella, varicella, and hepatitis B are viruses placing the fetus at risk for congenital defects.

4. *Answer:* A
   Rationale: Mental retardation, seizure medications, and neural tube defects such as spina bifida markedly increase the risk for disorders of the fetus' central nervous system and congenital anomalies.

5. *Answer:* B
   Rationale: The major risks associated with hypothyroidism are to the fetus, not the mother. Marfan syndrome, systemic lupus erythmatosus, and severe diabetes can cause life-threatening complications in the mother.

6. *Answer:* A
   Rationale: Exposure to cats is more of a concern than dogs, because of the prevalence of toxoplasmosis in cats. Exposure to pesticides and fertilizers used in nonorganic farming place the developing fetus at risk. Hot tubs increase the risk of neural tube defects. Daycare increases the risk of Janet's exposure to CMV and parvovirus B19.

7. *Answer:* C
   Rationale: Couple C has the most risk factors: conflict between the parents regarding child-rearing, nonattendance at preparatory classes, and an unplanned pregnancy within the context of social drinking. Couple A is very young and has limited resources based on Jody's eligibility for WIC. However, she is enrolled already in the program to assure her good nutrition during pregnancy. They have an extensive social support network. Adoption at an early age is not associated with problems in parenting. Couple B have accepted their unplanned pregnancy and attended preparatory classes. However, there are poor relationships with the grandparents and the couple has unrealistic expectations for life after the baby's birth. Couple D is positive about having the baby, has the support and involvement of the grandparents, and has prepared well for the baby's arrival. Their most obvious stressor is a return to graduate studies for both parents at the same time as the baby arrives.

8. *Answer:* C
   Rationale: The parent's adoption as a young infant is not highly correlated with problems in parenting. The experiences of neglectful parenting, exposure to domestic violence, and time in foster care are clearly associated with high-risk parenting.

9. *Answer:* B
   Rationale: Experience caring for young children helps the parent have more accurate expectations for the child's behavior and development and lower the risk for parent anger and frustration with the young child. An unplanned pregnancy increases the risk of fetal exposure to teratogens and the risk for challenges to the family's adjustment to parenthood. Eligibility for TANF and WIC suggests that there is a deficit of basic resources in the family. Consultation with a geneticist suggests that there is a history of serious congenital anomalies or inheritable diseases in the family history.

BIBLIOGRAPHY

American Academy of Pediatrics (AAP). (1996). Health supervision for children with Marfan syndrome. *Pediatrics, 98*(5), 978-982.

American Academy of Pediatrics (AAP). (1997). Breastfeeding and the use of human milk. *Pediatrics, 100*(6), 1035-1039.

American Academy of Pediatrics (AAP). (1998). Tobacco, alcohol, and other drugs: The role of the pediatrician in prevention and management of substance abuse. *Pediatrics, 101*(1), 125-128.

American Academy of Pediatrics (AAP). (1999a). Circumcision policy statement. *Pediatrics, 103*(3), 686-693.

American Academy of Pediatrics (AAP). (1999b). Human immunodeficiency virus screening. *Pediatrics, 104*(5), 128.

American Academy of Pediatrics (AAP). (2000a). Changing concepts of sudden infant death syndrome: Implications for infant sleeping environment and sleep position. *Pediatrics, 105*(3), 58-361.

American Academy of Pediatrics (AAP). (2000b). Fetal alcohol syndrome. *Pediatrics, 106*(2), 358-361.

American Academy of Pediatrics (AAP). (2001a). Care of adolescent parents and their children. *Pediatrics, 10*(2), 429-434.

American Academy of Pediatrics (AAP). (2001b). Health supervision for children with Down syndrome. *Pediatrics, 107*(2), 442-449.

American Academy of Pediatrics (AAP). (2001c). Tobacco's toll: Implications for pediatricians. *Pediatrics, 10*(4), 794-798.

American Academy of Pediatrics (AAP). (2001d). The prenatal visit. *Pediatrics, 10*(6), 1456-1458.

American Academy of Pediatrics (AAP). (2001e). Alcohol use and abuse: A pediatric concern. *Pediatrics, 108*(1), 185-189.

American Academy of Pediatrics (AAP). (2003a). Oral health risk assessment timing and establishment of the dental home. *Pediatrics, 111*(3), 1113-1116.

American Academy of Pediatrics (AAP). (2003b). Family-centered care and the pediatrician's role. *Pediatrics, 112*(3), 691-696.

American Academy of Pediatrics (AAP). (2004a). Postexposure prophylaxis in children and adolescents for nonoccupational exposure to human immunodeficiency virus. *Pediatrics, 111*(6), 1475-1489.

American Academy of Pediatrics (AAP). (2004b). Human milk, breastfeeding, and transmission of human immunodeficiency virus type 1 in the United States. *Pediatrics, 112*(5), 1196-1205.

American Academy of Pediatrics (AAP). (2004c). Hospital stay for healthy term newborns. *Pediatrics, 113*(5), 1434-1436.

American Academy of Pediatrics (AAP). (2004d). Prenatal screening and diagnosis for pediatricians. *Pediatrics, 114*(3), 889-894.

Barash, J.H., & Weinstein, L.C. (2002). Preconception and prenatal care. *Prim Care, 29*(3), 519-542.

Brent, R., Oakley, G., & Mattis, D. (2000). The unnecessary epidemic of folic acid, preventable spina bifida and anencephaly. *Pediatrics, 106*(4), 825-827.

Briggs, G.G., Freeman, R.K., & Yaffee, S.J. (2002). *A reference guide to fetal and neonatal risk: Drugs in pregnancy and lactation* (6th ed.). Philadelphia: Lippincott Williams & Wilkins.

Brundage, S.C. (2002). Preconception health care. *Am Fam Physician, 65*(12), 2507-2514.

Chacko, M.R., Anding, R., Kozinetz, C.A., et al. (2003). Neural tube defects: Knowledge and preconceptional prevention practices in minority young women. *Pediatrics, 112*(3), 536-542.

Champagne, C.M., Madianos, P.N., Lieff, S., et al. (2000). Periodontal medicine: Emerging concepts in pregnancy outcomes. *J Int Acad Periodontol, 2*(1), 9-13.

De Weerd, S., van der Bij, A.K., Cikot, R., et al. (2002). Preconception care: A screening tool for health assessment and risk detection. *Prev Med, 34*(5), 505-511.

Gabbe, S.G., Niebyl, J.P., & Simpson, J.L. (Eds.). (2002). *Obstetrics: Normal and problem pregnancies.* (4th ed.) (Online). Philadelphia: Churchill Livingstone.

Gueorguieva, R.V., Sarkar, N.P., Carter, R.L., et al. (2003). A risk assessment screening test for very low birth weight. *Matern Child Nurs J, 7*(2), 127-136.

Hauck, F.R., Herman, S., Donovan, M., et al. (2003). Sleep environment and the risk of sudden infant death syndrome in an urban population: The Chicago infant mortality study. *Pediatrics, 11*(5), 1207-1214.

Hindmarsh, P.C., Geary, M.P., Rodeck, C.H., et al. (2000). Effects of early maternal iron stores on placental weight and structure. *Lancet, 356*(9231), 719-723.

Hobbins, D. (2003). Full circle: The evolution of preconception health promotion in America. *J Obstet Gynecol Neonatal Nurs, 32*(4), 516-522.

Holzman, C., Bullen, B., Fisher, R., et al. (2001). Pregnancy outcomes and community health: The POUCH study of preterm delivery. *Paediatr Perinatal Epidemiol, 15*(Suppl. 2), 136-158.

Jackson-Allen, P.L., & Vessey, J.A. (2004). *Primary care of the child with a chronic condition.* (4th ed.). St. Louis: Mosby.

Jeffcoat, M.K., Geurs, N.C., Reddy, M.S., et al. (2001). Periodontal infection and preterm birth: Results of a prospective study. *J Am Dent Assoc, 132*(7), 875-880.

Koch, R., Hanley, W., Levy, H., et al. (2003). The maternal phenylketonuria international study: 1984-2002. *Pediatrics, 112*(6), 1523-1135.

Korenbrot, C., Steinberg, A., Bender, C., & Newberry, S. (2002). Preconception care: A systematic review. *Matern Child Health J, 6*(2), 75-88.

Lederman, S.A., Akabas, S.R., Moore, B.J., et al. (2004). Summary of presentations at the conference on preventing childhood obesity, December 8, 2003. *Pediatrics, 14*(4), 1146-1173.

Li, R., Zhao, Z., Mokdad, A., Barker, L., & Grummer-Strawn, L. (2003). Prevalence of breastfeeding in the United States: The 2001 national immunization survey. *Pediatrics, 111*(5), 1198-1201.

Lopez, A., Dietz, V.J., Wilson, M., et al. (2000). Preventing congenital toxoplasmosis. *MMWR Recomm Rep, 49*(RR-2), 59-68.

Lu, M.C., Prentice, J., Yu, S.M., et al. (2003). Childbirth education classes: Sociodemographic disparities in attendance and the association of attendance with breastfeeding initiation. *Matern Child Health J, 7*(2), 87-93.

Mahajan, S.D., Singh, S., Shah, P., et al. (2004). Effect of maternal malnutrition and anemia on the endocrine regulation of fetal growth. *Endocr Res, 30*(2), 189-203.

Maloni, J.A., Albrecht, S.A., Kelly-Thomas, K., et al. (2003). Implementing evidence-based practice: Reducing risk for low birth weight through pregnancy smoking cessation. *J Obstet Gynecol Neonatal Nurs, 32*(5), 676-682.

McFarlane, J., Parker, B., & Cross, B. (2001). *Abuse during pregnancy: A protocol for prevention and intervention.* (2nd ed.). White Plains, NY: March of Dimes Birth Defects Foundation.

Mone, S.M., Gillman, M.W., Miller, T.L., et al. (2004). Effects of environmental exposures on the cardiovascular system: Prenatal period through adolescence. *Pediatrics, 113*(4), 1058-1069.

Moos, M.K. (2003). Preconceptional wellness as a routine objective for women's health care: An integrative strategy. *J Obstet Gynecol Neonatal Nurs, 32*(4), 550-556.

Muchowski, K., & Paladine, H. (2003). Importance of preconception counseling. *Am Fam Physician, 67*(4), 701-702.

Naimi, T.S., Lipscomb, L.E., Brewer, R.D., & Gilbert, B.C. (2003). Binge drinking in the preconception period and the risk of unintended pregnancies: Implications for women and their children. *Pediatrics, 111*(5), 1136-1141.

National Association of Pediatric Nurse Practitioners (NAPNAP). (2000). Position statement on prevention of tobacco use in the pediatric population. *J Pediatr Health Care, 14*(3), 29A-30A.

National Association of Pediatric Nurse Practitioners (NAPNAP). (2001). Position statement on breastfeeding. *J Pediatr Health Care, 15*(5), 22A.

National Association of Pediatric Nurse Practitioners (NAPNAP). (2003). Position statement on the PNP's role in supporting infant and family well-being during the first year of life. *J Pediatr Health Care, 17*(3), 19A-20A.

National Institutes of Health (NIH) (2001). National Institutes of Health consensus development conference statement: Phenylketonuria: Screening and management, October 16-18, 2000. *Pediatrics, 108*(4), 972-982.

National Human Genome Research Institute. (2006). Learning about Tay-Sachs disease. Retrieved on May 9, 2006, from http://www.genome.gov/10001220.

Peters, V., Liu, K-L., Dominquez, K., et al. (2003). Missed opportunities for perinatal HIV prevention among HIV-exposed infants born 1996-2000, pediatric spectrum of HIV disease cohort. *Pediatrics, 111*(5), 1186-1191.

Postlethwaite, D. (2003). Preconception health counseling for women exposed to teratogens: The role of the nurse. *J Obstet Gynecol Neonatal Nurs, 32*(4), 523-532.

Rodier, P.M. (2004). Environmental causes of central nervous system maldevelopment. *Pediatrics, 113*(94), 1076-1083.

Sablock, U., Lindow, S.W., Arnott, P.I.E., & Masson, E.A. (2002). Prepregnancy counselling for women with medical disorders. *J Obstet Gynaecol, 202*(6), 637-638.

Saltzman, L.E., Johnson, C.H., Gilbert, B.C., & Goodwin, M.M. (2003). Physical abuse around the time of pregnancy: An examination of prevalence and risk factors in 16 states. *Matern Child Health J, 7*(1), 31-42.

Tiedje, L.B. (2003). Psychosocial pathways to prematurity: Changing our thinking toward a lifecourse and community approach. *J Obstet Gynecol Neonatal Nurs, 32*(5), 650-658.

Watkins, M.L., Rasmussen, S.A., Honein, M.A., et al. (2003). Maternal obesity and risk for birth defects. *Pediatrics, 111*(5), 1152-1158.

Widaman, K.F., & Azen, C. (2003). Relation of prenatal phenylalanine exposure to infant and childhood cognitive outcomes: Results from international maternal PKU collaborative study. *Pediatrics, 112*(6), 1537-1543.

Yu, S.M., Park, C.H., & Schwalberg, R.H. (2002). Factors associated with smoking cessation among U.S. pregnant women. *Matern Child Health J, 6*(2), 89-97.

18 Care of the Newborn Before Hospital Discharge

DANA K. ING

Select the best answer for each of the following questions:

1. During the physical examination of a 1-hour-old newborn, his parents share with you their concern over their son's Apgars which were 2, 6, and 9 at 1, 5, and 10 minutes of life. They ask you if their son is going to be "mentally retarded." Your response to their question should be based upon what additional information?
   A. Cord blood gases, presence of abnormal neurologic signs, and any other organ dysfunction.
   B. Initial blood glucose, temperature, and color.
   C. The degree of resuscitation required at delivery, presence of meconium-stained amniotic fluid, and initial temperature of newborn.
   D. Cord gases, initial temperature, and blood glucose.

2. A nursery nurse calls to notify you that a newborn under his care has had a temperature of 36.2° C for the last 4 hours despite interventions to warm the infant. The infant, born at 36 weeks gestation, weighs 2.3 kg. The nurse describes the infant to also have no interest in breastfeeding, and is tachypneic and lethargic. What additional information should be a priority at this time?
   A. Chest x-ray.
   B. Blood glucose.
   C. Blood type and Coombs' test.
   D. Complete blood count.

3. During Emma's routine 2-week post-delivery visit, you notice that her eyes are red and draining a thick, yellow discharge. You notice that her mother refused the administration of the 0.5% erythromycin ointment following her birth. You are concerned because eye prophylaxis is administered to prevent conjunctivitis and potential complications from a bacterial infection. Eye prophylaxis is routinely administered to newborns to prevent infection from which bacteria?
   A. Group B streptococcus.
   B. Gonorrhea.
   C. *Staphylococcus aureus.*
   D. *Escherichia coli.*

4. Patrick, a 2-day-old newborn, comes into the early discharge follow-up program. During his physical examination, you notice blood oozing from his umbilical stump and his circumcision site. What additional information should be a priority at this time before proceeding with your plan of care?
   A. Apgars, admission glucose level, and cord gases.
   B. Complete blood count, blood type, and Coombs' test.
   C. Did he receive vitamin K and is he being breastfed.
   D. Did he receive his hepatitis B vaccination.

5. During the discharge physical examination of David, a 36-hour-old infant born at 37 weeks gestation, you recommend that he be seen within 24 to 48 hours following discharge because he has slight yellow color to his face. He is being breastfed. His parents, who are first-time parents, question why they need to bring him back so soon. Your best response is based upon your understanding

that infants at higher risk for developing hyperbilirubinemia are those:
- A. Born at less than 38 weeks gestation and are breastfeeding.
- B. Born to first-time mothers.
- C. Demonstrating signs of jaundice within the first 36 hours of life.
- D. Who are discharged before 48 hours of age.

6. While examining an infant's head, you notice an area of swelling that is well-demarcated and does not cross the suture lines. This finding is caused by the rupture of blood vessels that traverse the skull to the periosteum, commonly known as:
- A. Craniosynostosis.
- B. Fractured skull.
- C. Cephalhematoma.
- D. Caput succedaneum.

7. Which of the following conditions places infants at risk for hypoglycemia resulting from inadequate glucose production?
- A. Hypothermia, large for gestational age, polycythemia.
- B. Small for gestational age, infant of an insulin-dependent diabetic mother.
- C. Hypothyroidism, adrenal insufficiency, Rh incompatibility.
- D. Polycythemia, infant of an insulin-dependent diabetic mother, galactosemia.

8. During a routine 2-week newborn follow-up examination, you notice that Kyle still has his umbilical cord. Upon further inspection, you note no odor, erythema, or purulent drainage, but rather clear fluid draining from the umbilical cord. What is the most likely cause of this drainage?
- A. Bacterial infection.
- B. Patent urachus.
- C. Omphalocele.
- D. Umbilical cyst.

9. Kelly, a 48-hour-old term newborn born via cesarean section for frank breech presentation, is ready for discharge. During the discharge physical examination of this newborn, you note positive Ortolani's sign of her hips. Your next priority for this infant should include which of the following?

- A. Ultrasound of the hips before discharge.
- B. Instruct the family how to triple-diaper their baby.
- C. Refer to an orthopedist.
- D. X-ray of the hips.

10. In the delivery room, an important step in stabilizing the newborn includes, but is not limited to, placing the infant on prewarmed blankets or towels to minimize heat loss. Which principle of heat transference is being applied during this practice?
- A. Convection
- B. Conduction
- C. Evaporation
- D. Radiation

11. You are called to evaluate a newborn who is 2 hours old. The nurse reports to you that this infant is sleepy and shows no interest in breastfeeding. A review of his history is unremarkable. On exam, he is sleeping, comfortable, has normal vital signs, and good tone and color. What should be your first priority given your review and examination?
- A. Do nothing at this time, because this is normal behavior for the second period of reactivity following birth.
- B. This is abnormal behavior for this newborn; order a CT scan.
- C. Instruct the nurse to feed this infant formula, since he shows no interest in breastfeeding.
- D. Obtain a complete blood count, blood glucose, and culture.

12. The parents of a term newborn boy ask you if you think they should consent to a circumcision for their newborn, Jake. As a nurse practitioner, the best response to this question should be based upon:
- A. What you decided for your own son.
- B. Understanding that you are there to provide accurate and unbiased information about circumcisions.
- C. The national trend for circumcision.
- D. The culture of this family.

13. The nursery nurse asks you to examine Scott because he shows no interest in breastfeeding, has not had any stool, and

now has a full abdomen. Scott is now 38 hours old. On examination, you note a respiratory rate of 65, a distended abdomen measuring 3 centimeters larger than at birth. He appears jaundiced and has had a bilious emesis. What condition is mostly likely causing Scott's symptoms?

  A. Feeding intolerance.
  B. Pyloric stenosis.
  C. Hirschprung's disease.
  D. Malrotation.

14. During the physical examination of a newborn, careful inspection of the back and spine reveals a deep dimple and hair tufts. Further evaluation is indicated because these findings are suggestive of what condition?

  A. Spina bifida occulta.
  B. Developmental dysplasia of the hip.
  C. Congenital meningitis.
  D. Imperforate anus.

15. During the inspection of a full-term, breech newborn's eyes and ears, you notice that the tops of the ears are approximately a centimeter below the position of the eyes. What is the significance of this finding?

  A. It is of no significance, since this is a normal finding.
  B. It is of no significance, since the infant was in breech position during his fetal life.
  C. It should warrant closer inspection of other body parts.
  D. It is a classic sign of hydrocephalus.

16. You are called to assess a newborn who is 10 minutes old. During your examination, you notice that the infant has a respiratory rate of 65 and remains cyanotic despite the oxygen that is being given to him by mask. What system should be your priority to assess next?

  A. Respiratory
  B. Cardiovascular
  C. Gastrointestinal
  D. Neurologic

17. During a discharge physical examination of a term newborn weighing 4.6 kg, now 30 hours old, you note that he nursed four times in the last 24 hours for 10 minutes on only one breast. On examination, he is noted to be a little jittery, has a respiratory rate ranging between 65 and 76, and his temperature has ranged between 97° and 97.2° Fahrenheit. Prenatal history is significant for maternal insulin-dependent diabetes and no history of drug use. His blood glucose levels after delivery were as follows: 40 at 1 hour of age and 55 at 2 hours. His blood glucose is now 50. What information should you obtain at this time?

  A. Another blood glucose immediately, because you suspect the blood glucose is lower than reported.
  B. Complete blood count, blood culture, electrolytes, and ammonia.
  C. Complete blood count, blood culture, and neonatal bilirubin.
  D. Complete blood count, blood culture, and serum calcium.

18. You are called to examine a newborn infant who is 15 minutes old. Apgars were 6 and 9 at 1 and 5 minutes, respectively. He received 30 seconds of positive pressure ventilation at delivery for poor respiratory effort. The infant is now breathing 80 times a minute with mild subcostal retractions and is intermittently grunting. His mucous membranes are pink and his hands and feet are blue-tinged and cold to touch. Upon auscultation of his chest, you note the following: Apical pulse of 140, regular rhythm, no murmur, and decreased breath sounds on the right side of his chest. What is the most likely cause of these symptoms?

  A. Persistent pulmonary hypertension.
  B. Congenital cardiac defect.
  C. Pneumothorax.
  D. Transient tachypnea of the newborn (TTN).

19. During a routine discharge exam of Matthew, a 48-hour-old newborn, his mother asks you about caring for her son's uncircumcised penis. She says that she was told to retract the foreskin with each diaper change. What recommendation would you give to her?

  A. The information she received is correct, so she should follow it to ensure that the foreskin retracts later in life.

B. At birth, the foreskin is not retractable and she should not force it to retract. Gently wash and dry the penis with each diaper change. The foreskin will loosen as her son grows.

C. Recommend that she have Matthew circumcised to avoid possible problems later in life.

D. Refer Matthew to a pediatric urologist because the foreskin should retract.

20. You are called to examine a 5-minute-old term newborn for respiratory distress. On examination, you notice that the newborn is cyanotic, grunting, tachypneic, and has a scaphoid abdomen. This newborn is demonstrating signs of what medical condition?

A. Meconium aspiration syndrome (MAS).

B. Respiratory distress syndrome (RDS).

C. Congenital diaphragmatic hernia (CDH).

D. Tracheoesophageal atresia (TEF).

21. Blood pressures are not usually obtained as part of the routine newborn vital signs. When are blood pressure measurements indicated in the normal newborn?

A. Inability to palpate pulses in the lower extremities.

B. Maternal history of chronic hypertension.

C. Newborn heart rate less than 120.

D. Hypoglycemia.

22. During a routine discharge examination of a 36-hour-old term female infant, the parents ask you about the "rash" on their newborn's skin. Upon examination, the "rash" appears as small, erythematous papules, some of which appear to be pustule-like, on the infant's trunk. There is a distinctive, diffuse, blotchy erythematous halo surrounding the vesicles. The parents verbalize that they are concerned that their newborn has acquired a skin infection while in the hospital and would like to speak to the unit's manager. The perinatal history is unremarkable and the newborn appears healthy and has been stable. What is the most likely cause of this "rash"?

A. Skin infection caused by *Candida albicans.*

B. Milia.

C. Herpes simplex.

D. Erythema toxicum.

23. All newborns discharged from the hospital should be placed in car safety seats that meet Federal Motor Vehicle Standards. What group of infants would you recommend car seat testing for prior to discharge?

A. Infants born greater than 41 weeks gestation weighing 4500 grams.

B. Infants less than 37 weeks and/or weighing less than 2500 grams.

C. Infants who will be traveling more than 60 minutes at a time.

D. All newborns should be tested prior to discharge.

24. During the physical examination of a 1-hour-old infant, you notice that he is not moving his left arm. He is able to bring his right arm into flexed position, but his left arm remains flaccid. The delivery record is significant for shoulder dystocia. How would you proceed with the rest of your examination?

A. Palpate the clavicles for crepitus, note what part of the left arm he is able or not able to move.

B. Immediately obtain an x-ray of the left arm.

C. Obtain blood glucose because the infant is large for gestational age.

D. Immediately show the family how to immobilize the infant's arm in a splint.

25. During a routine 2-week newborn checkup of Joshua, you notice that he has poor tone, a high-pitched cry, and has been described by his mother as "not interested in nursing." His mother reports that at times he "stiffens up." His mother also reports that his urine has a sweet smell. What additional information would be a priority for you, given Joshua's symptoms?

A. Blood glucose and complete blood count.

B. Results from the newborn metabolic screen.

C. Total and direct bilirubin.

D. Urinalysis and culture.

ANSWERS

1. **Answer:** A
Rationale: It is difficult to predict the neurologic outcome for any infant. By itself, a low Apgar score cannot predict the neurologic outcome, but requires additional information. Concern for neurologic injury is indicated in the presence of the following additional signs: Apgar score less than 3 for more than 5 minutes, profound metabolic acidosis, neurologic dysfunction, and multisystem organ dysfunction. Close developmental follow-up is indicated in these infants.

2. **Answer:** B
Rationale: Infants who are premature and small for gestational age are at risk for hypothermia because they have not accumulated adequate brown fat stores. In addition, infants who require resuscitation or are hypoglycemic are at risk for developing hypothermia. These infants require close monitoring of their glucose levels. If the infant continues to be hypothermic after euglycemia has been established, further studies are warranted and may include a complete blood count and blood culture.

3. **Answer:** B
Rationale: Eye prophylaxis such as 1% silver nitrate, 0.5% erythromycin ointment, and 1% tetracycline ointment are given to newborns to prevent neonatal gonorrheal bacterial conjunctivitis. Mothers who have tested negative for sexually transmitted diseases may choose to decline the administration of eye prophylaxis. Eye prophylaxis will not prevent the development of eye infections that occur later in the newborn period.

4. **Answer:** C
Rationale: Hemorrhagic disease of the newborn (HDN) occurs almost exclusively in breastfed infants because breast milk is deficient in vitamin K and commercial formula contains vitamin K. The classic symptoms of HDN occur 2 to 7 days after birth in breastfeeding infants and include generalized bleeding from the skin, umbilicus, circumcision site, and gastrointestinal tract. Vitamin K is routinely given to all newborns to prevent HDN from vitamin K deficiency. Other risk factors for HDN include maternal anticonvulsant and anticoagulant therapy, birth asphyxia, and prolonged labor.

5. **Answer:** A
Rationale: Infants at higher risk for developing hyperbilirubinemia are particularly those who are breastfed and born at less than 38 weeks of gestation. Infants of this group require closer monitoring. Appropriate follow-up should be based upon time of discharge and risk assessment. Parents need to be provided with written and verbal information about newborn jaundice.

6. **Answer:** C
Rationale: Cephalhematomas are caused by rupture of blood vessels that traverse the skull to periosteum. This type of head trauma typically presents as well-demarcated swellings on the head and do not cross suture lines. Complications such as skull fracture, intracranial hemorrhage, and hyperbilirubinemia require close monitoring and additional treatment. It may take up to 3 months for reabsorbtion of the cephalhematoma.

7. **Answer:** A
Rationale: Term infants at risk for hypoglycemia from inadequate glucose production include the following: Large for gestational age, intrauterine growth-restricted, postmature, cold stress, perinatal asphyxia, polycythemia, and inborn errors of metabolism.

8. **Answer:** B
Rationale: The umbilical cord usually separates around 1 to 2 weeks of life. The persistent presence of the umbilical cord with clear fluid drainage could indicate a patent urachus, a canal connecting the fetal bladder with the allantois, a membranous sac that contributes to the formation of the umbilical cord.

9. **Answer:** C
Rationale: According to American Academy of Pediatrics' recommendations for the management of developmental dysplasia of the hip (DDH), all newborns with posi-

tive Ortolani's or Barlow's signs at birth or during the routine 2-week exam should be referred to an orthopedist. The recommendations do not include further radiologic studies or triple-diapering the newborn.

10. *Answer:* B
Rationale: Thermoregulation is critical to the well-being of newborns because at birth, newborns can lose up to 1° F of body heat per minute. Heat loss through conduction, the transfer of heat from the body to the objects in contact with the body, can be prevented by using warmed blankets.

11. *Answer:* A
Rationale: Following delivery, newborns go through different periods of reactivity. The first period of reactivity begins at birth and lasts about 30 minutes. The second period is a period of sleep when infants typically fall into deep sleep, will have heart rate and respiratory rate within normal range, and may have temperature that is slightly below normal. This period lasts between 2 to 4 hours and is then followed by a second period of reactivity when the infant is awake and interested in feeding.

12. *Answer:* B
Rationale: The practitioner's responsibility in this situation is to provide accurate and unbiased information about circumcisions (i.e., benefits and potential risks). The discussion with the parents should provide them with the opportunity to discuss and ask questions about circumcisions. The practitioner should also explore the cultural and religious beliefs and practices of the family.

13. *Answer:* C
Rationale: Hirschprung's disease is a condition of absence of parasympathetic innervation to the distal intestine with absence of ganglionic cells in the submucosal and myenteric plexuses of the colon. Hirschprung's disease should be suspected in the newborn who does not pass meconium within 24 to 48 hours of birth. An abdominal x-ray will typically show diffuse intestinal and bowel dilation with absence of air in the rectum. The diagnosis is confirmed by rectal biopsy, which demonstrates absence of ganglionic cells. Surgery is the treatment for Hirschprung's disease.

14. *Answer:* A
Rationale: The physical examination of all newborns should include careful inspection of the trunk and spine for pilondial sinus tracts, dimples, and hair tuft. The physical findings suggest the presence spina bifida occulta. Spina bifida occulta is the incomplete closure of the vertebral bones. The defect does not allow exposure of the spinal cord. Additional studies and referrals may be warranted to determine extent of defect and long-term consequences.

15. *Answer:* C
Rationale: The tops of the ears are normally parallel with the eyes. If the tops of the ears are below this position, it is considered lowest and may be associated with certain syndromes such as trisomy 21. The practitioner should closely inspect the infant for additional physical traits for the presence of a possible syndrome.

16. *Answer:* B
Rationale: The cardiovascular system should be assessed next, since this infant is demonstrating signs of possible congenital cardiac disease. The assessment should include, but not be limited to, capillary refill time, presence of a murmur, blood pressure, and pulse. This infant should be transferred to the intensive care unit for additional evaluation and referrals.

17. *Answer:* D
Rationale: Symptoms of hypoglycemia, such as poor feeding, jitteriness, and tachypnea, are also symptoms of sepsis, hypocalcemia, or drug withdrawal. In absence of a maternal history of drug use, the practitioner should evaluate the infant for sepsis and hypocalcemia.

18. *Answer:* C
Rationale: Signs and symptoms of respiratory distress in the newborn are often nonspecific. For this reason, careful review of the infant's history is imperative for deter-

mining the differential diagnosis. The most likely cause of the respiratory symptoms is a pneumothorax, given the infant's resuscitation history of positive pressure ventilation and the noted decreased breath sounds.

19. *Answer:* B
Rationale: At birth, the foreskin adheres to the penis and will not retract. The foreskin should not be "forced" to retract. As the child grows, the foreskin will loosen. The uncircumcised penis should be gently washed and dried with each diaper change.

20. *Answer:* C
Rationale: Infants with large CDH usually present with cyanosis, respiratory distress, scaphoid abdomen, decreased or absent breath sounds on the side of the hernia, and displaced heart sounds. Bag and mask ventilation is contraindicated in the presence of CDH. The infant will need to be intubated to prevent air from entering the intestines. A large-bore nasogastric tube attached to continuous suction should also be placed.

21. *Answer:* A
Rationale: Strong arm pulses and weak or absent lower extremity pulses suggest coarctation of the aorta (COA). Blood pressure measurements from all four extremities are recommended. A higher blood pressure of the upper extremities greater than 15 mm Hg is suggestive of COA. If COA is suspected, notify the pediatrician and/or cardiologist immediately. The infant will need an echocardiogram and possibly prostaglandin E1 to maintain patency of the ductus arteriosus.

22. *Answer:* D
Rationale: Erythema toxicum is benign skin condition that occurs only during the neonatal period in approximately 48% of newborns. The condition is characterized by eythematous papules, pustules, and vesicles that are surrounded by a distinctive, diffuse, blotchy, and erythematous halo.

23. *Answer:* B
Rationale: Preterm infants at less than 37 weeks gestation and/or those weighing less than 2500 grams are at risk for apnea, brady-

cardia, and oxygen desaturation. The American Academy of Pediatrics recommends that these infants be tested in the car seat they will be expected to sit in during transportation. The infants should be monitored for apnea, bradycardia, and oxygen desaturation for a time period longer than their expected duration of travel. Discharge should be delayed if the infant demonstrates apnea, bradycardia, or oxygen desaturation until the infant can pass the car seat test in an appropriate car safety seat or bed.

24. *Answer:* A
Rationale: Asymmetry of movement of the upper extremities is an abnormal finding in the newborn and can result from birth trauma during a delivery with shoulder dystocia. An infant born with shoulder dystocia is at risk of having a fractured clavicle and nerve injury. An x-ray of the shoulder is recommended if a fractured clavicle is suspected. It is also important to note the extent of movement, or lack of movement of the arm and hands, as well as the position of the hand and wrist. Prior to discharge, the pediatric nurse practitioner must also note whether movement has returned to the affected side. If movement has not returned before the infant is ready for discharge, the pediatric nurse practitioner should arrange for additional referrals.

25. *Answer:* B
Rationale: All states in the United States test for newborn metabolic disorders. The number of disorders tested may differ from state to state. However, the more common disorders such as maple syrup urine disease (MSUD), is tested in all 50 states. Some of the classical signs of metabolic disorders include lethargy and poor tone. MSUD is a metabolic disorder characterized by sweet-smelling urine resembling the smell of maple syrup. Prior to discharge, all infants should have this test done. In the event that the parents refuse this test, the parents must complete the appropriate forms documenting this refusal.

BIBLIOGRAPHY

American Academy of Pediatrics. (2001). Circumcision: Frequently asked questions. Retrieved May 9, 2005, from www.medem.com/MedLB/article_detaillb.cfm?article_ID=ZZZ13FOPIUC&sub_cat=0.

American Academy of Pediatrics & American Heart Association. (2005). Neonatal Resuscitation Program. Retrieved on May 9, 2006, from http://www.aap.org/nrp/nrpmain.html.

American Academy of Pediatrics Committee on Fetus and Newborn. (2004). Hospital stay for healthy term newborns (RE9539). *Pediatrics, 113*(5), 1434-1436.

American Academy of Pediatrics Committee on Fetus and Newborn, American Academy of Pediatrics Committee on Obstetric Practice, American College of Obstetricians and Gynecologists. (1996). Use and abuse of the Apgar score. *Pediatrics, 98*(1), 141-142.

American Academy of Pediatrics Committee on Genetics, Section on Endocrinology, Section on Urology. (2000). Policy statement: Evaluation of the newborn with developmental anomalies of the external genitalia. *Pediatrics, 106*(1), 138-142.

American Academy of Pediatrics Committee on Injury and Poison Prevention. (1999). Safe transportation of newborns at hospital discharge. *Pediatrics, 104*(4), 987-987.

American Academy of Pediatrics Committee on Injury and Poison Prevention and Committee on Fetus and Newborn. (1996). Safe transportation of premature and low birth weight infants. *Pediatrics, 97*(5), 758-760.

American Academy of Pediatrics Committee on Practice and Ambulatory Medicine, and Section on Ophthalmology. (2003). Policy statement: Eye examination in infants, children, and young adults by pediatricians. *Pediatrics, 111*(4), 902-907.

American Academy of Pediatrics. Committee on Quality Improvement, Subcommittee on Developmental Dysplasia of the Hip. (2000). Clinical practice guideline: Early detection of developmental dysplasia of the hip. *Pediatrics 105*(4), 896-905.

American Academy of Pediatrics. Joint Committee on Infant Hearing. (2000). Position statement: Principles and guidelines for early hearing detection and intervention programs. *Pediatrics, 106*(4), 798-817.

American Academy of Pediatrics. Provisional Committee for Quality Improvement and Subcommittee on Hyperbilirubinemia. (2004). Practice guideline: Management of hyperbilirubinemia in the newborn infant, 35 or more weeks gestation. *Pediatrics, 114*(1), 297-316.

American Academy of Pediatrics. Section on Breastfeeding. (2005). Policy statement: Breastfeeding and the use of human milk. *Pediatrics, 115*(2), 496-506.

American Academy of Pediatrics. Section on Ophthalmology. (2002). Policy statement: Red reflex examination of infants. *Pediatrics, 109*(5), 980-981.

American Academy of Pediatrics. Task Force on Circumcision. (1999). Circumcision policy statement. *Pediatrics, 103*(3), 686-693.

American Academy of Pediatrics. Vitamin K Ad Hoc Task Force. (2003). Controversies concerning vitamin K and the newborn. *Pediatrics, 112*(1), 191-192.

Benjamin, K. (2002). Scrotal and inguinal masses in the newborn period. *Adv Neonatal Care, 2*(3), 140-148.

Blackburn, S.T. (2003). *Maternal, fetal, & neonatal physiology: A clinical perspective.* (2nd ed.). St. Louis: Saunders.

Cantu, S. (2004). Circumcision. Retrieved on July 6, 2005, from www.emedicine.com/ped/topic1791.htm.

Cooper, S., & Ratnavel, R. (2005). Milia. Retrieved on March 31, 2006, from www.emedicine.com/DERM/topic265.htm.

Cranmer, H., & Shannon, M. (2005). Pediatrics: Hypoglycemia. Retrieved on July 6, 2005, from http://master.emedicine.com/EMERG/topic384.htm.

Donlon, C. & Furdon, S. (2002). Part 2: Assessment of the umbilical cord outside of the delivery room. *Adv Neonatal Care, 2*(4), 187-197.

Dubik, M. (2001). Apgar scores still useful. *AAP Grand Rounds, 5,* 50.

Fuloria, M., & Kreiter, S. (2002a). The newborn examination: Part I. Emergencies and common abnormalities involving the skin, head, neck, chest, and respiratory and cardiovascular systems. *Am Fam Physician, 65*(1), 61-68.

Fuloria, M., & Kreiter, S. (2002b). The newborn examination: Part II. Emergencies and common abnormalities involving the abdomen, pelvis, extremities, genitalia, and spine. *Am Fam Physician, 65*(1), 265-270.

Gore, A.I., & Spencer, J.P. (2004). The newborn foot. *Am Fam Physisican, 69*(4), 865-872.

Hunter, J. & Malloy, M. (2002). Effects of sleep and play positions on infant development: Reconciling developmental concerns with SIDS prevention. *Newborn Infant Nurs Rev, 2*(1), 9-16.

Hutcheson, J., & Snyder, H.M. (2004). Ambiguous genitalia and intersexuality. Retrieved March

31, 2006, from www.emedicine.com/PED/topic1492.htm.

National Eye Institute. (1999). Clinical trial of eye prophylaxis in the newborn. Retrieved July 6, 2005 from www.nei.nih.gov/neitrials/viewStudyWeb.aspx?id=19.

Noerr, B. (2001). State of the science: Neonatal hypoglycemia. *Adv Neonatal Care, 1*(1), 4-21.

St. John, E.B. (2005). Hemorrhagic disease of the newborn. Retrieved July 6, 2005, from www.emedicine.com/ped/topic966.htm.

Tappero, E. & Honeyfield, M.E. (2003). *Physical assessment of the newborn* (2nd ed.). Santa Rosa, CA: NICU Ink Book.

Thureen, P., Deacon, J., Hernandez, J., & Hall, D. (2005). *Assessment and care of the well newborn* (2nd ed.). St. Louis: Saunders.

Yan, A.C. (2006). Erythema toxicum. Retrieved March 31, 2006, from http://www.emedicine.com/PED/topic697.htm.

Young-Wardell, C.D., & Fuchs, D. (2003). Biobehavioral assessment of the infant. *J Am Acad Child Adolesc Psychiatry, 42*(6), 746-747.

NOTES

SHIRLEY A. ALVARO

Select the best answer for each of the following questions:

1. Mary, a 6-month-old infant, comes into the clinic for a well child checkup. Her mom wants to know the average normal sleep patterns for 6-month-olds. The best response is:
   A. 8 hours at night and 7 to 8 hours during the day.
   B. 10 hours at night and 6 to 8 hours during the day.
   C. 8 hours and night and 2 to 3 hours during the day.
   D. 10 hours at night and 4 to 5 hours during the day.

2. Which of the following newborn infants are at risk for hearing loss?
   A. A 36-week gestation infant with a birth weight of 5 pounds 6 ounces.
   B. A term newborn with Apgars of 2 at 5 minutes and 5 at 5 minutes.
   C. A term infant born to a mother who took ampicillin for an ear infection 24 weeks into her pregnancy.
   D. A newborn with atrial septal defect.

3. Ben is a 3-day-old infant coming into the clinic for his first checkup. He was born 4 weeks prematurely. His mother had very sporadic prenatal care and the history is questionable, though the mom states she is "healthy" and ate well during her pregnancy, she just went into labor "early." The infant presents with mucotaneous lesions on his lips, ear, and face. Your differential diagnosis would include:
   A. Hepatitis B.
   B. Herpes simplex virus (HSV).

   C. Milia.
   D. Neonatal acne.

4. Melissa is a 7-day-old infant who comes into the clinic with her first-time mom. The mom's breasts are sore and cracking with a small amount of bleeding. She reports that she was positioning the baby correctly and has a good amount of milk supply. What is the BEST action?
   A. Check the baby's weight to see if there was weight gain/loss since discharge and consider referral to lactation consultant.
   B. Explain to the mom that it is "natural" to feel some discomfort the first few weeks of breast feeding and reassure her it will get better with time.
   C. Instruct the mom she may want to supplement her breastfeeding with formula to be sure the baby is satisfied and gains necessary weight as a growing infant.
   D. Encourage discontinuation of breast-feeding because both she and the infant are at risk for infection.

5. A developmentally appropriate 7-month-old should be able to:
   A. Wave bye-bye and play pat-a-cake.
   B. Speak in 2 to 3 word sentences.
   C. Scribble with a crayon.
   D. Walk well.

6. Mickey, a 7-day-old infant boy, is brought into the clinic for a diaper rash. The mom reports she changes the diaper at least eight times a day. She is a new mom and had understood that she probably only had to

change the diaper after feedings or if the infant seemed uncomfortable. The genital area is red with no satellite lesions. The mom is breastfeeding. What are the likely causes of this irritation?

A. *Candida albicans.*
B. Allergic contact dermatitis.
C. Irritant contact dermatitis.
D. Psoriasis.

7. Iron deficiency anemia is a concern during infancy and is associated with anemia, growth problems, and cognitive delay. Heme iron is important because:

A. It is from ingested meat and poultry and is released in the intestinal lumen and enters the enterocyte as an intact protein (metalloporphyrin).
B. It is made soluble by gastric acid in the stomach and is converted from ferric to ferrous form.
C. It can be readily absorbed in a droplet form for easy absorption.
D. Ferric reductase, a protein known as Dctb, takes part in the process of reducing ferric iron to ferrous iron.

8. Newborn screening is important to detect possible conditions that will interfere with normal growth and development. Normal thyroid (TSH) and free thyroxine (T_4) levels for a 6-week-old are:

A. Above 12 (TSH), 1.0 to 3.0 (free thyroxine).
B. Less than 5.5 (TSH), 0.7 to 1.7 (free thyroxine).
C. Less than 13.3 (TSH), 3.0 to 5.0 (free thyroxine).
D. 7 (TSH), 2.0 to 4.0 (free thyroxine).

9. A group of mothers are discussing their 8-month-old infants' developmental milestones. All of the mothers except one say their infants are exhibiting signs of separation anxiety. What might be an appropriate question to ask the mother whose child is not showing signs of separation anxiety?

A. How many siblings does your infant have?
B. Are you still breastfeeding?
C. Does the child attend daycare?
D. Where does the child sleep?

10. At what weight can a child be placed in a forward-facing infant restraint?

A. 10 pounds.
B. 15 pounds.
C. 20 pounds.
D. Infants should never be placed in a front-facing car seat.

11. In infancy, rhinoviruses are extremely common. What is the most efficient means of controlling the spread of this common pediatric condition?

A. Having the infant vaccinated against the disease.
B. Delaying daycare until at least 6 months old.
C. Considering alternative treatment such as Echinacea.
D. Frequent and proper handwashing.

12. Safety for the newborn cannot be stressed enough at the first well child visit. The primary areas that need to be addressed at the first visit are the following:

A. Crib safety, hot water heaters, car safety seats, smoke detectors, and sun exposure.
B. Home safety, ingestions, infant walkers, pet awareness.
C. Bed safety, hot liquid spills, loud noises, bright lights.
D. Pool safety, dealing with strangers, parental conflict.

13. The appropriate daily dosage of fluoride recommended by the American Dental Association and the Academy of Pediatrics for a 6-month-old infant whose water supply has less than 0.3 ppm of fluoride is:

A. 0.50 mg.
B. 0.25 mg.
C. 1.0 mg.
D. 0.1 mg.

14. Sarah is brought in for her 4-month-old visit by her dad. When asked how she was doing, he said "Fine, she is such a quiet baby. She likes to be held but doesn't really cry very much." All of the following are appropriate actions EXCEPT:

A. Perform a Denver II Developmental Screening Test.

B. Review the newborn screening examination results.
C. Determine if there is a family history of hearing loss.
D. Ask the father how many words Sarah verbalizes.

15. Christine, a 7-week-old infant, is brought in for "colic" and fussiness. Her mom reports she has tried everything to calm her, from rocking, walking in the stroller, to turning on the vacuum. She knows she is not "ill," she just wants her to get some sleep. The infant has been breastfed since birth. What is the BEST suggestion?
   A. Instruct the mother to avoid salty foods in her diet.
   B. Offering a bottle of ½ Karo syrup and ½ water 2 to 3 times per day would help satisfy her sucking needs and help to soothe the infant.
   C. Applying a warm-water bottle to her abdomen for 20 to 30 minutes may calm her uneasiness and help her rest.
   D. Tight or loose swaddling for 3 hours a day can help to reduce fussiness and reduces frequency and intensity of brainstem arousals.

16. From 9 to 11 months of age, the infant should be able to accomplish the following gross and fine motor activities:
   A. Crawls, pincer grasp, pull to stand, puts small toy in container but will not release.
   B. Creeps up stairs, pivots in sitting, stoops to recover.
   C. Colors with a crayon, throws a ball overhand.
   D. Holds a cup and spoon, turns pages.

17. According to the American Academy of Pediatric Dentistry, the first visit to the pediatric dentist should be:
   A. When all the primary teeth have erupted, which is usually at age 2 to 2½ years.
   B. When at least four upper and four lower teeth have erupted.
   C. When the first primary tooth erupts, but no later than 12 months of age.

D. Before the child starts preschool, at around 3 to 4 years of age.

18. Louise, a 2-month-old infant, is brought in for her well child visit. On the physical examination, you notice a white spot in the left eye while attempting to illicit the red reflex. You make a referral to a pediatric ophthalmologist. This finding is suggestive of:
   A. Glaucoma.
   B. Retinoblastoma.
   C. Blindness from possible gonococcus infection.
   D. Ptosis.

19. In infants, lead levels greater than _____ mcg/dl require follow-up.
   A. 1
   B. 2
   C. 5
   D. 10

20. Which of the following statements about safety in infants is TRUE?
   A. Hot water thermostats should be kept at 150° Fahrenheit.
   B. Use of walkers with parental supervision is safe.
   C. Buckets and bathtubs are the most frequent location for drowning in children younger than 1 year of age.
   D. Car seats that have been in a car accident are safe to reuse.

21. To avoid the risk of SIDS, parents should be instructed to:
   A. Remove all pillows and soft toys from the crib.
   B. Place the infant on his or her stomach to sleep.
   C. Have the infant sleep in the parents' bed for the first 4 weeks of life.
   D. Avoid pacifiers at sleep time.

22. Sandie, the mother of a breastfed 2-week-old, comes into the clinic because she is worried about the newborn's stool. She describes the stool as soft, yellow, with little seed-like things in it. What would be the most appropriate action for the pediatric nurse practitioner?

A. Take a sample and send it to the lab for culture.
B. Refer to the gastroenterologist.
C. Take a sample and send it to the lab for ova and parasites.
D. Reassure Sandie that this is normal for a breastfed newborn.

23. Natasha is bringing her infant, Joey, into the clinic for a 5-month visit. Which of the following newborn reflexes may still be present?
A. Stepping.
B. Plantar grasp.
C. Rooting.
D. Tonic neck.

24. Natasha asks about when she should begin feeding Joey solid food. The BEST response would be that solid foods:

A. Should have begun at age 3 months; let me get you a schedule for feeding.
B. Should begin at 12 months of age; we can discuss this at your 9-month visit.
C. Can begin between 4 and 6 months of age; the first foods should be infant cereal.
D. Should begin at 4 months of age; let me demonstrate how to add cereal to your baby bottle.

25. When should Natasha expect Joey to get his first tooth?
A. 6 months.
B. 9 months.
C. 12 months.
D. 15 months.

NOTES

ANSWERS

1. *Answer:* D
   Rationale: Six-month-old infants sleep an average of 10 hours during the night and 4.25 hours during the day.

2. *Answer:* B
   Rationale: Low Apgar scores have been associated with newborn hearing loss. Infants are also at risk for hearing loss if they: are born less than 1500 grams, have a family history of hearing loss, had intrauterine infections, have ear or craniofacial anomalies, have bacterial meningitis or respiratory distress, physical features of syndromes, or received ototoxic medications.

3. *Answer:* B
   Rationale: The incidence of neonatal HSV is estimated at 1 per 3,000 to 20,000 live births. Approximately 20% to 40% of infants born with HSV are born prematurely. Three-fourths of neonatal infections are caused by HSV-2 and 25% are the result of HSV-1.

4. *Answer:* A
   Rationale: Breastfeeding is a codependent relationship. The infant's ability to breastfeed affects the mother's milk supply. Maternal problems affect the infant's ability to receive adequate milk for growth. All concerns must be addressed promptly to avoid rapid downward spiral toward premature weaning.

5. *Answer:* A
   Rationale: A child speaks in 2 to 3 word sentences at 18 to 24 months, scribbles at 12 to 18 months, and walks well at 11 to 15 months.

6. *Answer:* C
   Rationale: Rash in the diaper area is usually caused by irritant contact dermatitis. Prolonged exposure to urine and feces triggers the skin breakdown. Diaper-wearing is associated with an elevated skin pH, which further activates feces enzymes. Prevention is the best medicine. More frequent diaper changes can prevent prolonged exposure to wetness and fecal enzymes. Newborns may urinate every 30 minutes and breastfed babies in the first several weeks of life also defecate several times a day.

7. *Answer:* A
   Rationale: Heme iron is about two to three times more absorbable than nonheme iron. In determining a patient's iron nutrition, one needs to consider measuring hemoglobin level to determine the iron-containing protein in circulating red blood cells. Hemoglobin cannot be made without iron. Other iron-related proteins may also be ordered such as ferritin and total iron binding capacity.

8. *Answer:* B
   Rationale: Newborn screening requirements vary by state but one most common is thyroid testing. There are two main tests, thyroid stimulating hormone (TSH) and free thyroxine (T_4). The testing screens for thyroid and pituitary disorders. TSH and T_4 must be measured together. Normal TSH values for older than 4 weeks is 5.5 and normal values for T_4 is 0.7 to 1.7.

9. *Answer:* C
   Rationale: Children who attend daycare have less pronounced separation anxiety.

10. *Answer:* C
    Rationale: Infants over 1 year of age and weighing at least 20 pounds can be placed in a front-facing child restraint.

11. *Answer:* D
    Rationale: The observation that hand-to-hand contact was an important mode of transmission of rhinovirus. Treatment of these infections is limited to symptomatic therapy. There is no clear evidence that zinc or Echinacea have any role in these infections. Interruption of transmission by handwashing remains the "only" method for prevention of rhinovirus infections.

12. *Answer:* A
    Rationale: Cribs need to have the slat distance less than 2 inches to prevent slippage or suffocation, mattress should be firm, babies need to be on their backs or sides, and

the rails "up" at all times. Hot water heaters should be set at less than 120° F; appropriate car safety seats should be in the back seat and facing backwards if baby is less than 20 lbs.; batteries should be checked regularly in smoke detectors throughout the home; avoid all exposure to sun if younger than 6 months of age, and use appropriate sunscreens and clothing for 6-month-old and older infants.

13. *Answer:* B
Rationale: Dietary supplements are recommended by the AAP and the Dental Association for infants and children without access to fluoridated water. The appropriate daily dose for places with less than 0.3 ppm of fluoride in the water supply: Birth to 2 years, 0.25 mg; 2 to 3 years, 0.50 mg; 3 to 13 yrs, 1.0 mg.

14. *Answer:* D
Rationale: The 4-month-old infant is usually cooperative and interactive. At 4 months, an infant does not say words. Behaviors such as mimicry of the parents' vocalizations and language stimulation are usually apparent. Babbling and cooing is present with turning to sounds or loud noises. The incidence of hearing loss is 3 per 1,000, 20 times greater than PKU. Universal newborn hearing screening is essential to confirm a diagnosis by 3 months of age because language development is significantly better when intervention begins before 6 months of age. Auditory brainstem response (ABR) or otoacoustic emissions (OAE) are both screening exams done on infants to determine hearing loss.

15. *Answer:* D
Rationale: The stated purpose of swaddling was to reduce newborn fussiness and crying and to restrict random arm and hand movements that often awaken a sleeping baby from nocturnal sleep. Modern swaddling during early infancy is said to promote restful sleep in the supine position, is easily accepted by most babies, reduces frequency and intensity of brainstem arousals during nocturnal sleep, reduces scratching of infant's face during periods of hunger or irritability, and reduces accidental rolling over to the supine position.

16. *Answer:* A
Rationale: From 9 to 11 months of age, the following are milestones—forward parachute, crawls, pincer grasp, pulls to stand, puts toy in container but will not release. Pivoting and walking begins at 12 to 14 months. Feeding self with utensils begins after 18 months, and holding a crayon and throwing a ball is begun after age 2 years.

17. *Answer:* C
Rationale: The well baby dental history should identify decay risk factors. The American Academy of Pediatric Dentistry recommends a visit to the pediatric dentist when the first primary tooth erupts but no later than 12 months of age. Before the first dental visit, oral health recommendations should be provided by the primary care provider. Early recognition of dental problems can prevent unnecessary pain and suffering to the pediatric patient.

18. *Answer:* B
Rationale: The pupil should be black on direct examination, and red when examined through the ophthalmoscope; if the red reflex looks pale or white, suspect retinoblastoma.

19. *Answer:* D
Rationale: Lead levels higher than 10 mcg/dl are considered high and require follow-up.

20. *Answer:* C
Rationale: Hot water thermostats should be kept at or less than 120° Fahrenheit. The use of walkers is not recommended for infants; a the number of injuries have occurred when the child and walker fell down stairs. Car seats that have been in a car accident are not safe to reuse.

21. *Answer:* A
Rationale: The risk of SIDS is reduced by having the infant sleep on his or her back; removing all blankets, pillows, and soft toys from the crib; avoiding sleeping in the same bed as the parents; and protecting from second-hand smoke. Pacifiers have not been associated with SIDS and may stint the upper airway, thus reducing the risk of SIDS.

22. *Answer:* D

Rationale: Breastfed newborn babies have frequent stools that are soft, sticky, and light yellow with a curd-like texture. The description of this newborn's stool is normal and the mother should be reassured.

23. *Answer:* D

Rationale: Stepping reflex disappears at 6 to 8 weeks and the plantar grasp disappears at 4 months. The rooting reflex disappears between 3 and 4 months. The tonic neck disappears between 4 and 6 months.

24. *Answer:* C

Rationale: Solid foods, usually single-grain cereals (rice), should begin between 4 to 6 months of age. New foods should be added to the diet weekly to detect the presence of food reactions or allergies.

25. *Answer:* A

Rationale: The first tooth eruption occurs at about 6 months of age; the lower central and lateral incisors are the first teeth to erupt.

BIBLIOGRAPHY

Agran, P.F., Anderson, C., Winn, D., Trent, R., et al. (2003). Rates of pediatric injuries by 3-month intervals for children 0 to 3 years of age. *Pediatrics, 111*(6 Pt 1), e683-e692.

American Academy of Pediatric Dentistry. (2002). Policy on the use of a caries-risk assessment tool (CAT) for infants, children and adolescents. Retrieved March 31, 2006, from www.aapd.org/members/referencemanual/pdfs/02-03/Caries%20Risk%20Assess.pdf.

American Academy of Pediatrics Section on Pediatric Dentistry. (2003). Oral health risk assessment timing and establishment of the dental home. *Pediatrics, 111*(5), 1113-1116.

American Academy of Pediatrics. (2005). Car safety seats: A guide for families - 2006. Retrieved April 2, 2006, from www.aap.org/family/carseatguide.htm.

American Academy of Pediatrics Clinical Report (2003). Hearing assessment in infants and children: Recommendations beyond neonatal screening. *Pediatrics, 111*(3), 436-440.

American Academy of Pediatrics Committee on Children with Disabilities. (2001). Developmental surveillance and screening of infants and young children. *Pediatrics, 108*(1), 192-196.

American Academy of Pediatrics Committee on Injury, Violence and Poison Prevention. (2001). Injuries associated with infant walkers. *Pediatrics, 108*(3), 790-792.

American Academy of Pediatrics Committee on Injury, Violence and Poison Prevention. (2004). Prevention of drowning in infants, children and adolescents. *Pediatrics, 112*(2), 437-439.

American Academy of Pediatrics Task Force on Sudden Infant Death Syndrome. (2005). The changing concept of Sudden Infant Death Syndrome: Diagnostic coding shifts, controversies regarding the sleeping environment, and new variables to consider in reducing risk. *Pediatrics, 116*(5), 1245-1255.

Ateah, C.A., Secco, L. & Woodgate, R.L. (2003). The risks and alternatives to physical punishment use with children. *J Pediatr Health Care, 17*(3), 126-132.

Bayley, N. (2005). Bayley scales of infant development-II. Available through Psychological Assessment Resources, Inc., at www3.parinc.com/products/product.aspO?Productid=BSID-II.

Beltrán-Aguilar, E.D., Barker, L.K., Canto, M.T., et al. (2005). Surveillance for Dental Caries, Dental Sealants, Tooth Retention, Edentulism, and Enamel Fluorosis, United States, 1988-1994 and 1999-2002. *MMWR, 54*(03), 1-44.

Berk, L.E. (2004). *Development through the lifespan* (3rd ed.). Boston: Allyn & Bacon.

Blackwell, P.B., & Baker, B.M. (2002). Estimating communication competence of infants and toddlers. *J Pediatr Health Care, 16*(1), 29-35.

Bricker, D., & Squires, J. (1999). *Ages & stages questionnaires: A parent-completed, child monitoring system* (2nd ed.). Baltimore: Paul H. Brookes.

Burns, C.E., Brady, M.A., Dunn, A.M., & Starr, N.B. (2004). *Pediatric primary care: A handbook for nurse practitioners* (3rd ed.). Philadelphia: Saunders.

Carey, W.B. (1998). Teaching parents about infant temperament. *Pediatrics, 102*(5), 1311-1316.

Chess, S., & Thomas, A. (1986). *Temperament in clinical practice*. New York: Guilford Press.

Colyar, M. (2004). Newborn screening tests. *Advance for Nurse Practitioners, 12*(10), 22.

Cunningham, M., Cox, E.O. (2003). The Committee on Practice and Ambulatory Medicine, & the Section on Otolaryngology and Bronchoesophagology. Hearing assessment in infants and children: Recommendations beyond neonatal screening. *Pediatrics, 111*(3), 436-440.

Dann, M.H. (2005). The lactation consult: Problem solving, teaching, and support for the breastfeeding family. *J Pediatr Health Care, 19*(1), 12-16.

Davis, K.F., Parker, K.P., & Montgomery, G.L. (2004a). Sleep in infants and young children: Part One: Normal sleep. *J Pediatr Health Care, 18*(2), 65-71.

Davis, K.F., Parker, K.P., & Montgomery, G.L. (2004b). Sleep in infants and young children: Part Two: Common sleep problems. *J Pediatr Health Care, 18*(3), 130-137.

Denver Developmental Materials, Inc. (2006). Denver-II. Retrieved May 11, 2006, from www.denverii.com/DenverII.html.

Dion, S., & Stadtler, A. (2002). Age-specific observations of the parent-child interaction. In M. Jellinek, B.P. Patel, & M.C. Froehle (Eds.). *Bright futures in practice: Mental health,* Vol. II. Tool Kit. Arlington, VA: National Center for Education in Maternal and Child Health.

Fluoride Recommendations Workgroup. (2001). Recommendations for using fluoride to prevent and control dental caries in the United States. *MMWR, 50*(RR14), 1-42.

Glassy, D., Romano, J., & the American Academy of Pediatrics Committee on Early Childhood, Adoption, and Dependent Care. (2003). Selecting appropriate toys for young children: The pediatrician's role. *Pediatrics, 111*(4), 911-913.

Gottesman, M.M. (1999). Enabling parents to "read" their baby. *J Pediatr Health Care, 13*(3), 148-151.

Green, M., & Palfrey, J.S. (Eds.). (2002). *Bright futures: Guidelines for health supervision of infants, children, and adolescents* (2nd ed., rev.). Arlington, VA: National Center for Education in Maternal and Child Health.

Hill, N.H., & Sullivan, L.M. (2004). *Management guidelines for nurse practitioners working with children and adolescents* (2nd ed.). Philadelphia: F.A. Davis.

Hornor, G. (2006). Ano-genital herpes in children. *J Pediatr Health Care, 20*(2), 106-14.

Kemper, A.R., Cohn, L.M., Fant, K.E., et al. (2005). Follow-up testing among children with elevated screening blood lead levels. *JAMA, 293*(18), 2232-2237.

Kochanska, G., Friesenborg, A.E., Lange, L.A., et al. (2004). Parents' personality and infants' temperament as contributors to their emerging relationship. *J Personal Social Psychol, 86*(5), 44-59.

Kube, D.A., Wilson, W.M., Petersen, M.C., & Palmer, F.B. (2000). CAT/CLAMS: Its use in detecting early childhood cognitive impairment. *Pediatric Neurol, 23*(3), 208-215.

Leung, A.K.C., & Lemay, J.F. (2004). Infantile colic: A review. *J Royal Soc Health, 124*(4), 162-266.

Lobo, M.L., Kotzer, A.M., Keefe, M.R., et al. (2004). Current beliefs and management strategies for treating infant colic. *J Pediatr Health Care, 18*(3), 115-122.

Ludington-Hoe, S.M., Cong, O., & Hashemi, F. (2002). Infant crying: Nature, physiologic consequences, and select interventions. *Neonatal Netw, 21*(2), 29-36.

McCarthy, P.L. (2004). The well child. In R.E. Behrman, R.M. Kliegman, & H.B. Jenson (Eds.). *Nelson textbook of pediatrics* (17th ed.). Philadelphia: Saunders.

Moon, R.Y. (2001). Are you talking to patients about SIDS? *Contemp Pediatr, 18*(3), 122-129.

Muscari, M.E. (2000). *Advanced pediatric clinical assessment: Skills and procedures.* Philadelphia: Lippincott Williams & Wilkins.

National Association of Pediatric Nurse Practitioners. (2001). *Breastfeeding.* Retrieved January 8, 2006, from http://www.napnap.org/index.cfm?page=10&sec=54&ssec=57.

National Association of Pediatric Nurse Practitioners. (2003). *The PNP's role in supporting infant and family well-being during the first year of life.* Retrieved January 8, 2006, from http://www.napnap.org/index.cfm?page=10&sec=54&ssec=70.

Pohl, C.A., & Renwick, A. (2002). Putting sleep disturbances to rest. *Contemp Pediatr, 19*(11), 74-94.

Poppell, S.L. (2002). Bed-sharing with infants. *MCN, Am J Matern Child Nurs, 27*(3), 193.

Schwartz, R.H., & Guthrie, K.L. (2006). Clinical practice primer: Musings on infant swaddling. *Infect Dis Child, 19*(6). Retrieved October 24, 2006, from http://www.idinchildren.com/200606/frameset.asp?article=clinical.asp.

Shea, K.M. (2003). Pediatric exposure and potential toxicity of phthalate plasticizers. *Pediatrics, 111*(6), 1467-1474.

Shields, B.J., & Smith, G.A. (2006). Success in the prevention of infant walker-related injuries: An analysis of national data, 1990-2001. *Pediatrics, 117*(3), e452-e459.

Soltis, J. (2004). The signal functions of early infant crying. *Behavioral and Brain Sciences, 27*(4), 443-458.

Turner, R.B. (2005). New considerations in the treatment and prevention of rhinovirus infections. *Pediatr Ann, 34*(1), 53-57.

20 Preterm Infant Follow-up Care

MARY ENZMAN HAGEDORN

Select the best answer for each of the following questions:

1. An infant born at 24 weeks gestation is brought to your office for a well child visit. The infant is now 16 weeks chronological age. Neuromotor development follows a predictable sequence in premature infants that progress to 40 weeks corrected gestational age. The pediatric nurse practitioner understands that:
   A. Muscle tone proceeds cephalocaudally.
   B. Perfection of primary reflexes proceeds caudocephally.
   C. There is symmetrical positioning of the lower extremities.
   D. Generalized hypotonia progresses to flexion.

2. The most common cause of sepsis in the neonate is:
   A. *Escherichia coli.*
   B. *Streptococcus pneumoniae.*
   C. Herpes simplex virus.
   D. Group B streptococcal (GBS) infection.

3. The most reliable assessment tool for physical and neurologic maturity of the preterm, seriously ill, or fragile neonate is the:
   A. Dubowitz Scale.
   B. Denver II.
   C. Ballard Gestational Aging Scale
   D. Brazelton Neonatal Behavioral Assessment Scale.

4. Neonates at greatest risk for acquiring a systemic infection include those:

A. With intrauterine growth retardation.
B. Born to a diabetic mother.
C. Born preterm and with very low birth weight.
D. Born postterm and small for gestational age.

5. The nurse practitioner examining a preterm neonate with possible sepsis should order the most sensitive laboratory indicator which is:
   A. Total white blood cell count.
   B. Absolute neutrophil count.
   C. Absolute band count.
   D. Absolute eosinophil count.

6. Infants with respiratory distress syndrome may develop respiratory compromise within the first few hours after birth. Which of the following signs represent the neonate's attempt to increase end-expiratory pressure in the earlier stages of respiratory distress syndrome?
   A. Tachypnea.
   B. Nasal flaring.
   C. Retractions.
   D. Expiratory grunting.

7. Chronic lung disease (CLD)/bronchopulmonary dysplasia (BPD) in premature infants is caused by:
   A. Respiratory distress and impaired gas exchange.
   B. Oxygen toxicity and barotraumas from pressure ventilation.
   C. Viral infections after birth.
   D. Bacterial infections after birth.

8. Which of the following infants are susceptible to respiratory syncytial virus (RSV) and bronchitis in the first year of life?
   A. Very low birth weight infants.
   B. Term infant with chronic rhinitis.
   C. Term infant with hypospadias.
   D. 38-week gestation infant with feeding problems.

9. The most common cause of apnea of prematurity is:
   A. Idiopathic.
   B. Gastroesophageal reflux.
   C. Tracheal malacia.
   D. Hypoxia.

10. The most common cardiac lesion in the premature infant is:
   A. Patent ductus arteriosus.
   B. Truncus.
   C. Transposition of great vessels.
   D. Aortic stenosis.

11. Necrotizing enterocolitis (NEC) is characterized by which of the following?
   A. A destructive infection of the small bowel.
   B. Abnormal air passage.
   C. Edema and bleeding into intestines.
   D. Frequent gastrointestinal infections.

12. Which of the following is the central factor responsible for respiratory distress syndrome in the newborn?
   A. Deficient surfactant production.
   B. Overproduction of surfactant.
   C. Pneumothorax.
   D. Absence of alveoli.

13. A newborn is diagnosed with retinopathy of prematurity (ROP). The pediatric nurse practitioner should know that:
   A. No treatment is currently available.
   B. Cryotherapy and laser therapy are effective treatments for preventing retinal detachment.
   C. Long-term sequelae result from the amount of oxygen toxicity to the optic nerve.
   D. Vitamins C and D are critical to the treatment of ROP.

14. Which of the following statements is MOST accurate about premature infants and genitourinary complications?
   A. Inguinal hernias are more common in male infants with a history of prematurity .
   B. Undescended testicles are not common in premature infants.
   C. Hypospadias is more common in premature infants.
   D. Hydroceles are less common in premature infants because of the small internal rings of the inguinal canal.

15. Factors that lead to anemia in premature infants include which of the following?
   A. Higher iron stores and lower erythropoietin production.
   B. Higher erythropoietin production and gastrointestinal bleeding.
   C. Frequent blood sampling and poor weight gain.
   D. Frequent blood sampling and lower iron stores.

16. The primary goal for families and infants in premature infant follow-up programs is:
   A. Regimented medical follow-up to prevent complications.
   B. Normalization of the family.
   C. Education and developmental follow-up in a controlled environment.
   D. Reinforcement of hospital discharge programs.

17. Preterm infants are predisposed to more frequent respiratory infections. What signs and symptoms would alert the pediatric nurse practitioner that a preterm infant is developing RSV?
   A. Wheezing, rhinorrhea, cough, low-grade fever.
   B. Stridor, drooling, high fever.
   C. Wheezing, tachycardia, high fever.
   D. Cough, rhinorrhea, intermittent fever.

18. Which of the following is true regarding hearing assessments for preterm infants?
   A. A repeat of the brainstem auditory-evoked response test is indicated every 6 months.

B. Brainstem auditory-evoked response should be repeated at 3 to 4 months of age.
C. Tympanometry is not indicated in the preterm infant.
D. An audiology visit is indicated every 6 months.

19. What is the LEAST accurate statement regarding immunizations in the preterm infant?
   A. The schedule is the same as for the term neonate.
   B. No live virus immunizations should be given because of the immaturity of the preterm infant's immune system.
   C. Synagist is indicated for preterm infants up to 2 years of age during the respiratory season.
   D. Influenza vaccine is indicated for preterm infants older than 6 months.

20. Gastroesophageal reflux (GER) often presents in the preterm infant with which of the following symptoms?
   A. Apnea, bradycardia, pneumonia, and worsening respiratory illness.
   B. Decreased apnea and tachycardia.
   C. Worsening respiratory illness and projectile vomiting.
   D. Apnea, bradycardia, and intermittent diarrhea.

21. Pharmacologic treatment of GER in the preterm infant may include all of the following medications EXCEPT:
   A. Furosemide.
   B. Metoclopramide.
   C. Ranitidine.
   D. Omeprazole.

22. The incidence of intraventricular hemorrhage (IVH) in very low birth weight infants is:
   A. 30% to 50%.
   B. less than 10%.
   C. over 50%.
   D. 17% to 59%.

23. Long-term neurologic sequelae of IVH include:
   A. Seizures, hydrocephalus, cerebral palsy, and developmental delays.
   B. Developmental delays, increased photosensitivity, and apnea.
   C. Seizures and cardiac defects.
   D. GER and seizures.

ANSWERS

1. *Answer:* D
   Rationale: Newborns born before 28 weeks gestation have complete hypotonia of the upper and lower extremities. As the neonate matures and nears term, the tone and posture are predominately flexion of the upper and lower extremities.

2. *Answer:* D
   Rationale: GBS infection is the leading cause of sepsis in neonates with an incidence of 1 to 8 cases per 100 live births.

3. *Answer:* C
   Rationale: The Dubowitz Scale is used to estimate gestational age. The Denver II is a screening tool evaluating fine motor and gross motor development, and social and language skills in healthy infants and children. The Ballard Gestational Aging Scale is used to assess the physical and neurologic maturity of the infant. The Brazelton Assessment Scale assesses neonatal behavior.

4. *Answer:* C
   Rationale: Multiple factors have been associated with the increased risk of infection during the neonatal period. The most important factors are preterm birth and maternal conditions that may predispose the neonate to infection. The more preterm the infant and the lower the birth weight, the higher the risk of infection and the more immature and ineffective the immune system.

5. *Answer:* B
   Rationale: When the presence of infection is recognized, the bone marrow begins to produce neutrophils, first in the immature form, to provide a defense against invading organisms.

6. *Answer:* D
   Rationale: The expiratory grunt is a useful mechanism that increases alveolar expansion to allow gas exchange. Tachypnea, nasal flaring, and retractions are later signs of respiratory distress.

7. *Answer:* B
   Rationale: Chronic lung disease (CLD)/bronchopulmonary dysplasia (BPD) is caused by oxygen toxicity and barotraumas. This condition is characterized by the development of respiratory distress and impaired gas exchange. Treatment for this condition is long-term supplemental oxygen therapy.

8. *Answer:* A
   Rationale: Very low birth weight infants are highly susceptible to RSV and bronchitis in the first year of life and can have catastrophic outcomes if this occurs.

9. *Answer:* A
   Rationale: About 23% of preterm infants will have apnea and most cases are idiopathic in origin.

10. *Answer:* A
    Rationale: The most common congenital heart defect in the premature infant is the patent ductus arteriosus.

11. *Answer:* A
    Rationale: NEC is a destructive infection of the small bowel and not an obstructive disease process of the bowel.

12. *Answer:* A
    Rationale: IRDS is a result of insufficient surfactant production.

13. *Answer:* B
    Rationale: Cryotherapy and laser therapy are critical treatments for prevention of retinal detachment.

14. *Answer:* A
    Rationale: The incidence of inguinal hernias in very low birth weight and extremely low birth weight infants is 30%, and 10% to 50% of these are bilateral.

15. *Answer:* D
    Rationale: Lower iron stores and frequent blood sampling are the leading causes of anemia in the premature infant. Compared to term infants, premature infants also have a lower erythropoietin production. A preterm

infant with anemia may show signs of tachycardia, poor feeding, low weight gain, and apnea with bradycardia.

16. *Answer:* B
    Rationale: The primary goal of infant follow-up programs is normalization.

17. *Answer:* A
    Rationale: The key signs that a preterm infant is developing RSV are: wheezing, rhinorrhea, cough, and low-grade fever.

18. *Answer:* B
    Rationale: Brainstem auditory-evoked response is recommended to be repeated at 3 to 4 months of age. Tympanometry and acoustic reflex should be tested at every visit with a preterm infant to determine presence of serous otitis and hearing loss.

19. *Answer:* B
    Rationale: There is no indication to restrict live virus vaccines in the preterm infant.

20. *Answer:* A
    Rationale: GER most commonly presents with increased apnea, bradycardia, pneumonia, or worsening BPD/CLD.

21. *Answer:* A
    Rationale: Furosemide is a diuretic and not used to treat GER. The three medications, Metaclopramide a GI smooth muscle stimulant, Omeprazole a gastric acid pump inhibitor, and Ranitidine a H_2 agonist, have been used to treat GER in the premature infant.

22. *Answer:* A
    Rationale: IVH in very low birth weight infants ranges from 30% to 50% with sequelae in 17% to 23%.

23. *Answer:* A
    Rationale: Neurologic sequelae includes seizures, hydrocephalus, cerebral palsy, and mental retardation, as well as developmental delays.

BIBLIOGRAPHY

Allen, E.C., Manuel, J.C., Legault, C., et al. (2004). Perception of child vulnerability among mothers of former premature infants. *Pediatrics, 113*(2), 267-273.

Ambalabanan, N., Nelson, K.G., Alexander, G., et al. (2000). Prediction of neurologic morbidity in extremely low birth weight infants. *J Perinatol, 20*(8), 496-503.

American Academy of Pediatrics Committee on Infectious Diseases and Committee on Fetus and Newborn. (2003). Revised indications for the use of palivizumab and respiratory syncytial virus immune globulin intravenous for the prevention of respiratory syncytial virus infections. *Pediatrics, 112*(6 Pt 1), 1442-1446.

American Academy of Pediatrics. Joint Committee on Infant Hearing. (2000). Position statement: Principles and guidelines for early hearing detection and intervention programs. *Pediatrics, 106*(4), 798-817.

Atkuri, L.V., & Ferguson, L.E. (2006). Pediatrics, pneumonia. Retrieved on April 1, 2006, from http://www.emedicine.com/emerg/topic396.htm.

Bensard, D., Calkins, C., Patrick, D., & Price, F. (2002). Neonatal surgery. In G. Merenstein & S. Gardner (Eds.). *Handbook of neonatal intensive care* (5th ed.). St. Louis: Mosby.

Centers for Disease Control and Prevention. (2006). 2000 growth charts: United States. Retrieved April 1, 2006, from www.cdc.gov/growthcharts.

Daley, H., & Kennedy, C. (2000). Meta-analysis: Effects of interventions in premature infant feeding. *J Perinatal Neonatal Nurs, 14*(3), 62-70.

Deloian, B. (2002). The premature infant. In J. Fox (Ed.). *Primary health care of infants, children, & adolescents.* St. Louis: Mosby.

Dzinkowkski, R.C. (2000). Symptoms and signs of cerebral palsy if present in infants and toddlers. Retrieved June 6, 2006, from www.geocities.com/aneecp/symptoms.htm.

Originally published as: Dzinkowkski, R.C., Smith, K.K., Dillow, K.A., & Yucha, C.B. (1996). Cerebral palsy: A comprehensive review. *Nurse Pract, 21*(2), 45-59.

Ehrenkranz, R.A., Younes, N., Lemons, J.A., et al. (1999). Longitudinal growth of hospitalized very low birth weight infants. *Pediatrics, 104*(2 Pt 1), 280-289.

Hagedorn, M., Gardner, S., & Abman, S. (2002). Respiratory diseases. In G. Merenstein & S.

Gardner (Eds.). *Handbook of neonatal intensive care* (5th ed.). St. Louis: Mosby.

Kilbride, H.W., Thorstad, K., & Daily, D.K. (2004). Preschool outcome of less than 801-gram preterm infants compared with full-term siblings. *Pediatrics, 113*(4), 742-747.

Kirmani, K.I., Lofthus, G., Pichichero, M.E., Voloshen, T., et al. (2002). Seven-year follow-up of vaccine response in extremely premature infants. *Pediatrics, 109*(3), 498-504.

March of Dimes PeriStats. (2006). Retrieved April 1, 2006, from www.marchofdimes.com/peristats/pdflib/195/99.pdf.

Meissner, H.C., Long, S.S., & American Academy of Pediatrics Committee on Infectious Diseases and Committee on Fetus and Newborn. (2003). Revised indications for the use of palivizumab and respiratory syncytial virus immune globulin intravenous for the prevention of respiratory syncytial virus infections. *Pediatrics, 112*(6 Pt 1), 1447-1452.

Nadeau, L., Tessier, R., Lefebvre, F., & Robaey, P. (2004). Victimization: a newly recognized outcome of prematurity. *Devel Med Child Neurol, 46*(8), 508-513.

National Eye Institute. (2005). Retinopathy of prematurity. Retrieved April 1, 2006, from www.nei.nih.gov/health/rop/index.asp#5.

Ritchie, S.K. (2002). Primary care of the premature infant discharged from the neonatal intensive care unit. *MCN, Am J Matern Child Nurs, 27*(2), 76-85.

Wood, N.S., Marlow, N., Costeloe, K., et al. (2000). Neurologic and developmental disability after extreme preterm birth. EPIcure Study Group. *N Engl J Med, 343*(6), 378-384.

NOTES

21 Child Abuse and Neglect

MARYANNE C. MURRAY

Select the best answer for each of the following questions:

1. According to the Federal Child Abuse Prevention and Treatment Act (CAPTA), child abuse and neglect are parent/caregiver acts of omission or commission which cause a child to suffer harm resulting in:
   A. Death, serious physical or emotional harm, sexual abuse, or exploitation.
   B. Death, psychiatric or physical disability, sexual confusion, or profiteering.
   C. Death, serious sexual abuse, physical sequelae, or sexual confusion.
   D. Death, serious depression, sexual abuse, academic disinterest, or physical pain.

2. Two-year-old Ann and her 9-month-old brother Cruz are brought to the pediatric clinic for their respective well child checks. Which of the following would alert you to search for evidence of neglect?
   A. The children have not had their baths today and their clothing bears remnants of their breakfasts.
   B. Ann and Cruz are both in the 95th percentile for weight and the 50th to 75th percentile for their height/length.
   C. Ann and Cruz have no socks, jackets, or hats despite the snowfall and subfreezing weather.
   D. Ann and Cruz have dropped from the 5th to the 10th percentile for weight to the 5th percentile for weight since their last well child checks 3 months ago.

3. Three-year-old Robert's mother brings him to the pediatric clinic for symptoms of upper respiratory infection. In the process of physical examination, Robert flinches as the stethoscope is placed for auscultation of the lungs. The pediatric nurse practitioner raises Robert's shirt and sees multiple contusions on his scapulae and over the spine, which could constitute evidence of:
   A. Parental noncompliance.
   B. Caregiver commission of abuse.
   C. Sibling rivalry.
   D. Robert's clumsiness.

4. After visualizing Robert's contusions, the pediatric nurse practitioner's first action should be to:
   A. Tell Robert's mother that she is abusing her son.
   B. Call child protective services.
   C. Call the police.
   D. Ask how the injuries were incurred.

5. Which statement is true regarding gender-related statistics on the issue of child maltreatment?
   A. Females are more likely than males to be victimized.
   B. Males are more likely than females to be victimized.
   C. Older female siblings are more likely than their younger male siblings to be victimized.
   D. There is no difference between females and males in the rates of victimization.

6. The most prevalent form of child maltreatment in severe cases requiring child protective services' attention is:
   A. Sexual abuse.

B. Neglect.
C. Physical abuse.
D. Emotional abuse.

7. Historically, child maltreatment is:
A. A new phenomenon in the past generation.
B. Evident in literature of the past century.
C. An invention of the ancient Romans to deal with unwanted children.
D. Probably a phenomenon since before recorded history.

8. A landmark case which set precedent for terminating parental rights of child abusers was the case of:
A. Oliver Twist in 1839.
B. David Copperfield in 1851.
C. Estella Havisham in 1861.
D. Mary Ellen McCormick in 1874.

9. The strategy by which this legal precedent was set to protect abused children was:
A. Intervention by the Society for the Prevention of Cruelty to Animals on the basis that a child could be considered an animal.
B. Assistance by the Red Cross who championed the causes of people victimized by tragedy.
C. Support from the American Civil Liberties Union who argued that the child's rights were being violated.
D. A decree issued by the World Council of Churches who decried all child-rearing practices which demeaned the dignity of children and/or their parents.

10. In 20th-century America, literature on "Battered Child Syndrome" was published and mandatory reporting laws were created in all 50 states in the:
A. 1920s.
B. 1940s.
C. 1960s.
D. 1980s.

11 A new risk to the well-being of children came about in the late 20th century and early 21st century with the popularity of home computers and Internet connections. Use of Internet chat rooms without adequate parental supervision has made children and youths vulnerable to many evils, the MOST dangerous of which is:
A. Exposure to predators who try to arrange in-person meetings for devious purposes.
B. Opportunities to cheat on homework.
C. Term papers available for purchase.
D. Materials which are inappropriate for the age of the receiving child.

12. In comparison to parents and caregivers who do not abuse or neglect children, those with the following traits are more likely to be perpetrators of abuse or neglect:
A. Older, experienced, nondrinking, churchgoing adults who have strict behavioral expectations.
B. Younger, experienced, nondrinking adults with significant stressors.
C. Older, inexperienced, substance-abusing adults with low-stress lifestyles.
D. Younger, inexperienced adults with substance abuse problems and high stress.

13. Research has revealed certain characteristics of children who are statistically more likely to be abused than those who lack these traits. Among these high-risk factors are:
A. Eagerly anticipated birth, preferred gender, named after a beloved relative, and hyperactivity.
B. Pregnancy achieved after high-tech conception, financial resources depleted, and precipitate delivery.
C. Unwanted pregnancy and difficult delivery, congenital anomalies, and unusual temperament.
D. Problem pregnancy, sunny disposition, and easy bonding with parent.

14. Long-term sequelae of child maltreatment include:
A. Personality disorders, mood disorders, reactive attachment disorder, and mood disturbances.
B. Reactive personality disorder, mood attachment disorder, mood disturbances, and diminished earning potential.

C. Reactive mood disturbances, diminished earning potential, personality disorders, and career role confusion.
D. Reactive attachment disorder, career role confusion, diminished earning potential, and personality disturbance.

15. Which of these children's presentations should alert a provider to the likelihood of abuse?
A. Two-month-old with contusions on her scapulae.
B. Eighteen-month-old with contusions on his forehead.
C. Three-year-old with contusions on her shins.
D. Four-year-old with abrasions on bilateral knees.

16. Angelina is a 12-year-old female whose mother brings her to the clinic for an exam after Angelina told her earlier today that an adult male new to the neighborhood was "messing with her." Angelina's mother's first reaction was to bring Angelina to the clinic, and she expressed great concern that the child may have "lost her virginity." No call to the police has been made as of this time. As you plan your care, you are aware that:
A. You do not want to call the police because there is a chance you could be wrong about this being abuse; Angelina may have consented to sexual activity with this man.
B. You must now perform a complete investigation including detailed interview about all related events, a physical examination, and photography of any injuries you may find, and you must hold this evidence in the chart until Angelina's mother decides what she wants to do about it.
C. You are very upset that Angelina's mother has failed to supervise her adequately, so you make the police report with some embellishment, knowing that you are immune to prosecution for false reporting.
D. You are a mandated reporter and required by law to report to the police

whenever you have reasonable suspicion, based on your training and experience, to believe that abuse or neglect may have occurred.

17. Because Angelina indicates she is having a great deal of discomfort "down there," and she is very fearful of exposing her "privates" to anyone, you consider the appropriate course of action and:
A. Insist that she immediately disrobe for you to conduct an examination, hoping your memory will serve you well in remembering what sorts of things to look for.
B. Refer her to a local gynecologist; you place the call and obtain an appointment for 3 weeks from now.
C. Refer her to the local hospital emergency department where they have a colposcope and the providers are experienced in working with such cases.
D. Advise Angelina's mother that Angelina has probably fabricated the story, as evidenced by her refusal to be examined.

18. According to the United States Department of Health and Human Services (2003) report, in confirmed cases of child abuse, what type of abuse is most frequently reported?
A. Neglect
B. Physical
C. Sexual
D. Emotional

19. Many non-organic causes of failure to thrive (FTT) are directly related to:
A. Maternal depression.
B. Infant sleep cycles.
C. Availability of high calorie, high fat, processed food products.
D. Unapproved child-rearing practices.

20. Examination of a young child's genitals should take place:
A. Only when the parents, caregivers, or police request it.
B. Whenever the child indicates someone has touched him or her.

C. Routinely as part of each physical exam.
D. Only when the genitalia are bleeding or painful.

21. Which statement is true regarding females and their hymens?
   A. Every girl is born with a hymen.
   B. Every hymen has an opening by the time of birth.
   C. Horseback riding may completely destroy a girl's hymen.
   D. Inflammation of the hymenal tissue is an absolute indicator of sexual abuse.

22. When following up on a possible or probable indicator of child sexual abuse in 5-year-old Annette, your examination includes:
   A. Visual inspection of the external genitalia being careful not to actually touch the labia.
   B. Visual inspection of the external genitalia with gentle separation of the labia majora.
   C. Visual inspection of the external genitalia and insertion of two fingers into the vagina to determine its compliance.
   D. Insertion of a pediatric speculum without inspection of the external genitalia.

23. Which 3-year-old patient presenting for a well child check would be of greatest concern to the pediatric nurse practitioner?
   A. European American Jane who has purple macular lesions on her scapulae.
   B. Asian American Tui who has multiple erythematous linear abrasions on her back.
   C. African American Donn'Tae who has three 1 to 2 cm nummular clusters of vesicular lesions on his left arm.
   D. Hispanic American Pedro who has irregularly shaped steel-blue macular lesions on his buttocks.

NOTES

ANSWERS

1. *Answer:* A
   Rationale: Sexual confusion, profiteering, and academic disinterest are not known to result from child maltreatment.

2. *Answer:* C
   Rationale: Lack of a daily bath or robust weight would not constitute neglect. A drop in weight percentile group may be a cause for concern and require intervention, but would not indicate neglect. Lack of clothing appropriate for the weather requires further investigation as it could cause serious bodily harm to the children.

3. *Answer:* B
   Rationale: If Robert was clumsy, it would more likely be reflected in contusions on his legs than his back. If his siblings were inflicting such contusions on him, caregiver supervision would be inadequate. Parental noncompliance is a distracter.

4. *Answer:* D
   Rationale: It is inappropriate to accuse a parent or caregiver of child maltreatment without investigating the cause and mechanism of the injuries. Calls to the police and child protective services may be warranted, but only after the parent and child are given an opportunity to explain how the injury occurred. If the story told is inconsistent with the injury or if the story changes, then the phone calls should be made to authorities.

5. *Answer:* D
   Rationale: The literature reveals child abuse cases are equally distributed by gender.

6. *Answer:* B
   Rationale: Neglect is the prevailing issue in the majority of case reports as well as child maltreatment fatalities.

7. *Answer:* D
   Rationale: Issues of child maltreatment have received more popular attention over the past century than in earlier times. Enduring of childhood hardships was a popular theme of nineteenth-century British and American literature. Roman history indicates infanticide was an acknowledged practice, but its origins are unknown and likely predate literature upon the subject.

8. *Answer:* D
   Rationale: Twist, Copperfield, and Havisham are all fictional characters created by Charles Dickens whose themes often included overcoming childhood hardships. Mary Ellen McCormick was a real child in New York. Her stepmother's beatings came to the attention of outsiders who sought to rescue the girl from this maltreatment.

9. *Answer:* A
   Rationale: The New York SPCA advocated for Mary Ellen McCormick because no laws existed to protect children at that time. Even today, children have relatively few legal rights compared with those of adults. The other answers are distracters.

10. *Answer:* C
    Rationale: It happened in the 1960s, with the 1961 publication of an article in the *Journal of the American Medical Association*. Between 1963 and 1968, all of the American states had enacted laws regarding mandatory reporting by health care providers.

11. *Answer:* A
    Rationale: News reports tell of children and youths who were lured into online "relationships" with adults who posed as the youths' peers and who persuaded the youths to take great personal risks, such as travelling long distances, without parental knowledge. Cheating and plagiarism, like many other dishonest activities, have been facilitated by the Internet, but generally do not pose direct risks to the well-being of children. Pornography, another risk, may cause psychological harm.

12. *Answer:* D
    Rationale: Perpetration of child maltreatment is correlated with youth and/or inexperience of parents, substance abuse, stress, depression, intimate partner violence, and experience of victimization in childhood.

13. *Answer:* C
    Rationale: Highly desired birth, gender, name association, high-tech conception, and precipitate delivery have not been correlated with child abuse victimization. Sunny dispo-

sition and easy bonding are protective factors.

14. *Answer:* A

Rationale: Personality disorders, mood disorders, reactive attachment disorder, and mood disturbances are the correct identifiers of the psychiatric issues which may result from child maltreatment. The other answers are fabricated diagnoses, e.g., mood attachment disorder.

15. *Answer:* A

Rationale: Developmental stages and mobility of the child aid in the determination of whether an injury could be self-inflicted or accidental. A 2-month-old baby does not have mobility sufficient to sustain an injury to the trunk. The other children mentioned have injuries consistent with their ambulatory skills.

16. *Answer:* D

Rationale: The pediatric nurse practitioner is a mandated reporter and must act on that mandate. Even if Angelina had agreed to sexual activity, the age difference between her and the alleged perpetrator would constitute criminal activity on his part. It would not be up to the parent to determine whether the police were to be contacted. A provider is immune to prosecution for reporting when she or he has reasonable suspicion, but a falsified report would not have immunity from consequences.

17. *Answer:* C

Rationale: When a pediatric patient needs such an exam and specialty forensic services are unavailable, a referral to the emergency department is appropriate, especially if there are acute injuries. It is not unusual for a child to resist examination of a painful body part, and modesty is naturally an issue for a 12-year-old girl.

18. *Answer:* A

Rationale: The United States Department of Health and Human Services (2003) reported that 61% of the cases of confirmed child abuse cases were neglect; physical abuse accounted for 19%, sexual abuse was 10%, and emotional abuse was 5%.

19. *Answer:* A

Rationale: Maternal depression is the root cause of many deficits in parenting. Impoverished environment may result from maternal depression. Food products, sleep cycles, and child-rearing practices are distracters.

20. *Answer:* C

Rationale: Examination of the young child's genitalia is a routine part of health surveillance.

21. *Answer:* A

Rationale: A hymen is present in every normal female baby. An imperforate hymen is an abnormality which requires surgical intervention. Option C is an old myth. Inflammation of the hymen (vulvovaginitis) has many causes.

22. *Answer:* B

Rationale: One cannot fully visualize the external genitalia without separating the labia majora. Visualization would occur before insertion of vaginal speculum.

23. *Answer:* A

Rationale: Jane's lesions on her scapulae are in an unusual place for contusions. Tui likely has undergone coining. Donn'Tae's vesicular clusters are probably impetigo. Pedro has Mongolian spots which are common to people with dark skin. It is important for the pediatric nurse practitioner to have knowledge of the ethnic and cultural customs in the community where he or she practices.

BIBLIOGRAPHY

Care, M. (2002). Imaging in suspected child abuse: What to expect and what to order. *Pediatr Ann, 31*(10), 651-659.

Christian, C.W., Lavelle, J.M., De Jong, A.R., et al. (2000). Forensic evidence findings in prepubertal victims of sexual assault. *Pediatrics, 106*(6, No. 1, Pt 1), 100-104.

Conway, M., Mendelson, M., Giannopoulos, C., et al. (2004). Childhood and adult sexual abuse, rumination on sadness, and dysphoria. *Child Abuse Negl, 28*(4), 393-410.

Daria, S., Sugar, N., Feldman, K., et al. (2004). Into hot water head first: Distribution of intentional and unintentional immersion burns. *Pediatr Emerg Care, 20*(5), 302-310.

Department of Health and Human Services (HHS) (U.S.). (2005). Administration on Children, Youth, and Families (ACF). Child maltreatment 2003 [online]. Washington (DC): Government Printing Office. Retrieved April 5, 2005, from www.acf.hhs.gov/programs/cb/pubs/cm03/index.htm.

Dubowitz, H. (Ed.) (1999). *Neglected children*. Thousand Oaks, CA: Sage Publications.

Dubowitz, H. (2002). Preventing child neglect and physical abuse: A role for pediatricians. *Pediatr Rev, 23*(6), 191-196.

Dubowitz, H., Giardino, A., & Gustavson, E. (2000). Child neglect: Guidance for pediatricians. *Pediatr Rev, 21*(4), 111-116.

Elvik, S.L. (1998). Child maltreatment. In T.E. Soud & J.S. Rogers (Eds.). *Manual of pediatric emergency nursing*. St. Louis: Mosby.

Feldman, K.W. (1997). Evaluation of physical abuse. In M.E. Helfer, et al. (Eds.). *The battered child* (5th ed.). Chicago: University of Chicago Press.

Flaherty, E.G., & Sege, R. (2005). Barriers to physician identification and reporting of child abuse. *Pediatr Ann, 34*(5), 349-356.

Giardino, A.P., & Finkel, M.A. (2005). Evaluating child sexual abuse. *Pediatr Ann, 34*(5), 382-394.

Hettiaratchy, S., & Dziewulski, P. (2004). ABC of burns: Pathophysiology and types of burns. *BMJ, 328*(7453), 1427-1429.

Hornor, G. (2004). Sexual behavior in children: Normal or not? *J Pediatr Health Care, 18*(2), 57-64.

Hornor, G. (2005). Physical abuse: Recognition and reporting. *J Pediatr Health Care, 19*(1), 4-11.

Jackson, S. (2004). A USA national survey of program services provided by child advocacy centers. *Child Abuse Negl, 28*(4), 411-421.

Kellogg, N. & the AAP Committee on Child Abuse and Neglect. (2005). The evaluation of sexual abuse in children. *Pediatrics, 116*(2), 506-512.

Kempe, C.H., Silverman, F.N., Steele, B.F., et al. (1962). Landmark article July 7, 1962: The battered-child syndrome. *JAMA, 251*(4), 3288-3294.

Leder, M., Knight, J., & Emans, S. (2001). Sexual abuse: Management strategies and legal issues. *Contemp Pediatr, 18,* 77-92.

Leder, M., Knight, J., & Emans, S. (2001). Sexual abuse: When to suspect it, how to assess for it. *Contemp Pediatr, 18,* 59-76.

Maguire, S., Mann, M., & Kemp, A. (2005). Are there patterns of bruising in childhood which are diagnostic or suggestive of abuse? A systematic review. *Arch Dis Child, 90*(2), 182-186.

McColgan, M.D., & Giardino, A.P. (2005). Internet poses multiple risks to children and adolescents. *Pediatr Ann, 34*(5), 406- 414.

Mudd, S., & Findlay, J. (2004). The cutaneous manifestations and common mimickers of physical child abuse. *J Pediatr Health Care, 18*(3), 123-129.

Nelms, B. (2003). Keeping children safe: Protecting children from sexual abuse. *J Pediatr Health Care, 17*(6), 275-276.

Oaksford, K., & Frude, N. (2003). The process of coping following child sexual abuse: A qualitative study. *J Child Sex Abus, 12*(2), 41-72.

Reece, R.M., & Sege, R. (2000). Childhood head injuries: Accidental or inflicted? *Arch Pediatr Adolesc Med, 154*(1), 11-15.

Rubin, D.M., Christian, C.W., Bilaniuk, L.T., et al. (2003). Occult head injury in high-risk abused children. *Pediatrics, 111*(6, Pt.1), 1382-1386

Scheid, J. (2003). Recognizing and managing long-term sequelae of childhood maltreatment. *Pediatr Ann, 32*(6), 391-401.

Schreier, H. (2002). Munchausen by proxy defined. *Pediatrics, 110*(5), 985-988.

Shanel-Hogan, K. (2004). What is this red mark? *J Calif Dent Assoc, 32*(4), 304-305.

Sinal, S., Petree, A., Harman-Giddens, M., et al. (2000). Is race or ethnicity a predictive factor in Shaken Baby Syndrome? *Child Abuse Negl,* 24(9), 1241-1246.

Spataro, J., Mullen, P., Burgess, P., et al. (2004). Impact of child sexual abuse on mental health: Prospective study in males and females. *Br J Psychiatry, 184,* 416-421.

Straus, M.A. (1994). Beating the devil out of them: Corporal punishment in American families. San Francisco: Jossey-Bass Publisher.

Thompson, S. (2005). Accidental or inflicted? *Pediatr Ann, 34*(5), 372-381.

Trenchs, V., Curcoy, A., Pou, J., et al. (2005). Retinal haemorrhages as proof of abusive head injury. *J Pediatr, 146*(3), 437-438.

Turner, J., & Reid, S. (2002). Munchausen's syndrome. *Lancet, 359*(9303), 346-349.

Tyler, K., Whitebeck, L., Hoyt, D., & Cauce, A. (2004). Risk factors for sexual victimization among male and female homeless and runaway youth. *J Interpers Violence, 19*(5), 503-520.

U.S. Department of Health & Human Services (HHS) (2003). Child maltreatment 2001: Reports from the states to the national child abuse and neglect data system. Washington, DC: U.S. Government Printing Office.

van As, A.B., Kalebka, R.R., van der Heyde Y. (2006). Animal attacks: A red herring of child abuse? *S Afr Med J, 96*(3), 184-186.

Walker, J., Carey, P., Mohr, N., et al. (2004). Gender differences in the prevalence of childhood sexual abuse and in the development of pediatric PTSD. *Arch Womens Ment Health, 7*(2), 111-121.

Westcott, H., & Jones, D. (1999). The abuse of disabled children. *J Child Psychol Psychiatry, 40*(4), 497-506.

22 Toddlers, Preschoolers, and School-agers

MARIAILIANA STARK

Select the best answer for each of the following questions:

1. NAPNAP recently released evidence-based guidelines for identifying and preventing overweight in children. Which of the following statements regarding nutrition and exercise for an infant is NOT correct?
   A. Breastfeeding throughout the first year of life is strongly encouraged.
   B. Delay introduction of solids until at least 9 months of age.
   C. Tummy time and floor time is encouraged.
   D. Counsel parents to avoid TV and all forms of screen time for children younger than 2 years.

2. Christa is a 2-year-old child who comes into the clinic for a well child exam. Which one of the following activities would NOT be an expectation for her age group?
   A. Build a tower of 10 blocks.
   B. Walk up stairs.
   C. Point to body parts.
   D. Put on clothing.

3. Willie is a 2-year-old child here at your clinic for his well child exam. His parents want to know when to start toilet training. Which of the following is NOT an indicator for toilet training readiness in a 2-year-old?
   A. The child is able to signal the need to toilet.
   B. The child can delay voiding for at least 2 hours.
   C. The child can follow one-step commands.
   D. The child can jump in place.

4. Routine blood pressure should be measured at well child visits, beginning at what age?
   A. 18 months.
   B. 2 years.
   C. 3 years.
   D. 4 years.

5. Which of the following statements is NOT correct regarding Early Childhood Guidelines for Nutrition and Activity?
   A. Parents are responsible for what, when, and where they eat.
   B. Children are responsible for whether they eat and how much they eat.
   C. Television viewing is recommended during mealtimes and bedtime.
   D. Limit fast foods to no more than 2 times week.

6. When performing a physical exam on a toddler, which aspect of the exam would you examine last?
   A. Head and eyes.
   B. Heart and lungs.
   C. Ears and mouth.
   D. Hips and extremities.

7. Which of the following is a common feature of 2-year-old behavior?
   A. Temper tantrums.
   B. Stranger anxiety.
   C. Interactive play.
   D. Fascinated with different parts of the body.

8. A mother is asking you at what age the anterior fontanelle usually closes. Your response is:

A. 2 to 4 months.
B. 4 to 6 months.
C. 9 to 18 months.
D. 2 to 3 years.

9. Which of the following statements is NOT included in the evidence-based guidelines for nutrition and activities related to the school-age child age group?
A. Limit 100% fruit juice to 4 to 6 oz. or less each day; avoid fruit drinks and soda.
B. Participate in 60 minutes of intermittent moderate to vigorous physical activity daily.
C. Limit television and screen time to less than 2 hours a day.
D. Skip breakfast if child is overweight.

10. Recommendations for a routine preventive health care exam of a 3-year-old include assessment of growth, development, and:
A. BMI for age and gender, blood pressure, vision and hearing screening, immunizations if behind, assess tuberculosis risk and give PPD if indicated, and lead screening.
B. Head circumference measurement and metabolic screening.
C. Vision and hearing screening, head circumference measurement, and urinalysis.
D. Head circumference, anemia screening, and hearing and vision screening.

11. A 4-year-old preschool female child has been waking up with nightmares for the last month. Her physical exam is without incident. Her medical history is significant for tympanostomy tubes at 3 years of age. She will be starting preschool this year and her family is expecting a new sibling next month. What is the best response to the family regarding her sleeping issues?
A. It is abnormal for healthy preschool children to have nightmares.
B. Preschool children have more night terrors.
C. Preschool children do not dream.

D. Nightmares are common during the preschool years and during times of stress.

12. Which of the following skills would be beyond the developmental level of the 4-year-old child?
A. Copies a circle.
B. Can say his or her first and last name.
C. Pedals a tricycle.
D. Can count 15 objects.

13. Role playing with the equipment during the course of the physical exam would be most beneficial for which of the following age groups?
A. Toddlers.
B. Preschool-age children.
C. Young school-age children.
D. Older school-age children.

14. Cara, a 4-year-old female child, presents for a well child visit. Her visual acuity using the Allen Picture Cards was 20/50 OD. The best course of action would be:
A. Referral to an ophthalmologist for evaluation.
B. Retest in 3 months.
C. Nothing at this time, because results are normal for this age.
D. Retest in 1 year.

15. You are performing a cover-uncover test on a 4-year-old child. The uncovered eye deviates in when the opposite eye is covered. This is considered:
A. Exotropia.
B. Esophoria.
C. Esotropia.
D. Exophoria.

16. Which of the following blood pressure measurements would be normal in a 4-year-old?
A. 60/40
B. 75/50
C. 90/60
D. 110/80

17. Which of the following issues or concepts is relevant to the school-age child?
A. Operational thinking.

B. Initiative.
C. Concrete operational thinking.
D. Separation-individuation.

18. Which of the following diagnoses is NOT more common among males?
    A. ADHD.
    B. Conduct disorder.
    C. Suicide.
    D. Failure to thrive.

19. Which one of the following statements is true regarding lying and stealing in the school-age child?
    A. They are highly correlated with later criminal behavior.
    B. The child will grow out of it.
    C. They are usually associated with deep psychological problems.
    D. Represent a transient behavior problem.

20. Physiologic splitting of the second heart sound during inspiration in a child:
    A. Is normal.
    B. Should be evaluated with an EKG and ultrasound.
    C. Is suggestive of an arterial septal defect.
    D. Should be referred to a cardiologist.

21. Which of the following is the most important history-taking question for a sports evaluation?
    A. Has the child ever had a head injury?
    B. Has the child ever fainted or lost consciousness during exercise?
    C. Does the child ever get short of breath with exercise?
    D. Has the child ever had prior surgeries?

22. A 9-year-girl old who weighs 70 lbs. is asking why she cannot sit in the front passenger seat of the family car. Your best response is:

A. The safest place for a child younger than 12 years old or under 80 lbs. is in the center of the back seat of a car.
B. Children traveling in automobiles with side-releasing air bags are considered safe.
C. Deactivation of the passenger side airbags is advised if the child sits in front.
D. Booster seats are not recommended for school-age children.

23. Which of the following statements is NOT true for the school-age child?
    A. They will grow an average of 2 inches per year and gain 4.5 to 6.5 lbs. per year.
    B. The skull and brain grow very slowly.
    C. The blood pressure increases and the heart rate and respiratory rate decrease.
    D. Ossification and mineralization of bones are complete at this age.

24. According to Erikson's stages of psychosocial development, the school-age child is developing a:
    A. Sense of industry.
    B. Sense of initiative.
    C. Superego.
    D. Sense of competence.

25. Which of the following statements regarding the school-age child is NOT true?
    A. Forty percent of deaths among school-age children result from unintentional injuries.
    B. The death rate from homicide has nearly doubled in children this age.
    C. Dental problems are the least identified health problem.
    D. Children between 5 and 14 years of age have the lowest health care expenditures.

ANSWERS

1. *Answer:* B
   Rationale: Early introduction of mixed feeding is associated with early, excessive weight gain in infancy and overweight in childhood. Infants do not require foods other than breast milk or formula until 4 to 6 months of age.

2. *Answer:* A
   Rationale: A 2-year-old child can walk up the stairs step by step, put on some article of clothing, and can point to body parts. Most 2-year-olds can stack only six blocks.

3. *Answer:* D
   Rationale: Anticipatory guidance about toilet training should be introduced early to prevent unrealistic expectations and encourage a child's successful accomplishment of this milestone. Successful training requires physiologic and psychologic readiness to toilet train. At the 2-year well child exam, the pediatric nurse practitioner can discuss signs of toileting readiness.

4. *Answer:* C
   Rationale: The American Academy of Pediatrics (AAP) recommends measuring blood pressure in children every year beginning at 3 years of age.

5. *Answer:* C.
   Rationale: Children who spend more time with television are more likely to be overweight than children who do not. The more time a child watches television, the less likely he or she is to develop early reading skills.

6. *Answer:* C
   Rationale: Conduct examination using noninvasive to invasive sequence, auscultate heart and lung sounds first, and examine ears and mouth last.

7. *Answer:* A
   Rationale: Temper tantrums are a common age-related behavior in 2 to 3 year olds. They are thought to occur as a result of the toddler's progression toward self-reliance and independence. Stranger anxiety occurs between 8 to 10 months of age. Toddlers play side by side, but interaction is minimal.

8. *Answer:* C
   Rationale: The anterior fontanelle closes between 9 and 18 months of age. Early closure usually leads to synostosis. Late closure is commonly seen with increased intracranial pressure, hypothyroidism, rickets, syphilis, Down syndrome, and osteogenesis imperfecta.

9. *Answer:* D
   Rationale: Eating breakfast helps ensure the child's steady metabolic rate throughout the day, which decreases the likelihood he or she will become overweight. Eating breakfast is associated with better school performance and behavior.

10. *Answer:* A
    Rationale: AAP and Bright Futures has recommended services that should be provided throughout the age span of the well child visits. At 3 years of age, the following are included: History and physical examination, blood pressure, vision and hearing, and developmental screen. If the child is at risk, the following screens are done: anemia, lead screen, UA, PPD, and cholesterol. Immunizations are given as needed for catch up. Anticipatory guidance is given.

11. *Answer:* D
    Rationale: Nightmares tend to occur during the toddler years and peak at 3 to 5 years of age. They occur more commonly during stressful events such as starting preschool and having a new sibling. Anticipatory guidance aimed at helping her through this transition period will help her cope and decrease her anxiety.

12. *Answer:* D
    Rationale: A 4-year-old should be able to pedal a tricycle, copy a circle, and give his or her full name. Usually at the age of 5 to 6 years, a child can count 10 objects.

13. *Answer:* B

Rationale: Preschool-age children respond more to verbal communication than toddlers and are beginning to perform some self-care tasks. Encounters with other people are becoming more interactive. The preschool-age child is beginning to express his or her feelings. Activities that minimize their anxieties will help in the transition of new experiences.

14. *Answer:* A
Rationale: The preschool child with a test result of 20/40 or below or those who have a two-line difference in result between the eyes should be referred to an ophthalmologist for evaluation.

15. *Answer:* C
Rationale: Esotropia is the inward turn of the eye when a child is unable to maintain alignment on an object of fixation because the muscles of the eye are not coordinated. The cover-uncover test is used to assess for strabismus, a defect in the position of the eyes in relation to each other.

16. *Answer:* C
Rationale: Routine blood pressure measurements should be started at 3 years of age. Blood pressures may vary with the child's height, weight, and gender. This blood pressure measurement is within the normal range for both male and female children.

17. *Answer:* C
Rationale: The major task in cognitive development of a school-age child is concrete thinking and adaptation to school. Children transition from a preoperational mode of thinking that uses intuitive problem solving to early concrete operational thinking. Concepts emerge in logical operations that include reversibility, conservation, classification, and seriation.

18. *Answer:* D
Rationale: ADHD, conduct disorder, and suicide have a higher reported incidence in the male gender.

19. *Answer:* D

Rationale: Lying and stealing are prevalent among 5 to 8 year old boys and are common transient developmental problems that may often result from developmental issues or external influences such as inconsistent discipline and inflexible, demanding environments.

20. *Answer:* A
Rationale: Physiologic splitting of the second heart sound during inspiration is normal. If it is heard both during inspiration and expiration, it may indicate atrial septal defect or pulmonic stenosis.

21. *Answer:* B
Rationale: The detection of potentially life-threatening conditions is one of the goals of the preparticipation sports physical exam. Fainting and/or passing out during exercise may indicate a potentially life-threatening cardiovascular condition.

22. *Answer:* A
Rationale: All new cars come equipped with air bags. When used with seat belts, air bags work well to protect older children and adults. Air bags are very dangerous for children in rear-facing car safety seats and to child passengers not properly positioned. All children up to age 13 years are safest in the back seat.

23. *Answer:* D
Rationale: The school-age child's bones are still immature and fractures of the growth plate can easily occur. Throughout childhood, the skeletal system matures as the epiphyses of the bones grow, become thinner, and eventually fuse.

24. *Answer:* A
Rationale: Erikson's theory states that the school-age child is in the stage of industry versus inferiority. Erikson believed that children in this stage are internally motivated to compete, achieve, and obtain recognition. However, children can feel inferior, develop a sense of failure, and lose interest in learning if their efforts to achieve are unsuccessful.

25. *Answer:* C

Rationale: Nearly 20% of children age 2 to 5 years have untreated caries and in low-socioeconomic areas, 80% of these children will remain untreated. Over twice as many children are without dental insurance as compared to those with medical insurance.

BIBLIOGRAPHY

American Academy of Pediatrics. (2003). Rates of pediatric injuries by 3 month intervals for children 0–3 years of age. *Pediatrics, 111*(6), e683-e692.

American Academy of Pediatrics, Committee on Nutrition. (1999). Calcium requirements of infants, children and adolescents. *Pediatrics, 104*(5), 1152-1157.

American Academy of Pediatrics Committee on Practice and Ambulatory Medicine. (2000). Recommendations for preventive pediatric health care. *Pediatrics, 105*(3), 645-646.

Carakushansky, M., O'Brien, K.O., & Levine, M.A. (2003). Vitamin D and calcium: Strong bones for life through better nutrition. *Contemp Pediatr, 20*(3), 37-53.

Centers for Disease Control and Prevention. (2005). CDC Childhood Lead Poisoning Prevention Program. Retrieved July 1, 2005, from www.cdc.gov/nceh/lead/lead.htm.

Glascoe, F.P., & Macias, M.M. (2003). How you can implement the AAP's new policy on developmental and behavioral screening? *Contemp Pediatr, 4*, 85-66.

Gottesman, M.M. (2002). Helping toddlers eat well. *J Pediatr Health Care, 16*(2), 92-96.

Green, M., & Palfrey, J.S. (Eds.). (2002). *Bright futures: Guidelines for health supervision of infants, children and adolescents* (2nd ed., rev.). Arlington VA: National Center for Education in Maternal and Child Health.

Green, M., Sullivan, P.D., & Eichberg, C.G. (2001). What to do with the angry toddler. *Contemp Pediatr, 18*(8), 65-84.

Instone, S.L. (2002). Developmental strategies for interviewing children. *J Pediatr Health Care, 16*(6), 304-305.

Marcus, S. (2005). Toxicity: Lead. Retrieved June 6, from www.emedicine.com/EMERG/topic293.htm.

National Association of Pediatric Nurse Practitioners (NAPNAP). (2006). Healthy Eating and Activity Together (HEAT[sm]) Clinical Practice Guideline: Identifying and Preventing Overweight in Childhood. Cherry Hill, NJ: NAPNAP.

Reilly, J.J., Armstrong, J., Dorosty, A.R., et al. (2005). Early life risk factors for obesity in childhood: Cohort study. *BMJ, 330*(7504), 1357.

Satter, E. (2000). *Child of mine: Feeding with love and good sense* (rev. ed.). Palo Alto, California: Bull Publishing.

23 Mental Health Promotion and Mental Health Screening for Children and Adolescents

DEBORAH SHELTON

Select the best answer for each of the following questions:

1. In formulating your diagnosis of attention deficit hyperactivity disorder (ADHD) in Matt, a school-aged child, you conduct a Global Assessment of Functioning. Assessment of Matt's mental function has the important goal of:
    A. Learning the unique functional characteristics and to diagnose signs and symptoms that suggest a mental disorder.
    B. Making a determination of need for inpatient treatment services required to keep Matt safe while in treatment.
    C. Providing a diagnostic classification that is reimbursable by Medicaid and private insurance.
    D. Assuring appropriate pharmacologic interventions are prescribed.

2. When you assess Sam, a 10-year-old child who is exhibiting a short attention span, you note that his history includes frequent moves. Your diagnosis is made more complicated by:
    A. The input of teachers, family members, and other professionals.
    B. Normal childhood development.
    C. The overabundance of evidence and research associated with childhood disorders.
    D. Developing practice guidelines and tougher reimbursement standards.

3. Psychotherapies provide important alternatives for those children who:

A. Have intact families that can manage the child's behavior with minimal intervention.
B. Cannot be treated in a less restrictive environment in the community.
C. Are diagnosed with an antisocial behavior disorder.
D. Are unable to tolerate medications, or when parents object to the use of medications.

4. Diagnoses to be considered for children who display inattentive, hyperactive, aggressive, and/or defiant behaviors would include:
    A. Attention deficit disorder, disruptive disorder, and/or oppositional defiant disorder.
    B. Major depression or bipolar disorder.
    C. Autism, Asperger's and/or Rett's disorder.
    D. Learning and communication disorders.

5. As a pediatric nurse practitioner, you understand the importance of parent-child attachment for positive mental health and normal growth and development. Important areas for your assessment of attachment would include:
    A. The parents' own attachment histories.
    B. Parenting skills.
    C. The infant's behavior toward strangers.
    D. Sibling response to the infant.

6. To support mental health in chronically ill children and adolescents, the environment should:
- A. Ignore safety standards in order to make it comfortable.
- B. Protect the child from memories of previous experiences.
- C. Provide capacity for active, passive, directed, and self-initiated play.
- D. Offer parenting classes so that parents do not feel guilty.

7. In your practice, you know that use of structured clinical interview questions are most appropriate for:
- A. Exploring the many different aspects of a child's functioning with parents and teachers.
- B. Asking parents or guardians about specific problems for diagnoses.
- C. Assuring high agreement between informants.
- D. Emergent themes from multiple informants.

8. As the pediatric nurse practitioner, you know that multiple informants are often used in assessing a child's behavior. You would expect what degree of cross-informant agreement between parents, teachers, and after-school care providers?
- A. High level of cross-informant agreement.
- B. Low level of cross-informant agreement.
- C. Low to moderate level of cross-informant agreement.
- D. Moderate to high level of cross-informant agreement.

9. Epidemiological trends in pediatric psychopharmacology reveal that:
- A. Twenty-one percent of children between the ages of 9 and 17 have a diagnosable mental health or addictive disorder, and of these, only 10% may have a medication-responsive psychiatric disorder.
- B. Antipsychotic medications are the medication class most often prescribed to youngsters.

- C. Research demonstrates that prescribing rates are uniform across health care providers.
- D. Treatment with multiple concurrent medications is favored by clinicians for children treated in outpatient settings.

10. Given that most psychiatric medications prescribed to children and adolescents are "off-label," which of the following statements is TRUE?
- A. If the clinician has a medically acceptable reason and a sound rationale for prescribing a drug to a child, the Federal Drug Administration (FDA) does not prohibit "off-label" use.
- B. FDA-approved drugs for approved indications are not approved for use when children are below the age limit for that drug.
- C. The FDA regulates prescribing practices as well as manufacturer advertising for medications.
- D. "Off-label" use of an approved drug does not increase the potential of liability for the clinician.

11. Carol, an 8-year-old, is diagnosed with obsessive compulsive disorder. Before prescribing sertraline, a selective serotonin reuptake inhibitor (SSRI), you would:
- A. Consider use of tricyclic antidepressants (TCAs) first, due to their low toxicity.
- B. Conduct a routine pediatric physical exam.
- C. Teach the patient and family that extensive lab testing is required to monitor plasma levels.
- D. Consider use of a monoamine oxidase inhibitor (MAOI) within 1 week if sertraline is ineffective.

12. Rick, a 14-year-old, has witnessed a car bombing. What comorbid conditions would you assess for?
- A. Disturbed thought patterns.
- B. Depression and substance abuse.
- C. Developmental disorder.
- D. Bipolar disorder.

13. Harry is referred to you by his parents for repeated and excessive aggression in school. Your initial comprehensive evaluation of the aggressive behavior suggests that Harry's aggressive behavior is adaptive. Your next step would be to:
   A. Determine the most appropriate medication to be used.
   B. Treat the underlying disorder.
   C. Examine options for societal, family, or school intervention.
   D. Adopt a target symptom approach to treating the aggression.

14. When monitoring the clinical response and side effects to medications in the treatment of Claire, an 11-year-old child who was referred to you by the school counselor for poor impulse control and violent outbursts, your initial action would be to:
   A. Suggest a punishment to be used in school.
   B. Obtain a baseline rating of aggressive behaviors to be followed.
   C. Prescribe a stimulant without determining the primary diagnosis.
   D. Use different rating scales each week to assure that you have correctly identified the type and cause of the aggression.

15. You are monitoring the progress of Sarah, a 14-year-old who has been diagnosed with major depressive disorder (MDD), during her first inpatient stay at a local children's psychiatric hospital. When teaching her parents about her disorder, you would be sure to tell them that:
   A. Sarah should have no difficulty returning to school and doing well.
   B. Suicidality is a more prominent feature in children younger than Sarah.
   C. Approximately 90% of major depressive episodes take 1 to 2 years to remit.
   D. It is unlikely that Sarah will experience another episode.

16. Carl, a 16-year-old high school student, has been referred to you after he "jokingly" made a statement to his teacher that he was going to kill himself. Your assessment indicates a high risk for suicide. Your initial action would be to:
   A. Report your findings to the principal.
   B. Refer Carl to a self-help group at the school.
   C. Recommend out-of-school suspension.
   D. Ensure his safety and notify his parents.

17. Liam, a 17-year-old high school senior, has reported feeling very anxious to his parents. They have brought him to your primary care practice because they have noticed a change in his behavior and a drop in his grades. Upon assessment, you note that there is no family history of anxiety disorders in biological relatives. You conduct a routine pediatric evaluation with special attention to:
   A. Mimic behavior.
   B. Use of over-the-counter medications and caffeine.
   C. Communication skills.
   D. Use of vitamins.

18. In response to the 1999 Surgeon General's Call to Action to Prevent Suicide, you are asked by the local public health department to make recommendations for development of a primary prevention program. Your plan would include:
   A. Encouraging healthy behaviors and coping skills for teens at a local high school.
   B. Incorporating suicide risk screening in primary care practices.
   C. Provide relapse prevention clinical services to people with depression.
   D. Develop a 2-minute educational commercial for the local public broadcast station regarding depression management.

19. A 17-year-old female is referred to you because of shortness of breath and feeling weak. Upon examination, you note that she is thin, walks with a waddling gait, and could not hold her hands above her head for more than a few seconds. She reports that she feels restless, has difficulty concentrating and poor memory. You might suspect a diagnosis of:

A. Depression.
B. Bulimia.
C. Hearing loss.
D. Seizure disorder.

20. A first-grader is referred to you for assessment because he does not follow directions, and has become defiant and uncooperative at school. He kicked his chair and it knocked one of his classmates over. He has been placed on an out-of-school suspension until his behavior is under control. Your initial assessment would be to:
A. Test sensory functioning (sight, hearing).
B. Blood screen for substance abuse.
C. Test for learning disability.
D. Assess for a seizure disorder.

21. Sam, a 2-year-old child, has been exhibiting excessively aggressive behavior. He hits anyone who is near him, throws his toys, has tantrums several times a day, and is generally perceived by his single mom as out of control. You would recommend which of the following psychosocial interventions?
A. Cognitive-behavioral therapy.
B. Conflict resolution training.
C. Behavior therapy.
D. Parent management training.

22. A 16-year-old is diagnosed with early onset schizophrenia and receives clozapine 12.5 mg twice a day as his initial dose. Three days later, he is brought to your office with symptoms of an acute dystonic reaction. Your initial action is to:
A. Stop his clozapine immediately.
B. Treat with diphenhydramine 25 to 50 mg orally.

C. Notify his prescribing psychiatrist.
D. Treat with benztropine 0.5 mg three times a day until symptoms remiss.

23. Singha is experiencing an extremely dry mouth, dry upper respiratory tract, dry skin, an elevated temperature, and is experiencing confusion. He has been prescribed a tricyclic antidepressant. You diagnose him with symptoms of anticholinergic toxicity, secondary to a drug-drug interaction. Your management of his toxicity would include:
A. IV for hydration, cardiac monitoring, ice bags to reduce hyperthermia.
B. Administer benztropine 1 mg IM and repeat in 30 minutes if needed.
C. Determine plasma levels for all medications.
D. Monitor and be prepared to provide supportive measures.

24. Mary is a 3-year-old whose parents are very upset about their daughter's apparent loss of bladder and bowel control. Upon taking a detailed history, you note that Mary has developed normally until this point. Her parents also comment that she seems to have greater difficulty with certain motor skills that she has had mastery over. A negative finding of your assessment of musculoskeletal and neurologic systems leads you to suspect which of the following developmental disorders?
A. Autism.
B. Childhood disintegrative disorder.
C. Rett's disorder.
D. Asperger's disorder.

ANSWERS

1. *Answer:* A
Rationale: Case formulation helps the clinician understand the child in the context of family and community. Diagnosis helps identify children who may have a mental disorder with an expected pattern of distress and limitation, course, and recovery. Both processes, case formulation and diagnosis, are useful in planning for treatment and supportive care. Both are helpful in developing a treatment plan.

2. *Answer:* B
Rationale: Many symptoms, such as outbursts of aggression, difficulty paying attention, fearfulness, shyness, or distress are normal in young children and may occur sporadically throughout childhood, particularly when interfering with habitual behaviors. Well-trained clinicians overcome this problem by determining whether a given symptom is occurring with an unexpected frequency, lasting for an unexpected length of time, or is occurring at an unexpected point in development.

3. *Answer:* D
Rationale: Psychotherapies are especially important alternatives for those children who are unable to tolerate, or whose parents prefer them not to take, medications. They also are important for conditions for which there are no medications with well-documented efficacy. They also are pivotal for families under stress from a child's mental disorder. Therapies can serve to reduce stress in parents and siblings and teach parents strategies for managing symptoms of the mental disorder in their child.

4. *Answer:* A
Rationale: Children who suffer from attention deficit disorder, disruptive disorder, and oppositional defiant disorder may be inattentive, hyperactive, aggressive, and/or defiant; they may repeatedly defy the societal rules of the child's own cultural group or disrupt a well-ordered environment such as a school classroom.

5. *Answer:* A
Rationale: Four important areas to be assessed to promote secure attachment between an infant and his or her parents include assessment of the parents' values and beliefs about parenting, their own attachment histories, the capacity for empathy and emotional availability, and their knowledge of infant temperament and communication. These assessments lead to promotion of the child's mental health through psychoeducational interventions with the parents. The goal is to engender cognitive and emotional states within the parent that will enhance the child's potential for a secure attachment.

6. *Answer:* C
Rationale: Dimensions of supportive physical environments are important to consider in fostering coping and resilience in children with disabilities or chronic disorders. Environments give powerful messages and structure behavior. Play is a normative method of expression for children.

7. *Answer:* B
Rationale: Structured questions are appropriate for querying parents about symptoms and criteria for psychiatric disorders, as defined in the DSM-IV-TR. Structured diagnostic interviews have a standardized set of questions and probes focusing on specific problems relevant for diagnoses.

8. *Answer:* C
Rationale: There is likely to be only low to moderate agreement between informants who are in different situations or different relationships with the same child. Low agreement between informants does not mean that one is right and the other is wrong, or that one has a truer picture of the child than does the other. Parents, for example, may know more than a teacher about many aspects of their child's functioning simply because they are the parents.

9. *Answer:* A
Rationale: Prescribing rates vary by provider and stimulant medications are among those most frequently utilized by children and adolescents. Concurrent medication

treatment is utilized most frequently in inpatient settings.

10. *Answer:* A

Rationale: The FDA does not regulate prescribing practices, only manufacturer advertising for medications. If the clinician has a medically sound reason and rationale for prescribing a drug to a child, the FDA does not prohibit "off-label" use. Thus, the clinician may prescribe FDA-approved drugs for non-FDA-approved indications. It is recommended that careful documentation in the medical record of the scientifically reasonable rationale for choosing a particular medication over another possible treatment may reduce the potential for liability.

11. *Answer:* B

Rationale: Routine examination, including height, weight, blood pressure, and heart rate need to be current, within 6 months of starting this medication.

12. *Answer:* B

Rationale: Children, adolescents, and adults with posttraumatic stress disorder (PTSD) commonly meet diagnostic criteria for other psychiatric disorders. PTSD rarely occurs in the absence of other psychiatric conditions. Comorbid disorders often found in people with PTSD include depression, substance abuse, other anxiety disorders, ADHD, and conduct disorder.

13. *Answer:* C

Rationale: An initial comprehensive evaluation of aggressive behavior aims to determine if the aggression as adaptive or maladaptive. If the aggression is adaptive—for example, in response to some understandable threat or dispute—psychiatric intervention may not be needed.

14. *Answer:* B

Rationale: Medication interventions for conduct disorder (CD); oppositional defiant disorder (ODD); and excessive, impulsive aggression are "off-label" uses, but have been found to be effective; however, it is important to carefully measure clinical response and side effects. When treating aggression with medication, the clinician should obtain a baseline rating of aggressive behaviors to be followed, obtain a baseline rating of medication side effects before medication titration begins, obtain a history of the behaviors from parents, teachers, and patient, and utilize a standardized clinical rating scale weekly to monthly to determine treatment response.

15. *Answer:* C

Rationale: Approximately 90% of major depressive episodes take 1 to 2 years to remit, the remaining 10% become chronically depressed. After successful treatment, relapse occurs in 40% to 60% of depressed patients within 5 years. Risk factors for recurrence include earlier age of onset, increased number of previous episodes, severity of the first episode, psychosis, developmental delay, and nonadherence to prescribed treatment.

16. *Answer:* D

Rationale: If suicide assessment indicates moderate to high risk, school-based practitioners must take immediate protective actions. These actions include informing the patient that you have a duty to report the suicidal thoughts/attempts, notify the parents, assess lethality and remove access to methods, and document your observations and actions.

17. *Answer:* B

Rationale: Specific medical factors and conditions that may mimic anxiety disorders include a need to evaluate use of medications, herbal supplements, assessment of drug abuse, over-the-counter medications, hypoglycemia, hyperthyroidism, cardiac arrhythmias, caffeine-induced anxiety, pheochromocytoma, migraine headache, and seizure disorder.

18. *Answer:* A

Rationale: Primary prevention activities are those that are aimed at interventions before pathologic changes have begun and during the natural history of susceptibility. Answer B refers to screening which is a secondary prevention strategy; C refers to tertiary prevention strategies; and D refers to education strategies.

19. *Answer:* B

Rationale: Bulimia affects women primarily, and commonly begins in adolescence. Self-induced vomiting, laxatives, and diuretics are sometimes used as aids to weight control resulting in serious medical problems. Complications due to depleted magnesium and potassium occur in approximately 25% of bulimic patients. Symptoms include restlessness, decreased concentration, and poor memory. Some bulimics resort to syrup of ipecac as a means for inducing vomiting because it is effective, cheap, and available without prescription. Ipecac is highly toxic to skeletal and cardiac muscles.

20. *Answer:* A

Rationale: It can be assumed that the cause for significant behavioral or psychologic symptoms in a child not under significant stress is most likely an organic problem. Children with visual and hearing problems develop behavioral problems out of stress and frustration.

21. *Answer:* D

Rationale: Effective psychosocial therapies for aggression and conduct problems emphasize interpersonal skills acquisition. Therapies that primarily encourage the expression of feelings are not effective in externalizing disorders. Cognitive-behavioral therapy (CBT) is useful with adolescents, conflict resolution and behavior therapy are appropriate for school-age children, and parent training is the focus for younger children between 2 and 6 years of age.

22. *Answer:* B

Rationale: Acute dystonic reactions are involuntary muscle spasms and contractions typically involving the muscles of the neck, jaw, mouth, and/or tongue. A period of maximum risk for acute dystonic reactions is within hours to 7 days following initiation of neuroleptics or atypical antipsychotic therapy. Compared to adults, children and adolescents may be particularly at risk to develop acute dystonic reactions upon exposure to antipsychotic medications. These symptoms are rapidly treated with anticholinergic and/or antiparkinsonian agents. Medications include diphenhydramine 25 to 50 mg orally, or diphenhydramine 25 mg IM for severe reactions; benztropine 1 to 2 mg orally, or benztropine 1 mg IM for severe reactions.

23. *Answer:* A

Rationale: Anticholinergic agents should be used cautiously with other medications known to have anticholinergic properties. Anticholinergic drug-drug interactions occur with a variety of drugs, including tricyclic antidepressants. Symptoms of anticholinergic toxicity include an extremely dry mouth, dry upper respiratory tract, dry skin, elevation of body temperature, confusion, delirium, hallucinations, disturbed memory, rapid heart rate, blush, and decreased sweating. Management of anticholinergic toxicity include: Supportive measures, adequate IV hydration, cardiac monitoring, gastric lavage or induced emesis in the conscious patient, monitor airway, and apply cold preparations to reduce hyperthermia.

24. *Answer:* B

Rationale: Onset of childhood disintegrative disorder occurs at 2 years or older, and must be differentiated from Rett's disorder (onset of deficits at 6 months to 2 years) and autism (onset of deficits before 38 months). To be diagnosed with childhood disintegrative disorder, a child must exhibit a loss of skills in two of the following areas: language, social or adaptive behavior, bowel or bladder control, play, and motor skills.

BIBLIOGRAPHY

ACT for Youth Downstate Center for Excellence, ACT for Youth Upstate Center of Excellence (2003). *A guide to positive youth development.* New York: Mount Sinai Adolescent Health Center.

American Medical Association (1994). *Guidelines for adolescent preventive services (GAPS).* Retrieved April 6, 2006, from www.ama-assn.org/ama/pub/category/1980.html.

Burke, R., & Herron, R. (2000). *Common sense parenting*, 2nd ed. Boys Town, NE: Boys Town.

Centers for Disease Control and Prevention. (1999). Suicide deaths and rates per 100,000. Retrieved October 15, 2004, from www.cdc.gov/nchs/data/hus/tables/2003.

Department of Health and Human Services (1999). *Mental health: A report of the surgeon general*. Rockville, MD: Department of Health and Human Services, Substance Abuse and Mental Health Services Administration, Center for Mental Health Services, National Institute of Mental Health. Retrieved on April 6, 2006, from www.surgeongeneral.gov/library/mentalhealth/toc.html#chapter3.

Glascoe, F.P. (2001). *Parents' evaluation of developmental status*. Nashville: Ellsworth & Vandemeer Press.

Jellinek, M. (2002). Pediatric Symptom Checklist. In M. Jellinek, (Ed.). *Bright futures in practice: Mental health*. Georgetown University: The National Center for Education in Maternal & Child Health. Retrieved on April 6, 2006, from http://www.brightfutures.org/mentalhealth/pdf/professionals/ped_sympton_chklst.pdf.

Kelleher, K.J., McInerny, T.K., Gardner, W.P., et al. (2000). Increasing identification of psychosocial problems: 1979–1996. *Pediatrics, 105*(6), 1313-1321.

Melnyk, B.M., Brown, H., Jones, D., et al. (2003). Improving the mental/psychosocial health of U.S. children and adolescents: Outcomes and implementation strategies from the National KySS Summit. *J Pediatr Health Care (Suppl), 17*(6), S1-S24.

Melnyk,B. M., Feinstein, N.F., Tuttle, J., et al. (2002). Mental health worries, communication, and needs of children, teens, and parents during the year of the nation's terrorist attack: Findings from the national KySS survey. *J Pediatr Health Care, 16*(5), 222-234.

Navon, M., Nelson, D., Pagano, M., & Murphy, M. (2001). Use of the pediatric symptom checklist in strategies to improve preventive behavioral health care. *Pediatric Serv, 52*(6) 800-804.

Pollack, C.L., & Kaye, D.L. (2002). Management and assessment of child mental health problems in the pediatric office. In D.L. Kaye, M.E. Montgomery, & S.W. Munson (Eds.). *Child and adolescent mental health*. Philadelphia: Lippincott Williams & Wilkins.

President's New Freedom Commission on Mental Health. *Interim report: Fragmentation and gaps in care for children*. Retrieved on April 6, 2006, from http://www.mentalhealth.samhsa.gov/publications/allpubs/NMH02-0144/gaps.asp.

Ryan-Wenger, N.A. (2001). Use of children's drawings for measurement of developmental level and emotional status. *J Child Fam Nurs, 4*(2), 139-149.

Satcher, D. (2003). *Mental health. A lifespan approach*. Keynote presentation. Rochester, New York: KySS Invitational Summit, March 29, 2003.

Shives, L.R., & Isaacs, A. (2002). *Psychiatric and mental health nursing*. Philadelphia: Lippincott.

United States General Accounting Office (GAO). (2003) *Report to congressional requesters: Child welfare and juvenile justice*. Retrieved April 6, 2006, from http://www.gao.gov/new.items/d03397.pdf.

U.S. Department of Health and Human Services. (2003). *Compendium of AHRQ Research Related to Mental Health* (AHRQ Pub. No. 03-0001).

U.S. Department of Health and Human Services. (2000). *Healthy People 2010*. Retrieved on April 6, 2006, from www.healthypeople.gov.

U.S. Department of Health and Human Services. (1999). *Mental health: A Report of the surgeon general—executive summary*. Rockville, MD: U.S. Department of Health and Human Services, Substance Abuse and Mental Health Services Administration, Center for Mental Health Services, National Institutes of Health, National Institute of Mental Health.

U.S. Department of Health and Human Services. (2006). Office of the Surgeon General. Retrieved on April 6, 2006, from http://www.surgeongeneral.gov/library/reports.htm.

Weitzman, M. (2003). Who is and who isn't providing mental health services to our nation's children. Invited presentation. Rochester, New York: National KySS Summit, March 28.

CHAPTER

24 Sports Participation: Evaluation and Monitoring

AMY K. FOY

Select the best answer for each of the following questions:

1. The fastest rise in sports participants has occurred in:
   A. High school girls and children younger than age 10.
   B. Boys younger than 6 years of age.
   C. Girls between the ages of 10 and 13.
   D. High-school boys.

2. Intrinsic motivation for sports participation include:
   A. Spend time with friends.
   B. Ribbons and trophies for rewards.
   C. Peer approval.
   D. Test ability against others.

3. Adult involvement with sports can have a positive influence on children if they:
   A. Encourage a competitive style of play when coaching.
   B. Teach the "no pain, no gain" philosophy.
   C. Role model a positive, respectful, courteous attitude based on positive reinforcement and consistency.
   D. Challenge the kids to work on advanced skills to improve their level of play.

4. Improved academic performance, lower body fat and improved strength result from:
   A. Watching sports.
   B. Participating in sports.
   C. Media influence.
   D. Peer pressure.

5. Cardiovascular benefits of exercise include:
   A. Improved mental clarity and sleep habits.
   B. Muscle strengthening and improved metabolism.
   C. Prevention of hypertension and increased endurance.
   D. Improved bone density and decreased incidence of stress fractures.

6. The most common injury among children playing sports is:
   A. Fracture.
   B. Sprain.
   C. Concussion.
   D. Compartment syndrome.

7. Which sport has the highest rate of injury among all high-school sports?
   A. Girls' cross country.
   B. Boys' basketball.
   C. Girls' tennis.
   D. Boys' wrestling.

8. Rehabilitation from injury is not complete until the athlete:
   A. Has regained 80% of range of motion, strength, and flexibility.
   B. Has no pain.
   C. Regains full range of motion, strength, and flexibility of the affected joint.
   D. Has undergone an MRI of the affected joint to ensure healing has taken place.

9. Protein requirements for athletes is:
   A. 5 g protein per kg of body weight per day.

B. 1 g protein per kg of body weight per day.
C. 0.5 g protein per kg of body weight per day.
D. 8 g protein per kg of body weight per day.

10. Inadequate carbohydrate intake may be associated with:
A. Cramping.
B. Nausea and heartburn.
C. Hyperactivity and jitters.
D. Fatigue and decreased performance.

11. An optimal diet for teen female athletes includes:
A. 1500 kcal/day with 40% protein.
B. 2000 kcal/day with 30% protein, 30% carbohydrates, and 30% fat.
C. A balanced diet of 3000 kcal/day in order to obtain at least 15 mg iron and 750 mg calcium.
D. 2000 kcal/day with 50% carbohydrates.

12. This nutritional source should be consumed 60 to 90 minutes before competition, within 30 minutes after vigorous exercise, and 2 hours later to enhance glycogen stores.
A. Carbohydrates
B. Protein
C. Potassium
D. Fat

13. A teen female needs 1200 mg of this nutrient. Excellent sources include dairy products, soy milk, orange juice, almonds, broccoli, and collards. This nutrient is:
A. Iron.
B. Potassium.
C. Magnesium.
D. Calcium.

14. A 15-year-old female gymnast comes into the clinic for a sports physical. After obtaining a thorough history, the pediatric nurse practitioner recognizes signs of female athlete triad syndrome. The gymnast complains of menstrual irregularities and shares that she only eats "fat-free" foods. She also states that she:

A. Has suffered two fractures in the past 12 months.
B. Only drinks skim milk.
C. Suffers from insomnia.
D. Suffers from occasional migraines.

15. A female athlete in your practice with a known history of an eating disorder and amenorrhea presents for a sports physical. The lab evaluation should include:
A. CBC with differential and thyroid profile.
B. Fasting blood glucose.
C. Hemoglobin and hematocrit and calcium level.
D. Urinalysis, estrogen, and progesterone levels.

16. As a pediatric nurse practitioner, you are a care provider for the regional highschool track meet. One of the runners fell and hit his head on the pavement. There was no loss of consciousness but he showed signs of transient confusion for about 10 minutes. You counsel his parents by explaining:
A. He suffered a Grade II concussion and needs immediate transport to a local emergency room.
B. He suffered a Grade I concussion and requires reexamination at 5-minute intervals at rest and with exertion.
C. He should be placed in a cervical spine immobilizer until a CT scan can be done.
D. He should be removed from the meet and refrain from playing any sports for 2 months.

17. A teen male lacrosse player is requesting to resume playing. He has an acutely enlarged spleen. The pediatric nurse practitioner should:
A. Council him to modify activity for 1 week and then resume play.
B. Put the teen on bed rest for 1 month or until the spleen's size decreases.
C. Advise no sports activity due to the potential of spleen rupture.
D. Allow him to resume playing the season.

18. A 5-year-old with Down syndrome is preparing to enroll in gymnastics. Prior to clearing her for participation, the pediatric nurse practitioner should order:
   A. Cervical spine radiographs to look for atlantoaxial instability.
   B. Urinalysis to look for proteinuria.
   C. CBC with differential to screen for leukemia.
   D. MRI of the head and neck to look for Arnold Chiari malformation.

19. A high-school football player admits to using anabolic steroids. You counsel him about the effects of the drug by explaining that it can lead to:
   A. Constipation.
   B. Early closure of growth plates.
   C. Dental caries.
   D. Aggression and acne.

20. The most popular nutritional supplement among young athletes is:
   A. Amphetamines.
   B. Ephedrine.
   C. Creatine.
   D. Caffeine.

21. A wrestler presents for a sports physical and complains of rapid weight loss in a short period and dizziness upon standing. You suspect he has been taking:
   A. Diuretics.
   B. Ephedrine.
   C. Epogen.
   D. Beta-blockers.

22. One of the athletes in your clinic complains of dizziness during exercise and frequent heart palpitations. You respond by:
   A. Encouraging adequate hydration before, during, and after sports activities.
   B. Advising eliminating any caffeine from his diet.
   C. Ordering a chest x-ray.
   D. Referring to a cardiologist to rule out cardiac disease or anomaly.

23. As a pediatric nurse practitioner, you advise parents of children interested in sports to:
   A. Focus on one sport year-round in order to excel.
   B. Begin team exposure around age 3 years.
   C. Balance sports with noncompetitive activities like art, music, or theater.
   D. Introduce a particular sport with one-to-one private lessons to allow the child to learn all the rules and skills of the game.

24. As a member of an athletic board of a private school, you recommend a curriculum for coaches that includes:
   A. Drama.
   B. Counseling kids about low-fat diets.
   C. Nonviolent conflict resolution.
   D. CPR training for athletes.

25. A school-age child with a BMI greater than the 95th percentile asks if he can participate in sports. Your response is to:
   A. Encourage sports participation, explaining the benefits of exercise.
   B. Discourage team sports and advise he focus on less competitive activities.
   C. Advocate for noncontact sports only.
   D. Develop a conditioning program for the child to work on for a few months and then move forward with sports if he is making progress with endurance and strengthening.

ANSWERS

1. *Answer:* A
   Rationale: According to *The Young Athlete* by J.D. Metzl and a *Newsweek* article by D. Noonan, the fastest rise in sports participation has been seen in high-school girls and children younger than age 10.

2. *Answer:* D
   Rationale: Testing one's abilities against others is an intrinsic factor motivating kids to participate in sports. The others listed are extrinsic factors.

3. *Answer:* C
   Rationale: Adults should be positive role models for the children and teach them good sportsmanship attitudes.

4. *Answer:* B
   Rationale: Participating in sports is the way to improve academic performance, lower body fat, and improve strength. The others do not provide these health benefits.

5. *Answer:* C
   Rationale: The others listed are health benefits but not cardiovascular benefits.

6. *Answer:* B
   Rationale: According to the 2005 CDC report on injury prevention, strains and sprains are the most common injuries among children playing sports.

7. *Answer:* A
   Rationale: According to the 2005 CDC report of injury prevention, girl's cross-country has the highest rate of injury among all high-school sports.

8. *Answer:* C
   Rationale: Rehabilitation is not complete until the athlete regains full range of motion, strength, and flexibility of the affected joint.

9. *Answer:* B
   Rationale: Intake of 1 g of protein per kg body weight per day is required for athletes.

10. *Answer:* D

Rationale: Inadequate carbohydrate intake can lead to fatigue and decreased performance.

11. *Answer:* C
    Rationale: A balanced diet of 3000 kcal/day is required to obtain the RDA benefits of 15 mg iron and 750 mg calcium per day.

12. *Answer:* A
    Rationale: These are the recommended times to consume carbohydrates, because this nutrient provides energy and enhances performance.

13. *Answer:* D
    Rationale: All foods listed are excellent sources of calcium.

14. *Answer:* A
    Rationale: The female athlete triad syndrome is consists of disordered eating, menstrual irregularities, and osteopenia or osteoporosis.

15. *Answer:* C
    Rationale: Amenorrhea and eating disorders lead to increased iron deficiency anemia and reduced calcium levels.

16. *Answer:* B
    Rationale: A Grade I concussion is defined as a head injury leading to transient confusion, inattention, no loss of consciousness, and mental status abnormalities that resolve within 15 minutes. Treatment for this involves examining immediately and at 5-minute intervals at rest and exertion.

17. *Answer:* C
    Rationale: An enlarged spleen is at risk for rupture during any sports activities.

18. *Answer:* A
    Rationale: Children with Down syndrome are at higher risk for atlantoaxial instability. Instability can be identified with cervical spine radiographs.

19. *Answer:* D
    Rationale: Anabolic steroids have many side effects, including aggression and acne.

20. *Answer:* C
Rationale: The most popular nutritional supplement is creatine with sales of more than $400 million annually.

21. *Answer:* A
Rationale: Hallmarks of diuretic abuse include excessive urination, rapid weight loss in a short period, and syncope due to orthostatic hypotension.

22. *Answer:* D
Rationale: Complaints of dizziness and heart palpitations during exertion warrant a cardiology evaluation to rule out cardiac etiology.

23. *Answer:* C
Rationale: It is important for adults to get their children involved in noncompetitive activities like art, music, and theater.

24. *Answer:* C
Rationale: According to Thompson (1995), a curriculum for coaches should include material about nonviolent conflict resolution, cooperation, physical and psychological child development principles, fitness, and sportsmanship.

25. *Answer:* A
Rationale: Sports participation for these children helps lead to regular exercise habits which is likely to persist through adulthood. Explaining the benefits of exercise can motivate them to continue participation.

BIBLIOGRAPHY

American Academy of Pediatrics, Committee on Sports Medicine and Fitness (2001). Medical conditions affecting sports participation. *Pediatrics, 107*(5), 1205-1209.

American Academy of Pediatrics, Committee on Sports Medicine and Fitness and Committee on School Health. (2001b). Organized sports for children and preadolescents. *Pediatrics, 107*(6), 1459-1452.

American Academy of Neurology. (1997). Practice parameter: The management of concussion in sports (summary statement). Report of the Quality Standards Subcommittee. *Neurology, 48*(3), 581-585.

American Academy of Orthopedic Surgeons. (2005). *Patient education library.* Retrieved July 21, 2005, from http://orthoinfo.aaos.org.

Ara, I., Vincente-Rodriquez, G., Jimenez-Ramirez, J., et al. (2004). Regular participation in sports is associated with enhanced physical fitness and lower fat mass in prepubertal boys. *Int J Obes Relat Metabol Disord, 28*(12), 1585-1593.

Armsey, T.D., & Hosey, R.G. (2004). Medical aspects of sports: Epidemiology of injuries, preparticipation physical examination, and drugs in sports. *Clin Sports Med, 223*(2), 255-279, vii.

Asplund, C.A., McKeag, D.A., & Olson, C.H. (2004). Sport-related concussion: Factors associated with prolonged return to play. *Clin J Sport Med, 14*(6), 339-343.

Berger, S., Kugler, J.D., Thomas, J.A., & Friedberg, D.Z. (2004). Sudden cardiac death in children and adolescents: Introduction and overview. *Pediatr Clin North Am, 51*(5), 1201-1209.

Bernhardt, D.L. (2004). *Concussion.* Retrieved on April 17, 2006, from http://www.emedicine.com/sports/topic27-Clinical.htm.

Bernhardt D.T., Gomez, J., Johnson, M.D., et al. (2001). Strength training by children and adolescents. *Pediatrics, 107*(6), 1470-1472.

Birch, K. (2005). Female athlete triad. *BMJ, 330*(7485), 244-246.

Centers for Disease Control and Prevention (2005). National Center for Injury Prevention and Control Activity Report: 2001. Retrieved June 6, 2006, from www.cdc.gov/ncipc/pub-res/unintentionalactivity/07-state-programs.htm.

Gittes, E.B. (2004). The female athlete triad. *J Pediatr Adolesc Gynecol, 17*(5), 363-365.

Halstead, M.E., & Bernhardt, D.T. (2002). Common infections in the young athlete. *Pediatr Ann, 31*(1), 42-48.

Harmon, K.G. (1999). Assessment and management of concussion in sports. *Am Fam Phys, 60*(3), 887-894.

Hass, C.J., Feigenbaum, M.S., & Franklin, B.A. (2001). Prescription of resistance training for healthy populations. *Sports Med, 31*(14), 953-964.

Lyznicki, J.M., Neilson, N.H., & Schneider, J.F. (2000). Cardiovascular screening of student athletes. *Am Fam Phys, 62*(4), 765-772.

Metzl, J.D. (2002). *The young athlete.* Boston: Little, Brown and Company.

Metzl, J.D., Small, E., Levine, S.R., & Gershel, J.C. (2001). Creatine use among young athletes. *Pediatrics, 108*(2), 421-425.

National Association of Pediatric Nurse Practitioners (NAPNAP) (2004). *Position statement on the prevention of tobacco use in the pediatric popula-*

tion. Retrieved on June 6, 2006, at http://www.napnap.org/Docs/pos-tobacco.pdf.

National Athletic Training Association. (2005). *Safety checklist for high school sports.* Retrieved July 21, 2005, from www.nata.org/publicinformation/files/safetychecklist.pdf.

National Institute on Drug Abuse (NIDA). (2000). *Steroid abuse and addiction.* Retrieved July 21, 2005, from www.nida.gov/research_reports/Steroids/AnabolicSteroids.html.

National Youth Sports Safety Foundation. (2005). *A primer for safety on youth sports.* Retrieved July 21, 2005, from www.nyssf.org/wframeset.html.

Noonan, D. (September 22, 2003). When safety is the name of the game. *Newsweek,* 64-66.

Novak, J. (2003). Cited by Wendy L. Bonifazi in "Quest for big muscles yields big problems." *Nurs Spect.* Retrieved June 6, 2006, from http://community.nursingspectrum.com/MagazineArticles/article.cfm?AID=12642.

Novak, J.C. (2001). PNPs: Activists in the local, national, and global arenas. *J Pediatr Health Care, 15*(5), 17A-18A.

Novak, J.C. (2002). The tobacco user's cessation helpline (TOUCH): A pilot study to developing effective interventions. *Purdue Nurse.* West Lafayette: Purdue University.

Peer, K.S. (2004). Bone health in athletes. Factors and future considerations. *Orthop Nurs, 23*(3), 174-181.

Sherman, R.T., & Thompson, R.A. (2004). The female athlete triad. *J School Nurs, 20*(4), 197-202.

Stollo, N.K. (2003). When competition is queen: Health issues in women athletes. *Adv Nurse Pract, 11*(7), 32-36, 39.

Story, M., Holt, K., & Sofka, D. (Eds.). (2002). *Bright futures in practice: Nutrition* (2nd ed.). Arlington, VA: National Center for Education in Maternal and Child Health.

Sullivan, J.A., & Anderson, S.J. (2000). *Care of the young athlete.* American Academy of Orthopedic Surgeons and the American Academy of Pediatrics. Elk Grove Village, IL: AAP Publishing.

Thompson, G.H. (2004). The neck. In R.E. Behrman, R.M. Kliegman, & H.B. Jenson (Eds.). *Nelson textbook of pediatrics* (17th ed.). Philadelphia: Saunders.

Thompson, J. (1995). *Positive coaching: Building character and self-esteem through sports, the Stanford experience.* Portola Valley, CA: Warde Publishers.

Vitulano, L.A. (2003). Psychosocial issues for children and adolescents with chronic illness: Self-esteem, school functioning and sports participation. *Child Adolesc Clin North Am, 12*(3), 585-592.

Wind, W.M., Schwend, R.M., & Larson, J. (2004). Sports for the physically challenged child. *J Am Acad Orthop Surg, 12*(2), 126-132.

25 Early Adolescents, Late Adolescents, and College-age Young Adults

NAOMI A. SCHAPIRO

Select the best answer for each of the following questions:

1. The leading causes of death for adolescents (ages 15 to 19) are:
    A. Accidents, congenital malformations, malignancies.
    B. Homicides, suicides, malignancies.
    C. Accidents, homicides, suicides.
    D. Malignancies, homicides, heart disease.

2. The Guidelines for Adolescent Preventive Services (GAPS) recommend yearly screenings for all adolescents to include:
    A. Psychosocial screening, blood pressure, and body mass index.
    B. Blood pressure, hemoglobin, complete physical examination.
    C. Complete physical examination, psychosocial screening, drug testing.
    D. Psychosocial screening, cholesterol screening, blood pressure.

3. You have recently seen Susanna, who is 15 years old, in your clinic, and have sent a confidential screen for sexually transmitted infections (STI). She has declined to share this information with her parents, but they are now requesting a complete copy of her medical records. Which response BEST describes your legal responsibilities?
    A. Federal regulations do not give her parents the right to access medical records related to sexual activity and STI testing.
    B. Federal regulations give her parents the right to access all of Susanna's medical records and override all state regulations.
    C. Federal regulations give her parents the right to access all of Susanna's medical records, but state regulations take precedence if they are more restrictive.
    D. Federal regulations give the individual health care provider discretion in releasing medical records related to confidential services.

4. Sandra Jones is a pediatric nurse practitioner employed by a school district to work in a high school. What regulations cover the privacy and confidentiality rules of her practice?
    A. Local regulations specific to the school district.
    B. Local regulations and HIPAA.
    C. FERPA and local regulations.
    D. FERPA, with HIPAA regulation of any third-party billing.

5. For most adolescent girls, menarche occurs between Tanner Stages (SMR):
    A. 1 and 2.
    B. 2 and 3.
    C. 3 and 4.
    D. 4 and 5.

6. Jonathan is 13 years old and has told you that some of his friends smoke cigarettes. He has a crush on a girl in his class. In counseling him to avoid tobacco use, which rationale is MOST likely to appeal to him?
    A. Tobacco is linked to increased rates of lung cancer.

B. Smoking cigarettes can stain his teeth and give him bad breath.
C. Tobacco increases his risk of dying from a heart attack.
D. Smoking cigarettes is expensive in the long run.

7. Which of the following traits best characterizes middle adolescents (14 to 16 years old)?
A. Concrete thinking, present orientation, and intense preoccupation with body image.
B. Long-range planning, adult cognitive abilities, developed individual values.
C. Intense peer group involvement, feelings of immortality, sexual experimentation.
D. Need for privacy, increased conflicts with parents, financial independence.

8. Which of the following teenagers is most likely to be interested in risk-taking behaviors?
A. An 11-year-old girl who is Tanner 2.
B. A 14-year-old girl who is Tanner 3.
C. A 12-year-old boy who is Tanner 2.
D. A 13-year-old girl who is Tanner 5.

9. Andre, who is 14 years old, is failing ninth grade. He has always enjoyed reading and received good grades in elementary school. His grades have gradually declined since sixth grade, with teachers often noting that he has trouble keeping track of his assignments and seems to daydream in class. This scenario is MOST consistent with:
A. Major learning disability.
B. Minor learning disability or attention deficit hyperactivity disorder.
C. Sudden trauma or major depression.
D. Frequent moves in elementary grades.

10. How do teen patterns of alcohol abuse differ from adult patterns of abuse?
A. Teens are more likely to feel guilty about excessive alcohol use than adults.
B. Teens are more likely to need an "eye-opener" than adults.

C. Teens are more likely to engage in binge drinking, rather than daily drinking.
D. Teens are more likely to seek help on their own for alcohol abuse than adults.

11. Marta, 16 years old, has come in for a well adolescent exam, and reports that she is applying for a job in a large department store that requires a urine drug screen of prospective employees. She drinks alcohol and smokes marijuana at parties, reportedly about twice a month. In counseling her about her drug use, which of the following is the most accurate statement?
A. Marijuana can be detected in urine drug screens up to 2 to 3 weeks after use.
B. Alcohol use has a profound effect on memory and motivation, even with occasional use.
C. Marijuana has a short half life in the body, and withdrawal effects can be felt within 1 week.
D. Alcohol use among high-school students is rare.

12. "Club drugs" include:
A. Acetaminophen, ibuprofen, and naproxen.
B. Ketamine, gamma hydroxybutyrate, and MDMA.
C. Oxycontin, codeine, and marijuana.
D. Testosterone, androstenedione, and erythropoietin.

13. Garvin, 17 years old, is seeing his regular pediatric nurse practitioner for a sports physical. While participating in a psychosocial screen, Garvin volunteers that he "hasn't had sex yet." What is the best INITIAL response to Garvin's statement?
A. Congratulate him for abstaining and move on to another topic.
B. Demonstrate condom use and give Garvin some condoms to take home.
C. Encourage Garvin to be screened for sexually transmitted infections.
D. Ask Garvin to clarify which behaviors are included in his definition of "sex."

14. Keiko, 16 years old, has been called back to her high-school health center for treatment of a positive Chlamydia result on a urine LCR test. Keiko insists that she and her boyfriend have been using latex condoms without difficulty 100% of the time, with no breaks or slips. If Keiko is reporting condom use accurately, which statement below BEST explains her positive Chlamydia result?
   A. Some teens are allergic to the latex used in most condoms.
   B. Even with perfect use, condoms to do not offer 100% protection against all STIs.
   C. They may have used a faulty condom.
   D. Many teens use condoms "late" in the encounter, after some genital contact has already occurred.

15. You are screening David, 14 years old, for sexual activity. Of the following statements, what is the BEST way to initiate this discussion with him?
   A. Ask him if any of his friends or acquaintances are starting to have sex.
   B. Ask him what he knows about sex.
   C. Ask him if he has a girlfriend.
   D. Ask him if he thinks he might have been exposed to a sexually transmitted infection.

16. A 17-year-old who is in your office for a checkup refuses to get undressed for the exam. Of all the possible explanations for this behavior, which one might require you to make an official report the day of the visit?
   A. The teen is embarrassed about being overweight.
   B. The teen has been sexually abused in the past.
   C. The teen has just gotten a tattoo without parental permission.
   D. The teen has extensive acne scarring on the back.

17. Which of the following statements about bullying is the most accurate?
   A. Girls are more likely to be bullied by physical contact than boys.
   B. African American children are most likely to be bullied.
   C. About 10% of sixth to tenth graders bully others "sometimes."
   D. Bullying is more likely in urban settings than in suburban or rural settings.

18. Jay has been brought to your office by his parents because he has recently started refusing to attend high school. Which of the following statements made on his psychosocial screen also put him at higher risk for suicidal ideation?
   A. Jay is a star player on a community soccer team.
   B. Jay has recently become involved with another boy at school and since then has reported one physical assault and frequent verbal harassment.
   C. Jay works 10 hours per week at a local coffee shop.
   D. Jay's parents were divorced 10 years ago, but have shared custody and celebrate some holidays together.

19. Which of the following interventions follows the principles of harm reduction?
   A. Treating a child with otitis media with high-dose amoxicillin.
   B. Urine screening for drug abuse.
   C. Setting up free shuttle services to and from school proms.
   D. Limiting the sale of alcohol to adults 21 and over.

20. Isabella, a high school senior, is in the clinic for her third pregnancy test in 4 months. Her pediatric nurse practitioner has given her two prescriptions for contraception which she has not filled. Which statement by the pediatric nurse practitioner is most consistent with a brief motivational interview approach?
   A. You'll never get to college if you don't start using birth control.
   B. Don't you know that condoms are not that effective for pregnancy prevention?
   C. Have you thought about abstaining from sex for a while?
   D. On a scale of 1 to 10, where 1 is not important and 10 is very important, how

important is it to you to use contraception?

21. Mark, 11 years old, is in your office with his father for a pre-camp physical exam. Mark's father notes that Mark is getting "fresh" at home, seems bored at school, and is unsupervised between 3:30 PM and 6:00 PM, when the father gets home from work. The father asks your advice about the best way to keep Mark from "getting into trouble, like some of the other kids in the neighborhood." Of the following, the best advice would be to:
   A. Encourage supervised after-school activities that will help Mark build some skills and follow any interests he might have, such as sports or music.
   B. Allow Mark some increased independence as an early adolescent.
   C. Accept Mark's attitude to school and some rude behavior at home as a normal part of adolescence.
   D. Take away all of Mark's privileges if he associates with neighborhood youth who are in trouble.

22. Jason is 18 years old and about to graduate from high school. Which of the following statements about Jason is most likely to be true?
   A. Jason has less impulse control than younger adolescents.
   B. Jason may lose his health insurance if he does not attend college full-time.
   C. Jason does not have adult confidentiality rights as long as he lives with his parents.
   D. Jason does not have comparable reasoning abilities to an older adult.

23. Cherisse, 15 years old, is seeing her pediatric nurse practitioner because of men-strual irregularities. In reviewing her chart, the pediatric nurse practitioner notices that Cherisse's weight has fluctuated widely over the last 2 years. Of the following topics, which are the most important for the pediatric nurse practitioner to cover in evaluating Cherisse for a possible eating disorder?
   A. Satisfaction with weight, drug use, sexual activity.
   B. Depression and suicidal ideation, sexual orientation, 24-hour diet recall.
   C. Drug use, history of sexual abuse, usual after-school activities.
   D. Satisfaction with weight, feeling that she should be dieting, number of diets in the past year.

24. Which statement about puberty is the most accurate?
   A. Girls are more likely than boys to reach full skeletal maturity in high school.
   B. In general, boys begin puberty earlier than girls.
   C. The growth spurt for girls begins earlier and lasts longer than for boys.
   D. Boys do not gain muscle mass after they have finished their skeletal growth.

25. Sara lived in foster care for several years before being placed with her grandmother in a new city. She is in tenth grade. Which of the following aspects of her life protects her from risk?
   A. Her recent move to a new city.
   B. Friendships with two girls who are at risk for dropping out of school.
   C. A basketball coach with whom she can talk about her problems.
   D. Occasional alcohol use at parties.

ANSWERS

1. *Answer:* C
   Rationale: According to the National Vital Statistics Report (Anderson, 2002), the leading causes of death for 15- to 19-year-olds overall are accidents, homicides, and suicides. Specific rankings vary by gender and ethnicity, and malignancies, heart disease, and congenital malformations are generally ranked fourth through sixth.

2. *Answer:* A
   Rationale: Guidelines for Adolescent Preventive Services (GAP) recommends a physical examination three times during adolescence, but recommends screening for height, weight, blood pressure, BMI, and psychosocial concerns yearly. Screening for anemia using hemoglobin or hematocrit is recommended twice during adolescence, and cholesterol screening for teens at particular risk. While screening for drug use via interview or questionnaire is part of yearly psychosocial screening, testing for drug abuse is not recommended as part of routine preventive services.

3. *Answer:* C
   Rationale: All 50 states allow adolescents to access some confidential services, although these vary widely from state to state. Current federal regulations do give parents the right to access all of a minor's medical records, but states that have more restrictive privacy laws can override this federal mandate, and some states do allow provider discretion in withholding sensitive information. In this volatile and sensitive legal area, pediatric nurse practitioners should be aware of current legal limits of confidentiality in their respective states.

4. *Answer:* D
   Rationale: Health records in a school district are covered by the Family Educational Rights and Privacy Act (FERPA), which allow school officials broader discretion in sharing information than HIPAA, and allows parents access to school-based health records. HIPAA applies to billing third parties, as in a school-based health center. Local regulations may affect policies regarding the extent of confidential services offered in the school, but not rules about privacy and disclosure. Pediatric nurse practitioners who are covered by both HIPAA and FERPA regulations should seek guidance as to their intersection.

5. *Answer:* C
   Rationale: Menarche (first menstrual period) begins between Tanner Stages 3 and 4, when the girl has reached 85% of her adult height, and generally within 4 years of thelarche (development of breast buds, a marker for Tanner 2). In general, the epiphyses close 2 years after menarche (Tanner 5).

6. *Answer:* B
   Rationale: As an early adolescent (ages 10 to 13), Jonathan is still thinking concretely about most life decisions and has little future orientation. A short-term consequence is most likely to appeal to him, especially one that affects an interest he has disclosed to you (his potential ability to attract a girl). While raising the price of cigarettes does decrease adolescent smoking overall, this rationale is unlikely to resonate with an early adolescent who has not yet begun to smoke, due to lack of future orientation.

7. *Answer:* C
   Rationale: Middle adolescence is characterized by intense peer group involvement, a sense of immortality, and increased risk-taking, as well as sexual experimentation. Present orientation, preoccupation with body image, and concrete thinking are characteristic of early adolescents, while long-range planning, adult cognitive abilities, and developed individual values are more characteristic of late adolescents. An increased need for privacy first surfaces in early adolescence but is characteristic of all teens; early adolescents have the highest frequency of arguments with their parents, and financial independence usually does not even begin until late adolescence.

8. *Answer:* D
   Rationale: Interest in risk-taking behaviors correlates better with sexual maturity rating than with chronological age, especially

for early developing adolescents. A 13-year-old girl who is Tanner 5 is more physically mature and appears "older" than most girls her age, possibly attracting older friends. The children in the other choices are not as physically mature and developing at an average rate relative to their peers.

9. *Answer:* B
   Rationale: Major learning disabilities and frequent moves in elementary grades are more consistent with a child who has always done poorly in school. Sudden trauma and major depression are more likely to be associated with a precipitous drop in grades. Children who experience a gradual decline in grades during middle school often have problems with organizing multiple subjects and assignments, consistent with executive function problems including ADHD.

10. *Answer:* C
    Rationale: According to the Youth Risk Behavior Surveys, about 30% of high-school students report five or more drinks at a time (binge drinking) in the past 30 days. The pattern of binge drinking at parties is more typical than daily use, even for adolescents with substance abuse problems. Physical dependence, typified by the need for a morning drink ("eye-opener") is relatively rare for adolescents, as are guilt feelings about drinking or attempts to quit. The typical adolescent in an alcohol dependence program has entered because of suspension from school or legal consequences.

11. *Answer:* A
    Rationale: Marijuana has a long half life, and withdrawal effects from regular use are often not felt until 6 weeks after cessation. While alcohol has many harmful effects, it is marijuana that most profoundly affects memory and motivation. According to the Youth Risk Behavior Surveys, about 80% of high-school students report some alcohol use.

12. *Answer:* B
    Rationale: "Club drugs," including a variety of stimulants, anesthetics, and hallucinogens, were originally associated with dances and raves, but are used in a variety of social settings. The OTC medications acetaminophen, ibuprofen, and naproxen can be overused, especially in combination cold and allergy medications, but are not generally abused in social settings. Narcotics and marijuana are sometimes taken in combination with club drugs. Testosterone, the testosterone precursor androstenedione, and erythropoietin are all used to enhance athletic performance.

13. *Answer:* D
    Rationale: Of 15- to 17-year-olds who have not had intercourse, up to 20% of boys have had oral sex experience. Ten to 15% of heterosexual adolescents engage in anal intercourse, and up to 4.5% of boys 15 to 19 years old have had same-sex experiences. It is typical for teens to define sex as just vaginal intercourse, so it is imperative for the pediatric nurse practitioner to elicit a more specific history. Congratulating the teen on abstinence, condom distribution, or STI test recommendations without clarifying his concept of "haven't had sex yet" would be premature.

14. *Answer:* D
    Rationale: While condoms do not offer 100% protection against infections such as herpes simplex and human papillomavirus, they are considered to be effective protection against gonorrhea and Chlamydia with perfect use. Some teens are allergic to latex, but Keiko has not reported any problems with condom use. It is possible for a condom to be faulty; however, they are subject to strict quality control in manufacture. A study of college students has reported that 38% use condoms "late" in the encounter, after initial penetration, which is the most likely explanation for Keiko's infection.

15. *Answer:* A
    Rationale: About one-third of ninth graders report having had intercourse on the Youth Risk Behavior Surveys, which do not ask about other types of sexual activity. For younger teens, it is often effective to ease into sensitive questions by asking about friends and acquaintances. Asking David about a girlfriend both presumes that he is hetero-

sexual and that any sexual exploration is in the context of an intimate relationship, while up to 4.5% of older teen boys report same-sex activity and many teens report that sexual activity can be part of a casual encounter. Asking teens what they know about a sensitive issue can be a conversation-stopper, while asking about exposure to STIs is an indirect and probably unproductive way of asking about sexual activity to a younger teen that is either still thinking concretely or else convinced that he is immune to risk.

16. *Answer:* B

Rationale: All 50 states require child abuse reports for sexual abuse while the adolescent is still a minor, even if the abuse occurred in the past. Unless the pediatric nurse practitioner has documentation that a report has already been made, a report would have to be filed after this visit. While the tattoo was probably not obtained legally and might put the teen at risk for blood-borne infections, it is not reportable in itself. Infections such as HIV or hepatitis B or C might require a Health Department report in the pediatric nurse practitioner's state, but definitive testing results would not be available the day of the visit.

17. *Answer:* C

Rationale: The Health Behavior of School-aged Children Survey estimates that 10.6% of sixth to tenth graders bully "sometimes." Girls are more likely to be bullied verbally than boys, and African American children are least likely to be bullied. No differences were found among urban, suburban, or rural settings.

18. *Answer:* B

Rationale: Over 40% of self-identified gay, lesbian, bisexual, or transgender youth do not feel safe at school, with almost half reporting daily verbal harassment and over 10% reporting physical assault. Studies have shown higher rates of suicidal ideation in gay and bisexual youth who have experienced harassment, particularly for boys. In general, playing sports is protective, as is working less than 20 hours per week. While divorce is considered an adverse childhood event that

increases risk for a variety of problems, the divorce is not recent, and having both parents involved and friendly mitigates any adverse effects.

19. *Answer:* C

Rationale: The principles of harm reduction involve a different approach to risky behavior such as substance abuse, neither a disease nor a criminal model, and a removal of barriers to services for individuals who are currently engaging in risky behavior. Even though alcohol and drug use are prohibited at school proms, their use is common, and the provision of free shuttle services decreases potential driving accidents in case substance use occurs. High-dose amoxicillin is a curative disease model approach to otitis media. Urine drug screening can be useful in treatment, but is an example of both criminal and disease model approaches, depending on the consequences of a positive test. Limiting the sale of alcohol is a legal approach.

20. *Answer:* D

Rationale: A motivational interview involves helping the patient to work through ambivalence and verbalize her own readiness to change, by having the patient give a number on a scale to both importance of change and confidence that she can change. The practitioner then encourages progress by having the patient elicit barriers to change and the first step to take. Giving the patient discouraging advice does not support behavior change. While it is true that condoms alone are not as effective as condoms combined with another form of contraception, Isabella may have some concerns about contraception we haven't heard yet. While abstinence is the most effective way to prevent a pregnancy and can be a good option for sexually experienced teens, in motivational interviewing the practitioner encourages the patient to come up with the solutions.

21. *Answer:* A

Rationale: Early adolescents do not have developed impulse control, nor do they have the future orientation that might help them avoid risky behavior. After-school hours are the times that adolescents are most likely to get into trouble. The best approach for a parent in the same situation as Mark's father is to keep Mark busy and supervised, and to help Mark develop some interests that may protect him from risky behavior in the future. While some rudeness is normal for early adolescents, there is no reason for Mark's father to lower his standards of acceptable behavior in the home. Staying away from teens that are engaging in risky behavior is an excellent idea, but it is most effectively accomplished by keeping Mark busy and supervised, rather than putting the onus on Mark (restrictions for failure to stay away).

22. *Answer:* B

Rationale: Both public and private health insurance policies are variable with respect to young adults, and Jason may be able to either keep his parents' health insurance or obtain insurance through his school if he attends college full-time; otherwise he is at risk of losing insurance support. At 18, Jason does have full confidentiality rights, although this may be more of a challenge to implement in a pediatric practice where his parents and the staff are used to fuller information-sharing than in an adult or family practice. Late adolescents generally have better impulse control than earlier adolescents. Cognitive development is not complete until age 20, but the main difference between the decision-making of late adolescents and older adults is life experience, not inherent reasoning ability.

23. *Answer:* D

Rationale: As the major risk factor for an eating disorder, questions about dieting are paramount. A complete psychosocial screen is part of any evaluation for eating disorders, but questions about drug use, sexual activity, sexual orientation, and even sexual abuse are not specific for eating disorders. An eating disorder should be part of the differential for an adolescent with menstrual irregularities and weight fluctuation.

24. *Answer:* A

Rationale: Girls begin puberty earlier than boys and have their growth spurt at earlier stage in puberty, in general complet-

ing their growth within 2 years of menarche. Boys begin their growth later, have increased growth over a longer period of time, and may not have completed their skeletal growth until ages 18 to 20. Young men have increased levels of testosterone as their epiphyses close, which accounts for an increase in muscle mass after skeletal growth is complete.

25. *Answer:* C

Rationale: Positive relationships with adults outside of the immediate family can be protective for youth, whether or not their families are stable. While Sara's move may eventually be a positive factor in her life, at the moment this disruption can be traumatic if she had to leave friends and other family members behind. Neither friendship with teens at risk for school failure nor alcohol use is protective.

BIBLIOGRAPHY

American Academy of Family Physicians, American Academy of Pediatrics, American College of Obstetricians and Gynecologists, and Society of Adolescent Medicine. (2004). Position Paper: Protecting adolescents: Ensuring access to care and reporting sexual activity and abuse. *J Adol Health, 35*(5), 420-423.

American Medical Association (AMA) Department of Adolescent Health. (1997). *Guidelines for adolescent preventive services (GAPS) recommendations monograph.* Chicago: AMA.

Anda, R.F., Chapman, D.P., Felitti, V.J., et al. (2002). Adverse childhood experiences and risk of paternity in teen pregnancy. *Obstet Gynecol, 100*(1), 37-45.

Anderson, R.N. (2002). Deaths: Leading causes for 2000. *Natl Vital Stat Rep, 50*(16), 1-85.

Anstine, D., & Grinenko, D. (2000). Rapid screening for disordered eating in college-aged females in the primary care setting. *J Adolesc Health, 26*(5), 338-342.

Boekeloo, B.O., Bradley, O., Jerry, J., et al. (2004). Randomized trial of brief office-based interventions to reduce adolescent alcohol use. *Arch Pediatr Adolesc Med, 158*(7), 635-642.

Bonny, A.E., Britto, M.T., Klostermann, B.K., et al. (2000). School disconnectedness: Identifying adolescents at risk. *Pediatrics, 106*(5), 1017-1021.

Bontempo, D.E., & D'Augelli, A.R. (2002). Effects of at-school victimization and sexual orientation on lesbian, gay, or bisexual youth's health risk behavior. *J Adolesc Health, 30*(5), 364-374.

Burstein, G.R., & Murray, P.J. (2003). Diagnosis and management of sexually transmitted disease pathogens among adolescents. *Pediatr Rev, 24*(3), 75-82.

Dailard, C. (March 2003). New medical records privacy rule: The interface with teen access to confidential care. *The Guttmacher Report on Public Policy*, 6-7.

Dennis, M., Babor, T.F., Roebuck, M.C., & Donaldson, J. (2002). Changing the focus: The case for recognizing and treating cannabis use disorders. *Addiction, 97*(Suppl 1), 4-15.

de Visser, R.O., & Smith, A.M. (2000). When always isn't enough: Implications of the late application of condoms for the validity and reliability of self-reported condom use. *AIDS Care, 12*(2), 221-224.

Dickey, S.B., & Deatrick, J. (2000). Autonomy and decision making for health promotion in adolescence. *Pediatr Nurs, 26*(5), 461-467.

English, A. (2000). Reproductive health services for adolescents: Critical legal issues. *Obstet Gynecol Clin North Am, 27*(1), 195-211.

Garofalo, R., & Harper, G.W. (2003). Not all adolescents are the same: Addressing the unique needs of gay and bisexual male youth. *Adolesc Med, 14*(3), 595-611.

Goldenring, J.M. & Rosen, D.S. (2004). Getting into adolescent heads: An essential update. *Contemp Pediatr, 21*(1), 64-80.

Gould, M.S., Greenberg, T., Velting, D.M., & Shaffer, D. (2003). Youth suicide risk and preventive interventions: A review of the past 10 years. *J Am Acad Child Adolesc Psychiatry, 42*(4), 86-405.

Grunbaum, J.A., Kann, L., Kinchen, S.A., et al. (2004). *Youth risk behavior surveillance - United States, 2003* [53 (SS-2)]: Morbidity and Mortality Weekly Report Center for Disease Control Surveillance Summaries.

Hickman, L.J., Jaycox, L.H., & Aronoff, J. (2004). Dating violence among adolescents: Prevalence, gender distribution, and prevention program effectiveness. *Trauma Violence Abuse, 5*(2), 123-142.

Kaiser Family Foundation. (2002). *Millions of young people mix sex with alcohol or drugs: With dangerous consequences*. Presented on February 7, 2002 at the conference titled "Dangerous liaisons: Substance abuse and sexual behavior." Sponsored by the National Center on Addiction and Substance Abuse at Columbia University, New York and the Kaiser Family Foundation. Press release retrieved on April 18, 2006, from http://www.outproud.org/pdf/CASANews-Release.pdf.

Klein, J.D., & Wilson, K.M. (2002). Delivering quality care: Adolescents' discussion of health risks with their providers. *J Adolesc Health, 30*(3), 190-195.

Lonczak, H.S., Abbott, R.D., Hawkins, J.D., et al. (2002). Effects of the Seattle Social Development Project on sexual behavior, pregnancy, birth and sexually transmitted disease outcomes by age 21 years. *Arch Pediatr Adolesc Med, 156*(5), 438-447.

Maradiegue, A. (2003) Minor's rights versus parental rights: Review of legal issues in adolescent health care. *J Midwifery Women's Health, 48*(3), 170-177.

Marlatt, G.A. (1996). Harm reduction: Come as you are. *Addict Behav, 21*(6), 779-788.

Mosher, W.D., Chandra, A., & Jones, J. (2005). *Sexual behavior and selected health measures: Men and women 15-44 years of age, United States, 2002*. Advance data from vital and health statistics; no 362. Hyattsville, MD: National Center for Health Statistics.

Muntner, P., He, J., Cutler, J.A., et al. (2004). Trends in blood pressure among children and adolescents. *JAMA, 291*(17), 2107-2113.

Muscari, M.E., & Berkstresser, M. (2001). The precollege examination: Fostering a healthy transition. *J Pediatr Health Care, 15*(2), 63-70.

Nansel, T.R., Overpeck, M., Pilla, R.S., et al. (2001). Bullying behaviors among US youth: prevalence and association with psychosocial adjustment. *JAMA, 285*(16), 2094-3000.

Nelson, T.F., Naimi, T.S., Brewer, R.D., & Wechsler, H. (2005). The state sets the rate: The relationship of college binge drinking to state binge drinking rates and selected state alcohol control policies. *Am J Public Health, 95*(3), 441-446.

Neumark-Sztainer, D., Story, M., Hannan, P.J., & Croll, J. (2002). Overweight status and eating patterns among adolescents: Where do youths stand in comparison with the Healthy People 2010 objectives? *Am J Public Health, 92*(5), 844-851.

Neumark-Sztainer, D., Wall, M.M., Story, M., & Perry, C.L. (2003). Correlates of unhealthy weight-control behaviors among adolescents: Implications for prevention programs. *Health Psychol, 22*(1), 88-98.

Pender, N.J., Murdaugh, C.L., & Parsons, M.A. (2002). *Health promotion in nursing practice* (4th ed.). Upper Saddle River, NJ: Prentice-Hall.

Radzik, M., Sherer, S., & Neinstein, L.S. (2002). Psychosocial development in normal adolescents. In L.S. Neinstein (Ed.). *Adolescent health care: A practical guide* (4th ed.). Philadelphia: Lippincott Williams & Wilkins.

Rosen, D.S., & Neinstein, L.S. (2002). Preventive health care for adolescents. In L.S. Neinstein (Ed.). *Adolescent health care: A practical guide* (4th ed.). Philadelphia: Lippincott Williams & Wilkins.

Saslow, D., Runowicz, C.D., Solomon, D., et al. (2002).American Cancer Society guideline for the early detection of cervical neoplasia and cancer. *CA: Cancer J Clin, 52*(6), 342-362.

Sexuality Information and Education Council of the United States (SIECUS). (2001). *Lesbian, gay, bisexual and transgender youth issues.* SIECUS Report, Volume 29, Number 4. Retrieved April 18, 2006, from www.siecus.org/pubs/fact/fact0013.html.

Shafer, M.A. (2000). With urine based screening, do sexually active adolescent girls still need annual pelvic examinations? No: recommending annual exams is not evidence based. *West J Med, 173*(5), 293.

Silverman, J.G., Raj, A., Mucci, L.A., & Hathaway, J.E. (2001). Dating violence against adolescent girls and associated substance use, unhealthy weight control, sexual risk behavior, pregnancy, and suicidality. *JAMA, 286*(5), 572-579.

Sindelar, H.A., Abrantes, A.M., Hart, C., et al. (2004). Motivational interviewing in pediatric practice. *Curr Probl Pediatr Adolesc Health Care, 34*(9), 322-339.

Strote, J., Lee, J.E., & Wechsler, H. (2002). Increasing MDMA use among college students: Results of a national survey. *J Adolesc Health, 30*(1), 64-72.

Tellier, P.P. (2002). Club drugs: Is it all ecstasy? *Pediatr Ann, 31*(9), 550-556.

Timperio, A., Salmon, J., & Ball, K. (2004). Evidence-based strategies to promote physical activity among children, adolescents and young adults: Review and update. *J Sci Med Sport, 7*(1), Suppl., 20-29.

U.S. Department Health & Human Services Public Health Service, Office of Assistant Secretary for Health. (2000). *Healthy People 2010: Conference Edition.* Washington, DC: HHS.

Wu, A.C., Lesperance, L., & Bernstein, H. (2002). Screening for iron deficiency. *Pediatr Rev, 23*(5), 171-177.

Zimmerman, M.A., Bingenheimer, J.B., & Notaro, P.C. (2002). Natural mentors and adolescent resiliency: A study with urban youth. *Am J Community Psychol, 30*(2), 221-243.

NOTES

Sexuality and Birth Control

JEAN B. IVEY

Select the best answer for each of the following questions:

1. The physiologic process which results in the initiation of puberty is the release of:
   A. FSH by the adrenal gland.
   B. LH by the ovaries and androgen by the testes.
   C. TRH, which stimulates TSH and prolactin.
   D. Estrogen and androgen by the testes and ovaries.

2. What events in puberty are related to the development of adolescent acne?
   A. The release of FSH.
   B. The release of TSH.
   C. Skin thickening and oil secretion.
   D. The production of inhibin B.

3. A 13-year-old is seen for a sports physical. What would be the appropriate approach when collecting a sexual history?
   A. "What has your mother told you about sex?"
   B. "You haven't had sex yet, have you?"
   C. "An important part of your development is your sexual development. Have you noticed changes in your body?"
   D. "Have you ever had hypospadias, epispadias, cryptorchidism, or microphallus?"

4. A female adolescent has the following characteristics: Breast buds with slight enlargement of the breast but no separation. Sparse, long, slightly pigmented, curly pubic hair along the labia. At what Sexual Maturity Rating (SMR, Tanner Stage) of development is this adolescent?
   A. Stage 0.
   B. Stage 2.
   C. Stage 4.
   D. Stage 1.

5. The toddler's sexual development focuses on:
   A. Rubbing or stroking the genitals.
   B. Playing "doctor" with peers.
   C. Covering the genitals, refusing to undress when strangers are present.
   D. Controlling defecation and urination.

6. At an annual exam for a 4-year-old, it would be appropriate for the pediatric nurse practitioner to discuss:
   A. Ways to stop masturbation.
   B. Protecting children from seeing adults undressed.
   C. Avoiding contact with gay or lesbian acquaintances.
   D. Modeling respectful, loving sexual behavior.

7. What issues would it be important and developmentally appropriate to discuss with a teenage male at Tanner Stage 2?
   A. Methods of birth control.
   B. Changes in his body, nocturnal emissions, and masturbation.
   C. Dating and serious relationships.
   D. Sexually transmitted diseases.

8. The mother of a 15-year-old tells the pediatric practitioner nurse that her daughter has told her that she is a lesbian. An appropriate response would be:

A. If she had one experience it doesn't make her a lesbian.
B. Do you believe her?
C. I wouldn't worry about it, she probably isn't being truthful.
D. Experimenting with sexuality is normal. How do you feel about her saying that?

9. An adolescent girl has a severe herpes infection in her pharynx and oral mucosa. She had said that she was not sexually active. Knowing that this type of herpes is sexually transmitted, what is the most likely explanation for this discrepancy?
A. This is probably some other viral infection not related to sexual contact.
B. Most adolescents don't consider oral sex to be sexual activity.
C. She is immunosuppressed.
D. She is probably got it from sharing straws, glasses, or lip gloss with friends.

10. What approach might be helpful when discussing pornography with adolescents?
A. Explain that they should never buy or look at pornographic images.
B. Get their parents to agree to block it from their home computers and explain that it is not appropriate for teens.
C. Discuss how it conveys negative attitudes and a lack of respect toward others.
D. Give them a copy of the laws about it and explain that it is wrong to look at or buy it.

11. Which of the following statement is TRUE regarding sexual activity in ninth- to twelfth-grade adolescent?
A. About 45% of ninth- to twelfth-grade adolescents have had sexual intercourse with four or more partners.
B. About 25% used a condom during the last sexual intercourse.
C. About 25% reported they got pregnant or got someone else pregnant.
D. About 45% of ninth- to twelfth-grade adolescents have had sexual intercourse.

12. In addition to advocating abstinence and condom use, what practice measures can help prevent sexually transmitted diseases and pregnancy in adolescents?
A. Availability of and information about contraceptives.
B. Getting teens to sign a pledge to not use alcohol or drugs.
C. Teaching tenth-grade students about the biology of reproduction.
D. Target low-income minority students for pregnancy prevention programs.

13. What is the common cause of failure or delayed physical development in an adolescent?
A. Type II diabetes.
B. Malnutrition.
C. Precocious puberty.
D. Sexually transmitted diseases.

14. Appropriate management of gynecomastia is:
A. Refer to endocrinology for a work-up.
B. Give testosterone supplements for a year.
C. Refer to a pediatric surgeon for excision of excess tissue.
D. Reassure that this is a temporary condition and will resolve without treatment.

15. Which hormone(s) cause the adolescent growth spurt in females?
A. Estrogen.
B. Androgens and thyroxin.
C. TSH and ACTH.
D. Gonadotropic hormones.

16. What stage of sexual maturation (Tanner Stage) is associated with the skeletal growth spurt in females?
A. Stage 1.
B. Stages 2 to 3.
C. Stage 5.
D. Stages 4 to 5.

17. A 6-year-old child with mild mental retardation and cerebral palsy comes to the clinic for a well child exam. Axillary hair and stage 2 pubic hair are present. What would be appropriate management for this child?

A. Explain to the parents that she needs sex education and that the school needs to be informed.
B. Prescribe a low-dose oral contraceptive.
C. Refer to endocrinology as soon as possible.
D. Prescribe monthly testosterone injections and monitor closely.

18. Selection of a method of birth control should be made by:
A. The health care provider based on his/her experience.
B. The parent of the adolescent since his/her insurance will pay for it.
C. The adolescent, who is the patient.
D. Jointly by the parent and child if possible.

19. Which of the following approaches might help an adolescent select a method of birth control?
A. Suggest that she try oral contraceptives for a month and see how she does.
B. Give her pamphlets describing the methods and side effects and tell her to come back when she decides.
C. Suggest that she talk to her mother about it.
D. Discuss her habits and lifestyle and compare methods that might be good for her.

20. Regardless of the method of birth control chosen, it is MOST important to stress that:
A. Adolescents should not be sexually active.
B. Condoms must also be used to prevent HIV and other STDs.

C. Weight gain is the usual side effect of most methods.
D. Oral contraceptives can't be used if the person is a smoker.

21. Depo Provera is often preferred by providers and teens because:
A. It is easier to remember so pregnancy is less likely.
B. It doesn't cause weight gain.
C. Periods are more regular.
D. Risk of STDs is decreased.

22. Transdermal contraceptives are:
A. Popular but ineffective if not removed and reapplied correctly.
B. Less effective than oral contraceptives.
C. More likely to cause weight gain.
D. Not recommended for nulliparous women.

23. Emergency contraception is:
A. Available by prescription only throughout the U.S.
B. Regulated by state laws and often not covered by health insurance.
C. Not appropriate for adolescent use.
D. Very likely to cause severe pain and bleeding.

24. An important part of family planning visits for sexually active teens is:
A. Ordering a pregnancy test prior to prescribing contraceptives.
B. Suggesting that she try abstinence prior to prescribing contraceptives.
C. Informing the parents about the teen's decision.
D. Explaining that as long as a pill is taken pregnancy is unlikely.

ANSWERS

1. *Answer:* C
    Rationale: At beginning of puberty, TRH causes the release of TSH and prolactin which simulate the onset of sexual development. The release of sex hormones is regulated by the anterior pituitary, including the release of FSH and LH. The anterior pituitary causes the release of these hormones. Estrogen and the androgens are released later in the process after stimulation by TSH and prolactin.

2. *Answer:* C
    Rationale: Skin thickening and oil secretion can result in skin pore plugging and overproduction of oil that is associated with acne. FSH stimulates sperm production. TSH initiates pubertal development but is not associated with acne. inhibin B is produced in the testicles and is associated with sperm production.

3. *Answer:* C
    Rationale: Asking if they had sex yet leads the adolescent to reply negatively and give the answer the provider wants, rather than facts. Exploring what others have told the adolescent is important, but should follow the exploration of sexual development. Option A gives the adolescent a chance to discuss whatever issues are important and the provider can follow up with appropriate questions to cover the other areas needed. Asking about disorders may affect sexuality and may be appropriate, but most adolescents won't know these terms and may be intimidated by this approach.

4. *Answer:* B
    Rationale: There is no Stage 0. When the characteristics differ (i.e., breasts in this case are closer to Stage 3 and genital development is closer to Stage 2), the lower stage is reported. Stage 4 characteristics are not present. Stage 1 characteristics are prepubertal.

5. *Answer:* D
    Rationale: The major developmental tasks for toddlers are gaining mastery with toileting. Playing doctor or refusal to undress with strangers is typical preschool behaviors.

Infants between 6 and 9 months discover their genitals and derive pleasure by stroking them.

6. *Answer:* D
    Rationale: Respectful loving sexual behavior is learned from role models. Masturbation is normal in preschoolers. Teaching a child where it is and is not appropriate is a better topic. Seeing adults undressed in appropriate places but clothed in others models appropriate behavior. Gay and lesbian acquaintances pose no threat to preschool children as role models.

7. *Answer:* B
    Rationale: At Tanner Stage 2, the first signs of puberty appear and it is important to discuss these issues. He is more likely to be concerned about his body and changes than sexual activity, although this information should be provided. He is probably not dating or in a serious relationship at this stage, although he probably has many questions about how to approach girls. While it is important for him to know about STDs, at Tanner Stage 2 he is probably more concerned about his body and the changes he is experiencing.

8. *Answer:* D
    Rationale: While one experience doesn't necessarily mean her daughter is a lesbian, this answer dismisses her concerns and assumes that this would be a negative outcome. Asking if the mother believes her daughter implies that the parent expects the teen to be deceptive/dishonest and implies that it probably isn't true. Saying she should not worry about it because she probably is not a lesbian conveys a negative attitude toward gay/lesbian lifestyles. Option D conveys the information but also gives the parent a chance to express feelings and concerns about the adolescent.

9. *Answer:* B
    Rationale: The pediatric nurse practitioner needs to ask specifically about oral sexual activity; many adolescents don't consider oral sex to be sexual activity. The most likely cause of infection is sexually transmitted herpes.

10. *Answer:* C

Rationale: Telling them not to look will make them feel guilty if they have done so, and blocking computers will probably make them more determined to see it. Option C provides the teen with a solid reason and they can understand and empathize with those who have been victimized. Providing information about the laws may not be effective because teens often find it an interesting challenge to circumvent laws.

11. *Answer:* D

Rationale: According to the 2001 Youth Risk Behavioral Survey, 45.6% of ninth- to twelfth-grade teens had sexual intercourse. Fifty-eight percent used a condom during their last sexual intercourse. About 5% reported they got pregnant or got someone else pregnant.

12. *Answer:* A

Rationale: Access to information is the most effective measure to prevent pregnancy and STDs. While drugs and alcohol play a part in impulsive behavior, such pledges can't be the mainstay of prevention. Tenth grade is too late to provide this information and have an effect on these problems. Targeting low-income minority students is discriminatory and ignores the fact that sexuality cuts across race and class lines.

13. *Answer:* B

Rationale: Malnutrition is a common cause of delayed or interruption of pubertal development due to inadequate amounts of body fat and nutrients. STDs and type II diabetes do not interfere with pubertal development. Precocious puberty is abnormally early pubertal development.

14. *Answer:* D

Rationale: Gynecomastia is not a condition requiring an endocrinology consult and giving testosterone is not an appropriate treatment. Surgery is not necessary. Ordinarily the condition resolves in a year or less, and appropriate reassurance is the best action.

15. *Answer:* B

Rationale: Androgens and thyroxin cause the growth spurt and development of secondary sexual characteristics. Estrogen does not cause the growth spurt. TSH and ACTH are involved in egg production. The gonadotropic hormones cause ovarian maturation and production of progesterone and estrogen.

16. *Answer:* B

Rationale: The growth spurt occurs during Tanner Stages 2 to 3. There is no growth spurt in Stage 1 and growth is slowed or complete by Stages 4 to 5.

17. *Answer:* C

Rationale: Secondary sexual characteristics occurring in a 6-year-old child are not normal and a referral should be made. Precocious puberty occurs when pubic and axillary hair occurs before 7 or 8 years in girls and before 9 years in boys.

18. *Answer:* D

Rationale: The health care provider can offer advice but should not decide for the patient. Parental involvement is helpful but the parent shouldn't make the final decision. The adolescent certainly should express his or her opinion and make the final decision in case of a conflict. But parental input would be helpful. The preferred method is a joint decision between parent and child.

19. *Answer:* D

Rationale: It would be better to involve her in the decision making. Written materials are good but a person-to-person discussion is better. She may not want her mother to know about her decisions. Discussing her lifestyle and habits would be the approach most likely to result in an informed choice.

20. *Answer:* B

Rationale: Other methods of birth control do not decrease the risk of STDs and HIV.

21. *Answer:* A

Rationale: The convenience of Depo Provera is a big advantage with teens. It is just as likely to cause weight gain as other methods. Amenorrhea is usual after a few months. STDs are not prevented by using Depo Provera.

22. *Answer:* A

Rationale: The teen must remember to apply a patch weekly for 3 weeks and then skip a week. Mistakes can result in pregnancy. Effectiveness depends on appropriate use but there is no difference between it and oral contraceptives. Parity isn't relevant for this method and they are not more likely to cause weight gain compared to other contraceptives.

23. *Answer:* B

Rationale: The FDA announced approval on August 24, 2006 for emergency contraception sales to those over 18 years of age over the counter. Girls aged 17 and under still require a prescription. State laws often regulate and affect availability of emergency contraception in local pharmacies. Adolescents are probably the population that most needs this option. Nausea and vomiting is the most frequent side effect, not pain and severe bleeding.

24. *Answer:* A

Rationale: Ordering a pregnancy test is prudent for a sexually active teen. A Pap smear and cultures are also indicated at an initial visit. Suggesting abstinence may be counterproductive and result in pregnancy in the sexually active adolescent. Notifying parents is not appropriate unless the state law requires such action. It is likely to destroy rapport and trust in the teen. It is important for oral contraceptives to be taken at about the same time of day to avoid pregnancy.

BIBLIOGRAPHY

Bethell, C., Lansky, D., Hendryx, M. (2000). *RWJF priority and program area performance indicators summary report*. Retrieved April 19, 2006, from http://www.markle.org/resources/facct/index.php.

Blythe, M.J. & Rosenthal, S.L. (2000). Female adolescent sexuality. *Adolesc Gynecol 27*(1), 125-139.

Dieben, T.O., Roumen, F.J., & Apter, D. (2002). Efficacy, cycle control and user acceptability of a novel combined contraceptive vaginal ring. *Obstet Gynecol, 100*(3), 585-593.

Escobar-Chavez, S.L., Torolero, S., Markham, C., & Low, B. (2004). Impact of the media on adolescent sexual attitudes and behaviors. Report submitted to the Centers for Disease Control and Prevention. Available at www.medinstitute.org/media/MediaExecSum.htm.

Faryna, E.L., & Morales, E. (2000). Self-efficacy and HIV-related risk behaviors among multiethnic adolescents. *Cultur Divers Ethnic Minor Psychol, 6*(1), 42-56.

Gilbert, L.K., Temby, J.R.E., Rogers, S.E. (2005). Evaluating a teen STD prevention Web site. *J Adolesc Health, 37*(3), 236-242.

Gold, R.B., & Sonfield, A. (2001). Reproductive health services for adolescents under the State Children's Health Insurance Program. *Fam Plan Perspect, 33*(2), 81-87.

Green, H.H., & Documet, P.I. (2005). Parent peer education: Lessons learned from a community-based initiative for teen pregnancy prevention. *J Adolesc Health, 37*(3 Suppl), S100-107.

Greydanus, D.E., Patel, D.R., & Rimsza, M.E. (2001). Contraception in the adolescent: An update. *Pediatrics, 107*(3), 562-573.

Grunbaum, J.A., Kann, L., Kinchen, S.A., et al. (2002). *Youth risk behavior surveillance—United States*, 2001. Retrieved June 6, 2002, from www.cdc.gov/mmwr/preview/mmwrhtml/ss5104a1.htm.

Hacker, K.A., Mare, Y., Strunk, N., & Horst, L. (2000). Listening to youth: Teen perspectives on pregnancy prevention. *J Adolesc Health, 26*(4), 279-288.

Jaccard, J., & Dittus, P.J. (2000). Adolescent perceptions of maternal approval of birth control and sexual risk behavior. *Am J Pub Health, 90*(9), 1426-1430.

Kaplowitz, P.B. (2003). Precocious puberty. Retrieved on June 6, 2006, from www.emedicine.com/ped/topic1882.htm.

Karofsky, P.S., Zeng, L., & Kosorok, M.R. (2000). Relationship between adolescent-parental communication and initiation of first intercourse by adolescents. *J Adolesc Health, 28*(1), 41-45.

Kollar, L.M. (2002). *New contraceptive options for adolescents*. Paper presented at the meeting of the National Association of Pediatric Nurse Practitioners Annual Nursing Conference, Orlando, FL.

Lonczak, H.S., Abbott, R.D., Hawkins, J.D., et al. (2002). Effects of the Seattle Social Development Project on sexual behavior, pregnancy, birth, and sexually transmitted disease outcomes by age 21 years. *Arch Pediatr Adolesc Med, 156*(5), 438-447.

Nelson, E.E., Leibenluft, E., McClure, E.B., & Pine, D.S. (2005). The social re-orientation of adolescence: A neuroscience perspective on the process and its relation to psychopathology. *Psychol Med, 35*(2), 163-174.

Nusbaum, M.R.H., & Hamilton, C.D. (2002). The proactive sexual health history. *Am Fam Physician, 66*(9), 1705-1712.

O'Sullivan, L.F., Meyer-Bahlburg, H.F.L., & Watkins, B.X. (2001). Mother-daughter communication about sex among urban African American and Latino families. *J Adolesc Res, 16*(3), 269-292.

Ozer, E.M., Park, M.J., Paul, T., et al. (2003). *America's adolescents: Are they healthy?* San Francisco: University of California, San Francisco, National Adolescent Health Information Center.

Plant, T.M. (2002). Neurophysiology of puberty. *J Adolesc Health, 31*(6S), 185-191.

Rogol, A.D., Roemmich, J.N., & Clark, P.A. (2002). Growth at puberty. *J Adolesc Health 31*(6S), 192-200.

Ryan, G. (2000a). Childhood sexuality: A decade of study. Part I—Research and curriculum development. *Child Abuse Negl, 24*(1), 33-48.

Ryan, G. (2000b). Childhood sexuality: A decade of study. Part II—Dissemination and future directions. *Child Abuse Negl, 24*(1), 49-61.

Santelli, J., Ott, M.A., Lyon, M., et al. (2006). Abstinence and abstinence-only education: A review of U.S. policies and programs. *J Adolesc Health, 38*(1), 72-81.

Savin-Williams, R.C., Cohen, K.M. (2004). Homoerotic development during childhood and adolescence. *Child Adolesc Psychiatr Clini North Am, 13*(3), 529-549, vii.

Vartanian, L.R. (2000). Revisiting the imaginary audience and personal fable constructs of adolescent egocentrism: A conceptual review. *Adolescence, 35*(140), 639-661.

NOTES

DIAGNOSIS AND MANAGEMENT OF COMMON ILLNESS IN CHILDREN AND ADOLESCENTS

Common Illnesses of the Head, Eyes, Ears, Nose, and Throat

PATRICIA JACKSON ALLEN

Select the best answer for each of the following questions:

1. All bacterial conjunctivitis:
    A. Must be treated with antibiotics to prevent complications.
    B. Is highly contagious requiring family education on prevention.
    C. Is more common than viral conjunctivitis.
    D. Is frequently caused by *M. catarrhalis*.

2. Aleshia, age 5 years, presents to your clinic with a 3-day history of itchy, inflamed eyes. Which of the following findings would be most supportive of the diagnosis of allergic conjunctivitis?
    A. Concurrent finding of atopic dermatitis.
    B. Concurrent finding of otitis media.
    C. Purulent drainage in one eye.
    D. Presence of enlarged tender cervical lymph nodes.

3. Laboratory analysis of neonatal ocular discharge would be positive for gram-negative intracellular diplococci for which of the following organisms?
    A. Chlamydia.
    B. *Haemophilus influenzae.*
    C. Adenovirus.
    D. Gonococcus.

4. Ms. Smith brings her 6-month-old daughter into the clinic for her well child checkup. When asked if she has any concerns regarding her daughter, she states "Her left eye tears all the time and has since birth. I went to urgent care once and the doctor gave me some antibiotic for her eye but that didn't seem to help." After completing your history and physical examination, you assess the infant to be healthy except for left dacryostenosis without evidence of infection. What education and counseling would you give the mother regarding your findings?
    A. Referral to an ophthalmologist is recommended since this condition has continued for 6 months.
    B. Another course of ophthalmic antibiotics is recommended to prevent infection while we wait for the tearing to stop.
    C. Spontaneous resolution almost always occurs by 12 months of age.
    D. The blockage in the tear duct was probably the result of a minor neonatal eye infection.

5. Justin is a 12-year-old boy brought in by his mother because of "swelling around his right eye for the past 24 hours." When evaluating Justin to determine whether he has a periorbital cellulitis or orbital cellulitis, which of the following findings would support the diagnosis of orbital cellulitis?
    A. History and evidence of a recent insect bite near the right eye.
    B. Proptosis of the right eye and decreased visual acuity.
    C. Induration, erythema, and tenderness around the right eye.
    D. History of being hit with a baseball in the right eye in the past 48 hours.

6. Heather, age 18 months, is found to have a positive cover-uncover test for her right eye during her well child examination.

Heather's mother reports she has noticed her daughter's "eye turning in when she is tired." Which of the following management plans would be appropriate at this time?

A. Refer to ophthalmology for evaluation and treatment.
B. Patch the right eye and tell mother to have the patch on 8 hours a day.
C. Schedule a return appointment in 2 months to reassess the eye.
D. Discuss with mother the need for surgery in the immediate future.

7. Joshua, age 6 months, has just been diagnosed with his first otitis media. The pediatric nurse practitioner wants to tell the mother of amendable risk factors that may decrease the risk of future otitis media. Which of the following factors is associated with increased ear infections?

A. Breastfeeding for the first 6 months of life.
B. Supine sleeping position.
C. Exposure to second-hand smoke.
D. Introduction of solids before 6 months of age.

8. Jessica is a 15-month-old child weighing 11 kg who attends full-time daycare and has just been diagnosed with her first symptomatic ear infection with fever for past 48 hours. There is no known history of drug allergies. Your treatment plan would include which of the following?

A. Tylenol for pain and fever and amoxicillin 400 mg orally twice a day for 10 days.
B. Auralgan (antipyrine and benzocaine) ear drops three times a day and Tylenol for pain and fever.
C. Amoxicillin-clavulanic acid 100 mg orally twice a day for 10 days and Tylenol for pain and fever management.
D. Amoxicillin 125 mg orally twice a day for 10 days and Auralgan for ear pain.

9. Alicia is 4 years old and was brought to the urgent care clinic by her mother because the school nurse called to report Alicia was complaining of left ear pain. The mother reports the child was well until last night when she started coughing and had a clear runny nose. There is no report of fever and Alicia appears in no acute distress and reports a level 4 on the Oucher Scale. Her left tympanic membrane is red without visible landmarks and movement on insufflation. Which of the following would be the most appropriate treatment plan at this time?

A. Tylenol for pain and fever and amoxicillin 250 mg orally twice a day for 10 days.
B. Auralgan (antipyrine and benzocaine) ear drops three times a day and Tylenol for pain and fever.
C. Amoxicillin-clavulanic acid 200 mg orally twice a day for 10 days and Tylenol for pain and fever management.
D. Amoxicillin 500 mg orally twice a day for 10 days and Auralgan for ear pain.

10. Timothy is a junior on the high-school swim team. He comes to the urgent care clinic today with a complaint of right ear pain for the past 2 days. He denies fever and symptoms of an upper respiratory infection. On examination, his external ear is painful when moved but not inflamed. The external canal is red, swollen, and tender with a white discharge. You are unable to see the tympanic membrane on the right ear but the left tympanic membrane appears normal. Your diagnosis would be:

A. Cholesteatoma.
B. Perforated tympanic membrane due to otitis media.
C. Foreign body in ear causing irritation and drainage.
D. Otitis externa.

11. Children with otitis media with effusion who are not at risk for developmental delay should:

A. Be placed on antihistamine therapy for 2 weeks to attempt to clear blocked eustachian tube.
B. Have a full course of high-dose amoxicillin to clear any underlying infection.
C. Have a 5-day course of prednisone to decrease inflammation.
D. Return to be reevaluated in 3 months for resolution of condition.

12. The primary diagnostic criteria for otitis media with effusion is:
   A. Minimal movement of tympanic membrane with pneumatic otoscopy.
   B. Convex tympanic membrane with no visible bony landmarks.
   C. A diffuse light reflex with red tympanic membrane.
   D. Abnormal audiogram showing hearing loss of 15 to 30 decibels.

13. Treatment of otitis externa is BEST accomplished by:
   A. Oral antibiotics to cover common organisms found in otitis externa.
   B. Removal of external ear drainage and application of topical antibiotics with a wick.
   C. Counseling parents not to remove ear drainage as this may damage the canal and lead to additional infection.
   D. Restrict water exposure to ears for 2 weeks to allow for drying and healing.

14. Common organisms found to cause otitis externa include:
   A. *Haemophilus influenzae, Streptococcus pneumoniae,* and adenovirus.
   B. *M. catarrhalis,* gram-negative enteric organisms, and herpes simplex.
   C. *Pseudomonas aeruginosa, Staphylococcus aureus,* and *Candida albicans.*
   D. *E. coli, Streptococcus pneumoniae,* and *Pirillus niger.*

15. John, age 5 years, has been diagnosed with a ruptured tympanic membrane as a result of otitis media 1 week ago that was treated with antibiotics. The plan of care should include:
   A. Referral to ENT for evaluation and treatment.
   B. Continued use of oral antibiotics to prevent infection until the membrane heals.
   C. Use of topical otic antibiotics to prevent infection until the membrane has healed.
   D. Education of parents on use of ear plugs to prevent water from entering the middle ear.

16. Ototoxicity due to medications results in which type of hearing loss?
   A. Conductive hearing loss.
   B. Sensorineural hearing loss.
   C. Mixed conductive and sensorineural hearing loss.
   D. Mild transitory hearing loss.

17. Allergic rhinitis has both an early and late phase with distinct pathophysiology and signs and symptoms. Which of the following is true about the late phase of allergic rhinitis?
   A. IgE-sensitized mast cells release prostaglandins, cytokines, and histamine.
   B. Leukotrienes are responsible for symptoms of sneezing and rhinorrhea.
   C. Nasal epithelium becomes infiltrated with inflammatory cells resulting in nasal congestion.
   D. Late phase symptoms of itching eyes and sneezing are the result of prostaglandin release.

18. Jennifer and Tate Johnson, ages 5 and 7 respectively, are brought to the clinic because of a 3 to 4 week history of sneezing, nasal congestion, rhinorrhea, and itchy eyes. The family moved a year ago from Arizona to New York. You have diagnosed allergic rhinitis. The mother says the children "have never had allergies before so couldn't this be a cold?" Which of the following information would support the diagnosis of allergic rhinitis?
   A. Low-grade fever off and on for the past 2 weeks.
   B. Asthma or atopic dermatitis in biological family members.
   C. Onset of symptoms late autumn and early winter.
   D. A history of sinusitis in both children.

19. Mrs. Johnson returns in a month and reports that Jennifer and Tate's allergy symptoms are limited to nasal rhinitis and congestion interfering with their activities of daily living. The most appropriate treatment would be:
   A. A safe first-generation antihistamine such as diphenhydramine.
   B. A systemic glucocorticoid in low dose to control the inflammatory process.

C. A second-generation glucocorticoid antihistamine such as fexofenadine.
D. Daily intranasal glucocorticoid during allergy season.

20. Sara, age 4 years, is brought to urgent care clinic with report of acute onset of 104° F temperature and difficulty swallowing. She appears anxious and is drooling. You suspect epiglottitis. Your immediate management plan would be:
A. Medical transportation to an emergency facility with anesthesiology notified.
B. Give an injection of ceftrioxone in the clinic and have the parents transport the child to the emergency department.
C. Obtain a CBC and blood cultures then transport child to the hospital for admission.
D. Obtain a rapid strep throat culture to rule out group A beta hemolytic infection.

21. Michael, age 13, is seen in clinic with acute onset of pharyngitis. Which of the following symptom clusters would be most consistent with group A beta hemolytic streptococcus infection?
A. Cough, nasal congestion, cervical lymphadenopathy.
B. Fever, headache, tender cervical lymphadenopathy.
C. Cough, fever, macular-papular rash on trunk.
D. Sneezing, rhinorrhea, exudates on tonsils.

22. You perform a rapid strep test on Michael and the results are positive. The most appropriate management plan would be:
A. Penicillin V 250 mg twice a day for 5 days and acetaminophen for fever and pain management.
B. Azithromycin for 5 days with ibuprofen for fever and pain management.
C. Penicillin V 500 mg twice a day for 10 days with either acetaminophen or ibuprofen for fever and pain management.
D. Cephalexin 500 mg twice a day for 10 days.

23. Matthew, age 10, is brought into the urgent care clinic with a swollen cervical lymph node that the mother reports has been there for a month. The lymph node is nontender and measures 2 cm in diameter. A review of his records indicates a previous positive group A beta hemolytic pharyngitis infection 1 month ago. The most appropriate management plan at this time would be
A. Immediate referral for biopsy and treatment.
B. Document size and characteristics of node and have child return in 2 weeks for reevaluation.
C. Repeat 10-day course of penicillin V.
D. Place PPD and obtain serology tests for toxoplasmosis and cytomegalovirus.

24. Which of the following children require immediate referral to otolaryngologist?
A. Two-year-old with a five-word vocabulary.
B. Two-year-old child with bilateral otitis media with effusion for 2 months.
C. A child with sudden hearing loss.
D. A child with history consistent with sleep apnea.

25. Which of the following statements is true about chalazions?
A. Chalazions are more common in children with eczema.
B. Chalazions are caused by obstruction of the meibomian glands of the upper and lower eyelids, causing a painless nodule.
C. Chalazions should be treated with either erythromycin or sulfacetamide 10% eye ointment.
D. Chalazions are caused by acute localized inflammation of one or more sebaceous glands of the eyelids, causing painful furuncle.

26. Which of the following terms describes an eye that deviates medially?
A. Exotrophia.
B. Esotrophia.
C. Hyperophia.
D. Hypotrophia.

ANSWERS

1. *Answer:* B
   Rationale: Bacterial conjunctivitis will usually heal on its own without complications. *N. gonorrhoeae* is the exception. Bacterial conjunctivitis is highly contagious and families must be given instructions on how to prevent or minimize transmission. Viral and allergic conjunctivitis are more common than bacterial causes for conjunctivitis. The most common causes of bacterial conjunctivitis are staphylococcus, streptococcus, and *Haemophilus influenzae.*

2. *Answer:* A
   Rationale: Allergic conjunctivitis is often associated with other allergic conditions such as asthma or atopic dermatitis. Otitis media is more often associated with conjunctivitis caused by *Haemophilus influenzae.* Purulent drainage is found more with bacterial infection and allergic conjunctivitis is most often bilateral. Conjunctivitis does not usually result in enlarged tender cervical lymph nodes.

3. *Answer:* D
   Rationale: Gram-negative intracellular diplococcus are diagnostic of *N. gonorrhoeae* infection and will not be present with infections caused by the other organisms.

4. *Answer:* C
   Rationale: Dacryostenosis is the result of cellular debris blocking the normal drainage system from the eye into the nose. It is not secondary to an infection. Ninety-five percent of infants with dacryostenosis will have spontaneous resolution by 12 months of age. Antibiotics are not necessary unless the eye drainage becomes purulent.

5. *Answer:* B
   Rationale: The diagnostic feature of orbital cellulitis is proptosis of the affected eye with visual changes. Trauma and insect bites are commonly associated with periorbital infections. Redness, swelling, and tenderness are common with both periorbital and orbital cellulitis.

6. *Answer:* A
   Rationale: Strabismus is a common cause of amblyopia and needs to be treated before loss of vision occurs. It is unknown if the current strabismus is due to weak eye muscles or refractive error, so the child must be seen by an ophthalmologist to decide the appropriate treatment. Patching may be indicated but not for 8 hours at a time.

7. *Answer:* C
   Rationale: Breastfeeding and supine sleeping positions are recommended. There is no known correlation with early introduction of solids and ear infections. Exposure to smoke in the environment is highly correlated with ear infections.

8. *Answer:* A
   Rationale: Jessica is a high-risk child for bacterial ear infections because of her age and attendance in daycare. She has had symptoms for 48 hours so should be treated. Since there is no history of recent antibiotic use, she should be started on high-dose (80-90 mg/kg/day) of amoxicillin and an antipyretic for fever and pain. Amoxicillin-clavulanic acid is not appropriate at this time and low-dose amoxicillin may not be sufficient to treat resistant organisms.

9. *Answer:* B
   Rationale: This child is not high-risk for bacterial otitis media and has only had symptoms for 24 hours. The mother should be told to manage pain with the ear drops and Tylenol and return to the clinic if symptoms persist for 2 more days or fever develops. No antibiotics are warranted at this visit.

10. *Answer:* D
    Rationale: Otitis externa is common in people with frequent water contact. It is painful and often results in a swollen canal obliterating the tympanic membrane. The discharge is often white and does not freely drain from the ear. Cholesteatomas do not usually result in pain although they may result in chronic ear drainage. Perforated tympanic membranes usually have a clear/yellow drainage that runs from the ear and

symptoms of acute pain with sudden relief; the external canal is not swollen.

11. *Answer:* D
Rationale: Otitis media with effusion is a common residual finding after otitis media and often takes 2 to 3 months to fully resolve. Watchful waiting is the most appropriate treatment. If unresolved in 3 months, then referral to an ENT for assessment and hearing evaluation is appropriate.

12. *Answer:* A
Rationale: Otitis media with effusion is a noninfectious collection of fluid in the middle ear. The fluid collection interferes with normal movement of the membrane by pneumatic otoscopy. This lack of movement may or may not interfere with hearing and the tympanic membrane usually looks yellow, concave, with or without bony landmarks visible.

13. *Answer:* B
Rationale: Topical antibiotics are the primary treatment modality for otitis externa. A wick is often used to assure application of the topical antibiotic to the entire length of the external ear canal. Ear drainage may need to be gently removed to allow topical application. Ear plugs can be used if water exposure to the ears is necessary during the treatment phase.

14. *Answer:* C
Rationale: Organisms that thrive in warm, moist climates on the skin are most common for otitis media externa. Pseudomonas, *Staphylococcus aureus*, and *Candida albicans* all thrive in warm, moist settings on the skin.

15. *Answer:* D
Rationale: Ruptured tympanic membrane is not an uncommon side effect with otitis media. It does not require referral to ENT unless it happens repeatedly or fails to heal. Antibiotics are not necessary unless the child is symptomatic for infection. It is important to prevent fluid from entering the middle ear by using cotton swabs with petro-leum jelly during bathing or fitted ear plugs while swimming.

16. *Answer:* B
Rationale: Ototoxicity resulting from medications results in sensorineural hearing loss due to damage to the cranial nerve VIII.

17. *Answer:* C
Rationale: The early phase of allergic rhinitis has histamine, prostaglandins, and cytokines released. Histamine causes the symptoms of sneezing and rhinorrhea. The late phase is characterized by nasal congestion.

18. *Answer:* B
Rationale: Jennifer and Tate are now exposed to new allergens since their move to New York. This move explains the lack of previous allergy symptoms. A family history of either atopic dermatitis or asthma would indicate an allergic family history and add support to the diagnosis. Fever is more consistent with an infective process as is onset of symptoms in late autumn and winter. A history of sinusitis is not informative because it could have been due to infection or allergies.

19. *Answer:* D
Rationale: Topical medication application, such as intranasal glucocorticoids, is preferable to systemic medication if the symptoms are limited to one system.

20. *Answer:* A
Rationale: It is possible this child has acute epiglottitis. Epiglottitis is a medical emergency and the child must be transported immediately via medical transport to a health care facility with skilled professionals who can perform an emergency intubation or tracheostomy. The clinician should not attempt to do any diagnostic tests or give medication because acute airway obstruction can occur at any time.

21. *Answer:* B
Rationale: Group A beta-hemolytic strep pharyngitis usually presents with fever, tender cervical lymphadenopathy, and possibly

headache or stomach ache. Other symptoms of URI are usually absent. Exudate on tonsils can be found with either viral or bacterial tonsillitis, so is not diagnostic of group A beta-hemolytic streptococcus pharyngitis.

22. **Answer:** C
    Rationale: The first-line drug of choice is penicillin unless there is a known resistance. The appropriate dose for an adolescent is 500 mg twice a day for 10 days. Fever and pain can be managed with either acetaminophen or ibuprofen.

23. **Answer:** B
    Rationale: The lymphadenopathy post-infection may last for 4 to 6 weeks. With a documented history of past infection the findings are within normal limits but need to be reevaluated to determine their resolution. If the node does not resolve or other symptoms develop, further evaluation is necessary.

24. **Answer:** C
    Rationale: The child with sudden hearing loss requires an immediate referral to an ENT to determine the cause. The others should be seen by an ENT but the referral is not an emergency.

25. **Answer:** B
    Rationale: Chalazions are caused by obstruction of the meibomian glands of the eyelids and usually resolve with warm compresses and good lid hygiene. Seborrheic blepharitis is associated with eczema. Acute inflammation of the sebaceous glands of the eyelids is associated with a painful furuncle.

26. **Answer:** B
    Rationale: An eye that deviates medially (inward) is referred to as *esotrophia*. Extrophia is an eye that deviates outward or laterally, hypertrophia is an eye that deviates upward, and hypotrophia is an eye that deviates downward.

BIBLIOGRAPHY

Allergic Rhinitis and Its Impact on Asthma (ARIA) Independent Expert Panel. (2001). Allergic rhinitis and its impact on asthma. *J Allergy Clin Immunol, 108*(5), S147-S334.

American Academy of Pediatrics (AAP) and the American Academy of Family Physicians (AAFP), Subcommittee on Management of Acute Otitis Media. (2004). Practice guideline on diagnosis and management of acute otitis media. *Am Fam Physician, 69*(11), 2713-2715.

American Academy of Pediatrics (AAP), American Academy of Family Physicians (AAFP), and American Academy of Otolaryngology—Head and Neck Surgery (AAO-HNS) Subcommittee on Otitis Media with Effusion. (2004). Practice guideline on diagnosis and management of otitis media with effusion. *Am Fam Physician, 69*(12), 2929-2931.

Auinger, P., Lanphear, B.P., Kalkwarf, H.J., & Mansour, M.E. (2003). Trends in otitis media among children in the United States. *Pediatrics, 112*(3), 514-520.

Aventura, M.L., Roque, M.R., & Aaberg, T.M. (2006). *Retinoblastoma.* Retrieved June 6, 2006, from www.emedicine.com/oph/topic346.htm.

Bisno, A.L., Gerber, M.A., Gwaltney, J.M., et al. (2002). Practice guidelines for the diagnosis and management of group A streptococcal pharyngitis (IDSA Guidelines). *Clin Infect Dis, 35*(2), 113-125.

Carr, M.M. (2004). *Inner ear, sudden hearing loss.* Retrieved April 21, 2006, from www.emedicine.com/ent/topic227.htm.

Cook, K.A., & Walsh, M. (2005). *Otitis media.* Retrieved on April 19, 2006, from http://www.emedicine.com/emerg/topic351.htm.

Curtis, T., & Wheeler, D.T. (2005). *Nystagmus, congenital.* Retrieved April 21, 2006, from www.emedicine.com/oph/topic688.htm.

Dhooge, I.J. (2003). Risk factors for the development of otitis media. *Curr Allergy Asthma Rep, 3*(4), 321-325.

Elder, M.A., Mellon, M.H., & Spector, S.L. (2002). The link between rhinitis and asthma. *Patient care for the nurse practitioner, November special edition.* Montvale, NJ: Thomson Medical Economics.

Givner, L.B. (2002). Periorbital versus orbital cellulitis. *Pediatr Infect Dis J, 21*(12), 1157-1158.

Howard, M.L. (2006). Middle ear, tympanic membrane, perforations. Retrieved on June 6, 2006, from http://www.emedicine.com/ent/topic206.htm.

Howell, R.M. (2005). *Corneal abrasion.* Retrieved June 6, 2006 from www.emedicine.com/EMERG/topic828.htm.

Jacobson, J., & Jacobson, C. (2004). Evaluation of hearing loss in infants and young children. *Pediatr Ann, 33*(12), 811-821.

Jones, W.S., & Kaleida, P.H. (2003). How helpful is pneumatic otoscopy in improving diagnostic accuracy? *Pediatrics, 112*(3), 510-513.

Kenna, M.A. (2004). Medical management of childhood hearing loss. *Pediatr Ann, 33*(12), 822-832.

McCormick, D.P., Chonmaitree, T., Pittman, C., et al. (2005). Nonsevere acute otitis media: A clinical trial comparing outcomes of watchful waiting versus immediate antibiotic therapy. *Pediatrics, 115*(6), 1455-1465.

Moeller, J.L., & Rifat, S.F. (2003). Identifying and treating uncomplicated corneal abrasions. *Physician Sports Med, 31*(8), 15-17.

Pelton, S.I. (2002). Acute otitis media in an era of increasing antimicrobial resistance and universal administration of pneumococcal conjugate vaccine. *Pediatr Infect Dis J, 21*(6), 599-604, 613-614.

Roland, P.S. (2006). *Cholesteatoma*. Retrieved June 6, 2006, from www.emedicine.com/ped/topic384.htm.

Roland, P.S. (2004). Inner ear, noise-induced hearing loss. Retrieved September 27, 2005, from www.emedicine.com/ent/topic723.htm.

Schroeder, A., & Darrow, D.H. (2004). Management of the draining ear in children. *Pediatr Ann, 33*(12), 843-853.

Silverman, M. A., & Bessman, E. (2005). *Conjunctivitis*. Retrieved on April 19, 2006, from http://www.emedicine.com/emerg/topic110.htm.

Woodall, B.S., & Meyers, A.D. (2005). *Nonallergic rhinitis*. Retrieved April 21, 2006, from www.emedicine.com/ent/topic402.htm.

Zagaria, M.A.E., & Buonanno, A.P. (2005). A patient-oriented approach to the management of allergic rhinitis. *Clin Rev, 15*(9), 58-70.

NOTES

28 Common Illnesses of the Pulmonary System

PATRICIA JACKSON ALLEN

Select the best answer for each of the following questions:

1. Elizabeth, age 5 years, is brought to the urgent care clinic by her father with a chief complaint of cough for 3 weeks. Which of the following positive family histories would be most consistent with a history of chronic cough?
   A. Asthma.
   B. Upper respiratory infections.
   C. Migraine headaches.
   D. Otitis media with effusion.

2. Upper respiratory tract infections are most often caused by:
   A. *Mycoplasma pneumoniae.*
   B. Adenovirus.
   C. *Haemophilus influenzae.*
   D. Rhinovirus.

3. Jennifer, age 3 years, is brought to clinic by her mother because of nasal drainage, cough, and fever of 102° F for the past 24 hours. Your diagnosis is an upper respiratory tract infection. Jennifer is fussy but in no acute distress. Your plan of care should include:
   A. Chest x-ray, viral cultures, and antiviral medication.
   B. Blood cultures, urine specific gravity, and amoxicillin.
   C. Supportive care for symptoms of fever, nasal drainage, cough.
   D. Chest x-ray, amoxicillin, cough medicine.

4. Jennifer's mother expresses concern regarding other family members "catching" Jennifer's illness. Which of the following would be appropriate education regarding contagion of upper respiratory tract infection?
   A. The child is contagious only when febrile and coughing.
   B. Good handwashing and covering cough with tissue is most important.
   C. All family members should be kept 5 feet or more away from Jennifer until her symptoms resolve.
   D. Jennifer will not be contagious 24 hours after she starts antibiotic therapy.

5. Manuel, a 9-month-old infant, has been hospitalized with laboratory-confirmed pertussis. Which of the following would be appropriate components of the management plan?
   A. Antibiotic treatment with Augmentin, immediate booster immunization with DTaP, oxygen as needed.
   B. Cough management with Robitussin DM, treatment with pertussis antitoxin, intensive care observation.
   C. Prophylactic treatment of close family members, antibiotics to control secondary pneumonia, liquid diet until coughing subsides.
   D. Treatment with erythromycin, prophylaxis of close contacts, report to state health department.

6. Sinusitis is an infrequent complication of upper respiratory infections and allergic rhinitis. Treatment for sinusitis includes:
   A. Short course of prednisone to reduce inflammation with decongestant to encourage drainage of sinuses.

B. Amoxicillin or erythromycin for 14 days, acetaminophen for fever or pain.
C. Increased fluids, hot showers, and decongestants or antihistamines.
D. Nasal inhaled steroids, decongestants, increased oral fluids.

7. Influenza A is a seasonal infection that can cause serious illness in young children and children with chronic respiratory conditions. Antiviral prophylactic drugs can diminish the severity of the infection. These medications are:
   A. Approved for infants and children of all ages.
   B. Are effective when given any time during the illness.
   C. Are dosed at 5 mg/kg/day for children less that 40 kg.
   D. Are effective for influenza A, B, and C.

8. Bronchiolitis is frequently caused by respiratory syncytial virus (RSV) and can be a serious respiratory infection in young children. Hospitalization is warranted if:
   A. Wheezing and respiratory distress result in oxygen saturation of less than 92%.
   B. Cough lasts less than 1 week with weight loss of 1 pound or more.
   C. Infant is under the age of 6 months.
   D. Respiratory rate is 50, pulse 120, and temperature 101.5° F in a 6-month-old infant.

9. Madison, age 2, is being seen in the emergency department for treatment of croup. Treatment for moderate croup includes:
   A. Antibiotic and antipyretic medications.
   B. Albuterol MDI with spacer every 4 hours until coughing ceases.
   C. Dexamethasone and oxygen supplementation.
   D. Robitussin for cough, increased oral fluids, and fever management.

10. Owen, age 4 years, is brought to the urgent care clinic by his mother who reports he has been listless, had a fever of 102° F, and a cough for the past 48 hours. Prior to these more acute symptoms, he had had symptoms of a cold for the previous week. You need to evaluate Owen for possible pneumonia. Which of the following signs and symptoms are most consistent with the diagnosis of pneumonia?
   A. Retractions, grunting, crackles on auscultation.
   B. Wheezing, cough, prolonged expiratory phase.
   C. Purulent nasal drainage, erythematous pharynx, mouth breathing.
   D. Barking cough, inspiratory stridor, grunting.

11. Common organisms causing pneumonia in newborn infants are:
   A. *Staphylococcus aureus*, pseudomonas, group A beta-hemolytic streptococcus.
   B. *Haemophilus influenzae, Staphylococcus pneumoniae*, herpes simplex.
   C. Mycoplasma, *Staphylococcus pneumoniae, Haemophilus influenzae*.
   D. Group B streptococci, gram-negative enteric bacilli, *Chlamydia trachomatis*.

12. The antibiotic of choice for a school-age child with suspected *Mycoplasma pneumoniae* would be:
   A. Amoxicillin.
   B. Penicillin.
   C. Macrolides.
   D. Cephalosporin.

13. Children infected with measles are contagious:
   A. As long as the rash is present.
   B. 3 to 5 days before the presence of a rash.
   C. Through respiratory droplets and secretions from the rash.
   D. During the febrile period of the illness.

14. The nurses in the newborn nursery request the pediatric nurse practitioner assess a newborn infant who appears to have difficulty feeding. The nurse practitioner determines tracheoesophageal fistula (TEF) must be ruled out. Which of the following tests should be ordered?

A. CAT scan with contrast dye.
B. Chromosome analysis.
C. Chest x-ray.
D. Barium swallow.

15. A 6-month treatment with INH, or rifampin for INH-resistant tuberculosis is required for:
A. All children with a 10 mm induration to Mantoux skin test.
B. Only children with a positive Mantoux test and positive chest x-ray for tuberculosis.
C. All children with positive Mantoux and previous history of Bacille Calmette-Guerin (BCG) vaccine.
D. All children with greater than 10 mm induration with Mantoux skin test and a history of positive risk factors.

16. Evan is a 2-month-old infant born at home and seen only once in the clinic for a newborn checkup at 3 days of age. According to his mother, he was doing well until 1 week ago when he started having difficulty feeding and "seemed to have trouble catching his breath." Possible causes of dyspnea in a young infant previously thought to be healthy include:
A. Diaphragmatic hernia.
B. Congestive heart failure due to patent ductus arteriosus.
C. Tracheoesophageal fistula.
D. Positive Coombs' test due to ABO incompatibility.

17. Pleural effusion is often associated with pulmonary infections caused by which of the following organisms?
A. *S. aureus, S. pneumoniae*.
B. *M. pneumoniae, M. catarrhalis*.
C. *H. influenzae*, staph epidermis.
D. *Pseudomonas aeruginosa*, group A streptococci.

18. Apnea in the newborn infant can be caused by obstruction in the airway, central nervous system abnormality, or a combination of both. Which of the following diagnoses is an example of obstructive apnea?
A. Apnea due to prematurity.
B. Choanal atresia.

C. CO_2 toxicity.
D. Increased intracranial pressure.

19. Common pharmacologic therapy for apnea of prematurity includes:
A. Albuterol.
B. Budesomide.
C. Amphetamines.
D. Caffeine.

20. Breath-holding spells are:
A. Most common in children over the age of 3 years.
B. Have been found to increase the risk of seizures in later life.
C. Used by children to manipulate caregiver behavior.
D. Involuntary events related to autonomic dysregulation.

21. Educating parents regarding breath-holding spells would include which of the following?
A. Protecting child from injury by lowering him or her to the floor before he or she falls.
B. The need to ignore the behavior, similar to the management of children with temper tantrum.
C. The importance of seeking counseling for parent-child interaction.
D. The need to insert a padded tongue depressor to prevent occlusion of the airway by the tongue.

22. Environmental factors associated with sudden infant death (SIDS) include:
A. Unsafe bedding.
B. Hypothermia.
C. Crowded living conditions.
D. Family poverty.

23. Choking on a foreign body such as food is a hazard especially in young children. Parents should be encouraged to do which of the following to reduce the hazard of choking?
A. Remove small items from the environment and evaluate toys for removable parts that may be inhaled.
B. Continue puréed or coarsely chopped foods until 24 months.

C. Feed the child all foods until 24 months when self-feeding should begin.

D. Remove all toys from child's crib so they cannot be inhaled while child is unattended.

24. Psychogenic cough is characterized by:

A. Repeated shallow cough mainly at night.

B. Productive cough with occasional vomiting.

C. Increased respiratory effort and rate.

D. Barking cough but not at night or during play.

25. Children with recurrent cough associated with a cold should:

A. Be prescribed a cough preparation to reduce the severity of cough.

B. Have menthol cream rubbed on their chest to reduce cough.

C. Be given acetaminophen before bedtime to reduce fever and pain associated with cold symptoms, thereby reducing cough.

D. Not be prescribed medications without evidence of their effectiveness.

NOTES

ANSWERS

1. *Answer:* A
   Rationale: Asthma is often associated with recurrent cough and has a strong family genetic pattern. Upper respiratory infections usually do not last for 3 weeks. Migraine headaches and otitis media with effusion are not associated with cough.

2. *Answer:* D
   Rationale: Upper respiratory tract infections are usually caused by viruses with rhinovirus being most common.

3. *Answer:* C
   Rationale: Treatment of upper respiratory tract infections is usually limited to symptom management. Laboratory tests are not usually necessary unless the child is in acute distress. Antibiotics are not appropriate, as most infections are caused by viruses.

4. *Answer:* B
   Rationale: Transmission of upper respiratory tract infections are best controlled by frequent handwashing and covering coughs to prevent respiratory droplet spread of the virus. Children are contagious before onset of symptoms and antibiotics are not given for viral infections.

5. *Answer:* D
   Rationale: Pertussis is treated with erythromycin and prophylaxis of close family and daycare contacts is recommended. Standard cough medications are not effective and there is no antitoxin preparation for pertussis. Administration of DTaP is not effective in treating an active infection.

6. *Answer:* B
   Rationale: Sinusitis is often caused by the same organisms that cause otitis media and should be treated with a 14-day course of antibiotics, usually amoxicillin or erythromycin. Steroids and decongestants have not been found to shorten the course of the illness.

7. *Answer:* C
   Rationale: Amantadine, rimantadine, and zanamivir are effective in diminishing the severity of influenza A only if given early in the course of the illness. They have not been approved by the FDA for children younger than 12 months of age and have no effect on influenza B or C. The standard dose is 5 mg/kg/day.

8. *Answer:* A
   Rationale: Infants who are unable to maintain oxygen saturation greater than 93% on room air are at high risk for respiratory failure and must be monitored and supported in a hospital setting. Cough with RSV often lasts more than a week and if oxygenation is WNL, it is not significant. Weight loss is common in young children during periods of illness. The vital signs listed in option D indicate a mild elevation in respiration, pulse, and temperature and by themselves do not warrant hospitalization.

9. *Answer:* C
   Rationale: Antibiotics are not used in treatment of croup unless secondary infections develop. Albuterol does not reduce the swelling of the larynx, so will not relieve the respiratory symptoms of croup. Robitussin is ineffective in treating the cough associated with croup, and young children with moderate croup may have difficulty taking extra oral fluids and may require intravenous fluids is they become dehydrated. Dexamethasone has recently been shown to reduce the symptoms and duration of croup and oxygen supplementation reduces the work of breathing.

10. *Answer:* A
    Rationale: Pneumonia is a lower respiratory infection resulting in inflammation and fluid collection in the bronchioles. Crackles, usually heard at the end of inspiration, are highly suggestive of pneumonia, as is increased work of breathing resulting in retractions and grunting. Wheezing, a barking cough, nasal discharge, and inflamed pharynx are more consistent with allergies and viral upper respiratory infections.

11. *Answer:* D
    Rationale: Newborns are exposed to a unique set of organisms as they pass through

the birth canal. These include all the organisms listed in answer D.

12. *Answer:* C
    Rationale: *Mycoplasma pneumoniae* is treated with the macrolide group of medications. Amoxicillin or cephalosporins are used for *H. influenzae*, and penicillin is used only for susceptible *S. pneumoniae*.

13. *Answer:* B
    Rationale: Children with measles are contagious during the early phase of the illness even before the rash develops. Respiratory droplet spread is the most frequent means of communication and the illness is not contagious via contact with the rash.

14. *Answer:* C
    Rationale: TEF can be accurately diagnosed with a chest x-ray. A CAT scan is not necessary and nothing should be given by mouth until it is determined how the fistula is attached to the trachea. Some chromosome abnormalities are associated with TEF so chromosome analysis may be done in the future but would not be diagnostic for the condition.

15. *Answer:* D
    Rationale: Children with a 10 mm induration and no risk factors or symptoms do not need to be treated with INH. Children with a positive PPD test of greater than 10 mm should be treated regardless of chest x-ray findings. All children who have been treated with BCG will have a positive PPD so only those with positive chest x-ray findings consistent with TB should be treated.

16. *Answer:* B
    Rationale: Diaphragmatic hernia and TEF would be identified at birth or shortly thereafter. Most ABO incompatibilities would also be evident early after birth. A heart defect may not be obvious at birth, but changes in blood flow with the increase in pulmonary pressure after birth may result in congestive heart failure over time.

17. *Answer:* A
    Rationale: The two most common organisms for pleural effusion are *S. aureus* and

S. pneumoniae, two organisms found in pneumonia and septicemia.

18. *Answer:* B
    Rationale: Apnea associated with prematurity, CO_2 toxicity, and intracranial pressure all are associated with CNS problems. Only choanal atresia is obstructive and requires surgery to correct.

19. *Answer:* D
    Rationale: Caffeine is used to stimulate the premature infant's nervous system to prevent apnea.

20. *Answer:* D
    Rationale: Breath-holding spells are most common in children from 6 to 24 months of age and are not voluntary but are the result of autonomic dysregulation leading to prolonged expiratory apnea. No long-term seizure problems have been identified.

21. *Answer:* A
    Rationale: Breath-holding spells may result in the loss of consciousness or seizure and a child may be injured during this process. Parents should be instructed in how to prevent injury and to observe the child during the episode. They should be told to never place anything in the child's mouth during these episodes. The episodes can be very frightening and parents need reassurance that their parenting is not the cause nor is the child able to control the episodes. Most children will outgrow the breath-holding spells by the preschool years.

22. *Answer:* A
    Rationale: Unsafe bedding has been strongly associated with SIDS. Hyperthermia has been associated also. Crowded living conditions and poverty are not directly associated with SIDS, but may present increased risks for other hazards such as parental substance abuse including smoking.

23. *Answer:* A
    Rationale: Children should be encouraged to eat table foods that are soft or cut into small pieces by 12 months of age. Certain foods are hazardous and should be avoided;

i.e., hard candy, peanuts, and grapes. As toddlers begin to explore, their environment must be evaluated for small items that could be put into the mouth. Toys without small removable parts can be safely placed in a child's crib for the child to play with upon waking.

24. *Answer:* D
    Rationale: Psychogenic cough is nonproductive honking or barking cough that is not continued at night and often resolves when the child is distracted. Repeated cough may evolve into a tic-like habit.

25. *Answer:* D
    Rationale: Standard cough and cold preparations have not shown evidence for effectiveness in controlling symptoms of cough. Unless the cough is severe, significantly interfering with feeding and sleep of the child, no medication should be given. Cough is protective, keeping the airway clear of secretions.

BIBLIOGRAPHY

Bocka, J. (2005). *Pediatrics, pertussis.* Retrieved June 19, 2006, from www.emedicine.com/emerg/topic394.htm.

Chang, A.K., & Barton, E.D. (2005). *Pneumothorax, iatrogenic, spontaneous and pneumomediastinum.* Retrieved on April 24, 2006, from http://www.emedicine.com/emerg/topic469.htm.

Fleming, D.M., Pannell, R.S., Elliot, A.J., & Cross, K.W. (2005). Respiratory illness associated with influenza and respiratory syncytial virus infection. *Arch Dis Child, 90*(7), 741-746.

Goodhue, C.J., & Brady, M.A. (2004). Respiratory disorders. In C.E. Burns, A.M. Dunn, M.A. Brady, et al. (Eds.). *Pediatric primary care: A handbook for nurse practitioners* (3rd ed.). Philadelphia: Saunders.

Holmes, R.L., & Fadden, C.T. (2004). Evaluation of the patient with chronic cough. *Am Fam Physician, 69*(9), 2159-2168.

Milioti, S., & Einspieler, C. (2005). The long-term outcome of infantile apparent life-threatening event (ALTE): A follow-up study until midpuberty. *Neuropediatrics, 36*(1), 1-5.

Patel, H., Platt, R., Lozano, J.M., & Wang, E.E. (2004). Glucocorticoids for acute viral bronchiolitis in infants and young children. *Cochrane Database Syst Rev, 3,* CD004878.

Ramadan, H.H. (2005). Pediatric sinusitis: Update. *J Otolaryngol, 34*(Suppl 1), S14-S17.

Russell, K., Wiebe, N., Saenz, A., et al. (2003). Glucocorticoids for croup. *Cochrane Database Syst Rev, 14,* CD001955.

Schwartz, M.W., Bell, L.M., Bingham, P.M., et al. (2005). *The 5 minute pediatric consult* (4th ed.). Philadelphia: Lippincott Williams & Wilkins.

Sharma, S., & Duerkson, D. (2006). Tracheoesophageal fistula. Retrieved June 19, 2006, from www.emedicine.com/med/topic3416.htm.

Smucny, J., Flynn, C., Becker, L., & Glazier, R. (2003). Beta$_2$-agonists for acute bronchitis. *Cochrane Database Syst Rev, 1,* CD001726.

Spiro, C.E. (2003). Evaluating chronic cough: A systematic approach. *Clin Rev, 13*(10), 52-57.

Spurling, G.K., Del Mar, C.B., Dooley, L., & Foxlee, R. (2004). Delayed antibiotics for symptoms and complications of respiratory infections. *Cochrane Database Syst Rev, 4,* CD004417.

Steiner, R.W.P. (2004). Treating acute bronchiolitis associated with RSV. *Am Fam Physician, 69*(2), 325-332.

Steinhorn, R.H. (2004). *Congenital diaphragmatic hernia.* Retrieved June 19, 2006, from www.emedicine.com/ped/topic2603.htm.

U.S. Food and Drug Administration. (2006). Influenza (flu) antiviral drugs and related information. Retrieved on April 21, 2006, from http://www.fda.gov/cder/drug/antivirals/influenza/.

29 Common Illnesses of the Cardiovascular System

JOYCE M. KNESTRICK

Select the best answer for each of the following questions:

1. Abby is 5 years old. She is brought to your office by her parents. The parents are concerned because Abby was playing soccer in a community league when she "passed out" while attempting to kick a goal. She quickly stood back up and attempted to continue to play before her parents pulled her out of the game. The child did not have any chest pain, shortness of breath, or palpitations. You suspect:
   A. Vasovagal syncope.
   B. Cardiac syncope.
   C. Postural orthostatic tachycardia syndrome (POTS).
   D. Convulsive syncope.

2. While performing a detailed cardiac examination on Abby, the pediatric nurse practitioner auscultates for heart sounds. She notes S_1 and S_2. These heart sounds are produced by:
   A. Opening of the atrioventricular (AV valve) which produces S_1 and opening of the semilunar valves which produces S_2.
   B. Closure of the AV valve which produces S_1 and closure of the aortic and pulmonic valves which produces S_2.
   C. Opening of the tricuspid valves which produces S_1 and closure of the AV valves which produces S_2.
   D. Mitral valve fluttering produces S_1 and the opening of the tricuspid valve produces S_2.

3. Jack, age 15, is brought to the clinic by his parents because he is complaining of "chest pain." The patient and his parents are very anxious. Jack is not short of breath and does not have chest pain at present. The pediatric nurse practitioner would obtain a:
   A. Cardiologist consult stat.
   B. Focused history from the patient to identify the cause of the chest pain.
   C. History from the parents of the chest pain so the child can rest.
   D. Complete family history to identify risk factors.

4. Jack's family history revealed that his father had a myocardial infarction (MI) at age 42 and has high cholesterol, and his paternal grandfather died at age 52 from a "heart attack." Jack is overweight and his blood pressure is 140/90 mm Hg. You draw a lipid profile and find his LDL is 130 mg/dl. You would:
   A. Repeat the lipid panel and recheck the LDL.
   B. Add more saturated fat to his diet.
   C. Start him on a statin medication.
   D. Counsel him on lifestyle changes and refer to a nutritionist.

5. What are the most common causes of chest pain in adolescents?
   A. Mitral valve prolapse from rheumatic fever and GI disturbances.
   B. Heart failure and cardiomyopathy.
   C. Musculoskeletal and idiopathic causes.
   D. Congenital heart disease and heart failure.

6. Allie, age 2, is brought to the clinic by her grandmother (Allie's guardian). The grandmother is concerned because Allie

"holds her breath until she turns pale." What additional information would you obtain from the grandmother?

A. Does anything trigger the episode, how long does it last, and does the child sleep afterward?

B. Does the child have a history of asthma and is she living in an older house?

C. Does the child have a fever, problems when running, and does the mother have anemia?

D. Was the child breastfed, does she have pica, and is she still taking a bottle?

7. The most common cause of secondary hypertension in a young child is:

A. Renal disease.

B. Coarctation of the aorta.

C. Idiopathic.

D. Obesity.

8. An elevated low density lipoprotein (LDL) level is significant because it:

A. Is responsible for the majority of plasma triglycerides when fasting.

B. Transports cholesterol from vessels to the liver for secretion in the bile.

C. Is the largest and highest in density and is formed in the intestine from fat.

D. Is atherogenic and directly associated with coronary disease when elevated.

9. Mark, age 12, has a blood pressure of 140/90 mm Hg. The pediatric nurse practitioner should:

A. Repeat the blood pressure on two additional and separate occasions.

B. Do an immediate cardiac work-up on the patient.

C. Consider this a normal reading.

D. Start the child on hydrochlorothiazide (HCTZ).

10. Mark is diagnosed with hypertension. Which laboratory tests would the pediatric nurse practitioner order for Mark?

A. Sedimentation rate, uric acid levels, and urine culture.

B. Drug screen, catecholamines, and uric acid levels.

C. BUN/creatinine, electrolytes, and complete blood cell count.

D. TSH, free testosterone, and BUN/creatinine.

11. Management of Mark's hypertension would include:

A. Avoiding fatty foods, fast foods, and all forms of exercise.

B. Attempting to maintain a normal weight, increase exercise, and moderate salt restriction.

C. Starting the child on an angiotensin-converting enzyme (ACE) inhibitor and a thiazide diuretic after the second visit.

D. Starting the child on a beta-blocker after the first visit.

12. Mark was eventually started on lisinopril (an ACE inhibitor) daily. The pediatric nurse practitioner would monitor:

A. Electrolytes periodically.

B. Heart rate.

C. Glycohemaglobin A1C.

D. Potassium and creatinine.

13. Mary, age 3, is brought to the office by her mother. Her mother reports that Mary has had a fever ranging from 101° F to 104° F. She took Mary to an urgent care center and was treated with antibiotics with no response. Mary's eyes are red bilaterally and her lips are red and cracked. You suspect:

A. Reye's syndrome.

B. Coxsackievirus.

C. Varicella.

D. Kawasaki syndrome.

14. The pediatric nurse practitioner tells Mary's mother that although the disease is self-limiting, treatment is essential to prevent:

A. Juvenile arthritis.

B. Coronary artery aneurysms.

C. Sterility.

D. The spread of the disease.

15. The goal of initial treatment of Mary's illness is to:

A. Decrease the risk of coronary occlusion.

B. Begin influenza immunization series.

C. Decrease systemic inflammation.

D. Increase the heart rate and cardiac output.

16. Mary is admitted to the hospital for treatment of her fever. The pediatric nurse practitioner knows that the following treatment will be started to shorten the fever and to decrease the risk of complications:
   A. Aspirin therapy.
   B. Intravenous antibiotics.
   C. Intravenous heparin.
   D. Intravenous immunoglobulin (IVIG).

17. Mary is later diagnosed with level-two risk for coronary artery disease. You explain to the parents that this means that Mary:
   A. Had a transient dilation with normalization of the echocardiogram in the past 8 weeks.
   B. Has a small to medium aneurysm in one coronary artery.
   C. Has never had any coronary abnormalities.
   D. Has coronary obstruction.

18. Rudy, age 10 months, is brought to the clinic by his parents. This mother is concerned because he is not eating well, seems to be sleeping more than usual, and is very fussy. His temperature is 99.1° F rectally, respirations are 20, he is diaphoretic, and his heart rate is 210 bpm. The pediatric nurse practitioner:
   A. Tells the mother that the pulse rate is normal, since the child has a fever.
   B. Listens to the heart rate for at least 10 seconds.
   C. Refers the child to a pediatric cardiologist.
   D. Tells the mother that a normal heart rate in an infant is 100 to 150 bpm.

19. Larry has a history of acute rheumatic fever (ARF). The pediatric nurse practitioner is following him for carditis. The pediatric nurse practitioner listens closely at the fifth intercostal space at the mid-clavicular line on the left side of the chest to hear closure of the:
   A. Tricuspid valve.
   B. Pulmonic valves.
   C. Aortic valve.
   D. Mitral valves.

20. Albert comes into the clinic with a fever of 103.6° F. He is complaining of joint pain and muscle weakness. On exam, he has swollen lymph nodes. According to the Jones' criteria, what other finding is needed to make the diagnosis of acute rheumatic fever?
   A. History of carditis.
   B. History of Lyme disease.
   C. History of group A streptococcal throat infection.
   D. History of juvenile arthritis.

21. The treatment of choice for acute rheumatic fever is:
   A. Erythromycin 800 mg orally twice a day.
   B. Cipro (ciprofloxacin) 500 mg orally twice a day.
   C. Benzanthine penicillin G IM.
   D. Depo-Medrol IV.

22. The pediatric nurse practitioner is examining a 2-year-old girl. The pediatric nurse practitioner hears a grade V systolic murmur. What are the characteristics of a grade V murmur? The murmur is:
   A. Heard without the stethoscope on the chest.
   B. Heard with the stethoscope partially on the chest.
   C. Heard with the diaphragm of the stethoscope.
   D. Barely audible with the bell of the stethoscope.

23. Harry has a history of Marfan syndrome. He presents to the emergency department with acute severe chest and back pain. This is an emergency because Marfan syndrome causes:
   A. Inflammation at the costochondral junction.
   B. Acute chest syndrome.
   C. Acute hypertension.
   D. Dissection of the aorta.

24. Cardiac chest pain in children is:
   A. Midpercodial and radiates to the left arm.
   B. Severe crushing pain that radiates to the back.
   C. Subcostal in nature.
   D. Often an emotional response.

ANSWERS

1. *Answer:* A
   Rationale: Vasovagal syncope is the most classic form of syncope and is exacerbated by anxiety, hyperventilation, and active use of the skeletal muscles. Cardiac syncope is associated with palpations, chest pain, and dyspnea. POTS is caused by acute anxiety, and has a 30 to 40 bpm heart rate increase, and exercise intolerance. Convulsive syncope is accompanied by acute pain, anxiety, and fear.

2. *Answer:* B
   Rationale: When the AV valve closes, it allows both ventricles to be filled simultaneously which produces S_1. When the aortic and pulmonic valves close, the second heart sound or S_2 is produced.

3. *Answer:* B
   Rationale: An accurate history from the child is the most important component of the clinical assessment to identify the cause of the pain. Parents may interpret the child's symptoms in light of their own experiences. Family history, although significant, should be done after the pain is assessed. The underlying cause of the chest pain should be assessed before a referral is made.

4. *Answer:* D
   Rationale: Lifestyle changes are the best method of cholesterol control in children, proper diet including a decrease in saturated fats and increase in exercise is recommended first, especially since his LDL is under 150.

5. *Answer:* C
   Rationale: Common causes of chest pain in children are musculoskeletal and idiopathic which are usually self-limited. Cardiovascular causes are less common but are serious if present. Adults have heart failure, GERD, and MVP as the most common causes.

6. *Answer:* A
   Rationale: "Pallid breath-holding spells" are often characterized by a trivial physical or emotional trauma that triggers a cry, pallor, and opisthotonoid posture; resolves after 1 minute, and is often followed by sleep.

7. *Answer:* A

Rationale: Renal diseases such as polycystic kidneys or glomerulonephritis are the most common secondary causes, followed by endocrine-induced hypertension.

8. *Answer:* D
   Rationale: LDL is responsible for the majority of plasma triglycerides; HDL transports cholesterol to be secreted. The largest and highest in density is triglycerides. LDL is associated with the increase risk of CAD.

9. *Answer:* A
   Rationale: A minimum of three readings with an average systolic BP of 140 mm Hg and a diastolic of 90 mm Hg establishes the diagnosis of hypertension. Two or more readings at separate times should be taken after the initial screening.

10. *Answer:* C
    Rationale: BUN and creatinine are used to assess renal function and CBC to assess for anemia; drug screen may be appropriate with suspected drug abuse. Catecholamine is used if a secondary cause is suspected.

11. *Answer:* B
    Rationale: Conservative management for high-normal elevation is indicated. Although medications may bring the pressure down, it is not an initial option.

12. *Answer:* D
    Rationale: To monitor kidney function, the pediatric nurse practitioner would check the potassium and creatinine level. Electrolytes should be monitored on diuretics.

13. *Answer:* D
    Rationale: Kawasaki syndrome is characterized by a prolonged fever not affected by antibiotics, red eyes, rash, erythematous and cracked lips, lymphadenopathy, and swollen and beefy-red hands and feet.

14. *Answer:* B
    Rationale: Kawasaki disease now surpasses acute rheumatic fever as the leading cause of acquired heart disease in the U.S. The incidence of coronary artery aneurysms is high in infants, but there has been a higher incidence in children older than 6 years, possibly related to late diagnosis.

15. *Answer:* C
    Rationale: The initial goal is to decrease system inflammation. Fever duration is a strong predictor of coronary outcome; the longer the fever, the increased risk of aneurysm.

16. *Answer:* D
    Rationale: IVIG shortens the duration of fever and decrease the risk of coronary artery aneurysms three- to five-fold.

17. *Answer:* A
    Rationale: Level 2 has transient dilation with normalization of measurement by 6 to 8 week echocardiogram, Level 1 has no coronary abnormalities, Level 3 has a small to medium aneurysm, and Level 5 has coronary artery obstruction.

18. *Answer:* C
    Rationale: The child is afebrile and the normal heart rate in a 10-month-old child is up to 180 bpm. This child has associated symptoms of SVT, along with poor feeding, pallor, and diaphoresis. The child should be referred, since the pediatric nurse practitioner would have a high suspicion of SVT.

19. *Answer:* D
    Rationale: Rheumatic fever can affect the mitral valve, so the pediatric nurse practitioner would listen for the opening and closing of the mitral valve.

20. *Answer:* C
    Rationale: According to the Jones' criteria, there should be two major manifestations which would include carditis, polyarthritis, Sydenham's chorea, erythema marginatum, and subcutaneous nodes; or one major and two minor manifestations (arthralgia, fever, elevated EDR, C-reactive protein, and prolonged P-R interval) and evidence of group A streptococcus infection.

21. *Answer:* C
    Rationale: Benzathine penicillin G is the antibiotic of choice for acute rheumatic fever. Erythromycin can be given if the child is allergic to penicillin.

22. *Answer:* B

Rationale: A murmur that is very loud and can be heard with the stethoscope partially off the chest wall is grade V. Grade VI is the loudest and heard with the stethoscope just moved from contact with the chest. Grade I is barely audible or faint with the bell of the stethoscope.

23. *Answer:* D
    Rationale: Dissection usually begins above the coronary ostia and extends the length of the aorta. It is estimated that around 10% of Marfan syndrome patients present with Type III dissections, and only rarely do dissections involve only the abdominal aorta.

24. *Answer:* A
    Rationale: Cardiac chest pain is usually acute and mid-pericardial, the pain can radiate to the left arm. Severe crushing pain radiating to the back is usually associated with aortic tears. Subcostal pain is generally chest wall related. The parents' experience with chest pain may influence symptoms.

BIBLIOGRAPHY

Baker, A.L., Gauvreau, K., Newburger, J.W., et al. (2003). Physical and psychosocial health in children who have had Kawasaki disease. *Pediatrics, 111*(3), 579-583.

Basso, C., Maron, B.J., Corrado, D., & Thiene, G. (2000). Clinical profile of congenital coronary artery anomalies with origin from the wrong aortic sinus leading to sudden death in young competitive athletes. *J Am Coll Cardiol, 35*(6), 1493-1501.

Belay, B., Belamarich, P., & Racine, A.D. (2004). Pediatric precursors of adult atherosclerosis. *Pediatr Rev, 25*(1), 4-16.

Blosser, C.G., & Freitas-Nichols, J. (2004). Cardiovascular disorders. In C.E. Burns, A.M. Dunn, M.A. Brady, et al. (Eds.). *Pediatric primary care: A handbook for nurse practitioners* (3rd ed.). Philadelphia: Saunders.

Burns, J.C., Shimizu, C., Shike, H., et al. (2005). Family-based association analysis implicates IL-4 in susceptibility to Kawasaki disease. *Genes Immun, 6*(5), 438-444.

Cheung, Y.F., Yung, T.C., Tam, S.C., et al. (2004). Novel and traditional cardiovascular risk factors in children after Kawasaki disease: Implications for premature atherosclerosis. *J Am Coll Cardiol, 43*(1), 120-124.

Chobanian, A.V., Bakris, G.L., Black, H.R., et al. (2003). Seventh report of the Joint National Committee on Prevention, Detection, Evaluation, and Treatment of High Blood Pressure. *Hypertension, 42*(6), 1206-1252.

Connolly, S.J., Sheldon, R., Thorpe, K.E., et al. (2003). Pacemaker therapy for prevention of syncope in patients with recurrent severe vasovagal syncope: Second Vasovagal Pacemaker Study (VPS II): A randomized trial. *JAMA, 289*(17), 2224-2229.

de Ferranti, S.D., Gauvreau, K., Ludwig, D.S., et al. (2004). Prevalence of the metabolic syndrome in American adolescents: Findings from the Third National Health and Nutrition Examination Survey. *Circulation, 110*(16), 2494-2497.

DiMario, F.J., Jr. (2001a). Breath-holding spells and pacemaker implantation. *Pediatrics, 108*(3), 765-766.

DiMario F.J., Jr. (2001b). Prospective study of children with cyanotic and pallid breath-holding spells. *Pediatrics, 107*(2), 265-269.

Evangelista, J.A., Parsons, M., & Renneburg, A.K. (2000). Chest pain in children: Diagnosis through history and physical examination. *J Pediatr Health Care, 14*(1), 3-8.

Flevari, P.P., Livanis, E.G., Theodorakis, G.N., et al. (2002). Baroreflexes in vasovagal syncope: Two types of abnormal response. *Pacing Clin Electrophysiol, 25*(9), 1315-1323.

Flynn, J.T. (2002). Differentiation between primary and secondary hypertension in children using ambulatory blood pressure monitoring. *Pediatrics, 110*(1), 89-93.

Fong, N.C., Hui, Y.W., Li, C.K., & Chiu, M.C. (2004). Evaluation of the efficacy of treatment of Kawasaki disease before day 5 of illness. *Pediatr Cardiol, 25*(1), 31-34.

Ganz, L., & Gugneja, M. (2005). *Paroxysmal supraventricular tachycardia*. Retrieved August 31, 2005, from www.emedicine.com/med/topic1762.htm#section~follow-up.

Goodhue, C.J., & Brady, M.A. (2004). Atopic disorders and rheumatic diseases. In C.E. Burns, A.M. Dunn, M.A. Brady, et al. (Eds.). *Pediatric primary care: A handbook for nurse practitioners* (3rd ed.). Philadelphia: Saunders.

Hamer, A.W., & Bray, J.E. (2005). Clinical recognition of neurally mediated syncope. *Intern Med J, 35*(4), 2160-2221.

Holman, R.C., Curns, A.T., Belay, E.D., et al. (2003). Kawasaki syndrome hospitalizations in the United States, 1997 and 2000. *Pediatrics, 112*(3), 495-501.

Hopkins, P.N. (2003). Familial hypercholesterolemia—Improving treatment and meeting guidelines. *Int J Cardiol, 89*(1), 13-23.

Inglefinger, J.R. (2004). Pediatric antecedents of adult cardiovascular disease—Awareness and intervention. *N Engl J Med, 350*(21), 2123-2126.

Institute for Clinical Systems Improvement (ICSI). (2004). *Lipid screening in children and adolescents.* Bloomington, MN: ICSI.

Kantoch, M.J. (2005). Supraventricular tachycardia in children. *Indian J Pediatr, 72*(7), 609-619.

Kapoor, W.N. (2003). Is there an effective treatment for neurally mediated syncope? *JAMA, 289*(17), 2272-2275.

Kelly, A.M., Porter, C.J., McGoon, M.D., et al. (2001) Breath-holding spells associated with significant bradycardia: Successful treatment with permanent pacemaker implantation. *Pediatrics, 108*(3), 698-702.

Kouakam, C., Vaksmann, G., Pachy, E., et al. (2000). Long-term follow-up of children and adolescents with syncope; Predictor of syncope recurrence. *Eur Heart J, 22*(17), 1618-1625.

Lane, S.E., Watts, R., & Scott, D.G. (2005). Epidemiology of systemic vasculitis. *Curr Rheumatol Rep, 7*(4), 270-275.

Lurbe, E., & Redon, J. (2002). Reproducibility and validity of ambulatory blood pressure monitoring in children. *Am J Hypertens, 15*(2 Pt 2), 69S-73S.

Lutwick, L.I., & Ravishankar, J. (2005). *Rheumatic fever*. Retrieved September 1, 2005, from www.emedicine.com/med/topic3435.htm.

Mansour, K.A., Thourani, V.H., Odessey, F.A. et al. (2003). Pectus deformities of the anterior chest wall. *Ped Resp Red, 4*(3), 237.

Maron, B.J. (2003). Sudden death in young athletes. *N Engl J Med, 349*, 1064-1075.

Marais, A.D., Firth, J.C., & Blom, D.J. (2004). Homozygous familial hypercholesterolemia and its management. *Semin Vasc Med, 4*(1), 35-42.

Massin, M. (2003). Neurocardiogenic syncope in children: Current concepts in diagnosis and management. *Paediatr Drug, 5*(5), 327-334.

McCrindle, B.W., Ose, L., & Marais, A.D. (2003). Efficacy and safety of atorvastatin in children and adolescents with familial hypercholesterolemia or severe hyperlipidemia: A multicenter, randomized, placebo-controlled trial. *J Pediatr, 143*(1), 74-80.

Miller, T.H., & Kruse, J.E. (2005). Evaluation of syncope. *Am Fam Phys, 72*(8), 1492-1502.

Morel, K., & Bye, M.R. (2000). Solving the puzzle of pediatric chest pain. *J Resp Dis Pediatr, 2*, 66-75.

Morgenstern, B. (2002). Blood pressure, hypertension, and ambulatory blood pressure monitoring in children and adolescents. *Am J Hypertens, 15*(2 Pt 2), 64S-66S.

Muntner, P., He, J., & Cutler, J.A. (2005). Trends in blood pressure among children and adolescents. *JAMA, 291*(17), 2107-2113.

National High Blood Pressure Education Program Working Group on High Blood Pressure in Children and Adolescents. (2004). The fourth report on the diagnosis, evaluation, and treatment of high blood pressure in children and adolescents. *Pediatrics, 114*(2 Suppl 4th Report), 555-576.

Newburger, J.W., & Fulton, D.R. (2004). Kawasaki disease. *Curr Opin Pediatr, 16*(5), 508-514.

Newburger, J.W., Takahashi, M., Gerber, M.A., et al. (2004). Diagnosis, treatment, and long-term management of Kawasaki disease: A statement for health professionals. From the Council of Cardiovascular Disease in the Young, Committee on Rheumatic Fever, Endocarditis and Kawasaki Disease. *Circulation, 110*(17), 2747-2771. (Also published in *Pediatrics*. (2004). *114*(6),1708-1733.)

Nicklas, T.A., von Duvillard, S.P., & Berenson, G.S. (2002). Tracking of serum lipids and lipoproteins from childhood to dyslipidemia in adults: The Bogalusa Heart Study. *Int J Sports Med, 23*(Suppl 1), S39-S43.

Pantell, R.H., & Goodman, B.W. (1983). Adolescent chest pain: A prospective study. *Pediatrics, 71*(6), 881-887.

Park, M.K., Menard, S.W., & Yuan, C. (2001). Comparison of auscultatory and oscillometric blood pressures. *Arch Pediatr Adolesc Med, 155*(1), 50-53.

Rhee, H. (2005). Relationships between physical symptoms and pubertal development. *J Pediatr Health Care, 19*(2), 95-103.

Saarel, E.V., Stefanelli, C.B., Fischbach, P.S., et al. (2004) Transtelephonic electrocardiographic monitors for evaluation of children and adolescents with suspected arrhythmias. *Pediatrics, 113*(2), 248-251.

Shulman, S.T. (2003). Is there a role for corticosteroids in Kawasaki disease? *J Pediatr, 142*(6), 601-603.

Soteriades, E.S., Evans, J.C., Larson, M.G., et al. (2002). Incidence and prognosis of syncope. *N Engl J Med, 347*(12), 878-885.

Varda, N.M., & Gregoric, A. (2005). A diagnostic approach for the child with hypertension. *Pediatr Nephrol, 20*(4), 499-506.

Wiegman, A., Rodenburg, J., de Jongh, S., et al. (2003). Family history and cardiovascular risk in familial hypercholesterolemia: Data in more than 1000 children. *Circulation, 107*(11), 1473-1478.

Williams, C.L., Hayman, L.L., Daniels, S.R., et al. (2002). Cardiovascular health in childhood: A statement for health professionals from the Committee on Atherosclerosis, Hypertension, and Obesity in the Young (AHOY) of the Council on Cardiovascular Disease in the Young, American Heart Association. *Circulation, 106*(1), 143-160.

Yildirim, A., Karakurt, C., Karademir, S., et al. (2004). Chest pain in children. *Int Pediatr, 19*(3), 175-179.

30 Common Illnesses of the Gastrointestinal System

LEIGH SMALL

Select the best answer for each of the following questions:

1. A 12-month-old is seeing the pediatric nurse practitioner for the first time for a well child checkup. Historical information is obtained from the mother about the child's weight gain trajectory and it is discovered that at birth, he weighed 7 pounds and 5 ounces and his head circumference was at the 50th percentile. Today he is 19 pounds and his head circumference is at the 15th percentile. Given what you know about normal growth in children, the best action that you should take would be:
   A. Tell this mother that the child's weight and height growth appear to be normal.
   B. Request the growth charts from the child's last primary care provider's office.
   C. Check the newborn screening results.
   D. Order a CBC with differential, lead level, a urinalysis, and a urine culture

2. Which of the following statements would contribute most to a pediatric nurse practitioner suspecting a diagnosis of colic in an infant?
   A. This is a bottle-feeding infant.
   B. This 6-week-old term infant has crying and fussy bouts of about 3 hours daily.
   C. This is a female infant.
   D. This 2-week-old infant has fussy periods for up to 2 hours on 2 days per week.

3. Joseph is a 3-week-old infant who was diagnosed with colic at 2 weeks of age. What is the best statement the pediatric nurse practitioner can make when the mother asks to change the infant's formula?
   A. "It has been proven that formula does not cause colic in infants. Let me demonstrate how to soothe Joseph."
   B. "You are probably overfeeding Joseph. How many ounces is he taking per day?"
   C. "Changes in formula are unlikely to affect his irritable behavior; however, we can try a new formula for a week and see if there is any change."
   D. "Joseph's irritability may be due to a gastrointestinal abnormality; I'll order an ultrasound to rule out problems such as malrotation and pyloric stenosis."

4. The best method to check for the first signs of dehydration in a child is:
   A. Look for the production of tears.
   B. Check for capillary refill greater than 3 seconds.
   C. Check for a reduced blood pressure and widening pulse pressure.
   D. Look at the lips to see if they are cracked.

5. A 5-week-old infant male presents in clinic with a week-long history of progressively increasing frequency of vomiting. This infant appears very tired and hungry. When fed sterile water he forcefully vomits non-bilious emesis. Your physical examination reveals a somewhat alert infant, who is thin with no tears. Other positive findings include a visible gastric wave and a small palpable

mass in the epigastric area. You are concerned about him and order lab work. Which of the following is most consistent with the diagnosis that you anticipate making?

A. 140 Na$^+$, 3.8 K$^+$, 92 Cl$^-$, 36 HCO$_3$.
B. 135 Na$^+$, 5.5 K$^+$, 99 Cl$^-$, 22 HCO$_3$.
C. 155 Na$^+$, 4.8 K$^+$, 87 Cl$^-$, 38 HCO$_3$.
D. 150 Na$^+$, 5.6 K$^+$, 102 Cl$^-$, 21 HCO$_3$.

6. A 7-month-old Hispanic infant comes in to your clinic due to reported episodes of screaming; however, he is alert, active, and playful when you see him. Your physical examination is benign except for a sausage-shaped mass in an otherwise soft, nontender abdomen. Just as his mother picks him up to leave he begins screaming inconsolably. What is the best course of action at this point?

A. Order a stat CBC with differential and blood cultures.
B. Order a stat barium enema to be given at a local emergency room.
C. Order an abdominal flat plate and check for free air.
D. Obtain a rectal swab and test for ova and parasites.

7. A 10-year-old female is brought to see you by her mother for a complaint of diarrhea. The girl reports that she has been having intermittent bouts of diarrheal stools with visible blood and mucus for 2 months. These episodes are accompanied with urgency and frequency. You note that her weight has decreased since her last visit one month ago by 5 pounds. What diagnosis are you LEAST likely to include in your differential list given this history?

A. Irritable bowel syndrome.
B. Infection.
C. Crohn's disease.
D. Ulcerative colitis.

8. Angela is a 12-month-old infant who has come to the clinic today due to persistent diarrhea, poor appetite, and fussiness. You notice when her diaper is removed during the examination that she has extra skin folds on her buttocks but her abdomen is both protuberant and tympanic when percussed. Additionally, her hair is thin and brittle and she is not able to easily pull herself up to a stand. The test that will most likely result in a diagnosis is:

A. A urine analysis.
B. A sweat test.
C. A CBC with differential.
D. Antiendomyseal antibody testing.

9. Which of the following conditions can present with chronic constipation?

A. Crohn's disease.
B. Hypercalcemia.
C. Ulcerative colitis.
D. Hypothyroidism.

10. The pediatric nurse practitioner is seeing an adolescent today for a follow-up on an acute but protracted episode of diarrhea. Her mother thinks that she does not look well even though her diarrhea has stopped. Her weight today is 94 pounds, down from her usual 100 pounds. Additionally, she is slightly tachycardic, mildly orthostatic, has dry mucous membranes, and has not voided for 6 hours. The best immediate action is:

A. Have her drink a half of a liter (16 ounces) of rehydration fluid hourly over the next 4 hours in the office.
B. Send her to the local emergency room for admission.
C. Have her drink a liter (33 ounces) of rehydration fluid hourly over the next 4 hours in the office.
D. Have her mother encourage her to drink lots of fluids and see her back in the morning.

11. A 4-month-old female has come to the clinic for a well child examination. The pediatric nurse practitioner notes that the infant preferentially holds her head to the right side and intermittently turns it further to the right side. When gentle pressure is applied, the infant is able to move her head freely in all directions. Other physical findings include arching behavior when placed in the supine position and intermittent dry coughing. What is the best course of action given these findings?

A. Refer to a pediatric neurologist for a potential underlying neurologic condition.
B. Observe in subsequent visits for other signs of strong child temperament and preference issues.

C. Refer to child developmental specialist for evaluation of her development.

D. Refer to a pediatric gastroenterologist for evaluation of gastroesophageal reflux.

12. An 18-month-old infant male presents for a well child visit. His mother reports that he drinks approximately 8 eight-ounce bottles a day of pasteurized whole cow's milk. His overall weight trajectory has been greater than the 95th percentile since he was 6 months old, although his head and height measurements remain between the 25th and 50th percentiles. His mother is concerned that he does not eat much food. The examination reveals a happy, overweight, pale infant male whose development is progressing and who is healthy. Which of the following laboratory values will be abnormal?

A. Serum sodium.
B. Hemoglobin.
C. Serum cholesterol.
D. Leukocyte count.

13. A previously well 14-year-old female has to be seen for complaints of abdominal pain and generalized malaise. The physical examination reveals fever of 105° Fahrenheit, pallor, posterior cervical shotty lymph nodes, splenomegaly, and abdominal tenderness. Her laboratory values are notable for elevated transaminase levels and lymphocytosis. The agent most likely to be responsible for these findings is:

A. Hepatitis B.
B. Hemolytic uremic syndrome.
C. Epstein-Barr virus.
D. Rubella virus.

14. An 8-year-old female comes to the office with a 6-hour history of periumbilical abdominal pain that is increasing in intensity and is accompanied with anorexia, nausea, and vomiting. Additionally, this child has a low-grade fever. The physical examination reveals guarding with generalized tenderness. The best thing to order given this clinical presentation would be:

A. A CBC with differential, sedimentation rate, lipase, and amylase.
B. A chest x-ray.
C. An abdominal flat plate (KUB).

D. An abdominal ultrasound.

15. What are the four most common causes of bacterial gastroenteritis in children?

A. Salmonella, *C. difficile*, *Shigella*, and *Campylobacter*.
B. Salmonella, *Campylobacter*, *Shigella*, and *E. coli*.
C. *Shigella*, *Giardia*, rotavirus, and salmonella.
D. Rotavirus, Norwalk, adenovirus, and salmonella.

16. Ralph is a 4-month-old infant male weighing 10 pounds and 7 ounces (4.76 kilograms) and has been determined to have a moderate degree of failure to thrive. The recommended calorie intake is 108 calories/kg of body weight for well children in this age group; therefore, the recommended calories per day that should be suggested to Ralph's mother would be:

A. 514 calories in 24 hours.
B. 622 calories in 24 hours.
C. 714 calories in 24 hours.
D. 771 calories in 24 hours.

17. Which of the following historical elements is NOT closely linked with irritable bowel syndrome?

A. Alternating periods of constipation and diarrhea.
B. Abdominal pain relieved by a bowel movement.
C. Hematochezia.
D. Abdominal distention and gas.

18. The preicteric phase of hepatitis B infection is most closely associated with:

A. Lethargy, lymphadenopathy, and nausea.
B. Right upper quadrant pain, fever, and vomiting.
C. Urticaria, fever, and right upper quadrant pain.
D. Arthritis, urticaria, and fever.

19. A 4-year-old presents with a history of painless, bright-red rectal bleeding intermittently for the last month. The physical examination, including the rectal exam, is entirely normal. The stool obtained on the rectal examination is guiac-positive. What is the most likely cause of this bleeding?

A. Gastric ulcers.
B. Malignancies.
C. Diverticulitis.
D. Polyps.

20. A 12-month-old infant comes in the office for an urgent visit. His mother has indicated that he has been very lethargic lately and there has been a 2-week history of acholic stools. He does not appear to be jaundiced or have hepatomegaly on examination; however, he does have an elevated urobilinogen. What would be the most accurate information to offer to this mother?
   A. All of the testing has been normal thus far, and so I would like to have you watch your child and call with any other problems and return in 2 weeks to follow up.
   B. These findings all suggest that there is rapid hemolysis or red blood cell breakdown occurring in your infant.
   C. These findings indicate that your infant may be suffering from an intrahepatic infection or problem in the liver.
   D. These findings indicate that your infant has an obstruction to the hepatic system and cannot excrete bile into the intestines.

21. The most likely diagnosis for a 6-year-old child with intense, recurrent, upper right quadrant abdominal pain episodes that follow meals but are not related to changes in bowel patterns is:
   A. Functional abdominal pain.
   B. Bladder infection.
   C. Ulcerative colitis.
   D. Cholecystistis.

22. A mother and her 4-month-old infant with chronic diarrhea and poor weight gain for 2 months come to the clinic for the results of a previously obtained stool culture. Which organism, if found on the culture results, would make the pediatric nurse practitioner include HIV into the differential diagnosis?
   A. Rotavirus.
   B. *Mycobacterium avium.*
   C. Yersinia.
   D. Salmonella.

23. An adolescent male with chronic epigastric pain that occurs primarily in the early morning and sometimes wakes him from sleep has come to be seen today by the pediatric nurse practitioner. The pain is not usually accompanied by vomiting and is relieved by eating. The physical examination is normal. Lab results include stool that is guiac-positive, a normal CBC with differential, and a slightly elevated sedimentation rate. What diagnosis should the pediatric nurse practitioner suspect?
   A. Functional abdominal pain.
   B. Appendicitis.
   C. Gastric ulcer.
   D. Hemorrhoids.

24. A pediatric nurse practitioner is seeing a 2-week-old infant male for a well child examination. The child is breastfeeding well and gaining weight appropriately. This mother indicates that he frequently becomes constipated, his abdomen becomes distended, and he is very irritable. The mother reports that she relieves these symptoms either by giving him a glycerin suppository or providing rectal stimulation just as she had been instructed to do in the hospital. He needed to have rectal stimulation in the hospital because his first stool had not occurred until 3 days of life. Following either of these techniques, he generally has an explosive stool accompanied by a large amount of gas and then seems to be fine for 3 to 4 more days. Given this history, which of the following would you suggest to determine the etiology of this problem most efficiently?
   A. Stool culture and ova and parasite analysis.
   B. Refer to a gastroenterologist for a rectal biopsy.
   C. Order a barium enema.
   D. Order a T_3 and TSH.

25. *Helicobacter pylori* infections in children are most frequently associated with which of the following?
   A. Gastric ulcers.
   B. Recurrent chronic abdominal pain.
   C. Chronic otitis media.
   D. Antral and duodenal ulcers.

ANSWERS

1. **Answer:** D

   Rationale: This infant has failed to triple his or her weight, is currently in the 3rd percentile, and has a slowing growth trajectory of the head circumference, suggesting that there is significant failure to thrive. While answers B and C are important to complete at some point, it is a greater priority to rule out anemia, lead toxicity, infection (chronic or subclinical), urinary infection, or kidney disorders as contributing causes of this child's poor growth.

2. **Answer:** B

   Rationale: Colic is diagnosed in infants when there are reports of excessive irritability, fussing or crying bouts of at least 3 hours a day, 3 or more days a week. This frustrating problem affects infant females and males equally and does not differentially affect bottle- or breastfeeding infants. Interestingly, this presents in the first 1 to 3 weeks of life in an abrupt or subtle onset and may last for up to 3 to 4 months of age.

3. **Answer:** C

   Rationale: Formula changes are not likely to result in changes in fussiness or irritability; however, approximately 5% of infants have been found to have carbohydrate sensitivities and/or protein allergies to some of the key components of cow's milk-based formula or soy formula. Therefore, children with marked irritability can be changed to a different formula with the trial lasting at least 1 week of duration [i.e., 1) cow milk-based, 2) soy based, 3) protein hydrolysate formulas], but parents should be cautioned that infant behaviors are not likely to change.

4. **Answer:** A

   Rationale: All of the responses are important signs and symptoms of dehydration that should be assessed; however, lack of tears is one of the first signs of those listed that suggest a child has moderate dehydration. The other options are all signs of severe dehydration.

5. **Answer:** B

   Rationale: The foremost diagnosis for this patient from a differential list developed for the symptom of persistent nonbilious vomiting is pyloric stenosis. This would result in a hypochloremic metabolic alkalosis due to the loss of hydrochloric acid from the stomach, without the loss of base from the duodenum. Therefore, the resultant lab values from an investigation of electrolytes should reveal and lowered chloride level and an elevated bicarbonate level. The sodium and potassium levels often remain within normal limits.

6. **Answer:** B

   Rationale: Intermittent crampy pain that produces episodic crying lasting approximately 20 minutes in a child who is in the second half of the first year of life is most likely to be caused from intussusception or a persistent or intermittent telescoping of one portion of the intestines down into the next distal bowel segment. This occurs most frequently in male infants between the age of 5 months and 1 year and may additionally result in emesis, currant jelly or bloody stools, lethargy, fever, and leukocytosis. Most frequently, the ileum is pulled into the colon by peristaltic action. There is often not a lead point in infants; however, if intussusception occurs in children older than 3 years, the lead point may be a polyp and this potential etiology should be investigated. A barium enema causes increased pressure on the distal bowel and reduces intussusception two-thirds of the time; therefore, this is diagnostic and therapeutic. Intussusception can result in impaired bowel circulation and, in some cases, necrosis resulting in a surgical emergency.

7. **Answer:** A

   Rationale: Infection, Crohn's disease, and ulcerative colitis are often the cause of bloody diarrhea and weight loss in children older than 4 years. Additionally, all three may result in urgency and frequency. Irritable bowel syndrome may result in alternating diarrhea and constipation; however, it is unlikely to be accompanied by weight loss or bloody stools.

8. **Answer:** D

   Rationale: Celiac disease most commonly presents in female children approximately 2 years of age. The typical presentation is an irritable child, with weight loss resulting in muscle wasting, accompanied with a bloated abdomen. Classical findings of biopsies of the intestinal mucosa include a flattening of the villi following chronic exposure to gluten products which results in bloating, increased gas production, diarrhea, explosive stool, and vomiting. Children are genetically predisposed to having this disease, thereby reinforcing the importance of a thorough and detailed family history.

9. *Answer:* D
   Rationale: Hypothyroidism can result in decreased gastric and peristaltic motility resulting in constipation. Additionally, hypercalcemia and diabetes mellitus can present with constipation due to the dehydration that can occur with both conditions. Crohn's disease and ulcerative colitis present with diarrhea.

10. *Answer:* C
    Rationale: This adolescent seems to be in the convalescent stage of this illness because the diarrheal portion of gastroenteritis has ended; however, this mother's concerns and your assessments indicate that she is suffering from a moderate level of dehydration. Her condition seems fairly stable but not enough to allow her to go home at this point. Oral rehydration is the best choice and moderate dehydration suggests that you should establish fluid replacement at 100 ml/kg of ideal body weight over 4 hours and reassess hourly.

11. *Answer:* D
    Rationale: Approximately 50% of 4-month-old infants are affected with gastroesophageal reflux. Spastic torticollis, hypotonia, arching in the supine position, marked irritability, and coughing can all be signs that there is gastroesophageal reflux that has resulted in the development of Sandifer's syndrome. Children with Sandifer's syndrome are frequently sent to neurologists to rule out an underlying seizure disorder; however, once the GER is successfully managed these symptoms often subside.

12. *Answer:* B
    Rationale: Cow's milk contains very little iron; therefore, children obtaining their primary nutrition from cow's milk intake also have a low intake of iron. As a result, the low iron intake has a negative effect on the production of hemoglobin. Additionally, a large intake of cow's milk has been associated with microscopic blood loss from intestines further complicating this issue of a low iron intake. The serum sodium and cholesterol and the leukocyte count are unrelated to this problem.

13. *Answer:* C
    Rationale: The child's age and clinical presentation are most suggestive of Epstein-Barr virus. Hepatitis B is unlikely to result in fever with elevated transaminase levels and splenomegaly with no other findings. Hemolytic uremic syndrome primarily occurs in infants and young children and is a disease involving a triad of symptoms including anemia, thrombocytopenia, and acute renal failure. Rubella virus begins as a facial rash that spreads to the trunk and limbs and may have co-occurring thrombocytopenia.

14. *Answer:* A
    Rationale: The priority differential diagnoses should include pyelonephritis, ruptured ovarian follicle, or ovarian torsion, inflammatory bowel disease, appendicitis, peptic ulcer disease, and pancreatitis. A CBC with differential, sedimentation rate, amylase, and lipase would most efficiently guide your decision-making process through this diagnostic challenge. Some of the other tests may be indicated after the results of the serum analysis.

15. *Answer:* B
    Rationale: The most common of bacterial causes of gastroenteritis in children include *Shigella*, salmonella, *E. coli*, *Campylobacter*, and *C. difficile*. The three common viral causes of gastroenteritis in children include adenovirus, rotavirus, and strains from the Norwalk group. Rates of adenovirus infections slightly increase in frequency during the summer months and the incidence of rotavirus increases in frequency in the winter months; however, the Norwalk group occurs year-round. Giardia is the most frequently occurring gastroenteritis of parasitic etiology.

16. *Answer:* D
Rationale: A child who has been diagnosed as failing to thrive should have an increased caloric intake of 150% of the normal calories recommended for that age group. The recommended caloric intake for 4-month-old infants is 108 calories/kilogram of body weight; therefore, this infant should receive 162 calories per kilogram of body weight or 771 calories each day. This would equate to 26 ounces of regular formula (30 calories per ounce) per day or a little greater than 4 ounces six times each day.

17. *Answer:* C
Rationale: Patients with irritable bowel syndrome (IBS) rarely present with hematochezia or bloody bowel movements. It is also rare that patients with IBS demonstrate systematic complaints such as fever, anorexia, and weight loss; however, these are all common complaints of patients diagnosed with an inflammatory bowel disease such as Crohn's disease or ulcerative colitis.

18. *Answer:* D
Rationale: The prodromal phase or pre-icteric phase of a hepatitis B infection follows the incubation period of 6 to 24 weeks. During this period of time, patients often experience general symptoms such as lethargy, anorexia, nausea, vomiting, and upper right quadrant abdominal pain. Some patients experience a mild fever, urticaria, and polyarthritis. This period can last for 2 days to 2 weeks and then frequently progresses to the icteric phase marked by bilirubinuria, pale stools, and jaundice.

19. *Answer:* D
Rationale: Juvenile gastrointestinal polyps frequently present as cases of painless rectal bleeding in otherwise well children less than 5 years of age without weight loss. The polyps are most commonly found in the rectum; although they may not be appreciated on rectal examination. A pediatric gastroenterologist will need to remove the polyps during an outpatient endoscopic procedure. These fleshy growths are most often singular, and not malignant or premalignant. Therefore, the singular polyps, to be differentiated from polypoid conditions with multiple pol-yps (i.e., Gardner's syndrome), are not associated with any cancerous conditions or predisposal to the development of cancer.

20. *Answer:* D
Rationale: An increase in unconjugated bilirubin is signaled as the unconjugated bilirubin, a breakdown product of hemoglobin (i.e., heme is converted to bilirubin), which cannot attach to glucuronide (conjugated bilirubin) found in the liver. Therefore, unconjugated bilirubin increases. If there is an intrahepatic inflammation or infection, the conjugated bilirubin will increase, the bilirubin will enter the small intestines and continue to color the stools, and the additional bilirubin will spill into the bloodstream, and be filtered by the kidneys causing the urobilinogen to increase. However, if there is an obstruction to the biliary collecting system, the serum conjugated bilirubin will increase resulting in an increased urobilinogen but the bile will not move into the gut and the stools will lack color or be "acholic" stools.

21. *Answer:* D
Rationale: The inflammation of ulcerative colitis usually occurs in the lower left quadrant and is frequently associated with changes in the frequency, urgency, and/or consistency of bowel movements. Pain from bladder infections is more likely to be lower mid-abdominal pain that can radiate to the lower back and is associated urinary frequency and urgency among many other symptoms. Localized pain is unlikely to be recurrent functional pain; therefore, this pain may be the result of cholecystitis.

22. *Answer:* B
Rationale: Rotavirus, Yersinia, and salmonella are all frequent causative agents of common gastroenteritis in children and would not raise suspicions of HIV infection; however, Mycobacterium species are rarely found in well children. Specifically, *Mycobacterium avium* is the etiologic agent of 95% of the infections found in children with AIDS. Therefore, an infant with FTT and generalized symptoms with a positive stool culture with *M. avium* is very likely infected with HIV.

23. *Answer:* C

Rationale: Nocturnal abdominal pain that is localized to the epigastric area and is relieved by eating is highly suggestive of a peptic ulcer. Finding blood in the stool (i.e., a positive guiac), and a mildly elevated sedimentation rate suggests that this is active ulceration that should be evaluated by a pediatric gastroenterologist conducting an upper endoscopy and then should be rigorously treated.

24. *Answer:* B

Rationale: In the case that an infant does not pass its first stool for greater than 48 hours, clinicians should consider Hirschprung's disease as one of the priority differential diagnoses. Hirschprung's disease is an obstruction to the colon related to an aganglionic section of large intestines usually found within first 3 to 5 cm of the rectal segment. A barium enema may provide an initial screen as it may identify a transition zone; however, this is not a reliable test to use with an infant younger than three months of age. While hypothyroidism may produce constipation, it generally does not result in failure to pass a stool in the first 48 hours. The clinical picture of an intestinal infection or presence of ova and parasites is very different and would not interfere with passing the initial bowel movement.

25. *Answer:* D

Rationale: H. pylori is a spirochete which most commonly burrows into the antral portion of the stomach and the duodenum. However, there only is a weak association with this organism and chronic recurrent abdominal pain and gastric ulcers.

BIBLIOGRAPHY

American Academy of Pediatrics Section on Breastfeeding. (2005). Breastfeeding and the use of human milk. *Pediatrics, 115*(2), 496-506.

Ammaniti, M., Ambruzzi, A.M., Lucarelli, L., et al. (2004). Malnutrition and dysfunctional mother-child feeding interactions: Clinical assessment and research implications. *J Am Coll Nutr, 23*(3), 259-271.

Berman, J. (July 1, 2003). Heading off the dangers of acute gastroenteritis. Retrieved April 28, 2006, from www.contemporarypediatrics.com/contpeds/article/articleDetail.jsp?id=111759.

Boynton, R.W., Dunn, E.S., Stephens, G.R., & Pulcini, J. (2003). *Manual of ambulatory pediatrics* (5th ed.). New York: Lippincott Williams & Wilkins.

Bullard, J., & Page, N.E. (2005). Cyclic vomiting syndrome: A disease in disguise. *Pediatr Nurs, 31*(1), 27-29.

Christensen, M.L., & Gold, B.D. (2002). *Clinical management of infants and children with gastroesophageal reflux disease: Disease recognition and therapeutic options.* Monograph from the symposium presented at the American Society of Health-System Pharmacists in Atlanta, GA, Dec. 9, 2002.

El-Baba, M.F. (2004). *Irritable bowel syndrome.* Retrieved April 28, 2006, from www.emedicine.com/ped/topic1210.htm.

Fox, J.A. (2003). *Primary health care of infants, children, & adolescents* (2nd ed.). St. Louis: Mosby.

Gold, B. (2003). Recurrent abdominal pain in children. Presented at Digestive Disease Week 2003, May 17-22, Orlando, FL, and reported by J. Rusk, in *Infect Dis Child*, July 2003, 39-40.

Hockenberry, M.J., Wilson, D., Winkelstein, M.L., & Kline, N.E. (2003). *Wong's nursing care of infants and children* (7th ed.). St. Louis: Mosby/Elsevier.

Kass, D.A., & Sinert, R. (2006). *Pediatrics: Pyloric stenosis.* Retrieved on April 28, 2006, from http://www.emedicine.com/EMERG/topic397.htm.

Krugman, S.D., & Dubowitz, H. (2003). Failure to thrive. *Am Fam Phys, 68*(5), 879-884.

Lobo, M.L., Kotzer, A.M., Keefe, M.R., et al. (2004). Current beliefs and management strategies for treating infant colic. *J Pediatr Health Care, 18*(3), 115-122.

Malaty, H.M., Abudayyeh, S., O'Malley, K.J., et al. (2005). Development of a multidimensional measure for recurrent abdominal pain in children: Population-based studies in three settings. *Pediatrics, 115*(2), 210-215.

Mason, D., Tobias, N., Lutkenhoff, M., et al. (2004). The APN's guide to pediatric constipation management. *Nurse Pract Am J Prim Health Care, 29*(7), 13-21.

Mast, E.E. (2004). Mother-to-infant hepatitis C virus transmission and breastfeeding. *Adv Exp Med Biol, 554*, 211-216.

Mulligan, S.A., Migita, D.S., Christakis, D.A., & Saint, S. (2003). *Saint-Frances guide to Pediatrics.* New York: Lippincott Williams & Wilkins.

National Center for Shaken Baby Syndrome (2006). *Period of PURPLE Crying.* Retrieved April 28, 2006, from http://dontshake.com/Subject.aspx?categoryID=1.

O'Brien, L.M., Heycock, E.G., Hanna, M., et al. (2004). Postnatal depression and faltering growth: A community study. *Pediatrics, 113*(5), 1242-1247.

Petersen-Smith, A.M. (2004). Gastrointestinal disorders. In C.E. Burns, A.M. Dunn, M.A. Brady, et al. (Eds.). *Pediatric primary care: A handbook for nurse practitioners* (3rd ed.). Philadelphia: Saunders.

Rowe, W.A. (2006). *Inflammatory bowel disease*. Retrieved April 28, 2006, from www.emedicine.com/med/topic1169.htm.

Rudolph, C.D., & Miranda, A. (2004). Treatment options for functional abdominal pain. *Pediatr Ann, 33*(2), 105-112.

Rudolph, C. D., Mazur, L. J., Liptak G. S., et. al. (2001). Guidelines for evaluation and treatment of gastroesophageal reflux in infants and children. *J Pediatr Gastroenterol Nutr, 32*(Suppl 2), S1-31.

Sears, C.L. (2005). Proper evaluation necessary before treating diarrhea. Presentation at the Clinical Infectious Disease Meeting, March 31-April 3, 2005, Orlando, FL. Reported by C.A. Richards in *Infect Dis Child*, July 2005, 56, 58.

Schwartz, M.W. (2003). *Clinical handbook of pediatrics* (3rd ed.). New York: Lippincott Williams & Wilkins.

Smart, S., & Cottrell, D. (2005). Going to the doctors: The views of mothers of children with recurrent abdominal pain. *Child Care Health Dev, 31*(3), 265-273.

Smink, D.S., Finkelstein, J.A., Peña, B.M.G., et al. (2004). Diagnosis of acute appendicitis in children using a clinical practice guideline. *J Pediatr Surg, 39*(3), 458-463.

Tucker, J. (2004). *Pediatrics: Appendicitis*. Retrieved April 28, 2006, from www.emedicine.com/EMERG/topic361.htm.

Turner, L.C. (2004). *Hepatitis A*. Retrieved April 28, 2006, from www.emedicine.com/ped/topic977.htm.

Walker, L.S. (2003). Age and gender effects on GI symptoms and somatization. Presented at Digestive Disease Week 2003, May 17-22, Orlando, FL, and reported by J. Rusk in *Infect Dis Child*, July 2003, 41, 43.

World Health Organization (WHO). (2000a). Hepatitis B fact sheet no. 204. Retrieved April 28, 2006, from www.who.int/mediacentre/factsheets/fs204/en/index.html.

World Health Organization (WHO). (2000a). Hepatitis C fact sheet no. 164. Retrieved April 28, 2006, from www.who.int/mediacentre/factsheets/fs164/en/index.html.

World Health Organization (WHO). (2005). Hepatitis E fact sheet no. 280. Retrieved April 28, 2006, from www.who.int/mediacentre/factsheets/fs280/en/index.html.

Youssef, N.N., Rosh, J.R., Loughran, M., et al. (2004). Treatment of functional abdominal pain in childhood with cognitive behavioral strategies. *J Pediatr Gastroenterol Nutr, 39*(2), 192-196.

31 Common Illnesses of the Reproductive and Urologic Systems

MARGARET MCNULTY AND MARIAILIANA J. STARK

Select the best answer for each of the following questions:

1. What factors do NOT affect the decision of how to obtain a urine specimen when urinary tract infection (UTI) is being considered?
   A. Toilet training abilities.
   B. Child's ability to cooperate.
   C. Severity of illness.
   D. The type of antibiotics being considered.

2. Malia is a 5-year-old who presents at your clinic after her mother reports that her urine is very bloody. Malia has been in good health. She has no reported rashes and is afebrile, although she did vomit once today and appears more tired than usual. She has had no history of UTI. Which of the following would NOT be included in your list of differential diagnoses for hematuria?
   A. Glomerulonephritis.
   B. Trauma.
   C. Benign recurrent hematuria.
   D. Inflammatory bowel disease.

3. What is the most common clinical presentation of infants and young children with a UTI?
   A. Skin rash.
   B. Irritability.
   C. Fever.
   D. Upper respiratory infection.

4. The most common causative organism for UTI in children is:
   A. *Escherichia coli.*
   B. Adenovirus.

   C. *Shigella.*
   D. *Streptococcus pneumoniae.*

5. What distinguishes lower from upper urinary tract bleeding?
   A. Temperature.
   B. Color of the urine.
   C. Location of abdominal pain.
   D. Presence of diarrhea.

6. Which of the following is NOT included in the risk factors for UTI?
   A. Sexual abuse.
   B. Poor hygiene.
   C. Infrequent voiding.
   D. Circumcised penis.

7. Acute bacterial pyelonephritis:
   A. Never presents with frequency, urgency, and dysuria.
   B. Occurs only in sexually active teenagers.
   C. Follows the ascending route of the UTI.
   D. Is not associated with fevers.

8. Hemolytic uremic syndrome (HUS) is one of the most common causes of acute renal failure in childhood. Which of the following conditions are associated with HUS?
   A. Hypotension and hematuria.
   B. Rectal prolapse with or without diarrhea.
   C. Microangiopathic hemolytic anemia, thrombocytopenia, and renal failure.
   D. Group A beta-hemolytic streptococcal infection.

9. Which of the following would NOT be included in the differential diagnosis for painful scrotal swelling?
    A. Hydrocele.
    B. Epididymitis.
    C. Testicular torsion.
    D. Hematocele secondary to trauma.

10. The management of a 12-year-old male child with acute scrotal pain and edema would include which of the following?
    A. Rest, ice, and scrotal support.
    B. Monitor closely with no intervention at this time.
    C. Immediate surgical referral.
    D. Pain management.

11. The most likely cause of proteinuria in a 14-year-old male who presents for a physical examination and no recent illnesses is which of the following?
    A. Acute nephritic syndrome.
    B. Orthostatic proteinuria.
    C. Exercise-induced proteinuria.
    D. Fever-induced proteinuria.

12. Which of the following is NOT true regarding cryptorchidism?
    A. About 20% of children will respond to hormonal therapy.
    B. The most common type is retractile testicles.
    C. Surgical orchidopexy remains the standard treatment.
    D. It only occurs unilaterally.

13. A mother and her 6-year-old son come into the clinic with a complaint of bedwetting. The history reveals the child wears "pull-ups" to bed each night and on most mornings the "pull up" is soaking wet. A diagnosis of primary nocturnal enuresis is confirmed. What would be the LEAST appropriate therapy at this point?
    A. Watchful waiting and reassurance that most children will outgrow bedwetting.
    B. Nighttime awakening for child to void during the night.
    C. Conditioning therapy with an alarm system.
    D. Imipramine therapy.

14. Painful genital bumps are associated with what condition?
    A. Herpes simplex.
    B. Genital warts.
    C. Labial adhesions.
    D. Vaginal candidiasis.

15. The Amsel criterion is used in the diagnosis of bacterial vaginosis. For the Amsel criteria, three of the following occur. Which of the following is NOT included in these criteria?
    A. Clue cells on saline wet prep.
    B. Vaginal pH of less than 3.
    C. Whiff test for positive volatile amines.
    D. Thin, homogenous discharge.

16. Which statement is NOT true of vulvovaginitis in prepubertal females?
    A. In childhood, 50% to 80% have nonspecific etiology.
    B. Most often associated with poor hygiene.
    C. Always associated with child abuse.
    D. 20% of girls with pinworms develop vulvovaginitis.

17. Which statement is NOT true about pinworm infections?
    A. Intense itching occurs in the rectal area.
    B. Infection occurs when eggs are ingested by the child.
    C. Bedding should be washed in hot water.
    D. Household contacts do not need to be treated.

18. Which statement regarding bacterial vaginosis (BV) is NOT true?
    A. Host factors include multiple sex partners, same-sex partners, douching, IUD use, and early sexual debut.
    B. Treatment of choice is oral or vaginal metronidazole.
    C. Sexual partner treatment is recommended.
    D. Recurrence rates are high.

19. The differential diagnosis of lower abdominal pain includes all of the following EXCEPT:

A. Pelvic inflammatory disease (PID).
B. Ectopic pregnancy.
C. Ovarian torsion.
D. Pinworm infestation.

20. Choose the statement that is NOT true.
   A. Smoking doubles the risk of follicular cysts.
   B. Ovarian cysts may occur in infancy.
   C. All masses are self-limiting.
   D. Refer growing cysts to gynecology.

21. The overall incidence of primary dysmenorrhea is:
   A. 10%.
   B. 25%.
   C. 50%.
   D. 80%.

22. Amy has a history of irregular menses with increased menstrual blood flow over the past few months. In addition to a CBC, what lab test would be appropriate at this time?
   A. PT and PTT.
   B. Fasting blood sugar.
   C. Lipid profile.
   D. Sedimentation rate.

23. Rebecca, a junior in the local high school, was diagnosed with fibroadenoma of the right breast. Which of the following statements is TRUE regarding this condition?

A. There is a low prevalence of fibroadenomas in teens.
B. This is a benign neoplasm.
C. Most will decrease in size without intervention.
D. No follow-up is necessary.

24. Which of the following statements is FALSE?
   A. There is an association between gynecomastia and the development of breast cancer.
   B. If mastitis occurs, breastfeeding can be continued.
   C. Mastalgia is treated with a supportive bra and analgesics.
   D. No treatment is required for an imperforate hymen with microperforation.

25. Labial adhesions:
   A. Can occur after irritation such as poor hygiene or sexual abuse.
   B. Occurs in 75% of all females 2 to 6 years of age.
   C. Can be treated with oral estrogen.
   D. Surgical separation is usually needed to resolve this condition.

ANSWERS

1. **Answer:** D
   Rationale: The method of obtaining a urine specimen is affected by the child's age, severity of illness, child's ability to cooperate, and toilet training abilities. The type of antibiotics being considered for treatment does not alter the method of obtaining a urine specimen. The colony count considered positive depends on the collection method; greater than or equal to 10,000 CFU for a catheterized specimen and greater than or equal to 100,000 CFU for clean-catch specimen. Bag specimens are only definitive when culture is negative.

2. **Answer:** D
   Rationale: The list for the differential diagnosis for hematuria is extensive. The most common causes of hematuria in clinical practice include UTI, trauma, benign recurrent hematuria, and glomerulonephritis.

3. **Answer:** C
   Rationale: Fever is the most common symptom in infants and children younger than 2 years of age. Symptoms of UTI in this age group are usually nonspecific and may include vomiting, poor feeding, or irritability.

4. **Answer:** A
   Rationale: Escherichia coli is the most common organism associated with UTIs. UTIs are usually caused by bacteria that ascend up the urethra into the bladder.

5. **Answer:** B
   Rationale: In general, brown-, tea-, or cola-colored urine suggest upper urinary tract bleeding. The bright-red blood suggests lower tract bleeding. The darker urine has had more time to become oxidized within the urinary tract.

6. **Answer:** D
   Rationale: Risk factors for UTIs include infrequent voiding, constipation, sexual abuse, pinworms, and poor perineal hygiene. Beginning in late infancy, UTI is more common in females compared to males.

7. **Answer:** C
   Rationale: Acute bacterial pyelonephritis is an inflammation of the ureters and kidneys. It is usually caused by bacteria that have ascended from the bladder after entering the urethra.

8. **Answer:** C
   Rationale: Hemolytic uremic syndrome is a heterogeneous group of similar entities. It is the most common cause of acute renal failure in childhood and is defined by a combination of microangiopathic hemolytic anemia, thrombocytopenia, and renal failure. Other symptoms include a sudden onset of oliguria, hypertension, pallor, lethargy, systolic flow murmur, bruising, and mild hematuria. Most (> 80%) HUS cases are caused by Shiga toxin-producing *Escherichia coli* 0157: H7.

9. **Answer:** A
   Rationale: Hydrocele is a nontender swelling of the scrotum due to collection of peritoneal fluid. Scrotal skin is normal. Testicular torsion is a twisting of the spermatic cord resulting in a sudden, unilateral pain with swelling and tenderness. Epididymitis is an inflammation of the epididymis resulting in sudden, unilateral testicular pain with erythema, swelling, and tenderness.

10. **Answer:** C
    Rationale: Testicular torsion, which presents with the prescribed symptoms, is a surgical emergency and should be immediately referred for surgical evaluation. Continued torsion could result in gangrene and/or loss of the testicle.

11. **Answer:** B
    Rationale: Thirty percent of cases of proteinuria are found on random urinalysis of children. The child excretes abnormal amounts of urinary protein when in the upright position, but excretes normal amounts of urinary protein when lying flat.

12. **Answer:** D
    Rationale: Cryptorchidism may be unilateral or bilateral. This condition can be due to a hyperactive cremasteric reflex (retractile

testicles), tension from external musculature (canalicular testicle), hormonal abnormalities (intraabdominal testicle), or problems during fetal development (ectopic or absent testicles).

13. *Answer:* D
Rationale: Imipramine is a tricylic antidepressant that was once used for the treatment of enuresis; however, it is rarely used today. Desmopressin acetate (DDAVP), a synthetic analogue of vasopressin, is effective for the treatment of enuresis. Pharmacotherapy is usually reserved for children older than 10 years who fail with other therapies.

14. *Answer:* A
Rationale: Labial adhesions and genital warts are nonpainful genital bumps. Apthosis and herpes simplex are painful. Vaginal candida infections do not cause any bumps.

15. *Answer:* B
Rationale: Amsel criteria for bacterial vaginosis includes three of the following: homogenous discharge, vaginal pH of greater than or equal to 4.5, positive whiff test, and clue cells on the wet prep.

16. *Answer:* C
Rationale: In prepubertal girls, vulvovaginitis is most often associated with poor hygiene and contact irritation. Sexual abuse must be a differential, but vulvovaginitis is not always associated with sexual abuse. History is important to rule out any suspicion of abuse.

17. *Answer:* D
Rationale: Treatment of the entire household is important to eliminate the spread of the pinworms once infestation has occurred. Oral anthelmintic medication, good handwashing, and washing bed linens and clothing in hot water are also indicated in the treatment of pinworms.

18. *Answer:* C
Rationale: Sexual partner treatment is not recommended in the treatment of bacterial vaginosis.

19. *Answer:* D

Rationale: Pinworms do not usually cause lower abdominal pain. In addition to PID, ectopic pregnancy, ovarian torsion, the differential diagnosis for lower abdominal pain might also include ovarian cyst and primary dysmenorrhea.

20. *Answer:* C
Rationale: All ovarian masses are not self-limiting. Conservative management over a 6-week period might be indicated if the mass measures 5 to 6 cm, but referral to gynecology is indicated if masses that are stable persist beyond 10 weeks or if masses are enlarging. Referral to the emergency department is always indicated if there are episodes of acute pain associated with the mass.

21. *Answer:* D
Rationale: Primary dysmenorrhea is very prevalent, with an overall incidence of 79.6%. The peak incidence is 1 to 3 years after menarche.

22. *Answer:* A
Rationale: CBC and PT, PTT are indicated with a history of increased menstrual blood flow. In addition, a Von Willebrand (VW) profile, platelets, and other lab tests might be indicated after a thorough history and physical exam is obtained.

23. *Answer:* C
Rationale: Fibroadenomas are common in teenage girls (especially black females) and accounts for 50% of breast masses in adolescent females. They are benign neoplasms. Only 2% will decrease in size without intervention and 32% will increase is size over a 5-year period. Follow-up is needed every 6 months or sooner if growth occurs.

24. *Answer:* A
Rationale: There is no relationship to the development of breast cancer with gynecomastia. Lactating women are encouraged to continue nursing. Breast pumping can also be used with mastitis. No treatment is needed in a case where a female has an imperforate hymen with microperforation. Mastalgia may occur premenstrually or during menstruation in adolescents and is treated with a supportive bra and analgesics.

25. *Answer:* A

Rationale: Labial adhesions are prevalent in 33% of prepubertal females. Local irritation or inflammation removes external layers of epidermis. The provider must obtain an accurate history and physical to rule out sexual abuse. Labial adhesions can be treated with topical application of estrogen twice a day for no longer than 2 weeks. Rarely, surgical intervention is required.

BIBLIOGRAPHY

American Academy of Pediatrics. (1999). Practice parameter: The diagnosis, treatment, and evaluation of the initial UTI in febrile infants and young children. *Pediatrics, 103*(4), 843-852.

American Academy of Pediatrics. (2003). Pinworm infection. In L.K. Pickering (Ed.). *Red Book: 2003 Report of the Committee on Infectious Diseases* (26th ed.). Elk Grove Village, IL: American Academy of Pediatrics.

Angel, C.A. (2004). Meatal stenosis. Retrieved May 1, 2006, from www.emedicine.com/ped/topic2356.htm.

Association for Genitourinary Medicine (AGUM), & Medical Society for the Study of Venereal Disease (MSSVD). (2002). National guideline on the management of vulvovaginal candidiasis. London: AGUM & MSSVD.

Bacon, J.L. (2002). Prepubertal labial adhesions: Evaluation of a referral population. *Am J Obstet Gynecol, 187*(2), 327-332.

Baker, L.A., Silver, R.I., & Docimo, S.G. (2001). Cryptorchidism. In J.P. Gearhart, R.C. Rink, & P.D.E. Mouriquand (Eds.). *Pediatric urology*. Philadelphia: Saunders.

Barakat, L.P., Smith-Whitley, K., Schulman, S., et al. (2001). Nocturnal enuresis in pediatric sickle cell disease. *J Dev Behav Pediatr, 22*(5), 300-305.

Brooks, L.J., & Topol, H.I. (2003). Enuresis in children with sleep apnea. *J Pediatr, 142*(5), 515-518.

Cantu, S. (2006). Phimosis and paraphimosis. Retrieved May 1, 2006, from www.emedicine.com/emerg/topic423.htm.

Centers for Disease Control and Prevention (CDC) (2004). Chlamydia screening among sexually active young female enrollees of health plans—United States, 1999-2001, *MMWR: Morb Mortal Wkly Rep, 53*(42), 983-985.

Centers for Disease Control and Prevention (CDC) (2006). Guidelines for treatment for sexually transmitted diseases. *MMWR Morb Mortal Wkly Rep, 55*, 1-94.

Cooper, C.S., Gallagher, B.L., & Carson, M.R. (2006). Prepubertal testicular and paratesticular tumors. Retrieved on May 1, 2006, from http://www.emedicine.com/ped/topic1423.htm.

Coste, J., Fernandez, H., Joye, N., et al. (2000). Role of chromosome abnormalities in ectopic pregnancy. *Fertil Steril, 74*(6), 1259-1260.

Cuckow, P.M., & Nyirady, P. (2001). Foreskin. In J.P. Gearhart, R.C. Rink, & P.D.E. Mouriquand (Eds.). *Pediatric urology*. Philadelphia: Saunders.

Davis, I.D., & Avner, E.D. (2004). Nephrology. In R.E. Behrman, R.M. Kliegman, & H.B. Jenson (Eds.). *Nelson textbook of pediatrics* (17th ed.). Philadelphia: Saunders.

Dogra, V., & Resnick, M.I. (2002). Ultrasonography of the scrotum. *J Ultrasound Med, 21*(8), 848.

Eiberg, H., Shaumburg, H.L., Von Gontard, A., & Rittig, S. (2001). Linkage study of a large Danish 4-generation family with urge incontinence and nocturnal enuresis. *J Urol, 166*(6), 2401-2403.

Elder, J.S. (2004). Anomalies of the penis and urethra. In R.E. Behrman., R.M. Kliegman, & H.B. Jenson (Eds.). *Nelson textbook of pediatrics* (17th ed.). Philadelphia: Saunders.

Enright, A.M., & Prober, C.G. (2002). Neonatal herpes infection: Diagnosis, treatment and prevention. *Semin Neonatol, 7*(4), 283-291.

Ersöz, H.O., Onde, M.E., Terekeci, H., et al. (2002). Causes of gynaecomastia in young adult males and factors associated with idiopathic gynaecomastia. *Int J Androl, 25*(5), 312-316.

Farhat, W., Bagli, D.J., Capolicchio, G., et al. (2000). The dysfunctional voiding scoring system: Quantitative standardization of dysfunctional voiding symptoms in children. *J Urol, 164*(3 Pt 2), 1011-1015.

Glazener, C.M.A., & Evans, J.H.C. (2005). Alarm interventions for nocturnal enuresis in children. *Cochrane Database Syst Rev,* 2:CD003637. Retrieved on May 1, 2006, from http://www.cochrane.org/reviews/en/ab002911.html.

Glazener, C.M.A., Evans, J.H.C., & Peto, R.E. (2006). Tricyclic and related drugs for nocturnal enuresis in children. *Cochrane Database Syst Rev,* 3: CD002117. Retrieved on May 1, 2006, from http://www.cochrane.org/reviews/en/ab002117.html.

Gloor, J.M., & Torres, V.E. (2001). Reflux and obstructive neuropathy. In R.W. Schrier (Series Ed.). *Atlas of diseases of the kidney* (Vol. 2, Ch. 8). CyberNephrology™ Center: Edmonton, Alberta, Canada. Retrieved May 1, 2006, from http://www.kidneyatlas.org/book2/adk2_08.pdf.

Haward, M., & Shafer, M.A. (2002). Vaginitis and cervicitis. In L.S. Neinstein (Ed.). *Adolescent health care: A practical guide* (4th ed.). Philadelphia: Lippincott Williams & Wilkins.

Herbst, R. (2003). Perineal streptococcal dermatitis/disease: Recognition and management. *Am J Clin Dermatol, 4*(8), 555-560.

Herrinton, L.J., Zhao, W., & Husson, G. (2003). Management of cryptorchidism and risk of testicular cancer. *Am J Epidemiol, 157*(7), 602-605.

Horner, N.K., & Lampe, J.W. (2000). Potential mechanisms of diet therapy for fibrocystic breast conditions show inadequate evidence of effectiveness. *J Am Dietetic Assoc, 100*(11), 1368-1380.

Jepson, R.G., Mihaljevic, L., & Craig, J. (2006). Cranberries for treating urinary tract infections. *Cochrane Database Syst Rev,* Cochrane Renal Group, 2. Retrieved on May 1, 2006, from http://www.cochrane.org/reviews/en/ab001322.html.

Joesoef, M.R., & Schmid, G. (June 2005). Bacterial vaginosis. *Clin Evidence,* (13):1968-1978.

Jordan, G.H., & Schlossberg, S.M. (2002). Surgery of the penis and urethra. In P.C. Walsh , A.B. Retik, E.D. Vaughan Jr., & A.J. Wein (Eds.). *Campbell's urology* (8th ed.). Philadelphia: Saunders.

Kazzi, A.A., & Roberts, R. (2004). Ovarian cysts. Retrieved December 20, 2004, from www.emedicine.com/EMERG/topic352.htm.

Khan, H.N., & Blamey, R.W. (2003). Endocrine treatment of physiological gynecomastia. *BMJ, 327*(7410), 301-302.

Kim, K.S., Torres, C.R., Yucel, S., et al. (2004). Induction of hypospadias in a murine model by maternal exposure to synthetic estrogens. *Environ Res, 94*(3), 267-275.

Kogan, S.J. (2001). The pediatric varicocele. In J.P. Gearhart, R.C. Rink, & P.D.E. Mouriquand (Eds.). *Pediatric urology.* Philadelphia: Saunders.

Kokoska, E.R., Keller, M.S., & Weber T.R. (2000). Acute ovarian torsion in children. *Am J Surg, 180*(6), 462-465.

Lane, W.M., & Robson, M. (2005). Enuresis. Retrieved on May 1, 2006, from www.emedicine.com/ped/topic689.htm.

Lee, P.A., & Coughlin, M.T. (2001). Fertility after bilateral cryptorchidism. Evaluation by paternity, hormone, and semen data, *Horm Res, 55*(1), 28-32.

Lethaby, A., Augood, C., & Duckitt, K. (2006). Nonsteroidal anti-inflammatory drugs for heavy menstrual bleeding. *Cochrane Database Syst Rev, (2)* CD000400. Retrieved on May 1, 2006 from http://www.cochrane.org/reviews/en/ab000400.html.

Lucanto, C., Bauer, S.B., Hyman, P.E., et al. (2000). Function of hollow viscera in children with constipation and voiding difficulties. *Dig Dis Sci, 45*(7), 1274-1280.

Luzzi, G.A., & O'Brien, T.S. (2001). Acute epididymitis. *Brit J Urol, 87*(8), 747-755.

MacKay, A.P., Fingerhut, L.A., & Duran, C.R. (2000). *Adolescent health chartbook. Health, United States, 2000.* Hyattsville, MD: National Center for Health Statistics.

Marcozzi, D. & Suner, S. (2001). Genitourinary emergencies: The nontraumatic acute scrotum. *Emerg Med Clin N Am, 19*(3), 547-568.

Marks, C., Tideman R.L., Estcourt, C.S., et al. (2000). Assessment of risk for pelvic inflammatory disease in an urban sexual health population. *Sex Transm Infect, 76*(6), 470-473.

McCarty, M.A., Garton, R.A., & Jorizzo, J., (2003). Complex aphthosis and Behçet's disease. *Dermatol Clin, 21*(1), 41-48.

Millet, A.V., & Dirbas, F.M. (2002). Clinical management of breast pain: A review. *Obstet Gynecol Surv, 57* (7), 451-461.

Milling, L.S., & Costantino, C.A. (2000). Clinical hypnosis with children: First steps toward empirical support. *Int J Clin Exper Hypnosis, 48*(2), 113-137.

Moore, K.N., Day, R.A., & Albers, M. (2002). Pathogenesis of urinary tract infections: A review. *J Clin Nurs, 11*(5), 568-574.

Morrow, M. (2000). The evaluation of common breast problems. *Am Fam Phys, 61*(8), 2371-2378.

Mycyk, M., & Moyer, P. (2004). Orchitis. Retrieved May 1, 2006, from www.emedicine.com/EMERG/topic344.htm.

Myziuk, L., Romanowski, B., & Brown, M. (2001). Endocervical gram stain smears and their usefulness in the diagnosis of *Chlamydia trachomatis. Sex Transm Infect, 77*(2), 103-106.

Neinstein, L.S., & Joffe, A. (2002). Gynecomastia. In L.S. Neinstein. (ed.). *Adolescent health care: A practical guide* (4th ed.). Philadelphia: Lippincott Williams & Wilkins.

Nelson, A.L., & Neinstein, L.S. (2002). Ectopic pregnancy. In L.S. Neinstein (Ed.). *Adolescent health care: A practical guide* (4th ed.). Philadelphia: Lippincott Williams & Wilkins.

Osuch, J.R. (2002). Breast health and disease over a lifetime. *Clin Obstet Gynecol, 45*(4), 1140-1161.

Patel, S.S., & Kazura, J.W. (2004). Enterobiasis *(Enterobius vericularis).* In R.E. Behrman, R.M. Kliegman, & H.B. Jenson (Eds.). *Nelson textbook of pediatrics* (17th ed.). Philadelphia: Saunders.

Penna, C., Fambrini, M., & Fallani, M.G. (2002). CO_2 laser treatment for Bartholin's gland cyst. *Int J Gynaecol Obstet, 76*(1), 79-80.

Porena, M., Costantini, E., Rociola, W., & Mearini, E. (2000). Biofeedback successfully cures detrusor-sphincter dyssynergia in pediatric patients. *J Urol, 163*(6), 1927-1931.

Rau, F.J., & Muram, D. (2001). Vulvovaginitis in children and adolescents. In J.S. Sanfilippo, D. Muram, J. Dewhurst, & P.A. Lee (Eds.). *Pediatric and adolescent gynecology* (2nd ed.). Philadelphia: Saunders.

Redsell, S.A., & Collier, J. (2001). Bedwetting, behavior and self-esteem: A review of the literature. *Child Care Health Devel, 27*(2), 149-162.

Rimsza, M.E. (2002). Dysfunctional uterine bleeding. *Pediatr Rev, 23*(7), 227-233.

Rowland, R.G., & Herman, J.R. (2002). Tumors and infectious disease of the testis, epididymis and scrotum. In J.Y. Gillenwater, J.T. Grayhack, S.S. Howard, & M.E. Mitchell (Eds.). *Adult and pediatric urology* (4th ed.). Philadelphia: Lippincott Williams & Wilkins.

Sakai, J., & Hebert, F. (2000). Secondary enuresis associated with obstructive sleep apnea. *J Am Acad Child Adolesc Psychiatry, 39*(2), 140-141.

Sanfilippo, J.S. (2004). Vulvovaginitis. In R.E. Behrman, R.M. Kliegman, & H.B. Jenson (Eds.). *Nelson textbook of pediatrics* (17th ed.). Philadelphia: Saunders.

Schack, L.E, & Nienstein, L.S. (2002). Herpes genitalis. In L.S. Neinstein (Ed.). *Adolescent health care: A practical guide* (4th ed.). Philadelphia: Lippincott, Williams & Wilkins.

Schneck, F.X., & Bellinger, M.F. (2002). Abnormalities of the testes and scrotum and their surgical management. In P.C. Walsh, A.B. Retik, E.D. Vaughan, & A.J. Wein (Eds.). *Campbell's urology* (8th ed.). Philadelphia: Saunders.

Shaikh, N., Hoberman, A., Wise, B., et al. (2003). Dysfunctional elimination syndrome: Is it related to early urinary tract infection or congenital vesicoureteral reflux? *Pediatrics, 112*(5), 1134-1137.

Shrier, L.A., Bowman, F.P., Lin, M., & Crowley-Nowik, P.A. (2003). Mucosal immunity of the adolescent female genital tract. *J Adolesc Health, 32*(3), 183-186.

Silber, S.J. (2001). The varicocele dilemma. *Human Reproduction Update, 7*(1), 70-77.

Smith, Y.R., Berman, D.R., & Quint, E.H. (2002). Premenarchial vaginal discharge: Findings of procedures to rule out foreign bodies. *J Pediatr Adolesc Gynecol, 15*(4), 227-230.

Strickland, J.L. (2002). Ovarian cysts in neonates, children and adolescents. *Curr Opin Obstet Gynecol, 14*(5), 459-465.

Terris, M.K. (2004). Urethritis. Retrieved December 20, 2004, from www.emedicine.com/med/topic2342.htm.

Thiedke, C.C. (2003). Nocturnal enuresis. *Am Fam Phys, 67*(7), 1499-1506.

Watson, M.C., Grimshaw, J.M., Bond, C.M., et al. (2003). Oral versus intravaginal imidazole and triazole anti-fungal treatment of uncomplicated vulvovaginal candidiasis. *BJOG Int J Obstet Gynaec, 109*(1), 85-95.

Wiesenfeld, H.C., Hillier, S.L., Krohn, M.A., et al. (2002). Lower genital tract infection and endometritis: Insight into subclinical pelvic inflammatory disease. *Obstet Gynecol, 100*(3), 456-63.

Wiesenfeld, H.C., Hillier, S.L., Krohn, M.A., et al. (2003). Bacterial vaginosis is a strong predictor of *Neisseria gonorrhoeae* and *Chlamydia trachomatis* infection. *Clin Infect Dis, 36*(5), 663-668.

Woo, Y.L., White, B., Corbally, R., et al. (2002). Von Willebrand's disease: An important cause of dysfunctional uterine bleeding. *Blood Coagul Fibrinolysis, 13*(2), 89-93.

Zacharia, T.T., Lakhar, B., Ittoop, A., & Menachary, J. (2003). Giant fibroadenoma. *Breast J, 9*(1), 53.

VICKI W. SHARRER

Select the best answer for each of the following questions:

1. Cynthia, a 14-year-old African American female, comes in for a physical examination. During her exam, thickening and darkening of the axillae are noted. What might this assessment finding indicate?
    A. Nothing; this is a normal finding in many African Americans.
    B. Insulin resistance and type 2 diabetes.
    C. Striae.
    D. Obesity.

2. Bryan, a 17-year-old male, presents with facial acne consisting of inflammatory lesions primarily on the face with comedonal papules and a few pustules. Which product should be prescribed first to treat the acne?
    A. Benzoyl peroxide.
    B. Erythromycin.
    C. Retinoid.
    D. Hormone therapy.

3. Sylvia, a 2-month-old infant, presents with a pruritic erythematous rash on her cheeks and scalp with oval patches on her trunk. A diagnosis of atopic dermatitis (AD) is made. What would be the most important intervention by the pediatric nurse practitioner at this time?
    A. Educate the parents about the chronic nature of AD.
    B. Discuss potential food sources to avoid.
    C. Discuss the avoidance of corticosteroids for treatment if possible.
    D. Emphasize the importance of consistent daily skin care.

4. A 6-year-old boy has been diagnosed with cellulitis of the foot following a puncture wound 2 days ago. He received his DTaP vaccine at age 5. He has had minimal fever and does not look toxic but has considerable pain with palpation of the site. Which of the following oral antibiotics would be most appropriate for treatment?
    A. Amoxicillin (Amoxil).
    B. Cephalexin (Keflex).
    C. Penicillin VK (Veetids).
    D. Trimethoprim/sulfamethoxazole (Bactrim).

5. Which of the following best describes Candida diaper dermatitis?
    A. Glazed, red plaques; may develop erosions; located on convex surface of perineum.
    B. Beefy red, sharply marginated, scaly plaques on convex surfaces of perineum.
    C. Excoriations, crusting, and lichenification; located mostly on convex surfaces of perineum.
    D. Salmon-colored scaly plaques; infant is asymptomatic.

6. Which of the following is appropriate education for the parent who has an infant diagnosed with Candida diaper dermatitis?
    A. Baby wipes should be avoided until the rash heals.
    B. Expose rash to air as much as possible to facilitate healing.
    C. Offer the infant yogurt at least once daily.
    D. Use cloth diapers instead of disposable until the rash clears.

7. The pediatric nurse practitioner is educating the parents of a child diagnosed with erythema infectiosum (EI), or fifth disease, in the clinic. Which of the following explanations takes priority?
   A. The child may return to school.
   B. Treatment is supportive.
   C. The rash may be precipitated by trauma, sunlight, heat, or cold.
   D. The child should avoid pregnant women.

8. A 4-year-old child presents to the clinic with a fever of 101° F; anorexia; fussiness; and vesicles on the buccal membranes, tongue, palms, and soles. What is the most likely diagnosis?
   A. Hand, foot, and mouth disease.
   B. Influenza.
   C. Varicella.
   D. Herpetic gingivostomatitis.

9. Which of the following is recognized as appropriate treatment for keratosis pilaris (KP)?
   A. Application of lubricants immediately after bathing.
   B. Topical corticosteroids.
   C. Frequent bathing.
   D. Nothing is effective for this condition.

10. A mother of a 3-year-old has questions about the care for her child who has just been diagnosed with molluscum contagiosum (MC). The pediatric nurse practitioner offers the following advice:
   A. There is low risk for communicability and the rash is self-limiting.
   B. The rash is highly contagious and the child should avoid contact with others.
   C. Systemic involvement is common and IV antibiotics will be ordered.
   D. The child will not be allowed to go back to preschool until he has been treated.

11. The pediatric nurse practitioner is examining a 2-week-old female who presents at the clinic with a chief complaint of a rash on her face. The pediatric nurse practitioner notes multiple pearly white papules, about 1

mm in diameter on the newborn's nose and cheeks. There is no redness or drainage. The infant is afebrile. What is the most appropriate course of action?
   A. Refer to the dermatologist.
   B. Order a topical antimicrobial medication such as Bactroban.
   C. Reassure the mother that this condition is benign and no treatment is necessary.
   D. Order systemic antibiotics, such as Keflex.

12. The pediatric nurse practitioner has diagnosed pediculosis capitis in an 8-month-old. Which of the following is the first line of treatment?
   A. Permethrin (Nix) Cream Rinse.
   B. Malathion (Ovide) 0.05%.
   C. Cover hair with mayonnaise overnight.
   D. Lindane 1% (Kwell).

13. A 17-year-old female presents to the clinic with a rash on her trunk that is a scaly, macular-papular with some pruritus; there are no lesions on the mucous membranes, palms, or soles. There is one round lesion that is much larger (about 3 cm in size) than the rest of the rash. It is salmon-colored with an erythematous border and appeared first. There have been no other signs of illness. The most likely diagnosis is:
   A. Keratosis pilaris.
   B. Pityriasis rosea.
   C. Seborrheic dermatitis.
   D. Tinea corporis.

14. Which of the following is correct regarding pityriasis rosea?
   A. It is teratogenic to a fetus.
   B. Sunlight increases the severity of the rash.
   C. Duration of the rash can be 3 to 4 months.
   D. Keflex will increase resolution of the rash.

15. Medication indicated for the treatment of pityriasis versicolor (tinea versicolor) is:
   A. Bactroban ointment.
   B. Keflex.

C. Selenium sulfide 2.5% lotion (Selsun).
D. Tetracycline.

16. The pediatric nurse practitioner is treating a 6-year-old patient suspected of having Rocky Mountain spotted fever. Which of the following is the most appropriate intervention?
A. Begin doxycycline immediately.
B. Defer treatment pending serologic confirmation of the diagnosis.
C. Discuss long-term sequelae with the parents.
D. Refer patient to orthopedist to treat and prevent joint degeneration.

17. Which of the following illnesses can result in significant congenital abnormalities?
A. Rubella (German measles).
B. Roseola.
C. Pityriasis rosea.
D. Scarlet fever.

18. Which of the following describes the rash of rubeola?
A. Discrete rose-pink macules approximately 2 to 3 mm in size; fade with pressure; most prominent on trunk; appearance after high fever falls.
B. Diffuse, fine erythematous macular-papular rash; begins on face and rapidly spreads to entire body; disappears by fourth day in same order that it appeared.
C. Deep red macular-papular rash; begins at hairline on forehead, behind ears, and at back of neck; spreads down from face and hairline over 3 days and later becomes confluent.
D. Progresses from crop of red macules to papules to vesicles that become umbilicated and then crust.

19. Which of the following is appropriate education for the adolescent taking griseofulvin for tinea capitis?
A. You must take the medication for 2 full weeks.
B. Take the medication with whole milk or ice cream.

C. You may not return to school until the lesion is completely healed.
D. You may return to school if you wear a cap during treatment.

20. A parent of a 12-month-old refuses to give their infant the vaccine for varicella stating that it would be better for her to get the disease. Which of the following is the best response by the pediatric nurse practitioner?
A. Chicken pox usually results in just a mild rash and provides lifelong protection.
B. Complications from chicken pox can include serious bacterial skin infections and can be fatal.
C. Only about 10% of children have residual scars from chicken pox.
D. If she gets chicken pox, there is a 50% chance she will develop shingles in the future.

21. What is the primary symptom of atopic dermatitis (AD)?
A. Allergic rhinitis.
B. Erythematous generalized dry skin.
C. Pruritus.
D. Erythematous weepy patches.

22. A 7-year-old presents to the clinic with complaints of not feeling well for about a week, and then developing a rash. The rash is on the arms, thighs, and trunk. The rash is erythematous and has a lace-like appearance. A diagnosis of fifth disease is made. An appropriate explanation to the parents by the pediatric nurse practitioner includes which of the following?
A. The child may not return to school until the rash is gone.
B. The child is thought to be no longer contagious once the rash appears.
C. The child will require cardiac evaluation for possible complications.
D. Transmission was most likely from contaminated water.

23. A school-age child presents to the clinic with a papular and pustular rash of the follicles on the upper thighs. What would be the most appropriate assessment question based on the appearance and location of the rash?

A. Have you eaten any new foods recently?
B. Have you been sleeping with any pets?
C. Is anyone in the family ill?
D. Have you been in a hot tub recently?

24. The pediatric nurse practitioner is treating a 10-month-old infant who has painful, grouped vesicles and ulcers on an erythematous base on the buccal mucosa, lips, and palate. The infant is drooling and has not been eating or drinking well and has been running a fever of 102° to 103° F. A diagnosis of gingivostomatitis is made. Which of the following is the most appropriate treatment for this infant?

A. Keflex for 7 days.
B. Ibuprofen and cool fluids for hydration.
C. Kaopectate and viscous lidocaine mixture to coat lesions.
D. Hospitalization for acyclovir administration.

25. Which of the following is true regarding the treatment of pediculosis?

A. Vinegar hair rinse may help loosen nits before combing.
B. The American Academy of Pediatrics recommends that manual removal of nits must be complete prior to school reentry.
C. Environmental disinfecting is essential as fomites have a major role in infestation.
D. Malathion 0.05% is highly effective and safe for infants and neonates.

NOTES

ANSWERS

1. *Answer:* B
   Rationale: This is a description of acanthosis nigricans and can be an indicator of insulin resistance and type 2 diabetes.

2. *Answer:* C
   Rationale: To minimize adverse effects, retinoids should be used before benzoyl peroxide; hormone therapy is only used in female patients; first-line therapy for all forms of acne includes a retinoid product and a topical antimicrobial, not an oral antimicrobial.

3. *Answer:* D
   Rationale: The most important issue is the teaching of daily proper skin care to control AD and prevent exacerbation of this chronic condition. Parents are taught to avoid irritants (harsh soaps, heat, wool clothing), not foods, and topical corticosteroids are used with rash flare-ups.

4. *Answer:* B
   Rationale: The most common organisms include group A beta-hemolytic streptococci and coagulase-positive staphylococci; cephalexin covers both these organisms and is indicated for bacterial infections of the skin; the other answers do not cover both organisms.

5. *Answer:* B
   Rationale: This is the classic description of Candida diaper dermatitis; answer A is a description of primary irritant diaper dermatitis; answer C is a typical of atopic diaper dermatitis; and answer D describes seborrheic diaper dermatitis.

6. *Answer:* B
   Rationale: Diapers create a dark, moist environment which can cause Candida to flourish; in combination with skin contact with urine and feces, the potential to develop or worsen diaper rash exists. Baby wipes may be used if the skin is not sensitive to the ingredients and research has not demonstrated that yogurt improves diaper rash. Disposable diapers are superior to cloth diapers as they have an agent that combines with liquid urine or stool to form a gel to keep liquid away from the infant's skin.

7. *Answer:* D
   Rationale: Complications from EI can be teratogenic when susceptible pregnant women are infected (occasional hydrops fetalis), although it is rare. Answers A, B, and C are true but not the priority explanation (most serious consequence).

8. *Answer:* A.
   Rationale: Influenza does not produce a rash. The rash of varicella is primarily on the trunk, face, scalp, palate, and neck and is in three stages: Papule, vesicle, and crusted lesion. Herpetic gingivostomatitis usually has high fever 104° to 105° F with no lesions on palms or soles.

9. *Answer:* A.
   Rationale: Steroids are not used for this condition, and frequent bathing is discouraged. Keratolytics are used for moderate to severe forms of KP.

10. *Answer:* A
    Rationale: Molluscum contagiosum (MC) is not highly contagious. MC is a benign, usually asymptomatic, skin disease with no systemic manifestations and the child with MC is not excluded from preschool/school.

11. *Answer:* C
    Rationale: This case describes a typical presentation of milia, which is present in up to 40% of newborns. Milia is the result of superficial inclusion cysts that will eventually resolve without treatment.

12. *Answer:* A
    Rationale: Nix is an over-the-counter product that has a low potential for toxic side effects and a high cure rate. Malathion is contraindicated in infants. Mayonnaise is not standard practice, although anecdotally has been described. Lindane 1% is available by prescription and is indicated primarily for failure of other therapies as there are many contraindications and precautions.

13. *Answer:* B
    Rationale: This is a classic description of pityriasis rosea with Herald patch.

14. *Answer:* C
Rationale: Pityriasis rosea is not teratogenic. Exposure to sunlight may relieve itching and enhance resolution of the rash; the etiology is thought to be viral and antibiotics are not indicated.

15. *Answer:* C
Rationale: Pityriasis rosea is thought to be yeast or yeast-like fungus; answers A, B, and D are antibiotics and are not indicated.

16. *Answer:* A
Rationale: Antibiotics should be started with suspicion of a Rocky Mountain spotted fever diagnosis. Discussion of the long-term sequelae is not a priority at this time and not indicated. Orthopedist referral is not appropriate; referral to a pediatrician is indicated if the patient presents with prominent CNS, cardiac, pulmonary, GI tract, and/or renal system involvement.

17. *Answer:* A
Rationale: Congenital rubella infection is associated with growth retardation, cardiac anomalies, ocular anomalies, deafness, cerebral disorders, and hematological disorders; the other disorders are usually benign.

18. *Answer:* C
Rationale: Answer A describes roseola infantum; answer B describes rubella; answer D describes varicella.

19. *Answer:* B
Rationale: High-fat foods enhance absorption of griseofulvin; this medication must be taken for 6 to 12 weeks. Patients may return to school if using topical treatment; for example, selenium sulfide shampoo to decrease shedding. Wearing a cap during treatment is not necessary.

20. *Answer:* B
Rationale: Children still die each year from varicella and should be protected with the vaccine; there is no way to know if her child will have a mild case or minimal scarring; there is a 10 % to 15% chance of developing herpes zoster infection (shingles) after varicella infection.

21. *Answer:* C
Rationale: Atopic dermatitis is known as the "itch that rashes"; secondary changes in the skin result from the trauma of scratching.

22. *Answer:* B
Rationale: Fifth disease is not believed to be infectious after the rash appears. Transmission is from contact with respiratory droplets, percutaneous exposure to blood or blood products, and transmission from mother to fetus.

23. *Answer:* D
Rationale: This describes a typical case of folliculitis due to bacterial infection associated with use of hot tubs.

24. *Answer:* B
Rationale: Treatment includes pain relief and maintenance of hydration with nonacidic, cool fluids; the child is too young to use viscous lidocaine, and no assessment findings indicate that hospitalization is necessary.

25. *Answer:* A
Rationale: Vinegar helps dissolve the adhesive substance holding the nit to the hair shaft. The AAP states that manual removal of nits is not necessary. Fomites do not have a major role in infestation; environmental disinfecting is often unnecessary. The use of malathion is contraindicated in infants and neonates.

BIBLIOGRAPHY

Akita, H., & Anderson, R.R. (June, 2004). Laser treatments in dermatology, CME #119. Retrieved May 9, 2006, from www.hmpcommunications.com/sa/displayArticleaa.cfm?articleID=article2755.

American Academy of Pediatrics Committee on Infectious Diseases (2003). *Red book.* Elk Grove Village, IL: American Academy of Pediatrics.

Baldwin, H.E., & Berson, D.S. (2005). *New perspectives in the management of acne, photo damage, and wound healing.* Cherry Hill, NJ: Elsevier.

Burns, C.E., Dunn, A.M., Brady, M.A., et al. (2004). *Pediatric primary care – a handbook for nurse practitioners* (3rd ed.). Philadelphia: Elsevier.

Conologue, D., & Meffert, J. (2005). Dermatologic manifestations of neurologic disease. Retrieved on May 11, 2006 from http://www.emedicine.com/DERM/topic549.htm.

Cooper, J.S. (2005). Warts, plantar. Retrieved May 9, 2006, from www.emedicine.com/emerg/topic641.htm.

Crowe, M.A. (2005). Molluscum contagiosum. Retrieved on May 5, 2006 from http://www.emedicine.com/PED/topic1759.htm.

Darmstadt, G.L., & Sidbury, R. (2004). The skin. In R.E. Behrman, R.M. Kliegman, & H.B. Jenson (Eds.). *Nelson textbook of pediatrics* (17th ed.). Philadelphia: Saunders.

Dohil, M.A. (2005). Moles, skin care and sun safety. Presentation at the Pediatric Dermatology for the Practitioner meeting in San Diego, March 18-19, 2005. Reported by L.J. Chamberlain in *Infect Dis Child, 6,* 48-49.

Dohil, M.A., & Eichenfield, L.F. (2005). A treatment approach for atopic dermatitis. *Pediatr Ann, 34*(3), 201-210.

Eichenfield, L.F. (2004). Consensus guidelines in diagnosis and treatment of atopic dermatitis. *Allergy, 59*(Suppl 78), 86-92.

Eichenfield, L., Honig, P.J., Harper, J., & Bikowski, J.B. (2004). Advances in the treatment of teen-age acne. *Infect Dis Child, 9*(Suppl.), 4-13.

Elston, D.M. (July 2005). Bites and stings: Be ready to respond quickly. *Clin Adv,* 24-32.

Frankowski, B.L., Weiner, L.B. & Committee on School Health the Committee on Infectious Diseases. American Academy of Pediatrics. (2002). Head lice. *Pediatrics, 110*(3), 638-643.

Gold, B., & Saavedra, J. (November 2004). Allergies are on the rise; focus on prevention. Reported by L. Riley in *Infect Dis Child,* 53.

Goldsmith, L.A., Lazarus, G.S., & Tharp, M.D. (1997). *Adult and pediatric dermatology: A color guide to diagnosis and treatment.* Philadelphia: F.A. Davis.

Hansen, R.C. (2004). Atopic dermatitis: Taming the "itch that rashes." *Contemp Pediatr Online,* July. Retrieved on May 9, 2006 from http://contpeds.adv100.com/contpeds/article/articleDetail.jsp?id=111753.

Levy, S.B. (2005). Sunscreens and photoprotection. Retrieved May 9, 2006, from www.emedicine.com/derm/topic510.htm.

Lutwick, L.I., & Seenivasan, M. (2005). Herpes simplex. Retrieved May 9, 2006, from www.emedicine.com/med/topic1006.htm.

Miller, T., & Frieden, I.J. (2005). Hemangiomas: New insights and classifications. *Pediatr Ann, 34*(3), 179-187.

Norman, R., & Wallace, K. (March 2005). A quick guide to five common skin diseases. *Clin Adv,* 24-30.

Opinion Research Corporation. (June 2005). TEEN CARAVAN® survey conducted in collaboration with the American Academy of Dermatology. *Infect Dis Child,* 50.

Paller, A.S., Nimmagadda, S., Schachner, L., et al. (2005). Fluocinolone acetonide 0.01% in peanut oil: Therapy for childhood atopic dermatitis, even in patients who are peanut sensitive. *J Am Acad Dermatol, 48*(4), 569-577.

Pannaraj, P.S., Turner, C.L., Bastian, J.F., & Burns, J.C. (2004). Failure to diagnose Kawasaki disease at the extremes of the pediatric age range. *Pediatr Infect Dis J, 23*(8), 789-791.

Parish, T.G. (2004). Inflammatory acne: Management in primary care. *Clin Rev, 14*(7), 40-45.

Rakel, R.E., Ault, K.A., Bocchini, J.A., Jr., et al. (2005). Combating human papillomavirus infection: Update on treatment and prevention. *Consultant, 45*(3), S5-S29.

Roberts, D.J., & Friedlander, S.F. (2005). Tinea capitis: A treatment update. *Pediatr Ann, 34*(3), 191-200.

Roberts, G., & Lack, G. (2005). Diagnosing peanut allergy with skin prick and specific IgE testing. *J Allergy Clin Immunol, 115*(6), 1291-1296.

Paller, A.S. (April 2005). New tools for managing pediatric psoriasis. Reported by M. Rosenthal in *Infect Dis Child,* 36..

Schwartz, M.W. (Ed). (2003). *The 5 minute pediatric consult.* Philadelphia: Lippincott Williams & Wilkins.

Shwayder, T. (2003). Five common skin problems—and a string of pearls for managing them. *Contemp Pediatr, Online,* July. Retrieved on May 11, 2006 from http://www.contemporarypediatrics.com/contpeds/article/articleDetail.jsp?id=111757.

Smolinski, K.N., & Yan, A.C. (2005). How and when to treat molluscum contagiosum and warts in children. *Pediatr Ann, 34*(3), 211-221.

Tharp, M.D. (2005). Atopic dermatitis today: A brief overview. *Pediatr News* (Suppl), 4-5.

Thiem, L.J. (2005). Body piercing: Clinical considerations. *Clin Rev, 15*(1), 30-35.

Trowers, A. (April 2005). Ethnicity in pediatric dermatology. Reported by M. Rosenthal in *Infect Dis Child,* 42-43.

Vernon, P. (2003). Acne vulgaris: Current treatment approaches. *Adv Nurse Pract, 11*(2), 59-62.

Zane, L.T. (September 2003). Tips to boost adherence to acne treatment. Reported by R. Finn in *Pediatr News,* 46.

CHAPTER

33 Common Illnesses of the Hematologic and Lymphatic Systems

ADELE E. YOUNG

Select the best answer for each of the following questions:

1. The American Academy of Pediatrics recommends the first screening for anemia in healthy children should occur:
   A. At birth.
   B. Between 9 and 12 months of age.
   C. At 2 years.
   D. Between 2 and 6 months of age.

2. A common cause of iron deficiency anemia in a young child is:
   A. Prolonged breastfeeding.
   B. Loss of blood.
   C. Consumption of large quantities of cow's milk.
   D. Consumption of large quantities of baby cereal.

3. A child diagnosed with transient erythroblastopenia of childhood would be expected to have the following laboratory results:
   A. Microcytic, microchromic, low serum iron.
   B. Elevated TIBC, hemoglobin of 7, reticulocyte count elevated.
   C. Macrochromic, macrocytic, decreased folic acid.
   D. Hemoglobin of 5, decreased reticulocyte count, neutropenia.

4. A 9-month-old infant is diagnosed with iron deficiency anemia. He has a hemoglobin of 9 and weighs 8 kg. The pediatric nurse practitioner should:
   A. Recommend an OTC vitamin with iron.

   B. Order on 0.6 ml of Fer-in-sol drops 75 mg (15 mg Fe/0.6 ml) three times a day.
   C. Order 1 ml of Feosol elixir (44/220 as sulfate mg in 5 ml) once a day.
   D. Recommend the child be given iron-fortified formula instead of breast milk.

5. A pediatric nurse practitioner has placed a child on iron supplementation to correct for iron deficiency anemia. Which of the following instructions should be provided to the family?
   A. Take with meals to avoid GI upset.
   B. Use a straw to avoid staining teeth.
   C. Expect pale yellow stools.
   D. Avoid giving with vitamin C as it decreases absorption.

6. The pediatric nurse practitioner has placed a child on iron supplementation for iron deficiency anemia. What is the most appropriate follow-up lab tests to order?
   A. Hemoglobin in 1 week.
   B. Reticulocyte count in 4 weeks.
   C. Hemoglobin in 4 weeks.
   D. Serum iron in 6 months.

7. Children who present with anemia should also be screened for increased:
   A. Lead levels.
   B. Mercury levels.
   C. Radon levels.
   D. Thiamine (B_1) levels.

8. An 8-year-old child newly arrived from Mexico is seen in the clinic with the complaint of fatigue and GI discomfort with

normal bowel movement. The child's hemoglobin is 9. The child's mother also reports a history of a low-grade fever and itchy papules between the toes of the right foot which have both resolved. As part of the differential diagnosis for this child, the pediatric nurse practitioner should consider:

A. Lactose intolerance.
B. Hookworm infestation.
C. Rotavirus infection.
D. Celiac disease.

9. Pernicious anemia is the result of a lack of:

A. Iron in the diet.
B. Exposure to sunlight.
C. Vitamin B_{12} in the diet.
D. Pancreatic enzymes.

10. A pediatric nurse practitioner is doing newborn nursery rounds. She observes mild jaundice in an infant less then 24 hours old. Which of the following would she consider as a cause for this?

A. Normal newborn hyperbilirubinemia.
B. Rh-positive fetus of an Rh-negative mother.
C. Rh-negative fetus of an Rh-positive mother.
D. Extrahepatic biliary atresia.

11. A 6-year-old child presents with generalized petechiae and purpuric rash. The mother is concerned because the child had Chinese food for the first time last night. The mother also reports that the child was sick with a fever and cough several weeks ago. The examination is otherwise normal. The most likely diagnosis is:

A. Henoch-Schönlein purpura.
B. Allergic reaction.
C. Viral exanthem.
D. Idiopathic thrombocytopenic purpura.

12. A child diagnosed with hemophilia type B (Christmas disease) would have a(n):

A. Prolonged PT (prothrombin time).
B. Decreased platelet count.
C. Decrease in factor VIII.
D. Increase in PTT (partial thromboplastin time).

13. An important part of comprehensive care for a child with hemophilia is:

A. Frequent blood transfusions.
B. Physical therapy.
C. Nonsteriodial antiinflammatory medication.
D. Dietary counseling.

14. An 8-year-old child presents with a 1-week history of fatigue and an increasingly sore throat and a history of a sibling with Epstein-Barr virus infection. On exam, you find widespread lymphadenopathy and mild hepatosplenomegaly. You order a rapid strep test and mono spot, which come back negative. The best course of action would be:

A. Treat with amoxicillin.
B. Repeat the mono spot in 1 week.
C. Order a hepatitis panel.
D. Treat with Augmentin.

15. An adolescent diagnosed with mononucleosis should avoid contact sports:

A. For 6 weeks.
B. For 6 months.
C. Until fatigue is gone.
D. Until hepatosplenomegaly has resolved.

16. A 5-year-old child presents with a warm, tender 3 to 4 cm epitrochlear lymph node. The mother reports that the child has had what she thinks are infected bug bites on his hand for about a week. The child lives on a farm with lots of animals and frequently plays outside. The exam is otherwise normal. Given this history, your most likely diagnosis is:

A. Cat-scratch disease.
B. Lyme disease.
C. Epstein-Barr virus.
D. Rocky Mountain spotted fever.

17. The normal life span of a red blood cell is:

A. 30 days.
B. 60 days.
C. 90 days.
D. 120 days.

18. An adolescent female comes to the clinic complaining of heavy menstruation

since she started her periods. When you question her, she also tells you that she has a history of nosebleeds that have been difficult to control. On exam, several bruises are noted. Which diagnosis should be considered?
A. Hemophilia type A.
B. Child abuse.
C. Von Willebrand disease.
D. Spontaneous abortion.

19. The recommended treatment for bleeding episodes for those with von Willebrand disease is:
A. Infusion of factor VIII.
B. Blood transfusion.
C. DDAVP intranasal inhalation.
D. Transfusion with von Willebrand factor.

20. The most likely way a child would acquire hookworm is:
A. Drinking contaminated water.
B. Walking barefoot on contaminated soil.
C. Sharing a toothbrush with a contaminated individual.
D. Inhaling contaminated air.

21. In mild hemolytic disease of the newborn, the treatment is:
A. Observation to ensure it does not get worse.

B. Transfusion to maintain RBC levels.
C. Phototherapy.
D. Exchange transfusion.

22. A 6-year-old child presents to the pediatric nurse practitioner in the emergency department with a cutaneous purpura rash mainly on the legs and buttocks, fever, and complaints of joint pain mostly in the knees and ankles. On examination, the pediatric nurse practitioner also notes some scrotal edema. On the basis of these findings, the most likely diagnosis is:
A. Henoch-Schönlein purpura.
B. Idiopathic thrombocytopenia purpura.
C. Testicular torsion.
D. Systemic lupus erythematosus.

23. The most serious complication of idiopathic thrombocytopenia purpura (ITP) is:
A. Renal disease.
B. Joint destruction.
C. Intracranial hemorrhage.
D. Osteolytic bone lesions.

24. The treatment of a child with the Henoch-Schönlein purpura includes:
A. IVIG.
B. NSAIDs.
C. High-dose corticosteroids.
D. Immune system modifiers.

ANSWERS

1. *Answer:* B
   Rationale: According to the American Academy of Pediatrics, the initial screening for anemia should occur between 9 and 12 months of age. Pediatric nurse practitioners should be aware of the recommendations for practice from professional organizations that set the standards of care in that field.

2. *Answer:* C
   Rationale: Cow's milk provides a poor source of iron in the diet. Children who are obtaining most of the calories in their diet from cow's milk are not eating enough iron-containing food. Baby cereal is iron-fortified and a good source of iron. Although breast milk contains less iron than formula, the iron is better absorbed and the amount is adequate. Loss of blood will decrease the RBC, resulting in anemia; however, this does not cause iron deficiency anemia.

3. *Answer:* D
   Rationale: The hematologic findings in transient erythroblastopenia of childhood are normochromic, normocitic, normal serum iron, normal TIBC, decreased hemoglobin, decreased reticulocyte count, and neutropenia.

4. *Answer:* B
   Rationale: The recommended dose of iron for a child is 3 to 6 mg/kg of elemental iron daily. This child weighs 8 kg, therefore he should get between 24 and 48 mg of elemental iron per day. The OTC vitamins with iron do not contain enough iron to provide appropriate therapy. Breast milk is an adequate source of iron, so there is no need to switch to formula.

5. *Answer:* B
   Rationale: To avoid staining the teeth, the dose of iron should be given through a straw or placed in the back of the infant's mouth. Iron absorption is enhanced by vitamin C and decreased if taken with food. Parents should be told that iron may cause the stools to turn a dark color.

6. *Answer:* C
   Rationale: There is unlikely to be an appreciable change in the hemoglobin level in 1 week. The reticulocyte count should increase in 3 to 4 days but this lab value would not be a helpful indicator at a month. Do not wait 6 months to evaluate your therapy.

7. *Answer:* A
   Rationale: Elevated lead levels can cause anemia because 99% of absorbed lead is bound to erythrocytes which interferes with critical heme synthesis. The other answers may be toxic but do not cause anemia.

8. *Answer:* B
   Rationale: Lactose intolerance does not cause anemia or fever. In the immigrant population, the pediatric nurse practitioner must consider a diagnosis of ova and parasites because parasites are common in the developing part of the world. Hookworm causes anemia due to blood loss from the intestine walls. Rotavirus causes more diarrhea and celiac disease presents with diarrhea with pale, loose, highly offensive-smelling stools.

9. *Answer:* C
   Rationale: Pernicious anemia is caused by a deficiency of Vitamin B_{12}. The most common cause for this deficiency is lack of vitamin B_{12} intake in the diet.

10. *Answer:* B
    Rationale: Jaundice in a neonate less than 24 hours old is not normal. An Rh-positive child of an Rh-negative mother would be at risk for hemolytic disease of the newborn because the maternal response to the foreign antigen results in the production of the IgG isotope that crosses the placental barrier. These antibodies attach to the fetal RBCs which causes hemolysis of the fetal RBCs, resulting in jaundice in the first 24 hours of life. Jaundice caused by biliary atresia presents in the first 2 to 3 days of life.

11. *Answer:* D
    Rationale: An allergic reaction or viral exanthems would not produce a petechiae/purpura rash. Henoch-Schönlein purpura is associated with fever and joint pain as well as a purpura rash over legs and buttocks. Idiopathic thrombocytopenic purpura is often associated with a history of a viral illness and presents with a generalized purpura and petechiae rash and an otherwise normal exam.

12. *Answer:* D
Rationale: The defect in hemophilia type B is in factor IX. The PT and platelet count is usually normal, but the PTT is two to three times normal.

13. *Answer:* B
Rationale: Children with hemophilia often experience bleeding into the joints. Without early and sustained physical therapy, the joints may become damaged and the child disabled. Children with hemophilia do not require blood transfusion; treatment includes infusions of replacement factor.

14. *Answer:* B
Rationale: The mono spot can be false negative, especially early in the disease process. A bacterial pharyngitis does not cause widespread enlarged lymph nodes. Treating a child with suspected mononucleosis with a penicillin antibiotic may cause a rash. Mild hepatomegaly is common finding in children with mononucleosis. There is no other symptom or history to suggest a diagnosis of hepatitis.

15. *Answer:* D
Rationale: A potential danger in a child who has an enlarged spleen playing contact sports is a rupturing of the spleen. Once the hepatosplenomegaly has resolved, the child can return to sports. The timing is individual to the child.

16. *Answer:* A
Rationale: This child has exposure to animals, so is vulnerable to possible bites. A kitten bite may often look like an infected bug bite. A single enlarged node near the site of puncture is the classic presentation of cat-scratch fever. Lyme disease presents with flu-like symptoms and the classic bull's-eye rash. Rocky Mountain spotted fever also presents with a rash. EBV has widespread lymph node enlargement, not a single node.

17. *Answer:* D
Rationale: The normal life span of a red blood cell is 120 days. If for any reason the life span is shortened, anemia may result due to the rate of destruction of RBCs being greater than the rate of formation of new RBCs.

18. *Answer:* C
Rationale: Von Willebrand disease is the most common of the inherited coagulation disorders. It is often diagnosed in adolescent females at the onset of menses due to heavy menstrual bleeding. Child abuse may cause bruising, but would not affect the menstrual cycles. A single episode of heavy bleeding may indicate a spontaneous abortion. Hemophilia type A would have had more of a history of bleeding and joint pain.

19. *Answer:* C
Rationale: DDAVP works by stimulating an increased release of von Willebrand factor. In severe cases of von Willebrand disease (type three), transfusions of vWf and factor VIII may be needed.

20. *Answer:* B
Rationale: Hookworm is contracted by direct contact with contaminated soil (larvae penetrate the skin and enter the bloodstream) or by accidental ingestion of contaminated soil.

21. *Answer:* C
Rationale: Phototherapy is usually sufficient to maintain bilirubin at a safe level in mild hemolytic disease. More aggressive methods such as exchange transfusion are required if the disease is more severe.

22. *Answer:* A
Rationale: The classic presentation of Henoch-Schönlein purpura is a purpuric rash, fever, joint pain, and scrotal edema. Testicular torsion would not have the rash or joint pain, and ITP does not normally present with fever. This is not the rash associated with SLE.

23. *Answer:* C
Rationale: The most serious complication of ITP is intracranial hemorrhage. ITP is a disease of the destruction of platelets and does not cause joint destruction, renal disease, or osteolytic bone lesions. The individual is at high risk for bleeds due to the decreased platelet count.

24. *Answer:* B
Rationale: NSAIDs are given to control the joint pain. Corticosteroids have not been

shown to change the course of the disease. IVIG and immune system modifiers are not helpful, as most children recover with no treatment.

BIBLIOGRAPHY

American Academy of Pediatrics Committee on Nutrition. (2004). *Pediatric nutrition handbook* (5th ed.). Elk Grove Village, IL: American Academy of Pediatrics.

American Academy of Pediatrics Committee on Practice and Ambulatory Medicine (2000). Recommendations for Preventative Pediatric Health Care, *Pediatrics, 105*(3), 645-646.

American Academy of Pediatrics (2003). *Red book: Report of the Committee on Infectious Diseases* (26th ed.). Elk Grove Village, IL: American Academy of Pediatrics.

American Association for Clinical Chemistry. (2004). The coagulation cascade. Retrieved May 11, 2006, from www.labtestsonline.org/understanding/analytes/coag_cascade/coagulation_cascade.html.

Bickley, L., & Szilagyi. P. (2004). *Bates' guide to physical examination & history taking* (8th ed.). Philadelphia: Lippincott.

Bossart, P. (2005). Henoch-Schönlein purpura. Retrieved May 11, 2006, from www.emedicine.com/emerg/topic845.htm.

Carley, A. (2003a). Anemia: When is it iron deficiency? *Pediatr Nurs, 29*(2), 127-133.

Carley, A. (2003b). Anemia: When is it not iron deficiency? *Pediatr Nurs, 29*(3), 205-211.

Centers for Disease Control and Prevention (CDC), National Center for Infectious Diseases. (2002). Epstein-Barr virus and infectious mononucleosis. Retrieved September 9, 2005, from www.cdc.gov/ncidod/diseases/ebv.htm.

Conrad, M.E. (2006). Anemia. Retrieved on May 12, 2006, from http://www.emedicine.com/med/topic132.htm.

Corbett, J.V. (2004*). Laboratory tests and diagnostic procedures with nursing diagnoses* (6th ed.). Stamford, CT: Appleton & Lange.

Glader, B. (2004). Iron deficiency anemia. In R.E. Behrman, R.M. Kliegman, & H.B. Jenson (Eds.). *Nelson textbook of pediatrics* (17th ed.). Philadelphia: Saunders.

Habal, R. (2004). Toxicity, lead. Retrieved May 11, 2006, from www.emedicine.com/MED/topic1269.htm.

Hermiston, M.L., & Mentzer, W.C. (2002). A practical approach to the evaluation of the anemic child. *Pediatr Clin N Am, 49*(5), 877-891.

Hockenberry, M., Wilson, D., Winkelstein, M., & Kline, N. (2003). *Wong's nursing care of infants and children* (7th ed.). St. Louis: Mosby.

Huang, L., & Miller, R. (2003). Transient erythroblastopenia of childhood. Retrieved September 9, 2005, from www.emedicine.com/ped/topic2279.htm.

Irwin, J.J., & Kirchner, J.T. (2001). Anemia in children. *Am Fam Phys, 64*(8), 1379-1386.

King, M.W. (2005). Medical biochemistry: Blood coagulation. Retrieved May 11, 2006, from http://web.indstate.edu/thcme/mwking/blood-coagulation.html.

Leung, A.K.C., & Chan, K.W. (2001). Evaluating the child with purpura. *Am Fam Phys, 64*(3), 419-428.

Leung, A.K.C., & Robson, W.L.M. (2004). Childhood cervical lymphadenopathy. *J Pediatr Health Care, 18*(1), 3-7.

Marcus, S. (2005). Toxicity, lead. Retrieved May 12, 2006, from www.emedicine.com/emerg/topic293.htm.

McCance, K.L., & Heuther, S.C. (2006). *Pathophysiology: The biologic basis for disease in adults and children* (5th ed.). St. Louis: Mosby.

Montgomery, R.R., & Scott, J.P. (2004). Hereditary clotting factor deficiencies (bleeding disorders). In R.E. Behrman, R.M. Kliegman, & H.B. Jenson (Eds.). *Nelson textbook of pediatrics* (17th ed.) Philadelphia: Saunders.

Montgomery, R.R., & Scott, J.P. (2004). Platelet and blood vessel disorders. In R.E. Behrman, R.M. Kliegman, & H.B. Jenson (Eds.). *Nelson textbook of pediatrics* (17th ed.) Philadelphia: Saunders.

Montgomery, R.R., & Scott, J.P. (2004). von Willebrand disease. In R.E. Behrman, R.M. Kliegman, & H.B. Jenson (Eds.). *Nelson textbook of pediatrics* (17th ed.) Philadelphia: Saunders.

Tam, A.B., & Hexdall, A. (2006). Hookworm. Retrieved on May 12, 2006, from http://www.emedicine.com/emerg/topic841.htm.

Tender, J., & Cheng, T.L. (2002). Iron deficiency anemia. In F.D. Burg., J.R. Ingelfinger, R.A. Polin, & A.A. Gershon (Eds.), *Gellis & Kagan's current pediatric therapy*. Philadelphia: Saunders.

Thiagarajan, P. (2004). Platelet disorders. Retrieved May 12, 2006, from www.emedicine.com/emerg/topic845.htm.

U.S. Department of Health and Human Services (HHS) and U.S. Department of Agriculture (USDA). (2005). *Dietary guidelines for Americans 2005*. Washington, DC: Government Printing Office.

Wagle, S., & Deshpande, P.G. (2003). Hemolytic disease of newborn. Retrieved on May 12, 2006, from http://www.emedicine.com/med/topic987.htm.

CHAPTER

34 Common Illnesses of the Musculoskeletal System

BARBARA HOYER SCHAFFNER

Select the best answer for each of the following questions:

1. A 10-year-old girl presents to the clinic with a complaint of right ankle pain after playing soccer the night before. She hops around the exam room as needed, bearing weight only occasionally using her toes only. She has decreased active ankle range of motion which improves with passive range of motion. Her mother reports a negative ankle x-ray from last night, unchanged swelling from last night after ice applied throughout the evening, but she is "walking on it more." You would assess the ankle as what grade ankle sprain?
   A. Grade I.
   B. Grade II.
   C. Grade III.
   D. Grade IV.

2. A 13-year-old girl presents for a routine physical. You elicit during your history that she has had lower back pain, on and off, for the last 3 to 4 months worse with spine hyperextension. Her mother states she knows it is caused by the gymnastics, as her older daughter also had this type of back pain at the same age and the sister is just fine. Today her back does not hurt, and she has full range of motion. You would:
   A. Order an x-ray of her back.
   B. Prescribe ibuprofen at any and all signs of back pain.
   C. Have her evaluated by a physical therapist.
   D. Have her change sports from gymnastics.

3. A 6-year-old male, small for stated age, presents complaining of "leg pains." The mother reports that the pain is becoming more frequent, worse at night, and does wake him up. Usually the pain is in his calves but sometimes also in his thighs. His physical examination shows no swelling, redness, or warmth with a steady gait and full active range of motion. You would suggest:
   A. Lower leg x-ray.
   B. Obtaining a sedimentation rate, rheumatoid factor, and antinuclear antibodies (ANA) level.
   C. Seventy-two hours of ibuprofen, given every 6 hours.
   D. Education and reassurance that this is typical and will resolve spontaneously.

4. Which child would be diagnosed with pathologic genu varum?
   A. 2-week-old with 15-degree bowlegs.
   B. 4-year-old with greater than 5-inch distance between knees.
   C. 30-month-old boy that has a newly developed knock-kneed appearance.
   D. 18-month-old girl with symmetrical bowlegged appearance.

5. What imaging study would be recommended for a 3-week-old who is noticed to have limited hip abduction and asymmetry of the thigh folds?
   A. X-ray.
   B. MRI.
   C. Ultrasound.
   D. No imaging study is necessary.

6. A 12-year-old boy has been prescribed ibuprofen 600 mg, 1 tablet every 6 hours as needed for pain from an ankle sprain. His mother calls the clinic and inquires if she can use OTC ibuprofen because it is less expensive. What information is most important in responding to the mother's concerns?
   A. Aspirin is just effective as ibuprofen at relieving pain.
   B. Brand-name preparations of ibuprofen are more effective than generic products.
   C. Three 200 mg generic over-the-counter ibuprofen tablets are equivalent to 600 mg prescription-strength ibuprofen.
   D. Acetaminophen and ibuprofen are essentially the same medication.

7. A 12-year-old obese African American male has complained of right anterior thigh pain intermittently for the past 6 weeks. His mom reports no history of trauma but notes "he is limping more and more." You note reluctance to walk at all, positioning of the right hip in an extreme external rotation and limited hip flexion on exam. You suspect:
   A. Osgood-Schlatter's disease.
   B. Septic arthritis.
   C. Toxic synovitis of the hip.
   D. Slipped capital femoral epiphysis.

8. A 15-month-old girl returns to the office with redness, swelling, and tenderness over her left knee. She has gradually decreased her independent walking. Two weeks ago, she fell and needed stitches in that same knee. The stitches were not removed when originally intended due to some excessive redness at the laceration site, but were removed 4 days ago. She is admitted for IV antibiotics to treat an infection caused most likely by:
   A. Group B streptococcus.
   B. *Klebsiella.*
   C. *Staphylococcus aureus.*
   D. *E. coli.*

9. Which treatments are appropriate for a male adolescent who has Osgood-Schlatter's disease?
   A. Activity modification and ice treatment as needed.

   B. Achilles stretching before activity and a knee brace during physical activity.
   C. Restriction from all sports activity until asymptomatic for 3 consecutive months.
   D. Ice and NSAIDs every day until full adult growth is achieved.

10. An 11-year-old girl is found to have a 15-degree curvature of the spine during a routine scoliosis exam. You would:
   A. Refer to orthopedic specialists.
   B. Refer to physical therapy for weekly treatments.
   C. Follow up every 3 to 4 months to monitor the degree of curvature.
   D. Arrange for placement in a Milwaukee brace, 23 out of 24 hours every day.

11. The parents of a 2½-week-old are very worried about the baby's stiff neck and "lump" on his neck." You diagnose the child with torticollis and the initial treatment includes:
   A. Bracing of the neck.
   B. Frequent repositioning of the infant's head.
   C. Pain control with acetaminophen with codeine.
   D. Preoperative testing for surgery within the week.

12. Which best describes Barlow's maneuver to assess an infant (less than 2 months of age) for developmental dysplasia of the hip (DDH)?
   A. With the infant supine, knees flexed, grasp the thigh and adduct while applying downward pressure.
   B. A clunk is heard while abducting the infant's thighs when in the supine position with knees flexed.
   C. Holding the infant in the standing position, one knee is higher than the other and the pelvis drops on the side unable to bear weight.
   D. With patient lying supine, flex both hips simultaneously to their limit, hold one hip flexed and lower the other leg, a positive sign would be the leg not lying flat.

13. Which would NOT be included in the differential diagnosis of limited arm movement in a 3-year-old?
   A. Brachial plexus injury.
   B. Subluxation of radial head.
   C. Fracture of the ulnar/radial bones.
   D. Fracture of the humerus.

14. What would be initial treatment for a toddler with upper arm/elbow pain and lack of movement of the arm when the physical examination reveals no swelling, redness, or bruising of the arm?
   A. X-ray of the ulna, radius, humerus, and elbow.
   B. Ice treatment and NSAIDs for the first 48 hours.
   C. Referral to orthopedic specialist.
   D. Closed reduction by applying pressure to the head of the radius with supination of the arm in 90-degree flexion.

15. A 17-year-old high school football player comes to your office after sustaining a knee injury on the field. He heard a "pop" of the knee when he tried to pivot to catch the football. He took acetaminophen last night and the trainer told him to keep it iced down. On examination, there is increased swelling and tenderness over the left knee. He has a positive Lachman's test with significant excursion and more movement of the left tibia when you draw it forward compared to the right tibia. What is your most likely diagnosis?
   A. Patellar fracture.
   B. Meniscus tear.
   C. Anterior cruciate ligament tear
   D. Posterior cruciate ligament tear.

16. Which symptom in a 10-year-old boy would most likely indicate a "Little League Elbow" injury?
   A. Gradual onset of elbow pain.
   B. Diffuse tenderness from mid-lower arm to mid-upper arm.
   C. Radiating pain to the shoulder.
   D. Increased pain with elbow hyperextension.

17. A 4-year-old boy presents with his mother who states that her son is beginning to "walk funny and seems less coordinated now." The noticed changes have occurred over the past 6 to 7 months. You would suspect muscular dystrophy with which reported history?
   A. Upper extremity weakness.
   B. History of delayed gross motor development.
   C. Persistent toe-walking with increasing reports of falling.
   D. Weak cough and frequent upper respiratory infections.

18. A patient presents with full range of motion against gravity and some resistance. You would grade their muscle strength as:
   A. 2.
   B. 3.
   C. 4.
   D. 5.

19. A positive bulge sign indicates:
   A. Medial collateral ligament tear.
   B. Torn meniscus.
   C. Herniated disk.
   D. Knee joint effusion.

20. A 2-week-old healthy baby presents with "in-pointing of the toes." On exam, the baby has an adduction of the forefoot that cannot be passively straightened. Your initial action would be:
   A. Refer to orthopedic specialist.
   B. Refer to physical therapy for passive stretching.
   C. X-ray the affected foot.
   D. Recheck the foot position at the 2-month checkup.

21. The appearance of flat-foot (pes planus):
   A. Resolves by adolescence.
   B. Is commonly seen in infants and toddlers.
   C. Is due to the absence of normal fat pads in the arch.
   D. Requires referral for surgical correction.

22. Included in the differential diagnosis for a patient with a painless limp would be:
   A. Juvenile rheumatoid arthritis (JRA).

B. Legg-Calvé-Perthes disease.
C. Slipped capital femoral epiphysis.
D. Leg length discrepancy.

23. Most common fractures in children occur in which area of the bone?
   A. Diaphysis.
   B. Cancellous bone.
   C. Epiphyseal plate.
   D. Compact bone.

24. Which child would NOT be able to return to the athletic field after a grade II ankle sprain?
   A. Can balance on one leg for 30 seconds with eyes closed.
   B. Strength of movement is 70% to 80% of the uninvolved ankle.
   C. Complains of pain only with active ankle range of motion.
   D. No tenderness on palpation of the affected ankle.

25. What is the most common site of osteosarcoma in adolescents?
   A. Tibia
   B. Fibula
   C. Femur
   D. Humerus

26. The parents of a 5-year-old recently diagnosed with muscular dystrophy (MD), wish to speak to you about the hereditary nature of the disease. As you prepare to answer their questions, you review that MD is:
   A. An X-linked recessive gene transmitted by unaffected female carriers.
   B. A recessive gene that requires that mother and father be carriers.
   C. A dominant sex-linked gene predominantly in white families from western Europe.
   D. A recessive gene that is known to skip a generation between transmission.

NOTES

ANSWERS

1. **Answer:** B
   Rationale: Sprains are rated on a scale of I to III. A level II sprain presents with decreased active ROM, moderate pain, moderate swelling, and difficult weight-bearing.

2. **Answer:** A
   Rationale: Although she is asymptomatic today, her history of gymnastics and lower back pain that becomes more painful with hyperextension could be a spondylitis which can be associated with other congenital spinal defects.

3. **Answer:** D
   Rationale: In the absence of abnormal physical findings and a history of traumatic injury, lower extremity pain in the school-age child that involves the muscles of the leg can be attributed to normal growth. There is no treatment for growing pains; education and reassurance that it is typical and will spontaneously resolve are appropriate.

4. **Answer:** B
   Rationale: Genu varum is an alignment of the knee with the tibia medially deviated in relation to the femur, giving a bowlegged appearance. It can be a part of normal development if symmetrical with less than a 5-inch distance between the knees with feet together in children 3 years or younger. Up to a 5-degree bowleg can be normal in newborns secondary to uterine position.

5. **Answer:** C
   Rationale: Ultrasound imaging is the most useful in infants under 4 months of age (but should not be used if the infant is less than 2 weeks of age because of a higher number of false-positive findings). An AP x-ray view of the pelvis is recommended at older ages.

6. **Answer:** C
   Rationale: All preparations of ibuprofen are essentially equivalent. To reduce the risk of Reye's syndrome, aspirin should not be given to children. Acetaminophen and ibuprofen, although both given frequently for pain, have different mechanisms of action; ibuprofen has more antiinflammatory actions.

7. **Answer:** D
   Rationale: Slipped capital femoral epiphysis is a displacement of the femoral head from the femoral neck, which presents with varying levels of pain frequently, reported in the thigh or knee. The child, usually a 9- to 15-year-old overweight/obese boy, will not bear weight and carries the affected leg in an externally rotated position. On exam, there are no signs of infection but limited flexion of the involved hip.

8. **Answer:** C
   Rationale: The reported symptoms are consistent with a diagnosis of septic arthritis of the knee. Given the previous signs of skin infection, the most likely organism causing the infection would be *Staphylococcus aureus*.

9. **Answer:** A
   Rationale: Osgood-Schlatter's disease is aseptic necrosis of the tibial tubercle below the knee and is considered an overuse injury occurring in adolescents during times of rapid growth. The condition is self-limiting. The pain, usually associated with knee extension, can be treated with activity modification, ice, NSAIDs, and a tibial band during periods of pain and/or increased activity. A strengthening of the quadriceps can be helpful in minimizing knee pain.

10. **Answer:** C
    Rationale: Scoliosis is most commonly noted during adolescence, more commonly in girls. A curvature less than 20 degrees is considered mild scoliosis and should be closely monitored every 3 to 4 months during growth spurts.

11. **Answer:** B
    Rationale: Initial treatment for torticollis is gentle massage and repositioning. For severe cases, bracing might be necessary. Parents should be reassured that the prognosis is excellent with early diagnosis and treatment.

12. **Answer:** A
    Rationale: Barlow's maneuver tests for developmental dysplasia of the hip (DDH). Barlow's and Ortolani's maneuvers are used for infants less than 2 months of age. Barlow's maneuver involves adduction of the

thigh while applying downward pressure, a positive maneuver would be a palpable dislocation of the femoral head, a "click" sound is considered to be benign.

13. *Answer:* A
Rationale: A brachial plexus injury involves damage to the brachial plexus and nerves C5 to C7 and T1 most commonly due to traumatic stretching of neck and shoulder during birth, and is found in newborns. There is noted paralysis or limited movement of the limb and absent or incomplete reflexes (biceps, Moro, grasp) on the affected side.

14. *Answer:* D
Rationale: When a child under the age of 4 years presents with no signs of traumatic injury to the arm but lacks movement and pain, the most likely diagnosis is a subluxation of the radial head (nursemaid's elbow) common in this age group because of the immature radial head and annular ligament. One to two attempts at closed reduction is recommended before x-ray.

15. *Answer:* C
Rationale: The Lachman's test is the standard test that with increased laxity (increased excursion) demonstrates an anterior cruciate ligament (ACL) tear. The mechanism of injury and hearing a "pop" of the knee is also consistent with an ACL tear.

16. *Answer:* A
Rationale: "Little League Elbow" presents with pain in elbow that develops over time, usually from overuse—excessive overhand throwing of a ball. Symptoms include decreased elbow ROM, mild flexion contracture, point tenderness, swelling, and decreased performance in throwing a ball.

17. *Answer:* C
Rationale: Muscular dystrophy usually presents in the preschool years with a gradual disappearance of motor skills that originally developed on a normal sequence and time. Muscle weakness presents initially in the lower extremities with report of "walking funny," clumsiness, persistent toe-walking, and Gower's sign.

18. *Answer:* C

Rationale: Muscle strength is graded on a 0 to 5 scale, with 0 = no evidence of contractility, 1 = slight contractility, no movement, 2 = full range of motion, gravity eliminated, 3 = full range of motion against gravity, 4 = full range of motion against gravity, some resistance, and 5 = full range of motion against gravity, full resistance.

19. *Answer:* D
Rationale: Bulge sign is performed by placing the ball of the hand over medial patella, milk fluid distally from suprapatellar pouch, and repeating several times. Reappearance of the swelling indicates knee joint effusion.

20. *Answer:* A
Rationale: Adduction of the forefoot with the foot plantar flexed at the ankle are common signs of clubfoot. Successful serial casting and manipulation needs to begin as early as possible, immediate referral to orthopedic specialist is indicated.

21. *Answer:* B
Rationale: Flat-footedness (pes planus) is common in infants and toddlers and usually resolves by age 2 to 3 years. Pes planus is commonly due to a fat pad located in the arch of the foot, and treatment usually includes arch supports (orthotics) for shoes.

22. *Answer:* D
Rationale: Juvenile rheumatoid arthritis (JRA), Legg-Calvé-Perthes disease, and slipped capital femoral epiphysis all present with a painful limp.

23. *Answer:* C
Rationale: Most common fractures in children occur in the epiphyseal plate (growth plate) because this is the weakest part of the growing bone.

24. *Answer:* C
Rationale: "Return to play" criteria after a lower extremity injury includes full pain-free active and passive range of motion, lack of tenderness, strength of joint is 70% to 80% of the uninvolved side, and can balance on one foot for 30 seconds with eyes closed.

25. *Answer:* D

Rationale: Osteosarcoma is the most common malignant bone tumor in adolescents and young adults. Osteosarcoma most commonly affects the humerus, followed by the distal femur and proximal tibia.

26. *Answer:* A

Rationale: MD is an X-linked recessive gene transmitted by unaffected female carriers through the dystrophin gene. The absence of dystrophin in the muscle membrane leads to progressive skeletal and cardiac muscle damage.

BIBLIOGRAPHY

American Academy of Pediatrics, Committee on Infectious Disease (2003). *Red book: 2003 Report of the Committee on Infectious Diseases* (26th ed.). Elk Grove Village, IL: American Academy of Pediatrics.

Boyarsky, I., & Rank, C. (2004). Little League elbow syndrome. Retrieved on May 12, 2006, from www.emedicine.com/sports/topic62.htm.

Brady, M.A., & Burns, C.E. (2004). Musculoskeletal disorders. In C.E. Burns, A.M. Dunn, M.A. Brady, et al. (Eds.). *Pediatric primary care: A handbook for nurse practitioners* (3rd ed.). Philadelphia: Saunders.

Calmbach, W.L., & Hutchens, M. (2003). Evaluation of patients presenting with knee pain; Part II: Differential diagnosis. *Am Fam Phys, 68*(5), 917-922.

El-Bohy, A.A., & Wong, B.L. (2005). The diagnosis of muscular dystrophy. *Pediatr Ann, 34*(7), 525-530.

Family Practice Notebook.com. Retrieved on May 13, 2006 from http://www.fpnotebook.com.

Foot & Ankle Institute (2006). Retrieved on May 12, 2006 from http://www.footankleinstitute.com/Anklesprain.html.

Ganel, A., Dudkiewicz, I., & Grogan, D.P. (2003). Pediatric orthopedic physical examination of the infant: A 5-minute assessment. *J Pediatr Health Care, 17*(1), 39-41.

Gore, A.I., & Spencer, J.P. (2004). The newborn foot. *Am Fam Phys, 69*(4), 865-872.

Goyal, S., Roscoe, J., Ryder, W.D., et al. (2004). Symptom interval in young people with bone cancer. *Eur J Cancer, 40*(15), 2280-2286.

GP Notebook.com. Retrieved on May 13, 2006 from http://www.gpnotebook.co.uk.

Hashkes, P.J., Gorenberg, M., Oren, V., et al. (2004). "Growing pains" in children are not associated with changes in vascular perfusion patterns in painful regions. *Clin Rheumatol, 24*(4), 342-345.

Hong, E. (2003) An approach to knee pain. Patient care for the nurse practitioner. Retrieved on May 12, 2006, from www.patientcarenp.com/be_core/content/journals/n/data/2003.html.

Jarvik, J.G., & Deyo, R.T. (2002) Diagnostic evaluation of low back pain with emphasis on imaging. *J Intern Med, 137*(7), 586-597.

LaMontagne, L.L., Hepworth, J.T., Cohen, F., & Salisbury, M.H. (2004). Adolescent scoliosis: Effects of corrective surgery, cognitive-behavioral interventions, and age on activity outcomes. *Appl Nurs Res, 17*(3), 168-177.

Mayo Clinic. (2005). Sprains and strains. Retrieved on May 12, 2006 from http://www.mayoclinic.com/health/sprainsand-strains/DS00343/DSECTION=9.

Mehlman, C.T., & Cripe, T.P. (2005). Osteosarcoma. Retrieved May 12, 2006, from www.emedicine.com/orthoped/topic531.htm.

Mercuri, E., & Longman, C. (2005). Congenital muscular dystrophy. *Pediatr Ann, 34*(7), 560-568.

Nochimson, G. (2005). Legg-Calvé-Perthes disease. Retrieved on May 12, 2006, from www.emedicine.com/emerg/topic294.htm.

Rimando, M.P. (2005). Ankle sprain. Retrieved on May 12, 2006, from http://www.emedicine.com/pmr/topic11.htm.

Santarlasci, P.R. (2000). Weekend warrior: Common injuries in recreational athletes. *Adv Nurse Pract, 8*(4), 42-46.

Seidel, H.M., Ball, J., Dains, J.E., & Benedict, G.W. (2003). *Mosby's guide to physical examination* (5th ed.). St. Louis: Mosby.

Taft, E., & Francis, R. (2003). Evaluation and management of scoliosis. *J Pediatr Health Care, 17*(1), 42-44.

Weidner, N.J. (2005). Developing an interdisciplinary palliative care plan for the patient with muscular dystrophy. *Pediatr Ann, 34*(7), 547-552.

Whitelaw, C.C., & Schikler, K.N. (2004). Transient synovitis. Retrieved on May 12, 2006, from www.emedicine.com/ped/topic1676.htm.

Wolfe, M.W., Uhl, T.L., & McCluskey, L.C. (2001) Management of ankle sprains. *Am Fam Phys, 63*(1), 93-104.

Wong, B.L. (2005). Muscular dystrophies. *Pediatr Ann, 34*(7), 507-510.

35 Common Illnesses of the Neurologic System

RITAMARIE JOHN

Select the best answer for each of the following questions:

1. A 5-year-old presents with acute headache. On examination, there is the new onset of difficulty in upward gaze of both eyes. What is the most likely cause of this problem?
   A. Strabismus.
   B. Increased intracranial pressure.
   C. Congenital paresis of cranial nerve IV.
   D. Migraine headache.

2. A 3-month-old has flattening on the right side of the occipital area and full range of motion of the neck. The child is sleeping on his back. Which one of the following actions is appropriate?
   A. Ordering a three-dimensional CT of head.
   B. Positioning the head on the unaffected side.
   C. Doing a skull x-ray.
   D. Referring to a neurosurgeon.

3. A developmentally normal 6-month-old presents with a full but not bulging fontanelle and a progressive increase in head circumference. The MRI shows benign enlargement of subarachnoid space in the frontal area. This is consistent with:
   A. Hydrocephalus.
   B. External hydrocephalus.
   C. Macrocephaly.
   D. Neurofibromatosis.

4. A 14-year-old without any medical problems presents with a 1-day history of fever and severe headache. On exam, she has a temperature of 101.4° F, positive Brudzinski's sign, and positive Kernig's sign. She is diagnosed with presumptive meningitis. What is a possible long-term complication?
   A. Brain abscess.
   B. Encephalitis.
   C. Hearing loss.
   D. Subdural effusions.

5. An 18-month-old comes to the office after a seizure. The child had a fever of 102.4° F. Other than a history of fever, the history and exam are unremarkable. The child is playing with a toy during the visit. What is the next best step?
   A. Parental education and observation.
   B. Referral to ED for septic workup.
   C. Admission for 24 hours.
   D. Treatment with antiepileptic drugs.

6. An 11-year-old has a history of headache for a year. The pain is episodic and occurs at the end of the day in the right fronto-temporal region. What is an appropriate first step in the drug treatment for this child?
   A. Ibuprofen.
   B. Sumatripan.
   C. Calcium channel blocker.
   D. Cyproheptadine.

7. A 5-year-old has a normal posture, bluish coloration to the sclera, and looseness of the joints (hypermobility) without weakness. Which is the most likely diagnosis?
   A. Ehlers-Danlos syndrome.
   B. Iron deficiency anemia.
   C. Spinal muscular atrophy, type II.
   D. Duchenne's muscular dystrophy.

8. A 6-week-old has a history of a fall from a surface 3 feet off the ground 1 hour earlier. The infant is alert and cooing. There is only a small amount of swelling. What is the next best step?
   A. Skull x-ray or CT scan.
   B. MRI.
   C. Head ultrasound.
   D. Observation.

9. What disorder is associated with positional plagiocephaly in a 2-month-old?
   A. Microcephaly
   B. Macrocephaly
   C. Torticollis
   D. Strabismus

10. A 7-year-old child presents with a 2-year history of headaches at the end of the day associated with stress. Recently, the headaches are not relieved with acetaminophen, are located in the occipital area, and are worse when the child coughs or is active. The child's personality has become increasingly irritable. Which is the most likely diagnosis?
    A. Cluster headache.
    B. Chronic progressive headache.
    C. Tension headache.
    D. Migraine headache.

11. On exam, a 4-year-old has large calves with lumbar lordosis, and a waddling, clumsy gait. The family history is unremarkable. Which is the most likely diagnosis?
    A. Muscular dystrophy.
    B. A brain tumor.
    C. Charcot-Marie-Tooth disease.
    D. Essential hypotonia.

12. An 18-month-old patient presents with lumbar lordosis, delay in walking, and diminished reflexes. The family history is incomplete. Which of the following lab tests will be most helpful?
    A. CBC.
    B. Lactase dehydrogenase (LD).
    C. Creatine kinase (CK).
    D. Erythrocyte sedimentation rate.

13. A 6-year-old complains of headaches on arising in the morning before school for 2 months. On physical examination, there is a head tilt, past pointing, and difficulty in performing rapid, alternating hand movements. What is the most appropriate next step?
    A. CT with contrast.
    B. MRI with contrast.
    C. Lumbar puncture.
    D. Plain radiograph of the skull.

14. A 14-year-old gymnast complains that her right side feels different from her left side. She also has pain in her neck which increases with coughing or sneezing. On examination, she has strength differences between her biceps, but has equal leg strength. There is mild tenderness in the lower cervical vertebra. The rest of the exam is unremarkable. Which of the following is the most likely cause?
    A. Myopathy.
    B. Neuropathy.
    C. Nerve root compression.
    D. Psychologic disturbance.

15. An 8-week-old presents with an acute onset of moving less and seemingly slipping out of the mother's arms when held. On exam, the infant is uninterested in her environment, has significant head lag, and is quiet. The temperature is normal. Which of the following tests should be ordered?
    A. Neonatal metabolic screen.
    B. Stool sample for *Clostridium botulinum*.
    C. Thyroid screen.
    D. Liver function tests.

16. A 19-month-old presents 1 hour after a fall off of a 3-foot stepladder. His past medical history is unremarkable. He vomited one time after the fall. On exam, there is a large right parietal hematoma. He is crying during the entire exam, but is quiet when not being examined. What is the most appropriate next step?
    A. Observation.
    B. Skull x-ray.
    C. CT of the head.
    D. MRI with contrast.

17. A 10-year-old complains of mild, late afternoon, nonpulsating pain in the frontal area with minimal photophobia. The physical exam is normal. Which is the most likely diagnosis?

A.   Cluster headache.
B.   Common migraine.
C.   Tension headache.
D.   Complicated migraine.

18.   A 9-year-old presents with complaints of feeling dizzy with nausea, and ringing in the ear. Which of the following tests would be helpful in evaluating this patient?
A.   Gower's maneuver.
B.   Kernig's sign.
C.   Brudzinski's sign.
D.   Tandem Romberg test.

19.   A right-hand–dominant 14-year-old has 30 café au lait spots and axillary freckling. He presents with a history of worsening headaches and difficulties with language. What is the most likely cause of the problem?
A.   Brainstem tumor.
B.   Right-sided cerebellar tumor.
C.   Left-sided cerebral tumor.
D.   Right-sided cerebral tumor.

20.   A 7-year-old has a cerebellar tumor. What set of symptoms can be expected?
A.   Intentional tremors, ataxia, head titubations.
B.   Growth retardation, precocious puberty, visual field defect.
C.   Intellectual changes, seizures, and contralateral hemiparesis.
D.   Focal headache, seizures, hyperreflexia, focal signs.

21.   A 15-year-old has familial essential tremors. He is embarrassed by his problem and wants to be treated. Which of the following treatments is the most appropriate?
A.   Stimulant.
B.   Beta-adrenergic blocker.
C.   Selective serotonin reuptake inhibitor.
D.   Anxiolytic.

22.   A normal 4-week-old has very brief, jerky bilateral movements only associated with going to sleep, and the movements stop when the child is awakened. What should be the first course of action?
A.   Referral to a pediatric neurologist.
B.   Reassurance to the parents.
C.   Referral for MRI.
D.   Referral for a CT scan.

23.   A 14-year-old presents with history of 2 months eye blinking as a 4-year-old. His parents recently divorced. His chief complaint today is a 1-month history of intermittent twitch of the upper eyebrow. The exam is normal. What should be the next course of action?
A.   Reassurance.
B.   Clonidine.
C.   Neurology referral.
D.   Psychiatric referral.

24.   A 6-year-old has a tumor compressing the brainstem. What set of symptoms can be expected?
A.   Word retrieval difficulties, seizures, hemiparesis.
B.   Ocular palsies, diplopia, and nystagmus.
C.   Intellectual changes, seizures, hearing loss.
D.   Visual field defects, precocious puberty, seizure.

25.   A 9-year-old presents with paresis of the right side of the face. On physical examination, the corner of the mouth droops, but he is able to close the right eye. Which is the most likely diagnosis?
A.   Peripheral eighth nerve palsy.
B.   Peripheral seventh nerve palsy.
C.   Central fifth nerve palsy.
D.   Central seventh nerve palsy.

ANSWERS

1. *Answer:* B

Rationale: Congenital paresis of cranial nerve IV causes an inability to look toward the outer aspect of the nose. Migraine headaches would not cause paresis of upward gaze. Strabismus can be vertical but would usually involve one eye. The nuclei of cranial nerves II to XII lie in the brainstem. The top of the brainstem or midbrain is the anatomic site for the vertical gaze center. The third ventricle is just above the midbrain. When hydrocephalus develops or a shunt is not working, the third ventricle becomes enlarged and it compresses the vertical gaze center.

2. *Answer:* B

Rationale: Positioning the child's head on unaffected side is the first recommended step. Skull x-ray may not show craniostenosis. While three-dimensional CT can show craniostenosis, it exposes the child to unnecessary radiation. If the practitioner is uncertain about the cause of the abnormal head shape, then a referral to a pediatric neurosurgeon can be made.

3. *Answer:* B

Rationale: External hydrocephalus is a benign enlargement of subarachnoid space in the frontal or frontoparietal region; the infant presents with a full but pulsatile anterior fontanelle with normal ventricles. With external hydrocephalus, the head size rapidly increases to 90% and then parallels the growth curve. The normal developmental status and lack of changes in the ventricles is not consistent with hydrocephalus. If the child has macrocephaly only, the MRI will not show fluid collection in the subarachnoid space. Neurofibromatosis may be present, but there is nothing in the history or physical consistent with this diagnosis.

4. *Answer:* C

Rationale: The mortality rate for meningitis is from 4% to 10%, with seizures being a common complication affecting one-third of patients. Subdural effusions are present in about one-third of complications and are asymptomatic and resolve without treatment.

Brain abscess is an uncommon complication and is more likely in the newborn period. The most common neurologic sequela of meningitis is hearing impairments occurring in up to 35% of patients. Speech impairments, learning disabilities, and behavioral problems are long-term complications of bacterial meningitis.

5. *Answer:* A

Rationale: According to both AAP and the Practice Committee of the Child Neurology Society, it is not appropriate to use antiepileptic drugs following a simple seizure. In the face of a normal neurologic exam, the child does not need admission to the hospital or a complete septic workup. Patients with a simple febrile seizure and a normal examination do not need CT scan or MRI. Parental education and observation is the next best step in this scenario.

6. *Answer:* A

Rationale: Analgesics such as acetaminophen and ibuprofen can be effective first-line drugs in children with intermittent headaches. Sumatriptan or ergotamine have vasoconstrictive properties and can be used early in the course of migraine. Cyproheptadine is an antihistamine and is approved for use in the prophylactic treatment of cluster and migraine headaches. Since the headaches are intermittent, starting with ibuprofen would be the best first step.

7. *Answer:* A

Rationale: Myopathy is a spectrum of disorders of muscle diseases that does not involve the central nervous system, peripheral nerves, or neuromuscular junction. It can result from inflammatory processes or a defect of muscle. Myopathies include Duchenne's muscular dystrophy, Becker's muscular dystrophy, Limb-Girdle muscular dystrophy, spinal muscular atrophy, inflammatory demyelinating neuropathies, Guillain-Barré syndrome and other rare disorders of neuromuscular junction. Children with myopathies will have lumbar lordosis and are weak in comparison to other children. Iron deficiency anemia can cause blue sclera but does not cause joint hypermobility. Ehlers-Danlos syndrome is characterized by skin hyperextensibility, joint hypermobility, tissue fragility, easy bruising, bluish color of the sclera, and paper-thin scars. It is important to differentiate myopathies from joint hypermobility in the assessment of pediatric patient. The former will have weakness associated with it.

8. *Answer:* A
   Rationale: Children younger than 2 years of age have a higher risk of skull fracture after minor mechanism of injury and intracranial lesions may be harder to detect on clinical exam. Therefore, in assessing young infants, it is very important to completely evaluate the mechanism of injury and assess carefully for changes in mental state, motor skills, and social behavior. MRI is expensive and would not be the best first step in a well-appearing infant. A CT is useful for patients with severe head trauma or unstable multiple organ injuries. Skull radiographs are useful for identifying linear fractures but will not show intracranial bleeding. Both were listed as a choice, as it would depend on the child's condition along with the mechanism of injury. Head ultrasound is used to identify enlarged ventricles.

9. *Answer:* C
   Rationale: Positional plagiocephaly is related to positioning of the head and is associated with torticollis. Deformational flattening of the occipital area will cause frontal and temporal prominence. The lambdoidal suture is not closed prematurely, but the supine infant positioning causes external pressure on the skull resulting in flattening. Congenital torticollis may occur if the there is stretching of the sternocleidomastoid muscle with a localized hematoma. There may be a mass felt in the body of the muscle due to fibrosis with shortening of the muscle on the affected side. In a 2-month-old, strabismus would not cause head tilt. Microcephaly and macrocephaly do not cause positional plagiocephaly.

10. *Answer:* B
    Rationale: Tension headaches are described as a tightening, nonpulsating pain with or without associated photophobia or

phonophobia, but without nausea, vomiting, or exacerbation with activity. The presenting history is not consistent with the child's original headache pattern. Migraine headaches are recurrent headaches with symptom-free periods. They may be associated with visual, sensory, or motor aura; abdominal pain; nausea or vomiting; throbbing headache; unilateral location; relief after sleeping; positive family history. They are usually frontotemporal and bilateral in children. Cluster headaches are rarely seen before age 10 and are characterized by one to several attacks recurring each 24 hours. They have headache-free periods which may last from months to years. Occipital headaches are rare and require immediate evaluation. The presentation of this child is consistent with chronic progressive headache and warrants immediate imaging.

11. *Answer:* A
    Rationale: The musculoskeletal clinical features of Duchenne's muscular dystrophy include normal milestones until walking, clumsiness, waddling gait, weakness in climbing stairs, pseudohypertrophy of calf muscles and contractures of heel cords, an early complaint of leg pain, toe walking, contractures of biceps, neck, and Achilles tendon. The child with Charcot-Marie-Tooth disease has stork-like legs with high arches. Essential hypotonia may include a waddling gait but there would be no pseudohypertrophy of the calves. A brain tumor may cause clumsiness but also would not cause pseudohypertrophy of the calf muscles.

12. *Answer:* C
    Rationale: Creatine kinase (CK) is markedly elevated in Duchenne's muscular dystrophy. While the lactic dehydrogenase (LD) and the AST may be elevated, CK is the most useful marker of muscle disease. The CBC and erythrocyte sedimentation rate will be normal.

13. *Answer:* B
    Rationale: The child presents with signs of a posterior fossa tumor. A CT scan does not image the posterior fossa as well as an MRI. A lumbar puncture would not be done prior to scanning due to the focal neurologic

signs. A plain radiograph of the skull would be done to identify depressed and linear skull fractures, but would not be helpful with this child.

14. *Answer:* C

Rationale: An inflammatory process starts nerve root compression which results in nerve root swelling. The compression can occur from disk herniation. The history and physical exam are consistent with a nerve root compression. Patients with cervical radiculopathy may have sensory changes, weakness of the shoulders; myopathy is manifested by proximal weakness and involves the limb girdle. Neuropathy is distal weakness. With pain in the neck and weakness of the biceps, there is likely involvement of C3 to C5. With the history of being a gymnast and the consistent finding, it is unlikely that this is psychosomatic.

15. *Answer:* B

Rationale: Botulism is an acute problem caused by the toxins produced by *Clostridium botulinum*. Infants present with apathy listlessness, feeding poorly, decreased head control, weak cry and suck, and hypotonia with an absence of fever. Metabolic disorders and thyroid disease would not be an acute presentation. Liver function tests would not be as helpful in the diagnosis of this child.

16. *Answer:* C

Rationale: The mechanism of injury along with a parietal hematoma is of concern. The most common place for a hematoma following minor trauma is on the forehead. In a child under 2 years old who has a nonfrontal hematoma following a fall, CT would provide a good look at bone and provide information about intracranial bleeding. MRI would require sedation and is not readily available to most care providers. Observation would not be appropriate given the age of the child, the history, and the physical exam findings. MRI provides superior anatomic details compared with CT, but CT is actually superior in the detection of acute bleeding.

17. *Answer:* C

Rationale: Migraine headaches are classified into migraine with aura or without aura. Common migraine is migraine without aura and is the most common type of pediatric headache. Generally, migraine has a moderate-to-severe intensity with a pulsating quality. Complicated migraines are more severe and are accompanied by neurologic signs. Tension headaches occur later in the day and are generally milder. Cluster headache is characterized by one to several attacks within a 1-day period with several weeks to months of headache-free periods.

18. *Answer:* D

Rationale: A Romberg test is a test for both balance and equilibrium. Once a child is a preschooler, you can ask the child to stand up with his or her eyes closed and the hands at the sides. If you have him or her walk in tandem, he or she will fall to the affected side if vertigo occurs. Gower's maneuver is a test for weakness of the pelvic girdle. It is elicited by having the child sit on the floor and asking him or her to rise to standing. If the Gower's maneuver is positive, he or she will push off the floor with the arms, keeping the legs extended and stiff at the knee. Kernig's sign is elicited by laying the patient down on his or her back and flexing the patient's leg at both the hip and knee at a 90-degree angle. Pain and increased resistance to extending the knee is considered a positive sign. Brudzinski's sign is elicited by flexing the neck forward. The knee and hip should not move in response to this maneuver.

19. *Answer:* C

Rationale: Neurofibromatosis type I is autosomal-dominant and the diagnosis requires the presence of two or more of major criteria which include six or more café au lait spots, axillary or inguinal freckling, two or more cutaneous neurofibromas, one plexiform neurofibroma, an optic glioma, two or more iris Lisch nodules, or a first-degree relative with NF1. Brain tumors occur at a higher frequency. While optic gliomas, brainstem, and cerebellum are common sites, they can also be supratentorial. This child presents with signs localized to the language which are on the left side of the brain. The history of worsening headaches is also consistent with a possible CNS lesion.

20. *Answer:* C

Rationale: Cerebral tumors are characterized by intellectual changes, seizures, and contralateral hemiparesis. With tumors in the hypothalamic region, there may be growth retardation, precocious puberty, and visual field defects. With supratentorial tumors, there may be a focal headache, seizures, hyperreflexia, and focal signs depending on the location of the tumor. Intentional tremors appear with activity and get worse as the patient's hand approaches near to the target.

21. *Answer:* B

Rationale: Essential tremor has been linked to chromosome 3q13 and chromosome 2p2-22. There are several normal forms of tremors such as physiologic tremor and enhanced physiologic tremor that occur when the child is angry or fearful. Essential tremor should only be treated when there is functional disability or social embarrassment. Two first-line drugs that can be used to treat essential tremors include propranolol and primidone. Other drugs include clonazepam, gabapentin, topiramate, or botulinum toxin.

22. *Answer:* B

Rationale: Benign sleep myoclonus of infancy is associated with the newborn going to sleep. Benign sleep myoclonus occurs within a few days of birth. Rhythmic myoclonic bilateral movements appear as the child is going to sleep but stop when the child is awakened. This is the characteristic feature of benign sleep myoclonus of infancy. Generally it resolves by the third month of life. However it may be mistaken for neonatal epilepsy. Ultrasound is justified if there are doubts about the diagnosis but putting the child to sleep for an MRI or exposing him to radiation of CT is not warranted. This is not a sign of disease and therefore the parents can be reassured. Referral for MRI, CT, or neurologist is not indicated in a benign process that is normal in a normal newborn.

23. *Answer:* A

Rationale: Transient tic disorder includes multiple motor and/or vocal tics with a total duration of symptoms for less than 1 year.

Clonidine and guanfacine have been shown to be effective in milder cases of Tourette's syndrome (TD) with dopamine receptor antagonist, the drug used in severe TD. Children with tics need observation. The diagnostic criteria for transient tic disorder include that the tics occur for a minimum of 1 month but not longer that 12 months. In addition, the criteria for TD have never been met. In TD, there must never be a tic-free period of more than 3 consecutive months. A neurology or psychiatric referral is not indicated for a transient tic disorder and reassurance is the appropriate action.

24. *Answer:* B

Rationale: Brainstem tumors present with nausea, vomiting, diplopia, weakness, unsteady gait, headache, and drowsiness. Hydrocephalus is a common occurrence. Downbeating nystagmus can be seen can be seen with involvement of the medulla, and upbeating nystagmus is seem when there is involvement of the cranial nerve VI. Seizures are less commonly seen with brainstem involvement. Loss of language and word retrieval problems are more common in supratentorial tumors. Precocious puberty and visual field defects are seen with involvement of the midline tumors.

25. *Answer:* D

Rationale: Motor fibers in the cerebral cortex travel to the pons where the majority cross over to the facial nerve nuclei on the other side. Some fibers do not cross over and will innervate the frontalis muscle and the orbicularis oculi muscle. If there is a problem above the level of the facial nerve nucleus in one cerebral hemisphere, there will be weakness of only the lower face. The ability to close the eye via the orbicularis oculi muscle is preserved. This may be the presentation of vascular malformation or tumor. Most common cause is swelling and edema of the facial nerve as it goes through facial canal within the temporal bone. When the forehead muscles are involved, a lower motor lesion of the facial nerve or peripheral facial nerve is involved. The trigeminal nerve is the cranial nerve V. The trigeminal nerve has three divisions: ophthalmic, maxillary, and mandibular. The cranial nerve V provides sensory innervation to structures of the face, sinuses, and portions of the cranial vault, and the mandibular division innervates muscles of mastication. The physical assessment of cranial nerve V palsy would be loss of facial and intraoral sensation and weakness of jaw closure.

BIBLIOGRAPHY

Adams, M., & Hugkins, L. (2003). The importance of minor anomalies in the evaluation of the newborn. *NeoRev, 4*(4), 99-104.

American Academy of Pediatrics, (2003). Prevention and management of positional skull deformities in infants, *Pediatrics, 112*(1), 199-202.

Barness, E.G. & Barness, L.A. (2003). *Clinical use of pediatric diagnostic tests.* Philadelphia: Lippincott, Williams, & Wilkins.

Baumann, R. & Duffner, P. (2000). Treatment of children with simple febrile seizures: The AAP Practice parameter. *Pediatr Neurol, 23*(1), 11-17.

Baumann, R. (2005). Febrile seizures. Retrieved May 17, 2006, from www.emedicine.com/neuro/topic134.htm.

Berman, S. (2003). Abnormal head: size and shape. In S. Berman (Ed.). *Pediatric decision making* (4th ed.). Philadelphia: Mosby.

Bickley, L, & Szilagyi, P. (2003). *Bates' guide to physical examination and history taking.* Philadelphia: Lippincott, Williams & Wilkins.

Biggs, W. (2003). Diagnosis and management of positional head deformity. *Am Fam Phys, 67*(9), 1953-1956.

Bigger, W.D. (2006). Duchenne muscular dystrophy. *Pediatr Rev, 27*(3), 83-89.

Black, K.J., & Webb, H. (2005). Tourette syndrome and other tic disorders. Retrieved October 15, 2005, from www.emedicine.com/neuro/topic664.htm#targetL.

Bressman, S.B. (2004). Dystonia genotypes, phenotypes, and classification. *Adv Neurol, 94*, 101-107.

Burke, D., & Hauser, R.A. (2001). Essential tremor. Retrieved October 15, 2005, from www.emedicine.com/NEURO/topic129.htm.

Centers for Disease Control and Prevention. (2005). Notice to readers: Concussion tool kit for high school coaches, *MMWR Morb Mortal Wkly Rep, 54*(37), 934. See also: www.cdc.gov/ncipc/tbi/Coaches_Tool_Kit.htm.

Chavez-Bueno, S. & McCracken, G.H. (2005). Bacterial meningitis in children. *Pediatr Clin North Am, 52*(3), 795-810.

Cohen, M.M. (2000). Sutural pathology. In M.M. Cohen, & R.E. MacLean (Eds.). *Craniosynostosis: Diagnosis, evaluation and management* (2nd ed.). New York: Oxford University Press.

Cohen, M. & Duffner, P. (1999). Tumors of the brain and spinal cord including leukemic involvement. In K. Swaiman & S. Ashwal (Eds.). *Pediatric neurology: Principles and practice.* Philadelphia: Mosby.

Conologue, T., & Meffert, J. (2005). Dermatologic manifestations of neurologic disease. Retrieved October 24, 2005, from www.emedicine.com/derm/topic549.htm.

Cox, N., & Hinkle, R. (2002). Infant botulism. *Am Fam Phys, 65*(7), 1388-1392.

Darras, B., & Jones, H.R. (2000). Diagnosis of pediatric neuromuscular disorders in the era of DNA analysis, *Pediatr Neurol, 23*(4), 289-300.

Demorest, R., & Landry, G. (2003). A football player with a concussion. *Pediatr Case Rev, 3*(3), 127-140.

Dinolfo, E. (2001). Ataxia. *Pediatr Rev, 22*(5), 177-178.

Egger, J., Grossmann, G., & Auchterlonie, I.A. (2003). Benign sleep myoclonus in infancy mistaken for epilepsy. *Br Med J, 326*, 975-977.

Ellison, P. (2003). The clumsy child. In S. Berman (Ed.). *Pediatric decision making* (4th ed.). Philadelphia: Mosby.

Ellison, P., & Berman, S. (2003). Childhood weakness and paralysis. In S. Berman (Ed.). *Pediatric decision making* (4th ed.). Philadelphia: Mosby.

Frank, Y. & Pavlakis, S. (2001). Brain imaging in neurobehavioral disorders. *Pediatr Neurol, 25*(4), 278-287.

Gill, J., & Gieron-Korthals, M. (2002). What pediatricians and parents need to know about febrile convulsions. *Contemp Pediatr, 19*(5), 139-150.

Goldbloom, R.B. (2003). *Pediatric clinical skills* (3rd ed.). Philadelphia: Saunders.

Gupta, R., & Appleton, R.E. (2001). Cerebral palsy: Not always what it seems. *Arch Dis Child, 85*(5), 356-360.

Gupta, P., Foster, J., Crowe, S., et al. (2003). Ophthalmologic findings in patients with nonsyndromic plagiocephaly. *J Craniofac Surg, 14*(4), 529-532.

Habal, M., Leimkuehler, T., Chambers, C., et al. (2003). Avoiding the sequela associated with deformational plagiocephaly. *J Craniofac Surg, 14*(3), 430-437.

Handique, S., Das, R., Barua, N., et al. (2002). External hydrocephalus in children. *Indian J Radiol Imag, 12*(2), 197-200.

Haslam, R.H.A. (2005). Headaches. In R.E. Behrman, R.M. Kliegman, & H.B. Jenson (Eds.). *Nel-

son textbook of pediatrics (17th ed.). Philadelphia: Saunders.

Headache Classification Subcommittee of the International Headache Society. (2004). The International Classification of Headache Disorders (2nd ed.). *Cephalgia, 24*(Suppl. 1). Retrieved May 17, 2006, from http://216.25.100.131/ihs-common/guidelines/pdfs/ihc_II_main_no_print.pdf.

Henson, J. (2001). Spinal cord gliomas. *Curr Opin Neurol, 14*(6), 679-682.

Hershey, A.D., & Winner, P.K. (2005). Pediatric migraine: Recognition and treatment. *J Am Osteopath Assoc, 105*(Suppl. 4), 2S-8S.

Hirtz, D., Berg, A., Bettis, D., et al. (2003). Practice parameter: Treatment of the child with a first unprovoked seizure. *Neurology, 60*(2), 166-175.

Hunstad, D. (2002). Bacterial meningitis in children. *Pediatr Case Rev, 2*(4), 195-202.

Hutchison, B.I., Hutchison, L.A.D., Thompson, J.M.D., et al. (2004). Plagiocephaly and brachycephaly in the first two years of life: A prospective cohort study. *Pediatrics, 114*(4), 970-980.

Isaacson, J.E., & Vora, N.M. (2004). Differential diagnosis and treatment of hearing loss. *Am Fam Phys, 68*(6), 1125-1132.

Jallo, G.I., Freed, D., & Epstein, F. (2003). Intramedullary spinal cord tumors in children. *Childs Nerv Syst, 19*(9), 641-649.

Jallo, G. & Marcovici, A. (2005). Medulloblastoma. Retrieved on May 17, 2006, from http://www.emedicine.com/neuro/topic624.htm.

Jankovic, J. (2001). Medical Progress: Tourette syndrome. *NEJM, 345*(16), 1184-1192.

Johnston, M.V., & Kinsman, S. (2004). Microcephaly. In R.E. Behrman, R.M. Kliegman, & H.B. Jenson (Eds.). *Nelson textbook of pediatrics* (17th ed.). Philadelphia: Saunders.

Kanegaye, J.T., Soliemanzadeh, P., & Bradley, J.S. (2001). Lumbar puncture in pediatric bacterial meningitis: Defining the time interval for recovery of cerebrospinal fluid pathogens after parenteral antibiotic pretreatment. *Pediatrics,* 108(5), 1169-1174.

Kieran, M. (2000). Advances in pediatric neurooncology. *Curr Opin Neurol, 13*(6), 627-634.

Krauss, J., & Jankovic, J. (2002). Head injury and posttraumatic movement disorders. *Neurosurgery, 50*(5), 927-939.

Kumar, A. (2004). Meningitis, bacterial. Retrieved October 15, 2005, from www.emedicine.com/PED/topic198.htm.

Kuperman, S. Tics and Tourette's syndrome in childhood. *Sem Pediatr Neurol, 10*(1), 35-40.

Lampl, C. (2002). Childhood-onset cluster headaches, *Pediatr Neurol 27*(2), 138-140.

Landolfi, J. & Vendataramana, A. (2006). Brainstem glioma. Retrieved August 28, 2005 from http://www.emedicine.com/NEURO/topic40.htm.

Larsen, W.J. (2001). *Human embryology*. New York: Churchill Livingstone.

Lewis, D.W., Ashwal, S., Dahl, G., et al. (2002). Practice parameter: Evaluation of children and adolescents with recurrent headaches: Report of the Quality Standards Subcommittee of the American Academy of Neurology and the Practice Committee of the Child Neurology Society. *Neurology, 59*(4), 490-498.

Li, B.U.K., & Howard, J.C. (2002). New hope for children with cyclic vomiting syndrome. *Contemp Pediatr, 19*(3), 121-130.

Lipton, R.B., Bigal, M.E., Steiner, T.J., et al. (2004). Classification of primary headaches. *Neurology, 63*(3), 427-435.

Mack, K.J. (2006). Episodic and chronic migraine in children. *Semin Neurol, 26*(2), 223-231.

Malago, G.A. (2005). Cervical radiculopathy. Retrieved August 28, 2005 from http://www.emedicine.com/SPORTS/topic21.htm.

Marine, B.S. & Fine, K.S. (2006). *Blueprints Pediatrics* (4th ed.). Philadelphia: Lippincott, Williams, and Wilkins.

Menkes, J.H., & Sarnat, H.B. (2000). *Child Neurology* (6th ed.). Philadelphia: Lippincott Williams & Wilkins.

Millichap, J.G., & Yee, M. (2003). The diet factor in pediatric and adolescent migraine. *Pediatr Neurol, 28*(1), 1-14.

Moe, P., Levisohn, P., & Berman, S. (2003). In S. Berman (Ed). *Pediatric Decision Making*. Philadelphia: Mosby.

Moore, K.L., & Persaud, T.V.N. (2003). *The developing human: Clinically oriented embryology*. Philadelphia: Saunders.

National Institute of Neurological Disorders and Stroke (NINDS). (2005). NINDS infantile hypotonia information page. Retrieved October 15, 2005, from www.ninds.nih.gov/disorders/hypotonia/hypotonia.htm.

Olness, K. (1999). Managing headaches without drugs. *Contemp Pediatr,16*, 101-110.

O'Sullivan, J. & Lees, A. (2000). Nonparkinsonian tremors. *Clin Neuropharmacol, 23*(5), 233-238.

Pandolfo, M. (2003). Friedreich's ataxia. In H.R. Jones, D. De Vivo, & B. Darras, *Neuromuscular disorders of infancy, childhood, and adolescence: A clinician's approach*. Amsterdam: Butterworth-Heinemann.

Perriello, V.A., & Barth, J.T. (2000). Sports concussions: Coming to the right conclusions. *Contemp Pediatr, 17*(2), 132-142.

Persing, J., James, H., Swanson, J., Kattwinkel, J., and the American Academy of Pediatrics Committee on Practice and Ambulatory Medicine, Section on Plastic Surgery and Section on Neurological Surgery. (2003). Clinical report: Prevention and management of positional skull deformities in infants. *Pediatrics, 112*(1), 199-202.

Prober, C.G. (2004). Central nervous system infections. In R.E. Behrman, R.M. Kliegman, & H.B. Jenson (Eds.). *Nelson textbook of pediatrics* (17th ed.). Philadelphia: Saunders.

Ramelli, G.P., Sozzo, A.B., Vella, S., et al. (2005). Benign neonatal sleep myoclonus: An under-recognized, non-epileptic condition. *Acta Paediatr, 94*(7), 962-963.

Risko, W. (2006). Infant botulism. *Pediatr Rev, 27*(1), 36-37.

Roland, E. (2000). Muscular dystrophy. *Pediatr Rev, 21*(7), 233-237.

Rubin, D.H., Suecoff, S.A., & Knupp, K. (2006). Headaches in children. *Pediatr Ann, 35*(5), 345-353.

Sargent, L.A. (2000). *Tennessee Craniofacial Center textbook*. Chattanooga, TN: Erlanger Health Systems. Available at www.craniofacialcenter.com.

Sarnat, H. & Menkes, J. (2000). Neuroembryology, genetic programming and malformation of the nervous system. In J. Menkes & H. Sarnat (Eds.), *Child neurology*. Philadelphia: Lippincott, Williams and Wilkins.

Schlaggar, B., & Mink, J. (2003). Movement disorders in children. *Pediatr Rev, 24*(2), 39-51.

Schutzman, S. & Greenes, D. (2001). Pediatric minor head trauma. *Ann Emerg Med, 37*(1), 65-74.

Sheth, R.D., & Iskandar, B.J. (2005). Craniosynostosis. Retrieved on May 17, 2006, from www.emedicine.com/neuro/topic80.htm.

Shin, J. & Persing, J. (2003). Asymmetric skull shapes: Diagnostic and therapeutic considerations. *J Craniofac Surg, 14*(5), 696-699.

Smaga, S. (2003). Tremor. *Am Fam Phys, 68*(8), 1545-1552.

Smith, L.H. & DeMyer, W.E. (2003). Anatomy of the brainstem. *Sem Pediatr Neurol, 10*(4), 235-240.

Steiner, R.D., Shaefer, G.B., and Pepin, M. (2006). Ehlers-Danlos syndrome. Retrieved on August 8, 2006 from http://www.emedicine.com/ped/topic654.htm.

Stock, A. & Singer, L. (2004). Head trauma. Retrieved on August 8, 2006, from http://www.emedicine.com/ped/topic929.htm.

Taketomo, C., Hodding, J.H., & Kraus, D.M. (2004). *Lexi-Comp's pediatric dosage handbook*. Hudson, OH: Lexi-Comp.

Tonsgard, J. (2006). Clinical manifestations and management of neurofibromatosis type 1. *Semin Pediatr Neurol, 13*(1), 2-7.

Tunnessen, W. & Roberts, K. (1999). *Signs and symptoms in pediatrics*. Philadelphia: Lippincott, Williams, & Wilkins.

Uddin, M. & Rodnitzky, R. (2003). Tremor in children. *Semin Pediatr Neurol, 10*(1), 26-34.

Warren, S.M., Brunet, L.J., Harland, R.M., et al. (2003). *Nature, 422*(6932), 625-629.

Williams, S. & Wessel, H. (2002). Neurology. In B. Zitelli & H. Davis (Eds.). *Atlas of pediatric physical diagnosis*. Philadelphia: Mosby.

Wolf, S.M. & McGoldrick, P.E. (2006). Recognition and management of pediatric seizure. *Pediatr Ann, 35*(5), 332-344.

Wright, W. (2004). Impact of the nurse practitioner in the management of migraine. *Am J Nurse Pract, 8*(6), 64-76.

Zenel, J. (2000). An infant who has head trauma. *Pediatr Rev, 21*(6), 210-214.

Zitelli, B.J., & Davis, H.W. (2002). *Atlas of pediatric diagnosis* (4th ed.). St. Louis: Mosby.

DIAGNOSIS AND MANAGEMENT OF CHRONIC CONDITIONS IN CHILDREN AND ADOLESCENTS

CHAPTER

36 Asthma

TERRY A. BUFORD

Select the best answer for each of the following questions:

1. Which of the following statements about asthma prevalence is the most accurate?
   A. Prevalence is greater for boys compared to girls in all ethnic groups.
   B. Prevalence among African American children is higher than other ethnic groups.
   C. Overall prevalence does not differ overall by income or ethnic group.
   D. Prevalence is lower for children of European American descent than other ethnic groups.

2. John is a 3-year-old who is being evaluated for suspected asthma. Which of the following findings in his health history would increase the probability of an asthma diagnosis?
   A. Six upper respiratory infections in the first year of life.
   B. Daycare attendance.
   C. Exposure to household pets.
   D. Positive family history of asthma.

3. Beth is a 10-year-old who is seen in your office for suspected asthma. Which of the following findings in her symptom history would support this diagnosis?
   A. Wakes up coughing at night.
   B. Midsternal burning pain after meals.
   C. Breathes hard when running the mile.
   D. Snores loudly at night.

4. When completing Beth's physical examination, which of the following findings would be inconsistent with a diagnosis of asthma?
   A. Prolonged expiratory flow time.
   B. Clear breath sounds bilaterally.
   C. Digital clubbing.
   D. Boggy, edematous nasal mucosa.

5. Which of the following tests would be most specific to confirm the airway obstruction in Beth's case?
   A. Oxygen saturation.
   B. Spirometry.
   C. Chest x-ray.
   D. Peak expiratory flow measurement.

6. Carlos is a 4-year-old with asthma. He has been waking up with a cough about 2 nights per week, and having daytime wheezing 2 to 3 times per week. Based on this presentation, select the correct asthma classification for Carlos.
   A. Mild intermittent.
   B. Mild persistent.
   C. Moderate persistent.
   D. Severe persistent.

7. Richard is an 8-year-old with mild persistent asthma. Which of the following treatment regimens would be preferred for him?
   A. Daily montelukast.
   B. Daily low-dose inhaled corticosteroids.
   C. Daily bronchodilator therapy.
   D. Daily cromolyn sodium.

8. Abigail, a 3-year-old, presents to the clinic with an upper respiratory infection and wheezing. This occurred the past two times

she had "colds." Her father and older brother have allergies and asthma. You suspect that Abigail may also have asthma. Which of the findings would be most appropriate to confirm the diagnosis in Abigail's case?

A. Wheezing improves or ceases with bronchodilator therapy.
B. Office spirometry shows airway obstruction.
C. Both inspiratory and expiratory wheezes are present.
D. PA and lateral chest x-rays are normal.

9. Tammy is a 7-year-old who has mild persistent asthma. Her mother is concerned about her grades because she has missed so much school because of her asthma. Which of the following responses is most appropriate for Tammy's mother?

A. Children with chronic health problems such as asthma often miss more school than their peers.
B. Children with asthma need to avoid missing school unless their symptoms are severe.
C. Children with asthma need to restrict their school activities so that asthma attacks are avoided.
D. Children with well-controlled asthma generally do not miss more school than their peers.

10. Tammy takes Flovent 110 mcg, two puffs twice a day routinely for her moderate persistent asthma. Her mother says she wants to stop the medicine because Tammy has not had any symptoms for the past 3 months. Which of the following responses would be most appropriate?

A. Tammy's lack of symptoms is an indication that her asthma is well-controlled by the Flovent.
B. Tammy's daily controller medication should never be reduced.
C. Tammy's lack of symptoms indicates that she was misdiagnosed.
D. Tammy's asthma is intermittent and she does not need daily controller therapy.

11. Jose is an 11-year-old who developed a runny nose and low-grade fever yesterday.

Today, he has begun coughing and wheezing on expiration, although he no longer has fever. Jose has asthma and takes Flovent, 110 mcg, two puffs twice a day for his asthma. Which of the following actions should the nurse practitioner suggest Jose take first?

A. Take an additional two puffs of Flovent now and twice a day for the next 2 weeks.
B. Go to the urgent care center immediately.
C. Drink fluids, and then lie down and rest.
D. Use his albuterol inhaler, two puffs now and repeat every 20 minutes up to three times.

The next three questions relate to the following scenario:

Janet is a 16-year-old who has moderate persistent asthma. She weighs 50 kg. Her asthma action plan calls for Advair Diskus 250/50, one inhalation twice a day in her green zone.

12. Which of the following additional medications should she receive for quick relief of asthma symptoms?

A. Atrovent inhaler, two puffs every 4 hours as needed.
B. Pulmicort turbohaler, 200 mcg, one inhalation twice a day.
C. Albuterol inhaler, two puffs every 4 hours as needed.
D. Montelukast, 10 mg orally once daily.

13. Which of the following medications would be most appropriate to intensify her controller therapy for yellow-zone treatment?

A. Increase her Advair 250/50 to two inhalations twice a day.
B. Add Flovent 110 mcg, two puffs twice a day.
C. Add scheduled albuterol inhaler, four puffs every 4 hours.
D. Add theophylline once daily.

14. Which of the following medications would be most appropriate to add to Janet's asthma plan in order to provide red-zone treatment?

A. Theophylline 500 mg once daily for 1 month.
B. Prednisone 60 mg once daily for 5 days.
C. Montelukast 10 mg once daily for 1 month.
D. Albuterol inhaler, two puffs every 4 hours.

15. John is a 6-year-old who has mild persistent asthma and dust-mite allergy. His mother asks about the effectiveness of environmental measures to improve his asthma. Which of the following responses is most appropriate?
A. Reducing exposure to dust mites by any means has been shown to be very effective in reducing asthma symptoms.
B. Chemical agents are superior in reducing the effects of dust-mite exposure compared to other methods.
C. Neither chemical nor physical reduction in dust-mite levels has shown evidence of significant improvement in asthma symptoms.
D. Only physical removal of dust mites has demonstrated improvements in asthma symptoms.

16. Which of the following classes of medication is most effective in reducing chronic airway inflammation in asthma?
A. Methylxanthines.
B. Inhaled β-agonists.
C. Leukotrienes.
D. Inhaled corticosteroids.

17. Allan is a 2-year-old asthmatic getting his first prescription for inhaled corticosteroids. Which of the following drug delivery system(s) would be most appropriate for his age group?
A. Rotadisk or turbohaler.
B. Nebulizer or inhaler with spacer and face mask.
C. Nebulizer therapy only.
D. Discus or rotadisk delivery system.

18. During Allan's teaching, you instruct his mother to have him rinse his mouth well following administration of his inhaled corticosteroid. Which of the following describes the primary purpose of this activity?
A. To prevent development of thrush.
B. To prevent medication overdosage.
C. To prevent dental decay.
D. To prevent development of streptococcal pharyngitis.

19. Karen is a 10-year-old who receives steroid therapy via a metered dose inhaler with a spacer. Her mother asks why the spacer is needed. Choose the most appropriate response to her question.
A. Spacers allow more medication to be deposited into the airway rather than the pharynx.
B. Spacers prevent accidental spray into the eyes.
C. Spacers allow for multiple doses of the medication to be administered in one puff.
D. Spacers extend the medication's effective duration.

20. Jennifer is a 6-year-old who has mild persistent asthma. She is being seen in clinic in early November for a well child physical. She weighs 20 kg. Her last visit was 6 months ago, and her asthma has been well-controlled since then. Spirometry was performed at that time and showed an FEV_1 at 80% of predicted. Her last asthma exacerbation was in April during spring allergy season and was successfully managed with yellow-zone treatment. Today, Jennifer's physical examination is normal. Which of the following orders by the pediatric nurse practitioner would be most appropriate?
A. Obtain spirometry in the office today.
B. Give influenza vaccine today.
C. Obtain a chest x-ray today.
D. Give pneumococcal 23 valent vaccine today.

21. Jennifer's mother is thinking about using an herbal tea for asthma and wants to know if it would help Jennifer use less medication. Which of the following responses by the pediatric nurse practitioner is most appropriate?
A. Herbal remedies are used by lots of people with asthma.

B. Herbal remedies can be beneficial for children with asthma.

C. Herbal remedies are recommended for children over the age of 12 years.

D. Herbal remedies lack evidence of effectiveness for asthma.

22. Marcus is a 14-year-old who has mild persistent asthma. He is seen in clinic for a school physical. His mother asks you to write a note for him to use the elevator at school because of his asthma. Which of the following responses is most appropriate?

A. If Marcus's asthma is well-controlled, he should be able to participate in normal activity.

B. Marcus should definitely avoid stairs at school.

C. Marcus should pretreat with his albuterol inhaler before climbing the stairs at school.

D. Marcus should use his albuterol before school and at lunchtime regularly to manage his school activity.

23. Which of the following factors is a significant predictor of asthma mortality among children?

A. Family history of chronic asthma.

B. Onset of wheezing during infancy.

C. History of perennial environmental allergies.

D. Previous intensive care unit admission for asthma.

24. Which of the following best describes the correct technique for using a conventional metered dose inhaler?

A. Actuate the inhaler concurrent with a rapid inhalation and hold for 10 seconds.

B. Actuate the inhaler concurrent with a rapid exhalation and hold for 10 seconds.

C. Actuate the inhaler concurrent with a slow inhalation and hold for 10 seconds.

D. Actuate the inhaler concurrent with a slow exhalation and hold for 10 seconds.

25. Which of the following best explains the pathophysiology of chronic asthma symptoms?

A. Airway hyperresponsiveness.

B. Abnormal mucus secretions.

C. Fixed airway resistance.

D. Chronic airway inflammation.

ANSWERS

1. *Answer:* C
   Rationale: Prevalence is greater for boys in all ethnic groups except Puerto-Rican children. Prevalence does not vary by income or ethnicity, although black children have three times more hospitalizations and mortality than white children.

2. *Answer:* D
   Rationale: Positive family history of asthma is a major risk factor for childhood asthma. The other factors are not predicted risk factors.

3. *Answer:* A
   Rationale: Nighttime cough is a common presentation for asthma. Midsternal pain after meals is associated with gastric reflux. Nighttime snoring is associated with upper airway obstruction. Breathing hard during intensive exercise is normal.

4. *Answer:* C
   Rationale: Digital clubbing is not typically associated with asthma, and should raise suspicion about another cause, such as cystic fibrosis.

5. *Answer:* B
   Rationale: Office spirometry can be used to diagnose airway obstruction in a child who is old enough to cooperate with the testing. This should be attempted with children older than 4 years, but many are not able to cooperate effectively before the age of 7 years.

6. *Answer:* C
   Rationale: Moderate persistent asthma is characterized by having daily symptoms during the day and more than 1 night per week. This most closely fits the picture described. Asthma is mild if there are night symptoms no more often than two times per month. Severe asthma would include continual day symptoms and frequent night symptoms.

7. *Answer:* B
   Rationale: Daily low-dose corticosteroids are the preferred treatment for mild persistent asthma because the evidence shows that they are the best at preventing airway inflammation.

8. *Answer:* A
   Rationale: Asthma is primarily a clinical diagnosis, especially for a 3-year-old who is too young for office-based spirometry. Reversibility of wheezing in response to a bronchodilator is sufficient for a diagnosis.

9. *Answer:* D
   Rationale: The goal of asthma treatment is to control symptoms so that children are able to attend school and participate in normal activities.

10. *Answer:* A
    Rationale: The goal of antiinflammatory control medication is to prevent asthma symptoms, thus Tammy's lack of symptoms is a good sign that her therapy is effective. It may be possible to reduce her therapy by 25% after 6 months of good control.

11. *Answer:* D
    Rationale: Initial treatment of an asthma exacerbation should begin with a short-acting β-agonist. This may be repeated every 20 minutes for two more doses to gain immediate control of symptoms.

12. *Answer:* C
    Rationale: Quick relief of asthma symptoms is best obtained with a medication that treats airway hyperresponsiveness, such as albuterol, a β-agonist drug.

13. *Answer:* B
    Rationale: Although there are several options for increasing asthma treatment during an exacerbation, increasing the daily dose of inhaled steroid is the only option listed here that will address airway inflammation. Doubling the dosage of Advair would result in overdosage of the salmeterol component of that medication. Adding scheduled albuterol or theophylline would treat airway hyperresponsiveness but not the underlying inflammation.

14. *Answer:* B
    Rationale: Red-zone treatment should be "burst" therapy with an oral steroid for 4 to 10 days.

15. *Answer:* C
Rationale: Although both chemical and physical measures are available to reduce dust-mite exposure, a recent metaanalysis failed to show significant effects from either of these treatments.

16. *Answer:* D
Rationale: Current evidence indicates that inhaled corticosteroids are the most effective means of reducing chronic airway inflammation in asthma.

17. *Answer:* B
Rationale: Both a nebulizer or an inhaler used with a spacer and face mask can be effective for administering inhaled asthma medications to infants and young children.

18. *Answer:* A
Rationale: Deposition of inhaled steroid medication into the oropharynx has been associated with development of thrush. Rinsing the mouth after medication administration is an effective way to prevent this adverse reaction.

19. *Answer:* A
Rationale: Use of a spacer helps project the inhaled medication directly to the airway, by passing the oropharynx, and minimizing what is swallowed. This has been shown to increase the effectiveness of the administered dose.

20. *Answer:* B
Rationale: Annual influenza vaccine is recommended for children with asthma. Spirometry is recommended annually and whenever treatment is changed, and Jennifer had it done 6 months ago, with good results. There is no indication for a chest x-ray or for pneumococcal 23 valent vaccine today.

21. *Answer:* D
Rationale: Although herbal preparations are often used by families who have children with asthma, there is currently no systematic evidence that any are effective in treating this disorder.

22. *Answer:* A

Rationale: The goal of asthma therapy is minimal disruption and normal activity (at home and school) for children with the disease. If Marcus cannot walk the stairs at school, his asthma management needs to be adjusted to gain better control.

23. *Answer:* D
Rationale: Asthma mortality is associated with a history of intensive care unit admission for an acute exacerbation, history of previous intubation for asthma, and overreliance on inhaled bronchodilator therapy.

24. *Answer:* C
Rationale: Use of a conventional metered dose inhaler requires coordination of inhalation with actuation of the inhaler, even if a spacer is used. It is important to inhale slowly, and hold the breath for 10 seconds. Then the second inhalation should be taken in the same manner. For young children who use a spacer with mask, the mask eliminates the need to coordinate the breathing with actuation of the inhaler.

25. *Answer:* D
Rationale: Chronic asthma symptoms are primarily caused by airway inflammation.

BIBLIOGRAPHY

American Academy of Allergy, Asthma & Immunology (AAAAI). (2004). *Pediatric asthma: Promoting best practice.* Milwaukee: American Academy of Allergy, Asthma & Immunology.

American Academy of Allergy, Asthma & Immunology (AAAAI). (2000). *The allergy report: Diseases of the atopic diathesis* (vol. 2). Milwaukee: American Academy of Allergy, Asthma & Immunology.

Aronson, N., Lefervre, F., Piper, M., et al. (2001). Management of chronic asthma. Evidence report/technology assessment number 44 (AHRQ Publication No. 01-E044). Rockville, MD: Agency for Healthcare Research and Quality.

Bisgaard, H. (2000). Long-acting beta(2) agonists in the management of childhood asthma. A critical review of the literature. *Pediatr Pulmonol, 29*(3), 221-234.

Busse, P., & Busse, W. (2002). Pathogenesis of asthma. In R. Slavin & R. Reisman (Eds.). *Asthma.* Philadelphia: American College of Physicians.

Castro-Rodriguez, J., Holberg, C., Wright, A., & Martinez, F. (2000). A clinical index to define risk of asthma in young children with recurrent wheezing. *Am J Respir Crit Care Med, 162*(4 Pt 1), 1403-1406.

Centers for Disease Control and Prevention. (2006a). Current asthma prevalence percents by age: National Health Interview Survey, 2003. Retrieved April 17, 2006, from www.cdc.gov/asthma/NHIS/2003_5able3-1.htm.

Centers for Disease Control and Prevention. (2006b). Lifetime asthma population estimates by age: National Health Interview Survey, 2003. Retrieved April 17, 2006, from www.cdc.gov/asthma/NHIS/2003_table4-1.htm.

Centers for Disease Control and Prevention (2006c). Lifetime asthma population estimates by age: National health Interview Survey, 2003. Retrieved April 17, 2006, from www.cdc.gov/asthma/NHIS/2003_table1-1.htm.

Centers for Disease Control and Prevention. (2003). Key clinical activities for quality asthma care: Recommendations of the National Asthma Education and Prevention Program. *MMWR Morb Mortal Wkly Rep, 52*(RR6), 1-8. Retrieved June 5, 2005, from www.cdc.gov/mmwr/preview/mmwrhtml/rr5206a1.htm.

Gotzsche, P.C., Johansen, H.K., Schmidt., L.M., et al. (2004). House dust mite control measures for asthma. *Cochrane Database Syst Rev (4)*: CD001187.

Halterman, J., Montes, G., Aligne, C., et al. (2001). School readiness among urban children with asthma. *Ambu Pediatr, 1*(4), 201-205.

Huntley, A., & Ernst, E. (2000). Herbal medicines for asthma: A systematic review. *Thorax, 55*(11), 925-929.

Institute of Medicine (IOM). (2000). *Clearing the air: Asthma and indoor air exposures.* Washington, DC: National Academy Press.

Jones, C., Santanello, N.C., Boccuzzi, S.J., et al. (2003). Adherence to prescribed treatment for asthma: Evidence from pharmacy benefits data. *J Asthma, 40*(1), 93-101.

Kavuru, M., Melamed, J., Gross, G., et al. (2000). Salmeterol and fluticasone propionate combined in a new powder inhalation device for the treatment of asthma: A randomized, double-blind, placebo-controlled trial. *J Allergy Clin Immunol, 105*(6 Pt 1), 1108-1116.

Kieckhefer, G., & Ratcliffe, M. (2004). Asthma. In P.L. Jackson & J.C. Vessey (Eds.). *Primary care of the child with a chronic condition* (4th ed.). St. Louis: Mosby.

Kieckhefer, G., & Trahms, C. (2000). Supporting development of children with chronic conditions: From compliance toward shared management. *Pediatr Nurs, 26*(4), 354-363.

Knafl, K., Breitmayer, B., Gallo, A., & Zoeller, L. (1996). Family response to childhood chronic illness: Description of management styles. *J Pediatr Nurs, 11*(5), 315-326.

Leonard, P., & Sur, S. (2003). Interleukin-12: Potential role in asthma therapy. *BioDrugs, 17*(1), 1-7.

Liu, A.H., Spahn, J.D., & Leung, D.Y.M. (2004). Childhood asthma. In R.E. Behrman, R.M. Kliegman, & H.B. Jenson (Eds.). *Nelson textbook of pediatrics* (17th ed.). Philadelphia: Saunders.

Marguet, C., Couder, L., Le Roux, P., et al. (2001). Inhalation treatment: Errors in application and difficulties in acceptance of the devices are frequent in wheezy infants and young children. *Pediatr Allergy Immunol, 12*(4), 224-230.

Markham, A., & Jarvis, B. (2000). Inhaled salmeterol/fluticasone propionate combination: A review of its use in persistent asthma. *Drugs, 60*(5), 1207-1233.

Martinez, F. (2002). Development of wheezing disorders and asthma in preschool children. *Pediatrics,109*(2 Suppl), 362-367.

National Heart, Lung, and Blood Institute NHLBI (1997). Expert panel report II: Guidelines for the diagnosis and management of asthma (97-4051). Bethesda, MD: National Institutes of Health.

National Heart, Lung, and Blood Institute NHLBI (2002). NAEPP expert panel report: Guidelines for the diagnosis and management of asthma—update on selected topics 2002. Bethesda, MD: National Heart Lung and Blood Institute.

Ni Chroinin, M., Greenstone, I.R., Danish, A., et al. (2005). Combination of inhaled long-acting beta$_2$-agonists and inhaled steroids versus higher dose of inhaled steroids in children and adults with persistent asthma, *Cochrane Database Syst Rev,*(4): CD005533.

O'Byrne, P.M., Barnes, P.J., Rodriquez-Roisin, R., et al. (2001). Low dose inhaled budesonide and formoterol in mild persistent asthma: The OPTIMA randomized trial. *Am J Respir Crit Care Med, 164*(8), 1392-1397.

Peat, J., Toelle, B., & Mellis, C. (2000). Problems and possibilities in understanding the natural history of asthma. *J Allergy Clin Immunol, 106*(3 Suppl), S144-S152.

Samet, J., Wiesch, D., & Ahmed, I. (2001). Pediatric asthma: Epidemiology and natural history. In C.K. Naspitz, S.J. Szefler, D.G. Tinkelman, et al. (Eds.). *Textbook of pediatric asthma: An international perspective.* London: Martin Dunitz.

Shrewsbury, S., Pyke, S., & Britton, M. (2000). Meta-analysis of increased dose of inhaled steroid or addition of salmeterol in symptomatic asthma (MIASMA). *Br Med J, 320*(7246), 1368-1373.

Stempel, D.A., O'Donnell, J.C., & Meyer, J.W. (2002). Inhaled corticosteroids plus salmeterol or montelukast: Effects on resource utilization and costs. *J Allergy Clin Immunol, 109*(3), 433-439.

Suessmuth, S., Freihorst, J., & Gappa, M. (2003). Low-dose theophylline in childhood asthma: A placebo-controlled, double-blind study. *Pediatr Allergy Immunol, 14*(5), 394-400.

Szefler, S.J., Weiss, S., & Tonascia, J. (2000). Long-term effects of budesonide or nedocromil in children with asthma. *N Engl J Med, 343*(15), 1054-1106.

Taketomo, C.K., Hodding, J.H., & Kraus, D.M. (2005). *Pediatric dosage handbook.* (9th ed.). Hudson, OH: Lexicomp.

Taussig, L., Wright, A., Holberg, C., et al. (2003). Tucson children's respiratory study: 1980 to present. *J Allergy Clin Immunol, 111*(4), 661-675.

NOTES

Cerebral Palsy

LORI LEI LUNDBERG

Select the best answer for each of the following questions:

1. How many infants are born with cerebral palsy (CP) each year in the United States?
   A. 1,000
   B. 10,000
   C. 5,000
   D. 20,000

2. Which of the following signs are associated with cerebral palsy in an infant?
   A. Head lag at 2 weeks.
   B. Parachute reflex at 2 months.
   C. Inability to sit unsupported at 4 months.
   D. Moro reflex at 9 months.

The next five questions relate to the following scenario:

Sarah is a 14-year-old girl affected by spastic quadriplegic cerebral palsy with a seizure disorder, severe global developmental delay, and neuromuscular scoliosis. Sarah is completely dependent on others to provide all of her care needs.

3. Sarah has been fitted with a body brace so that she may be comfortably positioned upright. Routine care for Sarah would include:
   A. Sterilizing the brace with a strong detergent.
   B. Providing good skin care, especially over bony prominences.
   C. Keeping Sarah out of the brace as much as possible.

   D. Allow Sarah to sit unsupported in a chair with a soft back.

4. Sarah has developed a stage 2 pressure sore from the rubbing of the brace over her coccyx area. The wound appears clean without redness or drainage. She is afebrile and does not appear to be septic. Initially, the most appropriate action of the pediatric nurse practitioner would be to:
   A. Perform a complete skin assessment, including how mother has been caring for Sarah's wound.
   B. Refer Sarah for home health for administration of intravenous antibiotics.
   C. Recommend that Sarah continue to wear the brace, even though her wound is not yet healed.
   D. Contact the medical media department to photograph Sarah's wound for documentation into her clinical record.

5. Before Sarah receives her DTaP immunization, the pediatric nurse practitioner should assess her:
   A. Seizure disorder.
   B. Developmental level.
   C. CBC.
   D. Current medications.

6. Angel, Sarah's mother, is concerned that her daughter is becoming dehydrated because she is having a hard time eating and drinking fluids. Sarah's BMI is less that the 5th percentile for her age; reflecting a 12% body weight loss over the last 4 months. Mother should first be counseled to:

A. Limit the amount of protein in Sarah's diet.
B. Enroll in a cooking class to learn to prepare nutritious meals.
C. Provide Angel with a healthy diet plan for Sarah to promote optimal nutrition.
D. Schedule an appointment with the gastroenterologist for the placement of a feeding tube.

7. Sarah has recently been transitioned into the orthopedic unit of her community high school. Sarah is provided the services of occupational, physical, and speech therapy. Which is the most holistic approach to meeting Sarah's educational needs?
A. Initiate developmental screening and diagnostic testing.
B. Focus the attention away from Sarah's emotional development.
C. Formulate and implement an individual family service plan utilizing an interdisciplinary team.
D. Plan for as much isolation as possible, recognizing she needs her own personal space.

The next four questions relate to the following scenario:

Neemo is an 8-year-old boy with significantly involved spastic quadriparesis of unknown etiology. Neemo appears to have normal mentation. He has a good appetite but is unable to feed himself. Neemo receives outpatient physical therapy; however, he continues to have problems with his movement and posture.

8. Neemo walks with a scissoring gait. Scissoring results from:
A. An increased tone in the periacetabular muscles that control adduction and internal rotation of the hip.
B. Knee joint laxity.
C. Symmetrical muscle tone in the lower extremities.
D. Ankle contractures.

9. Neemo's x-ray examination confirms the presence of hip dislocations more than

one-third of the way out of the hip sockets. Therefore, surgical intervention consisting of bilateral varus derotational osteotomies (VDRO's) has been scheduled. This is a complex procedure where:
A. The angle of the femur (thigh bone) is changed surgically to place the head of the femur back into the hip socket and spica cast is applied.
B. Medication is injected into the hip socket to lubricate the joint, increasing its range of motion.
C. The femur is cut into and surgical rods inserted and a long leg cast applied.
D. The muscles surrounding the knees are permanently shortened to limit their mobility and knee immobilizers are applied.

10. In accordance with the primary care medical home model as advocated by the American Academy of Pediatrics, Neemo's primary care provider must be included in the perioperative evaluation process. The rationale for the assessment of Neemo's up-to-date immunization status, particularly regarding varicella, is that:
A. Neemo's immunity will be compromised after undergoing general anesthesia.
B. Neemo's comfort would be aggravated by the presence of varicella lesions under his hip spica cast.
C. Live virus vaccines can be safely administered to anyone, regardless of immunity status.
D. Varicella vaccine, if needed, can be given orally postoperatively.

11. Neemo's appetite is poor due to difficulty chewing his food. During the preoperative physical examination, the pediatric nurse practitioner notices several blackened teeth with surrounding swollen, reddened areas. Neemo has been referred a pediatric periodontist to:
A. Instruct Neemo in the proper method of oral hygiene.
B. Provide fluoride therapy.
C. Treat the oral infection prior to surgery.
D. Undergo oral surgery.

The following five questions relate to the following scenario:

Trevor is a 5-year-old boy affected by cerebral palsy secondary to an anoxic brain injury (near-drowning incident), which occurred at 18 months of age. Trevor is home-schooled by his mother. He is aware of his environment, sensitive to his surroundings, and communicates through a device that answers "yes" and "no" by his pushing a button. Review of plan of care for Trevor is that Botox injections will be administered into his quadriceps and hip adductor muscles.

12. Trevor's preadmission planning should include:
   A. Informing Trevor that he will receive several shots into his affected muscles.
   B. Asking him what color of cast he would like on his legs.
   C. Assuring Trevor that he will be given a painless anesthetic prior to the procedure so that he will not feel, or remember, receiving the shots.
   D. Telling Trevor that a side effect of Botox is excessive drooling, and this will make him feel embarrassed.

13. The desired effect of Botox is:
   A. Reducing the rigidity and stiffness of Trevor's weak muscles, improving range of motion and overall mobility.
   B. Spontaneous resolution of Trevor's spasticity.
   C. Reversing damage to Trevor's developing brain.
   D. Decreasing Trevor's ability to control his spastic muscles.

14. Trevor receives physical therapy services through a community-based program. Mother would like Trevor to continue these services after receiving Botox. The most appropriate response of the pediatric nurse practitioner to Trevor's mother would be:
   A. Physical therapy should be continued to help improve flexibility in Trevor's weak muscles.
   B. Physical therapy will not significantly improve Trevor's symptoms.
   C. Physical therapy services should be discontinued after the cessation of therapeutic effects from Botox treatment.
   D. Physical therapy would be of no benefit to Trevor, as he is unable to walk.

15. The following is a true statement regarding the administration of Botox:
   A. Trevor may be injected with another dose of Botox the day after the first injection, especially if the medication does not appear to act immediately.
   B. Trevor may have an injection of Botox whenever he needs it; it is considered to be a "long-term fix" for orthopedic problems.
   C. Trevor may have another injection of Botox in 6 to 9 months.
   D. The dose of toxin a child is to receive is calculated by body surface area.

16. Trevor and his family live in a three-bedroom apartment; all three bedrooms are located upstairs. The family has a limited income; however, the parents have been successful at obtaining necessary resources to assist Trevor in meeting his daily care needs. Trevor has two older siblings who carry Trevor and his wheelchair up and down the stairs. What anticipatory guidance could the pediatric nurse practitioner provide to the family?
   A. None, the family is coping well.
   B. Refer family to local and state agencies for assistance in finding adequate housing.
   C. Plan for replacement of Trevor's wheelchair in 4 to 5 years.
   D. Hire an architect to draw up plans for structurally modifying their rented home.

The next four questions relate to the following scenario:

James is a 7-year-old boy affected by spastic left hemiplegic cerebral palsy. His MRI reveals evidence consistent with a previous anoxic ischemic brain injury. James ambulates with a left "toe walk" due to a left equinus deformity and left inward tibial torsion.

17. Which of the following primary care examinations should be conduced on James more frequently than annually?
   A. Dental
   B. Hearing
   C. Vision
   D. Growth

18. In planning for surgery, the physician can obtain excellent information about the mechanics of James' gait by obtaining:
   A. Skeletal x-rays.
   B. MRI.
   C. CT with and without contrast.
   D. Gait motion analysis video.

19. James has a history of receiving Botox injections (at the ages of 4, 5, and 6), resulting in a significant decrease in spasticity. Which statement is true regarding James' history?
   A. Botox injections appear to have been effective in delaying orthopedic surgery on James left lower extremity.
   B. Botox therapy was a "failure" as a long-term fix for James' leg.
   C. Botox therapy should not be attempted again.
   D. Research has proven Botox safe for long-term use.

20. What is the purpose for prescribing Baclofen for a child with CP?
   A. Decrease anxiety.
   B. Decrease spasticity.
   C. Reduce muscle spasms.
   D. Reduce extrapyramidal reactions.

NOTES

ANSWERS

1. **Answer:** B
   Rationale: According the Centers for Disease Control and Prevention, National Center for Birth Defects and Developmental Disabilities, there are approximately 10,000 infants born each year with CP.

2. **Answer:** D
   Rationale: Normal neonates will have a head lag at 2 weeks. Parachute reflex should be present in healthy newborns at 2 months of age. Most developmentally intact infants will be able to sit unsupported at 6 months. However, in healthy infants, the Moro reflex is not present past 6 months of age.

3. **Answer:** B
   Rationale: Meticulous skin hygiene will enhance healthy skin integrity, minimizing the chance of skin breakdown and secondary infection to occur.

4. **Answer:** A
   Rationale: A thorough nursing assessment involves the collection and analysis of data. The planning and implementing of patient care follows based on this information.

5. **Answer:** A
   Rationale: According to the CDC, a child with uncontrolled seizure disorder should not receive DTaP vaccine. Her developmental level, CBC results, and current medications should not interfere with routine inactive vaccinations.

6. **Answer:** C
   Rationale: Adequate caloric intake through the provision of a well-balanced diet is essential for a person to thrive. Vitamins and minerals play an important role in the breakdown of food to be utilized as energy.

7. **Answer:** C
   Rationale: The formulation and implementation of an individual family service plan (IFSP) will identify the strengths of each member of the child's family of origin, and garner the expertise of the entire educational team to address the child's needs in the school setting.

8. **Answer:** A
   Rationale: Scissoring results from increased tone in the muscles that control adduction and internal rotation of the hip.

9. **Answer:** A
   Rationale: A varus derotational osteotomy (VDRO) is a surgical procedure where the angle of the femur is changed surgically to place the head of the femur back into the hip socket. Spica casting immobilizes the hip joint.

10. **Answer:** B
    Rationale: The outbreak of varicella vesicles under a cast or brace is an entirely preventable occurrence. Unless medically contraindicated, a child's immunization status should be documented and verified as "up to date" prior to admission to the hospital for any surgical intervention.

11. **Answer:** C
    Rationale: Most orthopedic surgeries are considered to be "elective" procedures. Therefore, an individual should be medically at his or her own "personal best" before admission to the hospital for surgery, without clinical signs of illness or infection.

12. **Answer:** C
    Rationale: The child has communicated that he is fearful of experiencing pain. Addressing this fear by assuring him that the will receive a painless anesthetic prior to the procedure so that he will not feel or remember receiving the shots is meant to address his (very real) anxiety.

13. **Answer:** A
    Rationale: The therapeutic effects of Botox include reducing the rigidity and stiffness of weak muscles and improving range of motion and overall mobility.

14. **Answer:** A
    Rationale: In conjunction with physical therapy, such as stretching exercises or gait training, Botox injections help to strengthen weak muscles and restore normal movement and function.

15. *Answer:* C

Rationale: An injection of Botox takes from 3 to 7 days to work. Positive results of Botox therapy are transient, but may last as long as 9 months. The dose of toxin a child is to receive is calculated by body weight.

16. *Answer:* B

Rationale: Planning for the child's future needs must take normal growth and development into account. As a child who is totally dependent in his or her care needs gets taller and heavier, an increased burden is placed on a caregiver's physical ability to care for the child. To enhance the health of the family as a unit, long-term planning should include that their place of residence be ADA accessible.

17. *Answer:* A

Rationale: Children with cerebral palsy tend to have poor oral hygiene and dental problems. Certain medications, such as Dilantin, can cause dental problems. Children with cerebral palsy should be referred to a dentist with experience in caring for children with developmental delays and should have routine visits every 6 months.

18. *Answer:* D

Rationale: Computerized gait motion analysis conducted prior to surgical orthopedic surgery has become common. Precise measurements obtained through videography offer detailed information relating to specific abnormalities of the affected lower extremity joint as well as the muscle activity that controls motion throughout all phases of the gait cycle.

19. *Answer:* A

Rationale: Fortunately, Botox therapy appears to have been effective in delaying more invasive orthopedic surgery for this child. Botox is not to be considered a "long-term fix" for orthopedic problems. Unfortunately, the long-term effects (greater than 5 years) of receiving injections are not known at this time.

20. *Answer:* C

Rationale: Baclofen reduces muscle spasms, diazepam reduces anxiety and muscle spasms, dantrolene sodium and botulinum A toxin reduce spasticity, and benztropine mesylate reduces extrapyramidal reactions.

BIBLIOGRAPHY

American Academy of Pediatrics, Committee on Infectious Diseases. (2000). *2000 Red book: Report of the committee on infectious diseases* (25th ed.). Elk Grove Village, IL: American Academy of Pediatrics.

Bjornson, K.F., & McLaughlin, J.F. (2001). The measurement of health-related quality of life (HRQL) in children with cerebral palsy. *Eur J Neurol, 8*(Suppl. 5), 183-193.

Boop, F.A., Woo, R., & Maria, B.L. (2001). Consensus statement on the surgical management of spasticity related to cerebral palsy. *J Child Neurol, 16*(1), 68-69.

Boyd, R.N., & Hays, R.M. (2001). Current evidence for the use of botulinum toxin type A in the management of children with cerebral palsy: A systematic review. *Eur J Neurol, 8*(Suppl. 5), 1-20.

Butler, C., & Campbell, S. (2000). Evidence of the effects of intrathecal baclofen for spastic and dystonic cerebral palsy. AACPDM Treatment Outcomes Committee Review Panel. *Dev Med Child Neurol, 42*(9), 634-645.

Centers for Disease Control and Prevention, National Center for Birth Defects and Developmental Disabilities. (2002). *Cerebral palsy among children*. Retrieved May 20, 2006, from www.cdc.gov/ncbddd/factsheets/cp.pdf.

Cooley, W.C., & American Academy of Pediatrics Committee on Children with Disabilities. (2004). Providing a primary care medical home for children and youth with cerebral palsy. *Pediatrics, 114(4),* 1106-1113.

Demott, K. (2001). *E. coli* infection quadruples risk of cerebral palsy. *OB GYN News, 36*(18), 1.

Desloovere, K., Molenaers, G., Jonkers, I., et al. (2001). A randomized study of combined botulinum toxin type A and casting in the ambulant child with cerebral palsy using objective outcome measures. *Eur J Neurol, 8*(Suppl. 5), 75-87.

Dizon-Townson, D.S. (2001). Preterm labour and delivery: A genetic predisposition. *Paediatr Perinat Epidemiol, 15*(Suppl. 2), 57-62.

Dolk, H., Pattenden, S., & Johnson, A. (2001). Cerebral palsy, low birthweight and socioeconomic deprivation: Inequalities in a major cause of childhood disability. *Paediatr Perinat Epidemiol, 15*(4), 359-363.

dos Santos, R., Masiero, D., Novo, N.F., & Simionato, M.R. (2003). Oral conditions in children with cerebral palsy. *ASDC J Dent Child, 70*(1), 40-46.

Drummond, P.M., & Colver, A.F. (2002). Analysis by gestational age of cerebral palsy in singleton births in northeast England 1970-1994. *Paediatr Perinat Epidemiol, 16*(2), 172-180.

Edgar, T.S. (2001). Clinical utility of botulinum toxin in the treatment of cerebral palsy: Comprehensive review. *J Child Neurol, 16*(1), 37-46.

Feldman-Winter, L.B., Krueger, C.J., Neyhart, J.M., & McAbee, G.N. (2002). Public perceptions of cerebral palsy. *J Am Osteopath Assoc, 102*(9), 471-475.

Fennell, E.B., & Dikel, T.N. (2001). Cognitive and neuropsychological functioning in children with cerebral palsy. *J Child Neurol, 16*(1), 58-63.

Ferrari, F., Cioni, G.E., Roversi, C., et al. (2002). Cramped synchronized general movements in preterm infants as an early marker for cerebral palsy. *Arch Pediatr Adolesc Med, 156*(5), 460-468.

Flynn, J.M., & Miller, F. (2002). Management of hip disorders in patients with cerebral palsy. *J Am Acad Orthop Surg, 10*(3), 198-209.

Gibson, C.S., MacLennan, A.H., Goldwater, P.N., & Dekker, G.A. (2003). Antenatal causes of cerebral palsy: Associations between inherited thrombophilias, viral and bacterial infection, and inherited susceptibility to infection. *Obstet Gynecol Surv, 58*(3), 209-220.

Graham, H.K. (2001). Botulinum toxin type A management of spasticity in the context of orthopaedic surgery for children with spastic cerebral palsy. *Eur J Neurol, 8*(Suppl. 5), 30-39.

Griffin, H.D., Fitch, C.L., & Griffin, L.W. (2002). Causes and interventions in the area of cerebral palsy. *Infant Young Child, 14*(3), 18-24.

Henderson, R.C., Lark, R.K., Gurka, M.J., et al. (2002). Bone density and metabolism in children and adolescents with moderate to severe cerebral palsy. *Pediatrics, 110*(1, Pt 1), e5.

Henderson, R.C., Kairalla, J., Abbas, A., & Stevenson, R.D. (2004). Predicting low bone density in children and young adults with quadriplegic cerebral palsy. *Dev Med Child Neurol, 46*(6), 416-419.

Houlihan, C.M., O'Donnell, M., Conaway, M., & Stevenson, R.D. (2004). Bodily pain and health-related quality of life in children with cerebral palsy. *Dev Med Child Neurol, 46*(5), 305-310.

Hutton, J.L. & Pharoah, P.O. (2002). Effects of cognitive, motor, and sensory disabilities on survival in cerebral palsy. *Arch Dis Child, 86*(2), 84-91.

Johnston, M.V. (2004). Cerebral palsy. In R.E. Behrman, R.M. Kliegman, & H.B. Jenson (Eds.). *Nelson textbook of pediatrics* (17th ed.). Philadelphia: Saunders.

Kim, D.S., Choi, J.U., Yang, K.H., & Park, C.I. (2001). Selective posterior rhizotomy in children with cerebral palsy: A 10-year experience. *Childs Nerv Syst, 17*(9), 556-562.

Koman, L.A., Smith, B.P., & Balkrishnan, R. (2003). Spasticity associated with cerebral palsy in children: Guidelines for the use of botulinum A toxin. *Pediatr Drugs, 5*(1), 11-23.

Liptak, G.S., O'Donnell, M., Conaway, M., et al. (2001). Health status of children with moderate to severe cerebral palsy. *Dev Med Child Neurol, 43*(6), 364-370.

McLaughlin, J., Bjornson, K., Temkin, N., et al. (2002). Selective dorsal rhizotomy: Metaanalysis of three randomized controlled trials. *Dev Med Child Neurol, 44*(1), 17-25.

Molenaers, G., Desloovere, K., De Cat, J., et al. (2001). Single event multilevel botulinum toxin type A treatment and surgery similarities and differences. *Eur J Neurol, 8*(Suppl. 5), 88-97.

Murphy, N.A., Irwin, M.C., & Hoff, C. (2002). Intrathecal baclofen therapy in children with cerebral palsy: Efficacy and complications. *Arch Phys Med Rehab, 83*(9), 1721-1725.

National Institute of Neurological Disorders and Stroke (NINDS). (2001). Cerebral palsy: Hope through research. Retrieved May 20, 2006, from www.ninds.nih.gov/disorders/cerebral_palsy/detail_cerebral_palsy.htm.

Nehring, W.M. (2004). Cerebral palsy. In P.L. Jackson & J.A. Vessey (Eds.). *Primary care of the child with a chronic condition* (4th ed.). St. Louis: Mosby.

Nolan, J., Chalkiadis, G.A., Low, J., Olesch, C.A., Brown, T.C. (2000). Anaesthesia and pain management in cerebral palsy. *Anaesthesia, 55*(5), 32-41.

Raymond, G.V. (2002). Abnormal mental development. In D.L. Rimoin, J.M. Connor, R.E. Pyeritz, & B.R. Korf (Eds.). *Emery and Rimoin's principles and practice of medical genetics* (4th ed.). New York: Churchill Livingstone.

Reddihough, D.S., Baikie, G., & Walstab, J.E. (2001). Cerebral palsy in Victoria, Australia: Mortality and causes of death. *J Paediatr Child Health, 37*(2), 183-186.

Rosenbaum, P. (2003). Cerebral palsy: What parents and doctors want to know. *BMJ, 326*(7396), 970-974.

Rosenbaum, P.L., Walter, S.D., Hanna, S.E., et al. (2002). Prognosis for gross motor function in cerebral palsy: Creation of motor development curves. *JAMA, 288*(11), 1357-1363.

Sanger, T.D., Delgado, M.R., Gaebler-Spira, D., et al. (2003). Classification and definition of disorders causing hypertonia in childhood. *Pediatrics, 111*(1), e89-e97.

Schendel, D.E. (2001). Infection in pregnancy and cerebral palsy. *J Am Women's Assoc, 56*(3), 105-108.

Schendel, D.E., Schuchat, A., & Thorsen, P. (2002). Public health issues related to infection in pregnancy and cerebral palsy. *Ment Retard Dev Disabil Res Rev, 8*(1), 39-45.

Steinbok, P. (2001). Outcomes after selective dorsal rhizotomy for spastic cerebral palsy. *Childs Nerv Syst, 17*(1-2), 1-18.

Suzuki, J., & Ito, M. (2002). Incidence patterns of cerebral palsy in Shiga Prefecture, Japan, 1977-1991. *Brain Dev, 24*(1), 39-48.

Tasdemir, H.A., Buyukavci, M., Akcay, F., et al. (2001). Bone mineral density in children with cerebral palsy. *Pediatr Int, 43*(2), 157-160.

Thorogood, C., & Alexander, M.A. (2005). Cerebral palsy. Retrieved on May 20, 2006, from www.emedicine.com/pmr/topic24.htm.

Tilton, A.H., & Maria, B.L. (2001). Consensus statement on pharmacotherapy for spasticity. *J Child Neurol, 16*(1), 66-67.

White, H., Jenkins, J., Neace, W.P., et al. (2002). Clinically prescribed orthoses demonstrate an increase in velocity of gait in children with cerebral palsy: A retrospective study. *Dev Med Child Neurol, 44*(4), 227-232.

Wilson, B.A., Shannon, M.T., & Stang, C.L. (2005). *Nurse's drug guide 2005.* Upper Saddle River, NJ: Prentice-Hall.

Winter, S., Autry, A., Boyle, C., & Yeargin-Allsopp, M. (2002). Trends in the prevalence of cerebral palsy in a population-based study. *Pediatrics, 110*(6), 1220-1225.

Worley, G., Houlihan, C.M., Herman-Giddens, M.E., et al. (2002). Secondary sexual characteristics in children with cerebral palsy and moderate to severe motor impairment: A cross-sectional survey. *Pediatrics, 110*(5), 897-902.

Wu, Y.W., & Colford, J.M., Jr. (2000). Chorioamnionitis as a risk factor for cerebral palsy: A meta-analysis. *JAMA, 284*(11), 1417-1429.

NOTES

Childhood Cancer

SHARRON L. DOCHERTY

Select the best answer for each of the following questions:

1. Matthew is a 12-year-old who is being treated for a peripheral primitive neuroectodermal tumor of the pelvis. According to the International Classification of Childhood Cancers, which of the 12 categories would his cancer be grouped into?
   A. Malignant bone tumors.
   B. Sympathetic nervous system tumors.
   C. CNS and miscellaneous intracranial and intraspinal neoplasms.
   D. Soft-tissue sarcomas.

2. Matthew's mom asks you whether or not Matthew inherited this tumor from one of his parents. The most appropriate response would be:
   A. There is no data on genetics and cancer available at this time.
   B. Most childhood cancers are inherited and considered genetic.
   C. Most childhood cancers are not inherited but can be considered genetic because they occur at the molecular level.
   D. We will know the answer once the testing is completed.

3. Which embryologic germ layer tissue is responsible for the development of most childhood cancers?
   A. Mesoderm
   B. Endoderm
   C. Ectoderm
   D. Neuroderm

4. An early onset autosomal-dominant cancer predisposition syndrome that is associated with soft-tissue sarcomas, breast cancer, leukemia, osteosarcoma, and melanoma is:
   A. Von Hippel-Lindau disease.
   B. Li-Fraumeni syndrome.
   C. Retinoblastoma syndrome.
   D. Myelodysplasia syndrome.

5. Which of the following disorders have a strong association with acute lymphocytic leukemia or lymphoma?
   A. Ataxia-telangiectasia.
   B. Turner's syndrome.
   C. Klinefelter's syndrome.
   D. WAGR syndrome.

6. Which of the following cancers do children with AIDS have an increased risk of developing?
   A. Wilms' tumor.
   B. Brain tumor.
   C. Non-Hodgkin's lymphoma.
   D. Retinoblastoma.

7. Trey is a 9-month-old male who is brought to your office with a 1-week history of fever, malaise, and decreased appetite. Mom reports that she feels as though his "tummy is getting much bigger" and that she noticed the disposable diapers she recently bought no longer fit around his waist. On exam, you palpate a fixed abdominal mass that crosses the midline. Given Trey's age and physical findings, which cancer would you most likely suspect?
   A. Hodgkin's lymphoma.
   B. Wilms' tumor.

C. Rhabdomyosarcoma.

D. Neuroblastoma.

8. Melissa is a 15-year-old female who presents to your office with a painless, golf-ball sized lump in the inguinal region of her right thigh. She reports that over the past month she has awakened in the middle of the night feeling cold and sweaty. She also reports a weight loss of 5 pounds over the same time period. Given Melissa's age and historical findings, which cancer would you most likely suspect?

A. Hodgkin's lymphoma.

B. Rhabdomyosarcoma.

C. Acute lymphocytic leukemia.

D. Osteosarcoma.

9. Which of the following would be most appropriate initial diagnostic tests for Melissa's case?

A. X-ray and CT of right thigh.

B. CBC with differential, ESR, chest x-ray.

C. Abdominal ultrasound and ESR.

D. Urine for catecholamines and CBC.

10. You have been providing primary health care to Melissa over the past year as she has been undergoing treatment for her cancer. Her mother asks you when the she will be considered "cured of the cancer." The most appropriate response would be:

A. Melissa will be considered cured once she completes her treatment.

B. The medical community uses the term *cured* once a child is 5 years posttreatment and has not had any signs of cancer recurrence.

C. *Cured* is a very subjective term that is difficult to apply to children with cancer.

D. Once Melissa reaches adulthood, she will be considered cured of childhood cancer if she has not had any recurrence.

11. Which grouping of childhood cancers are more likely associated with the age group of birth through 1 year?

A. Neuroblastoma, retinoblastoma.

B. Acute lymphocytic leukemia.

C. Hodgkin's and non-Hodgkin's lymphoma.

D. Astrocytoma.

12. Mortality rates for childhood cancer have been on the decline since the late 1970s. Which type of childhood cancer continues to report higher mortality rates?

A. Acute lymphocytic leukemia (ALL).

B. Acute myelocytic leukemia (AML).

C. Retinoblastoma.

D. Wilms' tumor.

13. The role of the primary care provider in the diagnosis of a child with cancer can best be described as:

A. Ordering and interpreting diagnostic tests.

B. Performing diagnostic tests.

C. Counseling and education of child and parents around potential diagnosis.

D. Recognition of signs and symptoms and prompt referral to a pediatric cancer center.

14. The role of the primary care provider in the care of the child undergoing cancer treatment can best be described as:

A. Providing primary, preventive health maintenance to child throughout cancer treatment.

B. Administration of cancer treatment medications.

C. Screening for and administering treatment for any side-effects of cancer treatment.

D. The primary provider does not play a role until the child has completed cancer treatment.

15. Jeremy is undergoing treatment for AML. He is currently receiving high-dose chemotherapy that is aimed at removing the bulk of his leukemic cells. Which treatment stage is Jeremy currently in?

A. Induction.

B. Consolidation and intensification.

C. Maintenance therapy.

D. Precipitous therapy.

16. Autologous bone marrow transplantation uses stem cells from:

A. Umbilical cords.
B. Bone marrow of a related or unrelated donor.
C. The patient's own marrow which is reinfused following treatment.
D. An animal model.

17. Biologic response modifiers such as monoclonal antibodies are being used in the treatment of childhood cancer. They function mainly by:
A. Directly disrupting the growth and division of cancer cells.
B. Directly altering the genetic structure of cancer cells.
C. Placebo effect.
D. Using the innate immunologic defense mechanisms of the child to target cancer cells.

18. Miguel is an 8-year-old male who has just completed treatment for ALL that included chemotherapy. Miguel is currently in the 5th percentile for height and 10th percentile for weight. Miguel's father tells you that he used to be as tall as or taller than most children in his class. He asks you if Miguel will now always be the shortest one in his class. The most appropriate response is:
A. The effects of chemotherapy on growth are usually only temporary; he will most likely soon go through a period of catch-up growth.
B. Miguel will likely be the shortest one in his class because of his genetic predisposition.
C. Yes, because Miguel had ALL, he will now always be shorter than his classmates.
D. We can give Miguel hormones to help him grow.

19. Which mode of cancer treatment will have the most damaging effect on physical growth?
A. Chemotherapy.
B. Internal radiation.
C. Cranial radiation.
D. Biologic response modifiers.

20. Which of the following physical growth assessment guidelines should be followed for a child with cancer?

A. Height, weight, and BMI should be documented on standardized growth curves for all children every 2 months while the child is in therapy.
B. Height, weight, and BMI should be documented on standardized growth curves for all children every 2 months while the child is in therapy and for the first year after therapy.
C. Height, weight, BMI, and head circumference should be documented on standardized growth curves for all children every 2 months while the child is in therapy and for the first year after therapy.
D. Height, weight, and BMI should be documented on standardized growth curves for all children every 6 months while the child is in therapy and for the first year after therapy.

21. Mary is 14 years old and is 2 months into her treatment for AML. Mary appears withdrawn, has flat affect, and has been refusing social interactions with her friends. At her stage of cognitive development, she is most likely to be struggling with:
A. Feeling as though she deserved to get cancer because she had not been doing well in school.
B. Fearful that she is going to die.
C. Feeling a lack of control over her body and how the treatment is making her feel.
D. Anger at her parents for not preventing the cancer.

22. Which of the following 16-year-old children will be at the greatest risk for late effects of childhood cancer treatment?
A. Undergoing induction therapy for ALL.
B. Entering maintenance therapy for ALL.
C. Completed chemotherapy for ALL 5 years ago.
D. Completed chemotherapy for ALL when he was 2 years old.

23. Hazel is a 4-year-old female who completed immunosuppressive therapy treatment for a neuroblastoma 6 months ago. Her

mother has brought her to see you regarding her immunization status. You note she is due for her DTaP #5, IPV #4, and MMR #2. What would you give today?

A. Give Hazel all of her immunizations today.
B. Test Hazel's immunity for MMR and then treat accordingly.
C. Wait another 3 months and then resume Hazel's immunization schedule with inactivated vaccines.
D. Give Hazel her DTaP only today.

24. Children who have been treated for Hodgkin's disease should be given which of the following vaccinations 6 months following treatment?

A. Meningococcal
B. Varicella
C. MMR
D. Polio

25. Which of the following childhood cancers might be suspected for a child who presents with leukokoria?

A. Posterior fossa tumor.
B. Wilms' tumor.
C. Neuroblastoma.
D. Retinoblastoma.

NOTES

ANSWERS

1. *Answer:* D
Rationale: According to the ICCC classification system, depending upon the site in which they occur, primitive neurectodermal tumors (PNET) are classified as CNS and miscellaneous intracranial and intraspinal neoplasms or as soft-tissue sarcomas. Matthew's pelvic tumor would be considered a peripheral PNET tumor, and thus would fall into the soft-tissue sarcoma grouping.

2. *Answer:* C
Rationale: Childhood cancer can be considered genetic because it occurs at the molecular level, but most childhood cancers are not hereditary. Less than 10% of newly diagnosed childhood cancer cases can be attributed to inherited cancer susceptibility.

3. *Answer:* A
Rationale: Mesoderm is responsible for the development of the majority of types of tissues in which childhood cancer develops (e.g., muscle, connective tissue, bone, blood cells, testes).

4. *Answer:* B
Rationale: Li-Fraumeni syndrome is an early onset cancer predisposition syndrome that is associated with soft-tissue sarcomas, breast cancer, leukemia, osteosarcoma, melanoma, and cancer of the colon, pancreas, adrenal cortex, and brain.

5. *Answer:* A
Rationale: Ataxia-telangiectasia is associated with acute lymphocytic leukemia or lymphoma. Turner's syndrome and WAGR syndrome increase a child's risk for Wilms' tumor and ovarian cancer. Klinefelter's syndrome increases a child's risk for breast cancer.

6. *Answer:* C
Rationale: Children with AIDS have an increased risk of developing non-Hodgkin's lymphoma, Kaposi's sarcoma, and leiomyosarcoma.

7. *Answer:* D

Rationale: Neuroblastoma and Wilms' tumor are the most common intraabdominal tumors in children less than 1 year of age. Trey most likely has a neuroblastoma because his tumor crosses the midline (Wilms' tumors do not cross the midline), and because he has presented with a history of feeling systemic illness (fever, malaise, anorexia). Children with a Wilms' tumor often present with an abdominal mass but otherwise feeling well.

8. *Answer:* A
Rationale: The most common cancers in the 15- to 19-year old age group are Hodgkin's and non-Hodgkin's lymphoma. The most common symptoms of this cancer are a painless lump, recurrent fevers, cough, night sweats, dysphagia, and weight loss.

9. *Answer:* B
Rationale: Urine test for catecholamines is useful in the diagnosis of neuroblastoma. Although ultrasound and CAT scans may be indicated, the best initial tests would be a CBC, chest x-ray (to rule out mediastinal mass), and an ESR.

10. *Answer:* B
Rationale: Melissa will not be considered cured by the medical community until she reaches 5 years of disease-free survival.

11. *Answer:* A
Rationale: Neuroblastoma and retinoblastoma have a peak age at less than 1 year. Astrocytoma is fairly evenly distributed across the age groups. Acute lymphocytic leukemia has a peak incidence in the 1- to 4-year age group.

12. *Answer:* B
Rationale: With the exception of relapsed ALL, standard risk ALL has low mortality rates. AML continues to have higher mortality rates.

13. *Answer:* D
Rationale: Research shows a small likelihood that any single primary care provider will be involved in the diagnosis and referral of a child resulting in a confirmed diagnosis of cancer. Thus the diagnostic priorities shift

to identifying suspicious cases and making appropriate and prompt referrals.

14. *Answer:* A

Rationale: The primary provider plays a critical role in the care of the child undergoing cancer treatment through understanding the basic principles underlying childhood cancer treatment and providing the primary, preventive health maintenance and care of common acute illnesses to child and family throughout and following cancer treatment. The primary provider must refer any problems related to treatment or treatment side effects to the care providers at the childhood cancer treatment center.

15. *Answer:* A

Rationale: The stage of induction is described as intensive therapy that is used to remove the bulk of the disease in order to obtain remission. Consolidation, intensification, and maintenance therapy are used once the bulk of the disease has been removed and the patient is in remission.

16. *Answer:* C

Rationale: Autologous bone marrow transplant is defined as the reinfusion of a child's own bone marrow that had been removed before treatment.

17. *Answer:* D

Rationale: Biologic response modifiers are therapy directed at innate biologic systems (such as immunologic defense system) that are designed to destroy cells.

18. *Answer:* A

Rationale: When chemotherapy is given alone it may contribute to a temporary slowing of growth. Most children will experience catch-up growth once treatment is complete.

19. *Answer:* C

Rationale: Cranial radiation has been shown to most directly affect growth through damage to the endocrine glands responsible for growth-related hormone production.

20. *Answer:* B

Rationale: Height, weight, and BMI should be documented on standardized growth curves for all children every 2 months while the child is in therapy and for the first year after therapy. Head circumference should be documented and followed in children younger than 3 years of age.

21. *Answer:* C

Rationale: Children in the preoperational stage of development often feel as though their cancer is a form of justice for bad behavior. Once children reach the stage of formal operations they are more likely struggling with their inability to control the painful symptoms, treatments, or procedures.

22. *Answer:* D

Rationale: The younger the child was while undergoing childhood cancer treatment, the higher the risk for late effects.

23. *Answer:* A

Rationale: According to the Centers for Disease Control, live vaccines may be administered at or longer than 3 months after the termination of immunosuppressive therapy. Inactivated vaccines can be given at anytime; however, the immunosuppressed child may have a suboptimal response and should be revaccinated once immune competence is restored.

24. *Answer:* A

Rationale: Patients who have had Hodgkin's lymphoma are particularly susceptible to meningococcal disease.

25. *Answer:* D

Rationale: Leukokoria is the presence of a white reflex from the retina. This is an ominous sign for retinoblastoma.

BIBLIOGRAPHY

Alcoser, P.W., & Rodgers, C. (2003). Treatment strategies in childhood cancer. *J Pediatr Nurs, 18*(2), 103-112.

Areci, R.J., & Cripe, T.P. (2002). Emerging cancer-targeted therapies. *Pediatr Clin North Am, 49*(6), 1339-1368.

Arvidson, J., Lonnerholm, G., Tuvemo, T., et al. (2000). Prepubertal growth and growth hormone secretion in children after treatment for hematological malignancies, including autologous bone marrow transplantations. *Pediatr Hematol Oncol, 17*(4), 285-297.

Baggott, C., & Dragone, M.A. (2004). Cancer. In P.L. Jackson, & J.A. Vessey (Eds.). *Primary care of the child with a chronic condition* (4th ed.). St. Louis: Mosby.

Bergstrom, S.K. (2006). WAGR syndrome. Retrieved April 18, 2006, from http://www.emedicine.com/ped/topic2423.htm.

Bottomley, S.J., & Kassner, E. (2003). Late effects of childhood cancer therapy. *J Pediatr Nurs, 18*(2), 126-132.

Center for Disease Control and Prevention. (2006). National immunization program. Retrieved April 18, 200 from http://www.cdc.gov/nip/home-hcp.htm.

Chen, H. (2005). Klinefelter syndrome. Retrieved May 20, 2006, from www.emedicine.com/ped/topic1252.htm.

Cheung, N.K., & Rooney, C.M. (2002). Principles of immune and cellular therapy. In P.A. Pizzo & D.G. Poplack (Eds.). *Principles and practice of pediatric oncology* (4th ed.). Philadelphia: Lippincott Williams & Wilkins.

Feltbower, R.G., Lewis, I.J., Picton, S., et al. (2004). Diagnosing childhood cancer in primary care—A realistic expectation? *Brit J Cancer, 90*(10), 1882-1884.

Ferry, R.J., & Cohen, P. (2005). Beckwith-Wiedemann syndrome. Retrieved May 15, 2005, from www.emedicine.com/ped/topic218.htm.

Ganjavi, H., & Malkin, D. (August, 2002). Genetics of childhood cancer. *Clin Orthop Rel Res,* (401), 75-87.

Ghosh, S., & Jichici, D. (2005). Primitive neuroectodermal tumors of the central nervous system. Retrieved May 20, 2006, from http://www.emedicine.com/NEURO/topic326.htm.

Gulani, A. (2006). Von Hippel-Lindau disease. Retrieved May 20, 2006, from http://www.emedicine.com/OPH/topic354.htm.

Hasle, H., Clemmensen, I.H., & Mikkelsen, M. (2000). Risks of leukaemia and solid tumours in individuals with Down's syndrome. *Lancet, 355*(9199), 165-169.

Hudson, M.M., Mertens, A.C., Yasui, Y., et al. (2003). Health status of adult long-term survivors of childhood cancer: A report from the Childhood Cancer Survivor Study. *JAMA, 290,* 1583-1592.

Institute of Medicine. (2003). *Childhood cancer survivorship: Improving care and quality of life.* Washington, DC: The National Academies Press.

Jankovic, M., Spinetta, J.J., Martins, A.G., et al. (2004). Non-conventional therapies in childhood cancer: Guidelines for distinguishing non-harmful from harmful therapies: a report of the SIOP Working Committee on Psychosocial Issues in Pediatric Oncology. *Pediatr Blood Cancer, 42*(1), 106-108.

Jemal, A., Clegg, L.X., Ward, E., et al. (2004). Annual report to the nation on the status of cancer, 1975-2001, with a special feature regarding survival. *Cancer, 101*(1), 3-27.

Joswiak, S., Janniger, C.K., Kmiec, T., & Bernatowska, E. (2005). Ataxia-telangiectasia. Retrieved May 20, 2006, from www.emedicine.com/DERM/topic691.htm.

Kassner, E., Alcoser, P.W., & Hockenberry, M.J. (2002). Cancer in children. In K.L. McCance & S.E. Huether (Eds.). *Pathophysiology. The biologic basis for disease in adults and children* (4th ed.). Philadelphia: Mosby.

Liu, L. Krailo, M., Reaman, G.H., & Bernstein, L. (2003). Childhood cancer patients' access to cooperative group cancer programs: A population based study. *Cancer, 97*(5), 1339-1345.

Nagel, K., Eves, M., Waterhouse, L., et al. (2002). The development of an off-therapy needs questionnaire and protocol for survivors of childhood cancer. *J Pediatr Oncol Nurs, 19*(6), 229-233.

National Cancer Institute. (2005a). International classification of childhood cancer (ICCC). International Agency for Research on Cancer (IARC) Technical Report No. 29. Retrieved May 20, 2006, from http://seer.cancer.gov/iccc/iarciccc.html.

National Cancer Institute. (2005b). National Cancer Institute research on childhood cancers. Retrieved May 20, 2006, from http://cis.nci.nih.gov/fact/6_40.htm.

National Cancer Institute. (2005c). Surveillance, epidemiology and end results (SEER) modifications of the ICCC. Retrieved May 20, 2006, from http://seer.cancer.gov/iccc/seericcc.html.

National Cancer Institute. (2006). Late effects of childhood cancer therapies (PDQ®) Health Professional Version. Retrieved May 20, 2006, from www.nci.nih.gov/cancertopics/pdq/treatment/lateeffects/healthprofessional.

Oeffinger, K.C., & Hudson, M.M. (2004). Long-term complications following childhood and adolescent cancer: Foundations for providing risk-based health care for survivors. *CA Cancer J Clin, 54*(4), 208-236.

Pakakasama, S., & Tomlinson, G.E. (2002). Genetic predisposition and screening in pediatric cancer. *Pediatr Clin North Am, 49*(6), 1393-1413.

Plon, S.E., & Malkin, D. (2002). Childhood cancer and heredity. In P.A. Pizzo & D.G. Poplack (Eds.). *Principles and practice of pediatric oncology* (4th ed.). Philadelphia: Lippincott Williams & Wilkins.

Postellon, D. (2005). Turner syndrome. Retrieved May 20, 2006, from www.emedicine.com/ped/topic2330.htm.

Reaman, G.H. (2002). Pediatric oncology: Current views and outcomes. *Pediatr Clin North Am, 49*(6), 1305-1318, vii.

Ries, L.A.G., Harkins, D., Krapcho, M., et al. (Eds). (2006). *SEER Cancer Statistics Review, 1975-2003*, National Cancer Institute. Bethesda, MD, http://seer.cancer.gov/csr/1975_2003/ based on November 2005 SEER data submission, posted to the SEER web site, 2006.

Tarbell, N.J., & Kooy, H.M. (2002). General principles of radiation oncology. In P.A. Pizzo & D.G. Poplack (Eds.). *Principles and practice of pediatric oncology* (4th ed.). Philadelphia: Lippincott Williams & Wilkins.

Woodgate, R.L., & Degner, L.F. (2003). A substantive theory of keeping the spirit alive: The spirit within children with cancer and their families. *J Pediatr Oncol Nurs, 20*(3), 103-119.

Young, G., Toretsky, J.A., Campbell, A.B., & Eskenazi, A.E. (2000). Recognition of common childhood malignancies. *Am Fam Phys, 61*(7), 2144-2154.

Zebrack, B.J., & Zeltzer, L.K. (2003). Quality of life issues and cancer survivorship. *Curr Prob Cancer, 27*(4), 198-211.

NOTES

39 Cleft Lip and Palate

VICTORIA P. NIEDERHAUSER

Select the best answer for each of the following questions:

1. Cleft lip and palate occur in the developing embryo between:
   A. 1 to 3 weeks gestation.
   B. 3 to 12 weeks gestation.
   C. 12 to 18 weeks gestation.
   D. 18 to 24 weeks gestation.

2. A cleft lip that is one-sided and extends from the vermilion-cutaneous junction to two-thirds the height of the lip is classified as:
   A. Bilateral complete.
   B. Unilateral complete.
   C. Bilateral incomplete.
   D. Unilateral incomplete.

3. Upon examination of the oral cavity in Travis, a 2-day-old, the pediatric nurse practitioner observes a cleft uvula. The nursery nurses say that Travis takes a long time to feed. What should be the next action?
   A. Obtain a throat culture.
   B. Examine the hard and soft palate.
   C. Order a dietitian consultation.
   D. Palpate for cervical adenopathy.

4. Which of the following statements about the incidence and prevalence of cleft lip and palate is NOT true?
   A. In the United States, the incidence of cleft lip is higher than the incidence of cleft palate.
   B. Left unilateral clefts occur less frequently compared to right unilateral clefts.

C. Three percent of all cleft palates are submucosal cleft palates.
D. Cleft lips and palates occur more frequently in males.

5. Liza, a 16-year-old African American, is 24 weeks into her pregnancy. She has gestational diabetes that is well-controlled. She smokes 2 packs of cigarettes per day and she takes ibuprofen daily for back pain. Which of the following puts Liza's baby at risk for cleft lip and palate?
   A. African American race.
   B. Well-controlled gestational diabetes.
   C. Cigarette smoking.
   D. Daily ibuprofen.

6. Martha, a mother of a 9-month-old girl with a cleft lip and palate, asked the pediatric nurse practitioner why her daughter gets so many ear infections. The BEST response is:
   A. Infants with cleft lip and palate may have abnormal palate muscles or problems with their eustachian tubes that put them at risk for increased ear infections.
   B. The positive middle ear pressure causes an increase in ear infections in infants with cleft lip and palate.
   C. There is no relationship between increased ear infections and cleft lip and palate.
   D. There is an increase in the amount of bacteria in the throats and ear canals of infants with cleft lip and palate; this causes an increase in ear infections.

7. Jane is 26 weeks pregnant with her first baby. The ultrasound of the fetus done at

16 weeks gestation revealed a unilateral cleft lip. What advice should the pediatric nurse practitioner provide to Jane regarding breast-feeding her newborn?

A. Breastfeeding will likely cause an increase of ear infections in the newborn; therefore, it is not recommended.
B. Infants with cleft lip are likely to be successful at breastfeeding because the breast tissue will fill in the gap in the lip.
C. Newborn infants should be in a supine position when breastfeeding to allow for a better seal.
D. Breastfeeding will not be possible, as the newborn will not be able to suck at birth.

8. Primary care of the child with cleft lip and palate includes all of the following EXCEPT:

A. Monitoring growth.
B. Routine immunizations.
C. Evaluation of developmental milestones.

D. Encourage socialization in large day-care settings.

9. When is the ideal age for cleft lip repair surgery?

A. Immediately after delivery.
B. 2 weeks.
C. Between 2 and 6 months.
D. After 12 months.

10. The pediatric nurse practitioner is giving discharge instructions to parents of Sadie who just had her cleft lip repaired. For care of the suture line, Sadie's parents should:

A. Gently cleanse the suture line with half-strength hydrogen peroxide or saline.
B. Massage the suture line twice daily to prevent scarring.
C. Allow Sadie to get direct sunlight on her face for 2 hours each day.
D. Apply moisturizer cream to sutures three times daily.

NOTES

ANSWERS

1. *Answer:* B
   Rationale: Cleft lips and palates result from a failure of fusion of one or more of the five primordial prominences between 3 and 12 weeks gestation.

2. *Answer:* D
   Rationale: A unilateral incomplete cleft lip that is one-sided and extends from the vermilion-cutaneous junction to two-thirds the height of the lip. Bilateral cleft lip includes both sides and a complete cleft extends into the nasal cavity.

3. *Answer:* B
   Rationale: The pediatric nurse practitioner should examine the soft and hard palate because a subcutaneous cleft palate is often associated with a cleft uvula. Presence of a notch on the posterior border of the hard palate can be a sign of a submucosal cleft; an MRI can confirm the diagnosis.

4. *Answer:* B
   Rationale: In the United States, the incidence of cleft lips is 6 per 10,000 live births and cleft palates are 11 per 10,000 live births. The left unilateral cleft lips occur twice as frequently compared to the right unilateral cleft lips.

5. *Answer:* C
   Rationale: Compared to Asians, whites, Hispanics, and Native Americans, African Americans have the lowest incidence of cleft lip and palate. Cigarette smoking is a risk factor: maternal use of 20 or more cigarettes per day increases the risk of cleft lip and palate two-fold. Uncontrolled gestational diabetes also puts the fetus at risk for cleft lip and palate. Ibuprofen has not been associated with cleft lip and palate.

6. *Answer:* A
   Rationale: Infants with cleft lip and palate are at increased risk of chronic ear infections due to abnormal palate muscles or problems with their eustachian tubes and negative middle-ear pressure.

7. *Answer:* B
   Rationale: Breastfeeding should be encouraged in all infants, especially those infants with cleft lip and palate. The breast tissue is soft and will sometimes form the needed seal to enhance sucking. The protective immunity acquired with breastfeeding can decrease the incidence of ear infections in these infants. To prevent nasal regurgitation, these infants should be fed in a semi-upright position.

8. *Answer:* D
   Rationale: Avoiding large daycare settings will minimize exposures to respiratory and other infectious agents that can cause otitis media and other respiratory infections.

9. *Answer:* C
   Rationale: Most cleft lips are repaired between 2 and 6 months of age. Some health professionals go by the rule of 10s; at least 10 weeks, weighing at least 10 kg, and hemoglobin of at least 10.

10. *Answer:* A
    Rationale: Postoperatively, the suture line should be cleansed gently with half-strength hydrogen peroxide or normal saline. Exposing the wound to direct sunlight, applying moisturizer, and massaging the suture line are not standard care.

BIBLIOGRAPHY

Anastassov, G.E., & Joos, U. (2001). Comprehensive management of cleft lip and palate deformities. *J Oral Maxillofac Surg, 59*(9), 1062-1075.

Balasubrahanyam, G., Scherer, N.J., Martin, J., Michael, M. (1998). Cleft lip and palate: Keys to successful management. *Contemp Pediatr, 15*(ii), 133.

Bender, P.L. (2000). Genetics of cleft lip and palate. *J Pediatr Nurs, 15*(4), 242-249.

Broder, H.L., Smith, T.B., & Strauss, R.P. (2001). Developing a behavioral rating scale for comparing teachers' rating of children with and without craniofacial anomalies. *Cleft Palate Craniofac J, 38*(6), 560-565.

Centers for Disease Control and Prevention (CDC). (2006). Improved National Prevalence Estimates for 18 Selected Major Birth Defects—United States, 1999-2001. *MMWR, 54*(51 & 52), 1301-1305.

Chapple, J.R., & Nunn, J.H. (2001). The oral health of children with clefts of the lip, palate, or both. *Cleft Palate Craniofac J, 38*(5), 525-528.

Curtin, G., & Boekelheide, A. (2004). Cleft lip and palate. In P.L. Jackson & J.A. Vessey (Eds.). *Primary care of the child with a chronic condition* (4th ed.). St. Louis: Mosby.

Grow, J.L., & Lehman, J.A. (2002). A local perspective on the initial management of children with cleft lip and palate by primary care physicians. *Cleft Palate Craniofac J, 39*(5), 535-540.

Jones, K.L. (2005). *Smith's recognizable patterns of human malformation* (6th ed.). Philadelphia: Saunders.

Kapp-Simon, K.A. (2004). Psychological issues in cleft lip and palate. *Clin Plast Surg, 31*(2), 347-352.

Kirschner, R.E., & LaRossa, D. (2000). Cleft lip and palate. *Otolaryngol Clin North Am, 33*(6), 1191-1215.

Kreins, O. (1989). IAHSHAL. A concise documentation system for cleft lip, alveolus, and palate diagnoses. In O. Kriens (Ed.). *What is a cleft lip and palate? A multidisciplinary update*. Stuttgart, Germany: Thieme.

Kuehn, D.P., Ettema, S.L., Goldwasser, M.S., et al. (2001). Magnetic resonance imaging in the evaluation of occult submucous cleft palate. *Cleft Palate Craniofac J, 38*(5), 421-431.

Lidral, A.C., & Moreno, L.M. (2005). Progress toward discerning the genetics of cleft lip. *Curr Opin Pediatr, 17*(6), 731-739.

Moore, K.L., & Persaud, T.V.N. (2003). *The developing human: Clinically oriented embryology* (6th ed.). Philadelphia: Saunders.

Sandberg, D.J., Magee, W.P., & Denk, M.P. (2002). Neonatal cleft lip and cleft palate repair. *AORN J, 75*(3), 490-499.

Sheahan, P., & Blayney, A.W. (2003). Cleft palate and otitis media with effusion: A review. *Rev Laryngol Otol Rhinol, 124*(3), 171-177.

Spilson, S.V., Kim, H.J., & Chung, K.C. (2001). Association between maternal diabetes mellitus and newborn oral cleft. *Ann Plast Surg, 47*(5), 477-481.

Thigpen, J.L., & Kenner, C. (2003). Assessment and management of the gastrointestinal system In C. Kenner & J.W. Lott (Eds.). *Comprehensive neonatal nursing: A physiologic perspective*. Philadelphia: Saunders.

Wyszynski, D.F., Sarkozi, A., Vargha, P., & Czeilel, A.E. (2003). Birth weight and gestational age of newborns with cleft lip with or without cleft palate. *J Clin Pediatr Dent, 27*(2), 185-190.

Young, J.L., O'Riordan, M., Goldstein, J.A., & Robin, N.H. (2001). What information do parents of newborns with cleft lip, palate, or both want to know? *Cleft Palate Craniofac J, 38*(1), 55-58.

NOTES

40 Common Genetic Conditions in Children

IRMA LARA AND ROSE A. SALDIVAR

Select the best answer for each of the following questions:

1. The mother of a newborn child diagnosed with galactosemia asks you whether she will still be able to breastfeed. Your BEST answer would be:
   A. Breastfeeding is contraindicated in babies with galactosemia.
   B. You can continue with your plans to breastfeed.
   C. Bottle feed with your preferred commercial formula.
   D. You can breastfeed and supplement with formula.

2. Common causes of classic inborn error of metabolism (IEM) are:
   A. A defect in the lack of activity of a specific enzyme involved in amino acids, carbohydrates, and protein metabolism.
   B. A defect in the lack of activity of a specific enzyme involved in amino acid, carbohydrates, or lipid metabolism.
   C. A defect in the lack of activity of a specific enzyme involved in amino acids and carbohydrates metabolism.
   D. A defect in the lack of activity of a specific enzyme involved in amino acids, carbohydrates, or vitamin metabolism.

3. You are a pediatric nurse practitioner providing the mother of a child diagnosed with PKU with nutritional instruction about foods low in phenylanine. Which of the following foods are permitted?
   A. Milk, eggs, and chicken.
   B. Milk, meat, and beans.
   C. Orange juice, bananas, and potatoes.
   D. Orange juice, eggs, and turkey.

4. As the pediatric nurse practitioner providing well baby visits to Sally, the mother of a child with PKU, you must advise her that her child will need to be regularly monitored for which of the following?
   A. Plasma phenylalanine and hemoglobin levels.
   B. Plasma phenylalanine and hepatic levels.
   C. Plasma purified protein derivative and hemoglobin levels.
   D. Plasma prostatic acid and hepatic levels.

5. A newly diagnosed child with galactosemia may present with clinical symptoms of listlessness accompanied by:
   A. High blood sugar and tremors.
   B. High blood sugar and seizures.
   C. Low blood sugar and death.
   D. Lethargy and low blood sugar.

6. As the pediatric nurse practitioner, you instruct the parents of a child with galactosemia that the child must be provided with dietary supplements of what type of nutrient?
   A. Vitamin D.
   B. Selenium.
   C. Calcium.
   D. Vitamin C.

7. MSUD is rare, but relatively easy to detect. Usually detected by the first day of

life, the urine develops a characteristic smell of:

    A. "Musty" odor.
    B. "Sour" odor.
    C. "Burnt sugar" odor.
    D. "Fruity" odor.

8. A child diagnosed with MSUD has diet restrictions which require what type of modifications?

    A. High in amino acids, isoleucine, valine, and lysine.
    B. High in amino acids, lysine, isoleucine, and leucine.
    C. Low in amino acids, leucine, isoleucine, and valine.
    D. Low in amino acids, lysine, isoleucine, and valine.

9. While planning activities for school-age children with Down syndrome you must remember to take into consideration the children's:

    A. Willingness to participate.
    B. Chronological age.
    C. Developmental age.
    D. Gestational age.

10. The three classical physical features seen in children with fragile X syndrome are:

    A. Short narrow face, small ears, and enlarged testicles postpubescence.
    B. Long narrow face, prominent large ears, and enlarged testicles postpubescence.
    C. Long narrow face, small ears, and small testicles postpubescence.
    D. Short narrow face, prominent large ears, and enlarged testicles postpubescence.

11. The pediatric nurse practitioner who works in a specialty clinic for inherited disorders is evaluating a 6-year-old boy whose parents were referred by the school nurse due to poor attention span, speech delay, hyperactivity, and lack of age-appropriate social skills. Comments from his teacher also include that he is not able to complete his first-grade schoolwork. Which of the following diagnosis will you suspect?

    A. Down syndrome.
    B. Fragile X syndrome.
    C. Tay-Sachs disease.
    D. Klinefelter's syndrome.

12. What are two characteristic features of the newborn child with fetal alcohol syndrome?

    A. Short palpebral fissures and a small upper lip.
    B. Long palpebral fissures and a short upper lip.
    C. Long palpebral fissures and a long upper lip.
    D. Short palpebral fissures and a thin upper lip.

13. Which statement accurately reflects the most important indicator that a child is possibly presenting with an IEM disorder?

    A. Loss of a developmental milestone is evident within the first 3 months of birth.
    B. Most symptoms of the disorder develop after a change in diet has taken place.
    C. Progressive deterioration of the symptoms occurs after an initial period of apparent good health.
    D. Symptoms of developmental delay usually occur within 1 month of birth

14. Newborn screening policies vary from state to state. Two newborn screenings are universally mandated in all states. These screenings are:

    A. Galactosemia and sickle cell disease.
    B. PKU and congenital hypothyroidism.
    C. MSUD and PKU.
    D. Biotinidase deficiency and galactosemia.

15. Biotinidase deficiency may present itself with numerous clinical symptoms such as hypotonia, eczematous rash, alopecia, and seizures. Seizures for this genetic disorder can be described as:

    A. Generalized tonic-clonic.
    B. Infantile spasms.
    C. Not responsive to conventional therapies.
    D. Seizures in combination with other clinical symptoms of the disorder.

16. Galactosemia is a carbohydrate metabolism disorder where the body is unable to metabolize the simple sugar galactose. Removing lactose from the diet largely eliminates the toxic effects of the disease. Which of the following statements regarding dietary restrictions of this disorder is NOT accurate?
  A. All milk and milk-containing products must be avoided throughout the patient's lifetime.
  B. All lactose-free foods are also galactose-free.
  C. Infants may be fed soy or lactose-free formulas.
  D. Calcium supplementation will be required for an infant on soy formulas.

17. Gastrointestinal problems more commonly seen in a child with Down syndrome are Hirschsprung's disease and _____.
  A. Pyloric stenosis.
  B. Intussusception.
  C. Duodenal atresia.
  D. Gastroesophageal reflux.

18. The most common cause of mental retardation in the United States, approximately 1 to 2 out of 1000 births, is identified as:
  A. Down syndrome.
  B. Fetal alcohol syndrome.
  C. PKU.
  D. Congenital hypothyroidism.

19. You are the pediatric nurse practitioner providing home care instruction to the parents of a school-age child with MSUD. To assist the child with social acceptance by peers, parents should provide the school with:
  A. A list of acceptable snacks for special occasions, such as holidays and birthdays.
  B. Telephone numbers of specialty clinics for additional information on MSUD.
  C. A comprehensive nutritional book including portion size, calories, protein, and leucine content.
  D. A detailed schedule of activities in which the child is capable of participating without increasing risk of injury.

20. Down syndrome is an inherited congenital defect which results in mental retardation. This is the result of an extra chromosome which is found on which chromosomal number?
  A. Chromosome 3.
  B. Chromosome 22.
  C. Chromosome 21.
  D. Sex chromosome.

21. The second most common cause of genetically associated mental deficiencies is identified as:
  A. Trisomy 21.
  B. Trisomy 18.
  C. Fragile X.
  D. Turner's syndrome.

22. A 5-year-old boy has PKU. Which of the following foods on his lunch tray would you question?
  A. A dish of apples.
  B. A lettuce salad.
  C. Orange juice.
  D. Chocolate pudding.

23. A pediatric nurse practitioner holds a health education class for parents of children with PKU, galactosemia, and biotinidase deficiency. A common objective reinforced in this class on early and maintenance care is avoidance of:
  A. Obesity.
  B. Communicable diseases.
  C. Developmental delays.
  D. Milk products.

24. Galactosemia is a disorder of carbohydrate metabolism. Often classified as an inborn error of metabolism, the child is deficient in the liver enzyme galactose 1-phosphate uridyltransferase. Which diet restriction is required to avoid irreversible neurologic damage to the child?
  A. Wheat products.
  B. Milk products.
  C. Protein products.
  D. Lipid products.

ANSWERS

1. *Answer:* A
   Rationale: Breastfeeding is contraindicated in babies with galactosemia due the inability to digest lactose in milk.

2. *Answer:* B
   Rationale: Classic inborn error of metabolism (IEM) is caused by a defect in the activity of a specific enzyme involved in amino acids, carbohydrates, or lipid metabolism.

3. *Answer:* C
   Rationale: A child with PKU should avoid protein-rich foods.

4. *Answer:* A
   Rationale: Phenylalanine and hemoglobin levels should be closely monitored to ensure that the child is not becoming anemic because iron is found in protein-rich foods which are contraindicated in children with high phenylalanine.

5. *Answer:* D
   Rationale: Signs and symptoms of galactosemia are vomiting, low blood sugar, lethargy, irritability, convulsions, enlarged liver, and jaundice. If untreated, galactosemia leads to cirrhosis of the liver, cataracts, and mental retardation.

6. *Answer:* C
   Rationale: Infant's diet will be soy formula or other lactose-free formula so calcium supplementation is important because soy products are not rich in calcium.

7. *Answer:* C
   Rationale: Urine of a child with MSUD smells like maple syrup or burnt sugar.

8. *Answer:* C
   Rationale: Long-term management involves dietary restrictions of the three branched-chain amino acids (leucine, isoleucine, and valine).

9. *Answer:* C
   Rationale: Activities must be planned toward the developmental age of the child.

10. *Answer:* B
    Rationale: Physical features of a child with fragile X syndrome include high arched palate, long face, and large testicles in males. They have a characteristic "look" (long face and large ears).

11. *Answer:* B
    Rationale: Fifteen to twenty percent of children affected with fragile X syndrome may exhibit autistic-type behaviors, such as poor eye contact, hand flapping or odd gestures, and poor sensory skills. Speech and/or language delays are common features of fragile X syndrome.

12. *Answer:* D
    Rationale: The facial abnormalities of child with fetal alcohol syndrome include small eye opening, indistinct or flat philtrum, and thin upper lip.

13. *Answer:* C
    Rationale: Symptoms of an inborn error of metabolism become evident usually after some level of good health. In part, this is due to absence of or a build-up of an enzyme or metabolite. Symptoms may become present within the first week of life or thereafter.

14. *Answer:* B
    Rationale: Screening for PKU and congenital hypothyroidism are universally mandated in 51 jurisdictions. The next highest frequency tests are for galactosemia and sickle cell disease.

15. *Answer:* C
    Rationale: Seizures along with other clinical manifestations may not respond to conventional therapies. Seizures respond rapidly to pharmacologic dosing of biotin.

16. *Answer:* B
    Rationale: Some lactose-free foods still contain free galactose.

17. *Answer:* C
    Rationale: Hirschsprung's disease and duodenal atresia are gastrointestinal problems seen in 10% of Down syndrome children.

18. *Answer:* B

Rationale: Fetal alcohol syndrome occurs in approximately 1 to 2 out of every 1000 births.

19. *Answer:* A

Rationale: Social acceptance from peers is important. Most children at this age are aware of diet restrictions. Providing the school officials with a list of acceptable snacks allows the child to participate with peer activities. Options B and D will not assist the child developing peer acceptance. Option D provides more information than is necessary.

20. *Answer:* C

Rationale: Down syndrome, also referred to as trisomy 21, is identified with an additional chromosome on 21.

21. *Answer:* C

Rationale: Fragile X is the second most common cause of genetically associated mental deficiencies. Trisomy 21 (Down syndrome) is the most common.

22. *Answer:* D

Rationale: Milk products contain phenylalanine and should be avoided.

23. *Answer:* C

Rationale: Health instruction should include nutrition guidelines for specific disorders, regular pediatric care clinic visits, immunizations, and follow-up appointments with their specialty clinics as needed. Regular evaluations help detect developmental delays and provide avenue to strengthen these deficiencies.

24. *Answer:* B

Rationale: Lactose is the sugar found in milk. This is normally broken down in to galactose and glucose. Without the required enzyme, this breakdown cannot take place causing a build-up of galactose. Placing the child on a formula with milk substitute is required.

BIBLIOGRAPHY

American Academy of Pediatrics (AAP) Committee on Genetics. (2001). Policy Statement: Health supervision for children with Down syndrome. *Pediatrics, 107*(2), 442-449.

American Academy of Pediatrics (AAP) Committee on Genetics. (1996). Policy Statement: Health supervision for children with fragile X syndrome. *Pediatrics, 98*(2), 297-300.

American Academy of Pediatrics (AAP) Committee on Substance Abuse and Committee on Children with Disabilities. (2000). Policy Statement: Fetal alcohol syndrome & alcohol related neurodevelopmental disorders. *Pediatrics, 106*(2), 358-361.

Anadiotis, G.A., & Berry, G.T. (2006). Galactose-1-phosphate uridyltransferase deficiency (galactosemia). Retrieved May 21, 2006, from www.emedicine.com/ped/topic818.htm.

Anonymous. (1999). Health care guidelines for Down syndrome. *Down Synd Quart, 4*(3), 1-16.

Baloghova, J., & Schwartz, R.A. (2005). Homocystinuria. Retrieved May 21, 2006, from www.emedicine.com/ped/topic708.htm.

Bodamer, O.A., & Lee, B. (2006). Maple syrup urine disease. Retrieved May 21, 2006, from www.emedicine.com/ped/topic1368.htm.

Bosch, J.J. (2003). Health maintenance throughout the life span for individuals with Down syndrome. *J Am Acad Nurse Pract 15*(1), 5-17.

Difazio, M.P., & Davis, R.G. (2006). Biotinidase deficiency. Retrieved May 21, 2006, from www.emedicine.com/ped/topic239.htm.

March of Dimes. (2004). PKU. Retrieved May 21, 2006, from www.marchofdimes.com/professionals/681_1219.asp.

National Coalition for Health Professional Education in Genetics (NCHPEG). (2005). *Core competencies in genetics essential for all health-care professionals* (2nd ed.). Lutherville, MD: NCHPEG.

Philofsky, A., Hepburn, S.L., Hayes, A., et al. (2004). Linguistic and cognitive functioning and autism symptoms in young children with fragile X syndrome. *Am J Ment Retard AJMR, 109*(3), 208-218.

Roizen, N.J. (2002). Medical care and monitoring for the adolescent with Down syndrome. *Adolesc Med (Philadelphia), 13*(2), 345-358.

Roth, K.S. (2005). Galactokinase deficiency. Retrieved on May 21, 2006 from http://www.emedicine.com/ped/topic815.htm.

Weiner, D.L., & Wilkes, G. (2005). Inborn errors of metabolism. Retrieved on May 21, 2006 from http://www.emedicine.com/emerg/topic768.htm.

Williams, J. (2002). Education for genetics and nursing practice. *AACN Clin Issues, 13*(4), 492-500.

41 Common Mental Health Disorders in Children and Adolescents

DEBORAH SHELTON

Select the best answer for each of the following questions:

1. The domains most frequently assessed in children during a psychiatric assessment include:
   A. Likelihood of staying in therapy.
   B. Intelligence and cognitive functioning.
   C. Type of therapy to recommend.
   D. Behavior, but only if aggression is present.

2. A 16-year-old female junior in high school has been in trouble with school authorities since age 12 for petty theft. She has a history of truancy, and has most recently been expelled for smoking marijuana in the bathroom and setting fire to an abandoned house. She has been admitted to a psychiatric hospital for her behavioral problems. Her parents are unable to control her, and they state that she lies constantly, stays out all night without telling them where she is going, and is frequently angry with them when they try to intervene. You would consider which of the following diagnoses?
   A. Major depressive disorder.
   B. Conduct disorder.
   C. Oppositional defiant disorder.
   D. Bipolar disorder.

3. You are asked to reevaluate a child with oppositional defiant disorder and cooccurring learning disabilities and to develop a treatment plan. You base your treatment plan on:
   A. Medication use targeting symptoms of the primary diagnosis.

B. Working with the teacher to address the learning disability.
   C. Family behavioral therapy to interrupt coercive family processes.
   D. Building recreational activities into the child's daily schedule.

4. For the child who does not respond to a compliant-centered line of questioning, the strategy to be taken is:
   A. Stay with this tactic until the child gives in.
   B. Broaden the focus and ask the child to talk about more general aspects of life.
   C. Send the child away until he or she is ready to answer the questions.
   D. Don't include the child in the assessment.

5. One approach to the problem of aggression in psychiatrically referred juveniles is to consider aggression as a dimensional characteristic of patients that may be continuously present but in varying degrees across many different psychiatric disorders. With this dimensional approach to aggression, psychiatric medications are prescribed to:
   A. Target the primary diagnosis.
   B. Target aggression as a symptom.
   C. Target associated conditions, such as anxiety.
   D. Avoid dealing with the family.

6. The parents of a 3-year-old report that their son seems to be having difficulty with motor skills such as building blocks. Upon assessment, you find the child has more limited verbal skills than expected for his age

and is he has poor walking coordination. You would suspect which diagnosis?

A. Autistic disorder.
B. Asperger's disorder.
C. Childhood disintegrative disorder.
D. Rett's disorder.

7. The primary goal in treatment for a child diagnosed with autistic disorder is:

A. Advancement of normal development.
B. Assistance to families in coping with the disorder.
C. Long-term individual therapy.
D. Residential programming.

8. Carol, a first grader, is persistently refusing to go to school. She has always been a "clingy child," but this has become worse in the past 4 months. She follows her mother around the house and will not play unless her parents are in the room. Carol's mother reports that Carol has tantrums if she goes out to dinner with her husband. You might suspect that Carol is experiencing:

A. Separation anxiety.
B. Difficulty learning.
C. Early antisocial behavior.
D. Developmental delay.

9. According to the American Psychiatric Association DSM-IV Multiaxial Classification System (DSM-IV), which axis is considered psychosocial and environmental problems?

A. 1
B. 2
C. 3
D. 4

10. Mark, age 10, has had several major depressive disorder (MDD) episodes. His history shows that he had a rapid onset to his depression. Two of his mother's siblings have a history of depression. These episodes may be an early marker for:

A. Body dysmorphic disorder.
B. Trichotillomania.
C. Narcolepsy.
D. Bipolar disorder.

11. Peter, a 16-year-old, is expelled from school for repeated violations for disruptive behavior and breaking rules. He has a history of truancy and failing grades for several years, since the onset of these behaviors. Peter is unpopular with his peers, really doesn't have any friends, and spends a lot of time by himself. You would expect him to carry a diagnosis of:

A. Conduct disorder, adolescent onset.
B. Oppositional defiant disorder.
C. Unsocialized conduct disorder.
D. Delinquent.

12. David is a high-functioning 14-year-old boy diagnosed with autistic disorder. He has had individual and family therapy for several months. He is an awkward-looking adolescent who looks and acts younger than his chronologic age. His academic level is above average, but his social development is limited. He's just starting the seventh grade. You would recommend what type of treatment approach?

A. Group therapy.
B. Individual therapy.
C. Family therapy.
D. No further treatment.

13. Carla is a 16-year-old mildly depressed female who behaves immaturely for her age. She is struggling in high school, with attendance a major issue. In class, she disrupts the class process by a number of pranks to draw attention to herself. What type of group modality would be appropriate for Carla?

A. A psychotherapy group of both boys and girls with varied diagnoses.
B. A play therapy group of girls with mental health problems.
C. A school social club with both boys and girls from the same high school.
D. An activity psychotherapy group with other high school girls.

14. Mark is 8 years old and was referred by his pediatrician for evaluation because of serious weight loss without a medical cause. Upon examination, you note that Mark is extremely concerned about his weight and weighs himself daily. He complains he is too fat, and if he does not lose weight he cuts back on his food intake. He has lost 10 pounds in the past year and still thinks he's too fat. It

is clear he is underweight. The scales have been removed from the house by his parents, so Mark now counts calories. He checks and rechecks this frequently. Your primary diagnosis would be:

A. Bulimia.
B. Obsessive-compulsive disorder.
C. Anorexia nervosa.
D. Depression.

15. The treatment of eating disorders does not focus primarily upon pharmacologic interventions. Yet, pharmacologic interventions may be useful in treating target symptoms of obsessions and compulsions, high levels of anxiety, and depression. In considering the use of medications, you know that the compromised metabolism of many patients with eating disorders can put them at high risk for cardiac arrhythmias if:

A. Cyproheptadine (Periactin) is prescribed for anorexia nervosa.
B. Tricyclic antidepressants are prescribed for depressive features for anorexia nervosa.
C. High doses of fluoxetine are prescribed for bulimia nervosa.
D. Bupropion is prescribed for bulimia nervosa.

16. Patti, age 8, is an unusually quiet child who rarely smiles. She has been brought to the clinic with a history of sexual abuse for 2 years by her father. Since that time, she spends most of her time in her room alone watching television. She has difficulty falling asleep and reports nightmares about her father coming into her room. She fears that her father will come and attack her. She is generally irritable and often fights with siblings, and feels her mother "picks on her," and favors her siblings. Based on this history, the most likely diagnosis is:

A. Sleep disorder.
B. Posttraumatic stress disorder (PTSD).
C. Dysthymic disorder.
D. Depression, single episode.

17. Clinical assessment of a traumatized child should include information from the child and the nonabusing parent. This assessment places particular emphasis on:

A. Removal from the home.
B. Utilization of PTSD symptom inventories.
C. Putting the father in jail.
D. The current safety of the child.

18. Psychoeducational interventions are currently considered the mainstay of therapeutic treatment for the traumatized child or adolescent with a diagnosis of PTSD. A cognitive-behavioral therapeutic approach would work to:

A. Educate the traumatized child about the disorder.
B. Transform the child's self-concept from victim to survivor.
C. Assist the parents to manage their own trauma and emotional distress.
D. Desensitization to fear-inducing environmental stimuli that are reminders of the trauma.

19. The scientific body of literature that is emerging on the neurobiology of stress and trauma guide clinical pharmacology practice in PTSD. As a pediatric nurse practitioner, you know that the scientific work completed thus far:

A. Is based upon the adult population.
B. Suggests that the central nervous system is the primary neurobiological system that mediates the stress response.
C. Targets the immune system for psychopharmacologic interventions.
D. Does not support use of medication in children who are diagnosed with PTSD.

20. Portia, an 11-year old girl, thinks she is "going crazy." Over the past 2 months, she has awakened confused about where she is until she realizes that she is on the couch in the living room, or one of her sibling's bedrooms, when she knows she went to sleep in her own room. Her younger sister says that she has seen Portia looking like she is a "zombie," that she has done this several times, and that she did not answer when she called her. Portia fears she may have "amnesia" as she does not recall anything happening during the night. There is no history of

seizures, the electrocardiogram and physical exam are normal, Portia's mental status is unremarkable, and the family functions well. You would consider which diagnosis?
A. Sleepwalking disorder.
B. Sleep apnea.
C. Narcolepsy.
D. Disturbed nocturnal sleep.

21. Unusual arousal events during sleep occur most frequently in childhood because:
A. They are tied to deep stages of sleep.
B. Childhood is when the largest amount of slow-wave sleep occurs.
C. Children fall asleep rapidly and arousal events occur immediately.
D. Children nap frequently during the day.

22. Treatment of parasomnias in children focuses upon:
A. Prescribing benzodiazepines for the child with occasional sleepwalking.
B. Support to parents, including education about the nature of sleep.
C. Ensuring that the child does not nap during the day.
D. Informing the parents that sleepwalking is a precursor for a more serious mental disorder.

23. Paula, a 15-year-old, is brought to the clinic by her father after getting a call from the school counselor who was concerned that she was depressed and possibly suicidal. Her father also noticed that she seemed withdrawn and sad over the past month. Paula reports that her mood is much worse in the last 6 months, feeling depressed every day, all day long. She has lost interest in school and social activities. Paula is tired all the time and takes naps after school. At night she has trouble falling asleep, and trouble getting up in the morning. She reports increased feelings of anxiety and at times feeling "spacey." She is convinced she does not deserve to live and has considered killing herself with a kitchen knife when she does the dishes. She is diagnosed with major depressive disorder. As you consider prescribing antidepressant medication, you know that:
A. Asking about her suicidal ideas would reinforce her suicidality.

B. Close supervision for increased suicidality is needed for the first 4 weeks.
C. Her suicidal impulses are under control because she has not acted upon them.
D. Her father must be on the alert at all times because she could impulsively commit suicide.

24. Your assessment of a depressed adolescent reveals suicidal ideation, but the family support suggests that they can handle ambulatory treatment. Recommendations for management of the ambulatory suicidal patient include:
A. Medication should be withheld from the suicidal patient in all cases.
B. Minimize the number of medications available in the home to reduce the opportunity for overdose.
C. It is developmentally appropriate for parents to permit the teen to manage his or her medication.
D. The primary care provider does not need to consult with a child and adolescent mental health provider.

25. John, a 17-year-old with a history of depression, has been successfully treated with SSRIs. John has been compliant with this medication regimen, participates in regular therapy groups, and has been managing his depressive disorder well. However, at a high-school graduation party, he consumes alcohol and decides to experiment with cocaine when all of his friends goad him into trying it. Later that evening, when John gets home, his mother observes that he is acting drunk, tripping over his own feet. He also seems confused and shaky. Although she is concerned, it is not until he has a temperature and diarrhea that she decides to take him to the emergency room and call you, his pediatric health provider. You would suspect which of the following?
A. Central serotonin syndrome.
B. Acute dystonic reaction.
C. Neuroleptic-induced dyskinesia.
D. Akathisia.

ANSWERS

1. ***Answer:*** B
   Rationale: The domains most frequently assessed in children include current level of development; intelligence and cognitive functioning across a variety of processing abilities; academic achievement; personality, coping, and defensive strategies; type and severity of psychopathology; neuropsychologic dysfunction; and acquisition of adaptive or independence skills.

2. ***Answer:*** B
   Rationale: The repetitive and pervasive pattern of violating the basic rights of others and major age-appropriate social norms or rules indicates conduct disorder. Because the onset is after age 10, it would indicate adolescent onset type, which generally has a better prognosis than childhood onset type.

3. ***Answer:*** C
   Rationale: Oppositional defiant disorder is not considered to be medication-responsive. Treatment emphasizes parent management, behavioral training, and family behavioral therapy focused on interrupting coercive family processes. Psychopharmacologic interventions target associated comorbid disorders such as anxiety or depression.

4. ***Answer:*** B
   Rationale: When children do not respond to a standard, direct, compliant-centered line of questioning, even after several attempts, the clinician is advised to ask the child to talk about more general aspects of his or her life.

5. ***Answer:*** B
   Rationale: In the dimensional approach to aggression, psychiatric medications target aggression as a symptom of a disorder, rather than treating the disorder itself. This approach is analogous to the palliative treatment of pain or fever with medication, regardless of the underlying medical condition.

6. ***Answer:*** D
   Rationale: Some children with Rett's disorder receive an initial diagnosis of autistic disorder because of the marked disability in social interactions in both disorders, but the two disorders have some predictable differences. In Rett's disorder, a child shows deterioration of developmental milestones, head circumference, and overall growth. In autistic disorder, aberrant development is usually present from early on. In Rett's disorder, specific characteristic hand movements are always present. In autistic disorder, hand mannerisms may or may not appear. Poor coordination, ataxia, and apraxia are predictably part of Rett's disorder. Many people with autism have unremarkable gross motor function.

7. ***Answer:*** B
   Rationale: Autism marks a life-long pattern of disability. Approximately 75% of children with autism have mental retardation with marked deficits in reasoning, social understanding, and verbal tasks.

8. ***Answer:*** A
   Rationale: The essential feature of separation anxiety disorder is extreme anxiety precipitated by separation from parents, home, or other familiar surroundings. The distress is greater than that normally expected for the child's developmental level and cannot be explained by any other disorder.

9. ***Answer:*** D
   Rationale: According to the DSM-IV criteria, Axis 1 is psychological disorders, Axis 2 is personality disorders, Axis 3 is general medical conditions and Axis 4 is psychosocial and environmental problems.

10. ***Answer:*** D
    Rationale: The existence of major depressive episodes in prepubertal children may be an early marker for bipolar disorder. Rapid onset of depression, psychiatric symptoms while depressed, and a history of bipolarity in first-degree relatives are features thought to predict a bipolar course.

11. ***Answer:*** C
    Rationale: Criteria for the diagnosis of unsocialized conduct disorder includes the general criteria for conduct disorder, but also includes a clear poor relationship with the in-

dividual's peer group as shown by isolation, rejection, or unpopularity, and by lacking in close reciprocal friendships.

12. *Answer:* A
Rationale: Group therapy is an effective modality that can be structured in a variety of ways to address issues of interpersonal competence, peer relationships, and social skill. This modality can be modified to suit groups of children in various age groups and can focus on behavioral, educational, social skill, and psychodynamic issues.

13. *Answer:* D
Rationale: Developmentally, an activity therapy group is the recommended modality for pubertal children who do not have significantly disturbed personality patterns. Same-sex groups of no more than eight children are suggested to facilitate their engagement in a setting especially designed and planned for them.

14. *Answer:* C
Rationale: Although unusual for males, criteria for anorexia nervosa are met in that he refuses to maintain normal weight, and this has been going on for over a year. At a time when young boys this age are expected to gain 10 pounds, Mark has lost 10 pounds, putting him nearly 20 pounds underweight. Mark has other characteristic features of the disorder: fear of becoming fat and feeling fat even when obviously underweight.

15. *Answer:* B
Rationale: The compromised metabolism of many patients with anorexia can put them at high risk for cardiac arrhythmias if tricyclic drugs are used.

16. *Answer:* B
Rationale: The child's difficulties are most certainly related to the trauma of having been repeatedly sexually abused by her father. The stressor criterion for PTSD requires that the person has experienced, witnessed, or been confronted with an event that involves actual or threatened death, or injury, or threat to one's physical integrity. In addition, the diagnosis requires that the person's

response involve intense fear, helplessness, or horror. It is a reasonable inference that sexual intercourse with a child is experienced as a "threat to one's physical integrity," and Patti has reacted with intense fear.

17. *Answer:* D
Rationale: The safety of the child is always the first issue to be determined. Other areas for assessment include a description and history of exposure to the current trauma, history of prior trauma and adaptation, comorbid psychiatric conditions, parent and family functioning, and sources of comfort and support for the child.

18. *Answer:* D
Rationale: Desensitization to fear-inducing environmental stimuli that are reminders of the trauma, coupled with relaxation techniques and cognitive restructuring, have been used in the clinical treatment of childhood PTSD.

19. *Answer:* A
Rationale: It should be noted that most of the scientific work on the neurobiology of PTSD is based upon work with adult populations. There is a lack of empirical studies in pediatric PTSD.

20. *Answer:* A
Rationale: Episodes of arising from bed during sleep and walking about, appearing unresponsive during the episodes, experiencing amnesia for the episode upon awakening, and exhibiting no evidence of impairment in consciousness several minutes after awakening are characteristic of sleepwalking disorder.

21. *Answer:* B
Rationale: Arousal events during sleep are closely related to arousal behaviors emerging from deep slow-wave sleep. At the end of the deep sleep period, in the first half of the night, the transition to lighter stages of sleep is often accompanied by unusual arousal events. These events occur most frequently at the ages in childhood when the largest amount of slow-wave sleep occurs.

22. *Answer:* B

Rationale: Treatment of parasomnias (unusual arousal events during sleep) is generally supportive. Parents are often alarmed when they first encounter an arousal event in their child. Education about the nature of sleep, the disorder, and the favorable prognosis as the child matures can be very helpful. A 30 to 60 minute nap in the afternoon may decrease the child's need for delta sleep at night and decrease the frequency of arousal events. Benzodiazepines or tricyclic antidepressants are helpful for severe, dangerous, or frequent arousal events.

23. *Answer:* B

Rationale: Close clinical monitoring for increased suicidality is now recommended for youngsters initiating antidepressant therapies, including weekly face-to-face evaluation by the prescribing clinician over the first 4 weeks of treatment, every other week evaluation over the second month of treatment, and every 3 months thereafter, as indicated.

24. *Answer:* B

Rationale: The plan for management of the suicidal teen outside of a hospital includes minimizing the availability of extra medications by prescribing only enough to cover until the next appointment; having parents keep medications in a locked cabinet and to be involved in the medication management; removal of potentially lethal means of suicide such as firearms, knives, poisons, and pills; and developing a systematic plan for checking with the patient routinely to assess feelings and self-destructive urges.

25. *Answer:* A

Rationale: Drugs that increase the CNS serotonin neurotransmission and affect 5HT1A receptors may cause central serotonin syndrome (CSS). Symptoms may begin after an increase in serotonin drug monotherapy, but generally occur immediately or soon after combining medications that have a serotonergic mechanism of action. Medications associated with CSS include cocaine, which inhibits serotonin reuptake.

BIBLIOGRAPHY

American Academy of Child and Adolescent Psychiatry (AACAP). (2001). Summary of the practice parameters for the assessment and treatment of children and adolescents with suicidal behavior. *J Am Acad Child Adolecs Psychiatry, 40*(4), 495-499.

American Psychiatric Association. (1994). *Diagnostic and statistical manual of mental disorders (DSM-IV™),* (4th ed.). Washington, DC: American Psychiatric Association.

Brookman, R.R., & Sood, A.A. (2006). Disorders of mood and anxiety in adolescents. *Adolesc Med Clin, 17*(1), 79-95.

Emslie, G.J. & Mayes, T.L. (2001). Mood disorders in children and adolescents: Psychopharmacological treatment. *Biol Psychiatry, 49*(12), 1082-1090.

Frick, P.J. (2006). Developmental pathways to conduct disorder. *Child Adolesc Psychiatr Clin N Am, 15*(2), 311-331, vii.

James, A., Soler, A., & Weatherall, R. (2005). Cognitive behavioural therapy for anxiety disorders in children and adolescents. *Cochrane Database Syst Rev,* (4):CD004690.

Karnik, N.S., McMullin, M.A., & Steiner, H. (2006). Disruptive behaviors: Conduct and oppositional disorders in adolescents. *Adolesc Med Clin, 17*(1), 97-114.

Lyons, R.K, Dutra, L., Schuder, M.R., et al. (2006). From infant attachment disorganization to adult dissociation: Relational adaptations or traumatic experiences? *Psychiatr Clin North Am, 29*(1), 63-86, viii.

Melnyk, B.M., Feinstein, N.F., Tuttle, J., et al. (2002). Mental health worries, communication, and needs of children, teens, and parents during the year of the nation's terrorist attack: Findings from the national KySS survey. *J Ped Health Care, 16*(5), 222-234.

Melnyk, B.M., & Moldenhauer, Z. (1999). Current approaches to depression in children and adolescents. *Adv Nurse Pract, 7*(2), 24-29, 97.

Melnyk, B.M., Moldenhauer, Z., Veenema, McMurtrie, M.T., et al. (2001). The KySS (Keep Your children/yourself Safe and Secure) campaign: A national effort to decrease psychosocial morbidities in children and adolescents. *J Ped Health Care, 15*(2), 31A-34A.

Moldenhauer, Z., & Melnyk, B.M. (1999). Use of anti-depressants in the treatment of child and adolescent depression: Are they effective? *Pediatr Nurs, 25*(6), 643-646.

Nemeroff, C.B., & Vale, W.W. (2005). The neurobiology of depression: Inroads to treatment and new drug discovery. *J Clin Psychiatry, 66 Suppl 7,* 5-13.

Pelkonen, M., & Marttunen, M. (2003). Child and adolescent suicide: Epidemiology, risk factors, and approaches to prevention. *Paediatr Drugs, 5*(4), 243-265.

Pompili, M., Mancinelli, I., Girardi, P., et al. (2005). Childhood suicide: A major issue in pediatric health care. *Issues Compr Pediatr Nurs, 28*(1), 63-68.

Ryan, N.D. (2005). Treatment of depression in children and adolescents. *Lancet, 366*(9489), 933-940.

Ryan-Wenger, N.A. (2001). Use of children's drawings for measurement of developmental level and emotional status. *J Child Family Nurs, 4*(2), 139-149.

Scahill, L., Hamrin, V., & Pachler, M.E. (2005). The use of selective serotonin reuptake inhibitors in children and adolescents with major depression. *J Child Adolesc Psychiatr Nurs, 18*(2), 86-9.

Wagner, K.D. (2005). Pharmacotherapy for major depression in children and adolescents. *Prog Neuropsychopharmacol Biol Psychiatry, 29*(5), 819-826.

Waslick, B. (2006). Psychopharmacology interventions for pediatric anxiety disorders: A research update. *Child Adolesc Psychiatr Clin N Am, 15*(1), 51-71.

NOTES

CHAPTER 42

Congenital Heart Disease

KARI CRAWFORD

Select the best answer for each of the following questions:

1. A pediatric nurse practitioner is counseling a new mom who is devastated that her newborn has been born with a congenital heart defect. The mother is certain that the wine she had each night with meals, prior to knowing she was pregnant, caused this defect. In the discussion, the pediatric nurse practitioner should:
   A. Offer support and empathy knowing how guilty she must be feeling.
   B. Insist that was certainly not the case, because the baby's heart could have become malformed at any point during the pregnancy.
   C. Provide her with information on Alcoholics Anonymous.
   D. Offer support and reassurance that it is still not known what causes heart defects, but that it is unlikely that glasses of wine caused the defect.

2. Charlene is a 14-year-old first-time mom who brings her 1-month-old son to the clinic because she thinks "he doesn't act right. Last week, he was not breastfeeding well, was sweaty when he woke up, and he breathes real fast." Based on the history, the differential diagnosis should include:
   A. Congenial hyperthyroidism.
   B. Congenital heart disease.
   C. Feeding disorder.
   D. Hypothermia.

3. A 2-month-old infant with Down syndrome is being seen for the first time at the clinic. There are no previous medical records

available. The MOST important part of the history would include asking if he:
   A. Has been checked for diabetes.
   B. Has had rheumatic fever.
   C. Was evaluated for a congenital heart defect.
   D. Has problems with diarrhea.

4. The newborn examination on a child with Down syndrome should always include:
   A. Checking four-point blood pressures and femoral pulses.
   B. A cardiac ultrasound.
   C. An arterial blood gas.
   D. A repeat of the newborn screen.

5. One of the best ways to obtain an accurate cardiac assessment in a young child is to:
   A. Have the child lay flat on the exam table.
   B. Have the child sit on the exam table.
   C. Remove all anxiety-causing items prior to auscultation or delay painful procedures.
   D. Have the child sit in his parent's lap and attempt to distract with a toy or video.

6. While helping the local junior high school complete its annual sports physicals, the pediatric nurse practitioner notes a murmur in a 13-year-old male who wants to try out for basketball. The systolic murmur is a grade 2/6 heard best at the left sternal border. There is no radiation, clicks, or thrills. The teen has no symptoms of recurrent respiratory illnesses, syncope, or poor growth. The pediatric nurse practitioner should:

295

A. Send him to the nearest emergency room.
B. Refer to the cardiologist immediately.
C. Reassure the family that this is an innocent murmur and clear him for participation in basketball.
D. Do not allow him to participate in sports and encourage hydration.

7. A 7-year-old presents to the clinic with flu-like symptoms and a fever of 101.5° F. The pediatric nurse practitioner notes that the child has a murmur. This child is well-known to the pediatric nurse practitioner and there has been no previous documentation of a heart murmur in the past. The best action is:
   A. Document the murmur and have him return in 1 to 2 weeks for reevaluation.
   B. Stat referral to cardiology.
   C. Obtain an ECG and ECHO.
   D. Routine referral to cardiology.

8. While assessing a 5-year-old with a history of a ventricular septal defect (VSD) the pediatric nurse practitioner notes a thrill on palpation and can auscultate the murmur with the stethoscope partially off the chest. What grade is this murmur?
   A. 4
   B. 5
   C. 6
   D. 7

9. The most highly sensitive, specific, and cost-effective tool in the diagnosis of congenital heart disease is:
   A. Chest x-ray.
   B. Electrocardiogram.
   C. Echocardiogram.
   D. Cardiac catheterization.

10. Which child should NOT be allowed to participate in sports until further evaluation by a cardiologist?
   A. Healthy 15-year-old male of normal height and weight who has no previous history of cardiac events. Family history reveals an aunt and grandfather who had sudden death before age 35.
   B. Healthy 8-year-old female with a history of asthma well-controlled and

known to be exacerbated by seasonal allergies.
   C. Healthy 13-year-old Latino female whose mother has mitral valve prolapse.
   D. Healthy 16-year-old male with a repaired atrial septal defect at the age of 4.

11. A 15-year-old is brought to your office today by her mother who insists you tell her daughter it is dangerous for her to have a tattoo. This patient had a patent ductus arteriosus (PDA) closed when she was an infant. You tell them:
   A. Any child who has previous cardiac surgery should receive subacute bacterial endocarditis (SBE) prophylaxis for such procedures.
   B. It is extremely risky to have a tattoo, as it might cause bacteria from the tattoo needle to be spread to her old PDA closure scar.
   C. The dye used in tattoos can migrate to her heart valve and cause damage.
   D. You advise that they have an educated discussion about the risk and legal age for a tattoo, but that her PDA repair no longer poses a risk for SBE.

12. A 6-month-old with complete atrioventricular canal defect comes into the clinic. The pediatric nurse practitioner notes a consistent drop in weight over the last 3 months. Mom reports he drinks 1.5 to 2 oz every 4 hours and it takes him nearly an hour to finish the feeding. What is the most appropriate action?
   A. No changes at this time; this is normal growth for a cardiac baby.
   B. Refer to cardiology immediately upon completion of your visit.
   C. Change formula to 24 cal/oz and have them follow up with their cardiologist in the next week.
   D. Send the family to the local hospital for placement of a feeding tube.

13. Shock can occur in a infant with a single ventricle lesion, transposition of the great arteries, tetralogy of Fallot, or coarctation of the aorta if:
   A. The patent ductus arteriosus closes.

B. There is a large atrial septal defect.
C. The child gets dehydrated.
D. The foramen ovale closes.

14. A 7-year-old is being seen for a complaint of headaches and hypertension. An important differential for the pediatric nurse practitioner to consider is:
A. Patent ductus arteriosus.
B. Aortic insufficiency.
C. Coarctation of the aorta.
D. Interrupted aortic arch.

15. The majority of congenital heart lesions are related to:
A. Excessive smoking by mother.
B. Down syndrome.
C. Spontaneous mutations in the fetus.
D. Environmental factors and chromosomal abnormalities.

16. Which of the following is a maternal risk factor for congenital heart disease?
A. Maternal age younger than 40 years.
B. Rubella infection.
C. Maternal hypothroidism.
D. Bipolar disorder.

17. A newborn nursery nurse is caring for a cyanotic infant and places him on 100% oxygen. The infant's oxygen saturation goes from 85% to 88% and his PaO$_2$ remains in the 40s. She suspects this infant must:
A. Have a cardiac mixing lesion and is likely ductal-dependant.
B. Has a persistent patent ductus arteriosus.
C. Be in hypovolemic shock.
D. Need to have respiratory suctioning.

18. A 12-year-old male has come to the clinic for a sport physical. On assessment, you find he is greater than the 95th percentile for height and his arm span is greater than his height. The mother informs you that her father died at age 33 of an aortic aneurysm. Suspecting that this child might have Marfan syndrome, the pediatric nurse practitioner should:
A. Draw a PT and PTT screen.
B. Order thyroid studies.
C. Make referrals to cardiology and genetics.
D. Order a bone scan.

19. A new patient to the practice is being followed by cardiology for coronary aneurysm. The mom said he had an illness when he was toddler but she cannot remember the name. What is the most likely cause of the aneurysm?
A. Myocardial infarction.
B. Myocarditis.
C. Epstein-Barr virus.
D. Kawasaki disease.

20. Teens with the following family history should be further evaluated by a cardiologist prior to sports activities:
A. Unexplained sudden death at or before age 30.
B. Adult onset diabetes.
C. Asthma.
D. Arthritis.

21. A patient who is cyanotic will likely be worsened by:
A. Excessive sleep.
B. Anemia.
C. Alkalosis.
D. Light activity.

22. Which of the following congenital heart disease lesions is acyanotic?
A. Coarctation of the aorta
B. Truncus arteriosis
C. Ventricular septal defect
D. Pulmonary stenosis

23. A 3-month-old with known congenital heart disease comes into the clinic for a routine physical examination. The pediatric nurse practitioner notes no weight gain in the past 4 weeks. The child is taking milk-based formula (20 kcal/ounce) 1 to 2 ounces every 3 to 4 hours. The pediatric nurse practitioner should:
A. Increase the feedings of the current formula to 3 to 4 ounces every 1 to 2 hours.
B. Change the infant to a higher calorie formula (24-30 kcal/ounce).
C. Reassure the mother that the child will catch up and reschedule a weight check in 2 weeks.
D. Change the infant to a soy-based formula.

ANSWERS

1. *Answer:* D
   Rationale: Most causes of CHD are not identified. There are identified syndromes that are associated with certain heart defects; however, the etiology is thought to be both genetic and environmental. One percent of the population is born with congenital heart disease and parents are usually told the cause is unknown and it occurred before the mother knew she was pregnant.

2. *Answer:* B
   Rationale: Pulmonary vascular resistance drops in infancy during the first few days of life. This allows for infants with left to right shunts to easily send more blood to their lungs which will cause symptoms of heart failure. It is often true that even young mothers know their infants well enough to pick up on subtle changes; their concerns should be completely evaluated. The other choices would not present with feeding difficulties, fast breathing, and sweating.

3. *Answer:* C
   Rationale: Although it would be important to assess previous lab results, previous illnesses, and elimination patterns, the most important historical information would be asking about a history of a congenital heart defect. As high as 80% of children with Down syndrome will have a congenital heart defect.

4. *Answer:* A
   Rationale: Four-point blood pressures and lower extremity pulse checks may reveal a coarctation of the aorta. The others are not physical examination techniques.

5. *Answer:* D
   Rationale: The best assessments are obtained when the patient is in an environment where he or she feels safe. Sitting on exam tables away from family members can be frightening and crying will interfere with a good cardiac exam.

6. *Answer:* C
   Rationale: Murmurs are sounds of turbulence of blood flow across something and do not always indicate heart disease. Many murmurs in children and adolescents are be-

nign. The location, intensity, and timing of the murmur are also important features in determining the etiology of a murmur.

7. *Answer:* A
   Rationale: Murmurs can occur during changes in a patient's physiologic state such as febrile illness, anemia, or pregnancy and do not necessarily indicate pathology.

8. *Answer:* B
   Rationale: Grading criteria for murmurs are based on intensity and associated sounds. Murmurs greater than grade 5 can be heard with the stethoscope off the chest and are associated with a thrill.

9. *Answer:* C
   Rationale: The advancement of technology has pushed the ECHO to the forefront as one of the most useful noninvasive diagnostic tools. Chest x-ray and electrocardiograms may not be specific enough to determine the diagnosis. Cardiac catheterizations are expensive and involve greater risk.

10. *Answer:* A
    Rationale: Any patient who has a history in the family of young, unexplained death should have a further evaluation prior to sports participation to rule out arrhythmias.

11. *Answer:* D
    Rationale: SBE prophylaxis is used for nonrepaired lesions or corrected lesions with residual shunts as well as lesions that are only palliated. This patient would no longer need SBE prophylaxis.

12. *Answer:* C
    Rationale: This infant is likely in heart failure so increased demands will necessitate increased calorie needs. If he spends more than 30 minutes per feeding, he is likely burning the calories he is working so hard to take in. Increased-calorie formula allows for infants to eat less with more benefit. Follow-up with the cardiologist is also necessary for a cardiac child who is showing growth deceleration.

13. *Answer:* A
    Rationale: All of these conditions are potentially ductal-dependent lesions. Closure

of the communication in a ductal-dependent lesion will cause shock.

14. *Answer:* C
Rationale: Older children evaluated for hypertension may often have cardiac disease as opposed to renal disease; to evaluate hypertension, four-point blood pressures and femoral pulse examination are critical.

15. *Answer:* D
Rationale: The cause of most cardiac lesions is unknown but they are thought to be multifactorial.

16. *Answer:* B
Rationale: Risk factors for congenital heart disease include maternal age over 40, rubella, certain drug use during pregnancy, illegal drug use, alcohol ingestion, smoking, diabetes, PKU, and exposure to toxins.

17. *Answer:* A
Rationale: In the hyperoxia test, administration of 100% O_2 will not change PaO_2 in cardiac lesions; however, it will improve saturation for infants with pulmonary disease.

18. *Answer:* C
Rationale: Marfan syndrome is a hereditary disease that affects the connective tissue, including the blood vessels and heart. Ninety percent of people with Marfan syndrome have cardiac and blood vessel involvement. The two major conditions found in people with Marfan syndrome are mitral valve prolapse and aortic dilatation. Any patient with suspected Marfan syndrome should be referred to genetics and cardiology.

19. *Answer:* D
Rationale: One of the complications of Kawasaki disease is coronary artery aneurysm. Myocardial infarction, myocarditis, and Epstein-Barr virus do not cause coronary aneurysms.

20. *Answer:* A
Rationale: Children who have a family history of unexplained early deaths need to be evaluated by cardiology. Family history of asthma, arthritis, and/or diabetes is not an indication for cardiology referrals prior to playing sports.

21. *Answer:* B
Rationale: Hemoglobin transports oxygen, so cyanotic patients have increased oxygen-carrying capacity with higher hemoglobin levels. Sleep, alkalosis, and light activity should not increase cyanosis.

22. *Answer:* C
Rationale: A ventricular septal defect is a hole in the septum between the right and left ventricles. Oxygenated blood recirculates in the heart because the blood crosses the defect from the left to the right side of the heart.

23. *Answer:* B
Rationale: Children with CHD need more calories to grow. Increasing the number of feeding and the amount of feedings will tire the child. Soy-based formulas would not make a difference in growth.

BIBLIOGRAPHY

Allen, H.D., Clark, E.B., Gutgesell, H.P., & Driscoll, D.J. (2001). *Moss and Adams' heart disease in infants, children, and adolescents: Including the fetus and young adult* (Vol 1 & 2). Philadelphia: Lippincott Williams & Wilkins.

American College of Cardiology (ACC) and American Heart Association (AHA) (1997). Endocarditis prophylaxis information. Retrieved June 30, 2006, from www.americanheart.org/presenter.jhtml?identifier=11086.

Blosser, C.G., & Freitas-Nichols, J. (2004). Cardiovascular disorders. In C.E. Burns, A.M. Dunn, M.A. Brady, et al. (Eds.). *Pediatric primary care: A handbook for nurse practitioners* (3rd ed.). Philadelphia: Saunders.

Harris, M., & Valmorida, J. (2000). Neonates with congenital heart disease: An overview. *Neonat Network, 19*(5), 37-41.

Jackson, P., & Vessey, J. (2004). *Primary care of the child with a chronic condition* (4th ed.). St. Louis: Mosby.

Park, M. (2002). *Pediatric cardiology for practitioners* (4th ed.). St. Louis: Mosby.

Poddar, B., & Basu, S. (2004). Approach to a child with a heart murmur. *Indian J Pediatr, 71*(1), 63-66.

Schwartz, R.A., Richards, G.M., & Goyal, S. (2006). Clubbing of the nails. Retrieved May 21, 2006, from www.emedicine.com/derm/topic780.htm.

Smith, P. (2001). Primary care in children with congenital heart disease. *J Pediatr Nurs, 16*(5), 308-319.

43 Cystic Fibrosis

LOIS PANCRATZ

Select the best answer for each of the following questions:

1. Cystic fibrosis is an autosomal-recessive inheritance pattern disease also thought to be caused by a defect in the CF gene, cystic fibrosis transmembrane conductance regulator (CFTR), which:
   A. Is located on the long arm of chromosome 7.
   B. Encodes for lipids that function as a chloride channel.
   C. Is not regulated by cyclic adenosine monophosphate (cAMP).
   D. No mutations of the CF gene have been identified.

2. The most likely presentation of cystic fibrosis in a neonate would be:
   A. Meconium ileus or generalized swelling, jaundice.
   B. Steatorrhea.
   C. Wheezing and coughing.
   D. Recurrent or persistent pneumonia.

3. The ethnic group most frequently affected by cystic fibrosis is:
   A. Asian American.
   B. African American.
   C. Hispanic.
   D. White.

4. Mr. and Mrs. Jones are planning to start a family; however, they are concerned about the fact that Mr. Jones' brother has cystic fibrosis and decide to be tested. Testing indicates that both Mr. Jones and Mrs. Jones are carriers of cystic fibrosis. How would you help them understand the significance of the results?
   A. Tell them they have a 50% chance of the child having cystic fibrosis.
   B. Having children is not recommended in view of these results.
   C. They have a 25% chance of having a child with cystic fibrosis.
   D. Since this is a recessive gene, their chances are no more significant than noncarriers.

5. Signs and symptoms of cystic fibrosis vary widely by age. Approximately one-third of patients are diagnosed by:
   A. 6 years.
   B. 12 years.
   C. 2 months.
   D. 12 months.

6. The CFTR protein in patients with cystic fibrosis is involved with Cl⁻ conductance, consistent with the observation that 99% of patients with cystic fibrosis have:
   A. Low levels of sweat chloride.
   B. Elevated levels of sweat chloride.
   C. Normal levels of sweat chloride.
   D. Absent levels of potassium.

7. The respiratory epithelium of cystic fibrosis patients exhibits marked impermeability to chloride and excessive reabsorption of sodium. These alterations lead to:
   A. Excessively moist epithelium.
   B. Relative dehydration of the airway secretions.
   C. Resistance to infections.
   D. No significant clinical symptoms.

8. Most patients with cystic fibrosis (90%) also have:
   A. Abnormal liver function tests.
   B. Cholelithiasis.
   C. Pancreatic insufficiency.
   D. Anemia.

9. Maldigestion associated with cystic fibrosis results in secondary malabsorption manifested by:
   A. Steatorrhea.
   B. Melena.
   C. Clay-colored stools.
   D. Chronic diarrhea.

10. The definitive test for cystic fibrosis is:
   A. The sweat test.
   B. A sputum culture.
   C. A fecal fat test.
   D. A Chymex test for pancreatic insufficiency.

11. Mrs. Smith is concerned about her 4-day-old baby because her niece was diagnosed with cystic fibrosis. What is the best method in conjunction with DNA analysis and sweat test to assess for cystic fibrosis in a 4-day-old infant?
   A. Sweat test.
   B. CBC.
   C. Immunoreactive trypsin test (IRT).
   D. Pulmonary function test.

12. ENT manifestations of cystic fibrosis may include mucus-secreting salivary ducts which are enlarged and display focal plugging and dilatation of ducts as well as:
   A. Otitis media.
   B. Pharyngitis.
   C. Nasal polyps.
   D. Oral lesions.

13. Noncystic fibrosis conditions that produce elevated sweat electrolytes include all of the following EXCEPT:
   A. Diabetes.
   B. Adrenal insufficiency.
   C. Hypothyroidism.
   D. Malnutrition.

14. J.J. is a 14-year-old male with cystic fibrosis who is being seen for an acute episode of bronchitis. In choosing an antibiotic for J.J., you consider that in cystic fibrosis patients, the airways are frequently colonized by:
   A. Mycoplasma.
   B. *Staphylococcus aureus* and *Pseudomonas aeruginosa*.
   C. *Streptococcus pneumoniae*.
   D. *Klebsiella pneumoniae*.

15. Body systems typically affected by cystic fibrosis include ENT, respiratory, gastrointestinal, sweat glands, and all of the following EXCEPT:
   A. Ocular.
   B. Biliary tract.
   C. Musculoskeletal.
   D. Genitourinary.

16. When teaching parents who have a child with cystic fibrosis, it is important to note that the best method of preserving pulmonary function is to:
   A. Continuously administer low-flow oxygen.
   B. Administer bronchodilators on a regular basis.
   C. Perform chest physiotherapy with postural drainage, percussion, and vibration.
   D. Use maintenance antibiotic prophylactic therapy.

17. Gretchen is a 5-year-old with cystic fibrosis who is being seen today for her annual exam. She has been treated for the last 6 weeks with antibiotics and corticosteroids for a persistent episode of bronchitis. At today's visit you would:
   A. Give her immunizations as scheduled.
   B. Defer her immunizations until she has completed the corticosteroids.
   C. Defer her immunizations until she has completed the antibiotic.
   D. Defer any live immunizations; she may receive inactivated immunizations today.

18. In order to decrease the viscosity of respiratory secretions, the pediatric nurse

practitioner orders recombinant human de-oxyribonuclease (rhDNase), knowing the mechanism of action is that rhDNase:

A. Cleaves the extracellular DNA from the neutrophils in sputum to make it less viscous.
B. Corrects the defect in the CF gene on chromosome 7.
C. Has potent antibacterial action that prevents the growth of pseudomonas and staphylococci.
D. Has antibacterial, bronchodilator, and mucolytic actions.

19. Ann is a 13-year-old with cystic fibrosis who is in the office for her annual examination. Laboratory studies pertinent to this visit would include:

A. Electrolytes.
B. Lipid panel.
C. Glucose.
D. Urinalysis.

20. Nutritional considerations for the cystic fibrosis patient would include:

A. Low-fat, low-cholesterol diet.
B. Low-salt diet.
C. Low-calorie diet.
D. Vitamin A, D, E, and K replacements.

21. Antiinflammatory medications in cystic fibrosis patients are:

A. Contraindicated.
B. Used as to treat bacterial infections.
C. Used in low doses to decrease inflammation of the airways.
D. Used in high doses to decrease inflammation of the airways.

22. When ordering pancreatic enzyme replacements for cystic fibrosis patients, all of the following are true EXCEPT:

A. Enzyme dosage and product should be individualized for each patient.
B. Replacements fully correct stool fat and nitrogen losses.
C. Administration of large doses has been linked to colonic strictures requiring surgery.
D. Enzyme replacement should not exceed 10,000 units/kg/day.

23. Gastrointestinal symptoms related to GERD as a complication of cystic fibrosis may be improved by:

A. Clarithromycin.
B. Proton pump inhibitors.
C. Bentyl syrup.
D. Carafate.

24. Complications of cystic fibrosis would include all of the following EXCEPT:

A. Fungal vaginitis.
B. Rectal prolapse.
C. Pneumothorax.
D. Obesity.

25. The average life expectancy of patients with cystic fibrosis is:

A. 45.
B. 56.
C. 36.
D. 25.

ANSWERS

1. *Answer:* A
   Rationale: CFTR encodes for protein that functions as a chloride channel. More than 1400 mutations of CF gene have been identified. CFTR is regulated by cyclic adenosine monophosphate (cAMP).

2. *Answer:* A
   Rationale: Steatorrhea, wheezing, and coughing are more common in the infant; persistent pneumonia is more common in older children and adults.

3. *Answer:* D
   Rationale: Northern European descendents have a 1 in 30 chance of carrying the gene responsible for cystic fibrosis, African Americans 1 chance in 62, and Asian Americans 1 chance in 90.

4. *Answer:* C
   Rationale: The chance of a child having cystic fibrosis is 25%, of the child being a carrier 50%, and a 25% chance of having no evidence of the disease or carrier state with each pregnancy.

5. *Answer:* C
   Rationale: Median age of diagnosis is 14 months with one-third of the patients diagnosed at less than 2 months by positive family history, meconium ileus, and neonatal screening.

6. *Answer:* B
   Rationale: Cystic fibrosis patients have elevated levels of sweat chloride as CFTR is a chloride channel and substantially regulates epithelial chloride and possibly sodium transport.

7. *Answer:* B
   Rationale: Dehydration of the airway secretions results in impaired mucociliary transport and airway obstruction; this leads to chronic bronchial infections.

8. *Answer:* C
   Rationale: Inspissation of mucus in the pancreatic ducts and consequent autodigestion of the pancreas.

9. *Answer:* A
   Rationale: Large, fatty, floating, foul-smelling stools result. Melena (black, tarry stools) is most often associated with rectal bleeding, clay-colored stools exhibit an absence of bile pigment typical of hepatic disease. Chronic diarrhea may have many etiologies and is not specific to cystic fibrosis.

10. *Answer:* A
    Rationale: The definitive tests for cystic fibrosis are the sweat test and DNA analysis. The diagnosis is confirmed by a positive sweat test and the presence of two of the recognized CF mutations in DNA, one each on the maternally and paternally derived chromosome 7. An abnormal Chymex test for pancreatic insufficiency is a supportive laboratory test to diagnose cystic fibrosis. A fecal fat test is reliable but not diagnostic of cystic fibrosis, but may be ordered with an amylase or lipase to look at other aspects of pancreas and digestive function in the presence of a negative trypsin test. The IRT is not diagnostic by itself, as there are a fair number of false positives and problems other than CF and pancreatic dysfunction that can cause a positive IRT.

11. *Answer:* C
    Rationale: Newborns in the first weeks of life may not produce enough sweat for an accurate test; this test has relatively poor specificity because as many as 90% of the positives on initial screen are false positives. Most newborns with CF can be identified by determination of immunoreactive trypsinogen coupled with confirmatory sweat or DNA testing. Early testing and diagnosis is desirable as it may prevent early nutritional deficiencies; however, there is no evidence that early diagnosis improves pulmonary outcome.

12. *Answer:* C
    Rationale: Otitis media and pharyngitis are usually viral or bacterial in origin. Oral lesions are not specific to cystic fibrosis, although cheilosis at the corners of the mouth may develop as a result of vitamin B complex deficiency. The nasal mucosa may contain inflammatory cells, be edematous, and form

large or multiple polyps, usually form a base surrounding the ostia of the maxillary and ethmoid sinuses.

13. **Answer:** A
Rationale: While diabetes may produce a diaphoresis resulting in clammy skin, the sweat chloride is not necessarily elevated, as diabetics have normal sweat glands. The function of the sweat duct cells is to absorb rather than secrete chloride, salt is not retrieved from the isotonic primary sweat as it is transported to the skin surface; chloride and sodium levels are consequently elevated.

14. **Answer:** B
Rationale: These two organisms rarely infect the lungs of other individuals; however, there is evidence that the CF airway epithelial cells or surface liquids provide a favorable environment for attachment or induce adherence properties of these organisms.

15. **Answer:** A
Rationale: In 15% to 20% of newborn infants with CF, the ileum is completely obstructed by meconium. Eighty-five percent of affected children show evidence of malnutrition due to exocrine pancreatic insufficiency. Sexual development is often delayed, more than 95% of males are azoospermic, and adolescent females may experience secondary amenorrhea. Cervicitis and accumulation of tenacious mucus in the cervical canal has been noted.

16. **Answer:** C
Rationale: Daily chest physiotherapy with postural drainage, percussion, and vibration help to remove abnormally thick mucus from the bronchial tree. The problem in cystic fibrosis is with the epithelial cells and their secretions, so bronchodilators do not help. Antibiotics should be used during acute infections; frequent use of antibiotics during acute infections may cause resistance. To minimize resistance, avoid prophylactic use of antibiotics. Oxygen therapy may at times be necessary for hypoxemia, but should not be used continuously.

17. **Answer:** D
Rationale: Immunosuppression with corticosteroids is a contraindication for live attenuated immunizations. The pediatric nurse practitioner should consult with the National Immunization Program (www.cdc.gov) for the minimum wait intervals for live immunizations after corticosteroid therapy.

18. **Answer:** A
Rationale: rhDNase decreases the viscosity of sputum by digesting the neutrophil DNA; although rhDNase can reduce the frequency of infections, it does not have any antibacterial or bronchodilatory actions.

19. **Answer:** C
Rationale: According to guidelines for care from Cystic Fibrosis Foundation, blood glucose should be measured every year after age 13 because in adolescents and adults, a relative insulin deficiency may develop and hyperglycemia and CF-related diabetes may become symptomatic.

20. **Answer:** D
Rationale: Because of pancreatic insufficiency that results in malabsorption of fat-soluble vitamins, supplementation is recommended as well as a high-calorie diet.

21. **Answer:** D
Rationale: Corticosteroids are useful for the treatment of allergic bronchopulmonary reactive airway diseases by decreasing inflammation in high doses. They have no antibacterial properties, may result in growth retardation, cataracts, and abnormal glucose tolerance.

22. **Answer:** B
Rationale: Extracts of animal pancreas given with ingested food reduce but do not fully correct stool fat and nitrogen losses. The dose of enzymes required usually increases with age, but some teenagers and young adults may later have a decrease in their requirement.

23. **Answer:** B
Rationale: Proton pump inhibitors would alleviate symptoms of GERD. Bentyl

is an anticholinergic used in irritable bowel syndrome, clarithromycin is a macrolide antibiotic useful for treating *H. pylori* infections; carafate is useful adjunctive therapy in healing duodenal ulcers.

24. *Answer:* D

Rationale: Most CF patients have difficulty with malnutrition. Rectal prolapse occurs in 20% to 25% of individuals, fungal vaginal infections may occur as result of frequent antibiotic use, pneumothorax is encountered in less than 1% of children and teenagers, but is more frequently encountered in older adults and may be life-threatening.

25. *Answer:* C

Rationale: According to the Cystic Fibrosis Foundation, as of 2004 the average life expectancy was 36.8, with 95% of patients dying of respiratory failure.

BIBLIOGRAPHY

Abbott, J., & Hart, A. (March 2005). Measuring and reporting quality of life outcomes in clinical trials in cystic fibrosis: A critical review. *Health Qual Life Outcomes, 3*, 19.

Amin, R., Bean, J., Burklow, K., & Jeffries, J. (2005). The relationship between sleep disturbance and pulmonary function in stable pediatric cystic fibrosis patients. *Chest, 128*(3), 1357-1363.

Cystic Fibrosis Consortium. (2006). Database on CFTR gene. Retrieved on May 21, 2006, from http://www.genet.sickkids.on.ca/cftr/.

Cystic Fibrosis Foundation (2006). Clinical practice guidelines for cystic fibrosis—cystic fibrosis outpatient treatment map for patients, parents, and professionals. Retrieved on June 26, 2006, from http://www.rain.org~medmall/cysticfibrosis/index.html.

Cystic Fibrosis Foundation (2005). Patient registry annual data report, 2005. Retrieved May 21, 2006, from www.cff.org/publications/files/2002%20CF%20Patient%20Registry%20Report.pdf.

Davis, P. (2001). Cystic fibrosis. *Pediatr Rev, 22*(8), 257-263.

Gibson, R.L., Burns, J.L., & Ramsey, B.W. (2003). Pathophysiology and management of pulmonary infections in cystic fibrosis. *Am J Resp Crit Care Med, 168*(8), 918-951.

Grosse, S., Boyle, C.A., Botkin, J.R., et al. (2004). Newborn screening for cystic fibrosis: Evaluation of benefits and risks and recommendations for state newborn screening programs. *MMWR Morb Mortal Wkly Rep, 53*(RR13), 1-36.

Kulich, M., Rosenfeld, M., Goss, C.H., & Wilmott, R. (2003). Improved survival among young patients with cystic fibrosis. *J Pediatr, 142*(6), 631-636.

McMullen, A.H., & Bryson, E.A. (2004). Cystic fibrosis. In P.L. Jackson, & J.A. Vessey (Eds.). *Primary care of the child with a chronic condition* (4th ed.). St. Louis: Mosby.

Modi, A.C., & Quittner, A.L. (2003). Validation of a disease-specific measure of health-related quality of life for children with cystic fibrosis. *J Pediatr Psychol, 28*(8), 535-545.

Murray, N., & Brown, K.R. (2005). Cystic fibrosis. Retrieved June 26, 2006, from www.emedicine.com/ent/topic515.htm.

Peckham, D., & Littlewood, J. (2003). The sweat test. Retrieved on May 21, 2006, from http://www.cysticfibrosismedicine.com/htmldocs/CFText/sweat.htm.

Rosenfeld, M., Gibson, R.L., McNamara, S., et al. (2001). Early pulmonary infection, inflammation, and clinical outcomes in infants with cystic fibrosis. *Pediatric Pulmonol, 32*(5), 356-366.

Saiman, L., & Siegel, J. (2004). Infection control in cystic fibrosis. *Clin Microbiol Rev, 17*(1), 57-71.

Saiman, L., Marshall, B.C., Mayer-Hamblett, N., et al. (2003). Azithromycin in patients with cystic fibrosis chronically infected with *Pseudomonas aeruginosa. JAMA, 290*(13), 1749-1756.

Sharma, G. (2006). Cystic fibrosis. Retrieved June 26, 2006, from www.emedicine.com/PED/topic535.htm.

Diabetes Types 1 and 2

STEPHANIE BONNEY

Select the best answer for each of the following questions:

1. Which of the following is true about type 1 diabetes?
   A. Less than 10,000 children per year are diagnosed with type 1 diabetes.
   B. It occurs equally in all races.
   C. It occurs equally in girls and boys.
   D. The incidence of type 1 diabetes is expected to decrease over time.

2. Which is the most important factor in the development of type 1 diabetes?
   A. HLA genes are elevated.
   B. Infectious agents.
   C. Age.
   D. Stress.

3. Which of the following is first in the chain of pathophysiology in type 1 diabetes?
   A. Polyuria
   B. Polydipsia
   C. Polyphagia
   D. Hyperglycemia

4. A 12-year old-presents to your office with a 2-week history of polyuria, polydipsia, and polyphagia. She also is complaining of weakness, vomiting, and abdominal pain. Based on the signs and symptoms, which of the following is the most appropriate first action?
   A. Immediate referral to the emergency department.
   B. HLA.
   C. Urinalysis.
   D. Random plasma glucose.

5. An 11-year-old presents with signs of declining glucose tolerance. He most likely has:
   A. Prediabetes.
   B. Type 1 diabetes.
   C. Type 2 diabetes.
   D. Diabetes insipidus.

6. For children ages 6 to 12, the recommended Hb A1C range is:
   A. Less than 7.5.
   B. 7.5 to 8.
   C. Less than 8.
   D. Greater than 8.

7. A 10-year-old was recently diagnosed with type 1 diabetes. Which of the following is the most important to tell her family when giving anticipatory guidance?
   A. The time after diagnosis is the "honeymoon" and can last an unpredictable amount of time.
   B. Beta cell destruction is complete in 2 years.
   C. The need for insulin increases after diagnosis.
   D. The need for insulin decreases after diagnosis.

8. Which of the following insulins would be the most appropriate to give for a blood glucose of 300?
   A. Regular
   B. NPH
   C. Ultralente
   D. Lantus

9. For a 10-year-old boy newly diagnosed with type 1 diabetes, which would be

the most important to include in his teaching regarding his blood glucose monitoring?
- A. Continuous blood glucose monitoring devices are available.
- B. Blood glucose testing is usually done four or more times a day.
- C. His weight and height need to be observed.
- D. Blood glucose testing should be done weekly.

10. When teaching a newly diagnosed 11-year-old type 1 diabetic, the most important benefit of diet and exercise is:
- A. Lowering blood pressure.
- B. Gaining a sense of well-being.
- C. Lowering pulse.
- D. Maintaining weight and growth.

11. The parents of a newly diagnosed type 1 diabetic are asking about the factor that leads to long-term complications. You explain that it is:
- A. Hyperglycemia.
- B. Hypoglycemia.
- C. Infrequent infections.
- D. Unpredictable glucose control.

12. During an annual exam of a type 1 diabetic, the pediatric nurse practitioner notes capillary occlusion on fundoscopic exam. The most appropriate action is:
- A. Referral to an ophthalmologist.
- B. Schedule a recheck appointment in 1 month.
- C. Schedule a recheck appointment in 6 months.
- D. Schedule a routine examination in 1 year.

13. Which of the following is true about type 2 diabetes?
- A. Sixty percent of children with diabetes have type 2.
- B. It is found more in nonwhite ethnic groups.
- C. There is not usually a family history.
- D. It is usually diagnosed before age 10 years.

14. A 14-year-old obese Hispanic male presents with fatigue, nighttime enuresis,

and acanthosis nigricans. The most likely diagnosis is:
- A. Prediabetes.
- B. Type 1 diabetes.
- C. Type 2 diabetes.
- D. Diabetes insipidus.

15. A 16-year-old presents with obesity, acanthosis nigricans, and a father who has type 2 diabetes. What test would you recommend?
- A. Fasting blood glucose levels.
- B. HLA.
- C. Autoantibodies to insulin.
- D. Urinalysis.

16. The most important therapy in managing type 2 diabetes is:
- A. Insulin.
- B. Metformin.
- C. Diet.
- D. Exercise.

17. In providing anticipatory guidance to a 16-year-old newly diagnosed type 2 diabetic, which information is the most important to discuss?
- A. Hyperglycemia.
- B. Hypoglycemia.
- C. Frequent infections.
- D. Insulin resistance.

18. A 15-year-old obese female with poorly controlled type 2 diabetes presents with dyslipidemia and hypertension. These are signs of which of the following complications of type 2 diabetes?
- A. Metabolic syndrome.
- B. Polycystic ovary disease.
- C. Retinopathy.
- D. Neuropathy.

19. A 13-year-old male presents for a routine physical with weight loss. Blood test results show a fasting blood glucose of 150. He most likely has which of the following?
- A. Prediabetes.
- B. Type 1 diabetes.
- C. Type 2 diabetes.
- D. Diabetes insipidus.

20. Which of the following is a characteristic sign of type 2 diabetes?

A. Polydipsia.
B. Polyphagia.
C. Polyuria.
D. Acanthosis nigricans.

21. A 9-year-old boy presents with a 4-month history of weight loss and "difficulty holding his urine" as per his mother. A fasting plasma glucose is 150. Which of the following is the most appropriate diagnosis?
A. Prediabetes.
B. Type 1 diabetes.
C. Type 2 diabetes.
D. Diabetes insipidus.

22. The most important measure for treating a 9-month-old with type 1 diabetes includes which of the following?
A. Preventing hypoglycemia.
B. Positive reinforcement.
C. Preventing an erratic appetite.
D. Making diabetes schedule accommodating.

23. Which of the following is the most useful in managing type 1 diabetes in a 4-year-old?
A. Positive reinforcement.
B. Teaching benefits of the best control.
C. Making diabetes schedule accommodating.
D. Body image concerns.

24. Which of the following is important anticipatory guidance for the parents of a 9-year-old with type 1 diabetes?
A. Managing a child with an erratic appetite.
B. Teaching the child that there is no-one to blame for the diabetes.
C. Parents remain involved in the child's diet and insulin management.
D. Encouraging the child to be totally independent in diabetes care.

NOTES

ANSWERS

1. *Answer:* C
   Rationale: Type 1 diabetes occurs equally in boys and girls. Each year, more than 13,000 children are diagnosed with type 1 diabetes. It is more prevalent in whites than African Americans. The number of cases of type 1 diabetes is anticipated to increase over time.

2. *Answer:* A
   Rationale: In order to develop diabetes, there must be genetic vulnerability with HLA genes elevated. Infectious agents, age, and stress are also factors in developing type 1 diabetes.

3. *Answer:* D
   Rationale: The pancreas produces less insulin which leads hyperglycemia. This in turn leads to polyuria, polydipsia, and polyphagia.

4. *Answer:* A
   Rationale: Refer the child to the emergency department as she may have diabetic ketoacidosis (DKA), which is a medical emergency. The other tests are important in diagnosing type 1 diabetes when the child does not appear severely ill.

5. *Answer:* A
   Rationale: Prediabetes presents with declining glucose tolerance. Type 1 diabetes presents with a deceased amount of insulin. Type 2 diabetes presents with resistance to peripheral insulin. Diabetes insipidus presents with the kidneys being unable to preserve water.

6. *Answer:* C
   Rationale: An Hb A1C of less than 8 is recommended for children 6 to 12 years of age. For ages 13 to 19, an Hb A1C is recommended to be less than 7.5, and for under the age of 6 years, 7.5 to 8.5.

7. *Answer:* C
   Rationale: While the "honeymoon" phase and beta cell destruction are important to discuss with the family, it is more important to discuss insulin. Insulin needs grow after diagnosis, not decline.

8. *Answer:* A
   Rationale: For an elevated blood glucose, a short-acting insulin such as Regular insulin is the most appropriate to give. Long-acting insulins such as NPH, Ultralente, and Lantus are not appropriate to quickly lower blood glucose.

9. *Answer:* B
   Rationale: Continuous blood glucose monitoring devices are not precise. Weight and height do need to be observed, but it is more important to teach a child about the number of times blood glucose needs to be checked. Blood glucose needs to be checked at least four times a day.

10. *Answer:* D
    Rationale: While all of the other factors are benefits of diet and exercise, maintaining weight and growth is the most important. Weight loss can suggest inadequate blood glucose control.

11. *Answer:* D
    Rationale: Unpredictable glucose control leads to more complications which include hyperglycemia and hypoglycemia. Frequent infections are also a possibility.

12. *Answer:* A
    Rationale: Capillary occlusion on fundoscopic exam is an indication of diabetic retinopathy which requires urgent referral to an ophthalmologist.

13. *Answer:* B
    Rationale: Type 2 diabetes is more common in nonwhite ethic groups such as Hispanics, African Americans, and Native Americans. Type 2 diabetes is usually found in 30% to 40% of children with diabetes. There is usually a family history and it is usually diagnosed after age 10.

14. *Answer:* C
    Rationale: Type 2 diabetes can present with obesity, fatigue, nighttime enuresis, and acanthosis nigricans. Prediabetes presents with declining glucose tolerance. Type 1 diabetes presents with a deceased amount of insulin. Diabetes insipidus presents with the kidneys being unable to preserve water.

15. *Answer:* A
Rationale: Blood glucose levels should be done first to establish the diagnosis of type 2 diabetes. The other tests are secondary tests.

16. *Answer:* C
Rationale: Diet is the most important management of type 2 diabetes by eating a reduced-calorie diet regularly. Insulin may be required initially, and metformin may be necessary as maintenance therapy. Exercise is important along with diet.

17. *Answer:* D
Rationale: Insulin resistance is the most important complication of type 2 diabetes. It can lead to metabolic syndrome and polycystic ovary disease. Hyperglycemia, hypoglycemia, and frequent infections are complications of type 2 diabetes as well.

18. *Answer:* A
Rationale: Obesity, dyslipidemia, and hypertension are signs of metabolic syndrome which is connected to insulin resistance. Polycystic ovary disease, retinopathy, and neuropathy are other complications of type 2 diabetes.

19. *Answer:* B
Rationale: The diagnostic criterion for type 1 diabetes includes weight loss, and a fasting blood glucose of greater than 126, along with polydipsia, polyuria, and polyphagia.

20. *Answer:* D
Rationale: Acanthosis nigricans is a typical sign of type 2 diabetes. Polydipsia, polyphagia, and polyuria are all signs of type 1 diabetes.

21. *Answer:* B
Rationale: Weight loss, polyuria, and a fasting plasma glucose of 150 are all signs of type 1 diabetes.

22. *Answer:* A
Rationale: Preventing hypoglycemia is the most important management strategy in a 9-month-old. Positive reinforcement, preventing an erratic appetite, and making a diabetes schedule accommodating are important as the child grows older.

23. *Answer:* A
Rationale: Positive reinforcement is important for a preschooler in order to help the child develop self-confidence. Teaching the benefits of the best control of diabetes, making the diabetes schedule accommodating, and body image concerns are all important as the child grows older.

24. *Answer:* C
Rationale: With a 9-year-old it is important to have the parents remain involved with the diabetes care while encouraging independence. Managing a child with an erratic appetite and teaching the child there is no-one to blame for the diabetes are all tasks for younger children and their parents.

BIBLIOGRAPHY

Alemzadeh, R., & Wyatt, D.T. (2004). Diabetes mellitus in children. In R.E. Behrman, R.M. Kliegman, & H.B. Jenson (Eds.). *Nelson textbook of pediatrics* (17th ed.). Philadelphia: Saunders.

Beck, M.J., Evans, B.J., Quarry-Horn, J.L., & Kerrigan, J.R. (2002). Type 2 diabetes mellitus: Issues for the medical care of pediatric and adult patients. *South Med J, 95*(9), 992-1000.

Boland, E.A., & Grey, M. (2004). Diabetes mellitus (types 1 and 2). In P.J. Allen, & J.A. Vessey (Eds.). *Primary care of the child with a chronic condition*. St. Louis: Mosby.

Brosnan, C.A., Upchurch, S., & Schreiner, B. (2001). Type 2 diabetes in children and adolescents: An emerging disease. *J Pediatr Health Care, 15*(4), 187-193.

Centers for Disease Control and Prevention (CDC). (2005). Diabetes projects. From the National Center for Chronic Disease Prevention and Health Promotion. Retrieved April 10, 2005, from www.cdc.gov/diabetes/projects/cda2.htm.

Fagot-Campagna, A., Pettitt, D.J., Engelgau, M.M., et al. (2000). Type 2 diabetes among North American children and adolescents: An epidemiologic review and a public health perspective. *J Pediatr, 136*(5), 664-672.

Gale, E.A.M. (2002). The rise of childhood type 1 diabetes in the 20th century. *Diabetes, 51*(12), 3353-3361.

Hernandez, C.A., & Williamson, K.M. (2004). Evaluation of a self-awareness education session for youth with type 1 diabetes. *Pediatr Nurs, 30*(6), 459-454, 502.

Lueder, G.T., Silverstein, J., and American Academy of Pediatrics Section on Ophthalmology and Section on Endocrinology. (2005). Screening for retinopathy in the pediatric patient with type 1 diabetes mellitus. *Pediatrics, 116*(1), 270-273

Morales, A., She, J-X., & Schatz, D.A. (2004). Genetics of type 1 diabetes. In O. Pescovitz & E. Eugster (Eds.). *Pediatric endocrinology: Mechanisms, manifestations, and management.* New York: Lippincott Williams & Wilkins.

Olantunbosun, S., & Dagogo-Jack, S. (2006). Insulin resistance. Retrieved June 30, 2006, from www.emedicine.com/med/topic1173.htm.

Pinhas-Hamiel, O., & Zeitler, P. (2001). Type 2 diabetes: Not just for grownups anymore. *Contemp Pediatr, 18*(1), 102-125.

Roemer, J.B. (2004). Endocrine and metabolic diseases. In C.E. Burns, A.M. Dunn, M.A. Brady, et al. (Eds.). *Pediatric primary care: A handbook for nurse practitioners* (3rd ed.). Philadelphia: Saunders.

Silverstein, J., Klingensmith, G., Copeland, K., et al. (2005). Care of children and adolescents with type 1 diabetes. *Diabetes Care, 28*(1), 186-212.

Votey, S.R., & Peters, A.L. (2005). Type 2 diabetes: A review. Retrieved June 30, 2006, from www.emedicine.com/EMERG/topic134.htm#target1.

Votey, S.R., & Peters, A.L. (2006). Type 1 diabetes: A review. Retrieved April 10, 2005, from www.emedicine.com/EMERG/topic133.htm#target1.

White, J.J. (2005). The glycemic index: How useful is it? *Consultant, 45*(4), 558-560.

NOTES

45 Eating Disorders

KIERSTEN A. M. WELLS

Select the best answer for each of the following questions:

1. The mortality rate of patients with eating disorders is:
   A. 5% to 10%.
   B. 1% to 2%.
   C. 20% to 25%.
   D. 40% to 60%.

2. A 12-year-old patient with an eating disorder presents to clinic for her yearly sports physical. She has a heart rate of 40, a temperature of 35.6° C, a respiratory rate of 14, and a blood pressure of 95/45 mm Hg. Her height is 65 inches and weight is 84 lbs. You note a 15 lb. weight loss since her physical last year. What would be most appropriate at this time?
   A. Admit her to the hospital.
   B. Order an echocardiogram for low heart rate.
   C. Complete the physical and clear for sports if normal.
   D. Withhold her from playing sports and refer to dietitian.

3. The initial main goal of inpatient hospitalization of an eating disorder patient would be:
   A. Immediate weight gain to 50% on BMI growth charts.
   B. Acute medical stabilization.
   C. Three to six months of intensive inpatient therapy.
   D. Prepare him or her for immediate residential treatment.

4. Which statement is true about males with eating disorders?

A. In the United States, there are more male bulimics compared to females.
B. Bipolar disorder is the most common denominator for eating disorders in males.
C. Males comprise 10% of all eating disorder patients.
D. Eating issues are related to depression and body dysmorphic disorders.

5. What might be the nutritional findings in a teen with anorexia?
   A. Decreased vitamin D level, decreased essential fatty acids (EFAs), decreased thiamine.
   B. Increased vitamin D level, increased EFAs, decreased thiamine level.
   C. Hyperglycemia, elevated thiamine, decreased EFAs.
   D. Increased potassium, decreased EFAs, increased thiamine.

6. The factor that is most related to the initiation of cycles of disordered eating is:
   A. Parents with personality disorders (axis II) and obesity.
   B. Family history of bipolar disorder and anxiety.
   C. Vomiting and diuretic use.
   D. Desire to lose weight and dieting behaviors.

7. The most common initial eating disorder diagnosis is:
   A. Anorexia nervosa.
   B. Bulimia nervosa.
   C. Eating disorder not otherwise specified (EDNOS).
   D. Female athletic triad.

8. What laboratory values would you expect to find in your patient with anorexia who presents with an acute, substantial weight loss in a short time followed by weight gain?
    A. Low phosphorus, low potassium, low magnesium, low glucose.
    B. High potassium, low sodium, high glucose.
    C. Low calcium, high sodium, low protein.
    D. High magnesium, low glucose, high potassium.

9. A 13-year-old male patient with a known eating disorder presents to the clinic with stable vital signs, an ESR of 145, diarrhea, and a macular rash. What is the best action?
    A. Order a C reactive protein (CRP) to evaluate acute inflammation.
    B. Conduct other systems workups to rule out malignancies or inflammatory diseases.
    C. Refer to infectious disease clinic.
    D. Reassure parents this is a normal finding in teens who present with eating disorders.

10. A 16-year-old female patient with known laxative abuse presents with a blood pressure of 150/100 mm Hg, a serum bicarbonate level of 32, a potassium of 3.0, and a serum chloride of 82. What action should the pediatric nurse practitioner take first?
    A. Order a comprehensive laxative screen, a toxicology screen, and admit her to the hospital.
    B. Order antihypertensive medication and a complete blood count.
    C. Schedule for blood pressure recheck in 2 days.
    D. Order an echocardiogram to rule out congenital heart disease.

11. What is a common and effective evidence-based treatment for bulimia nervosa?
    A. Cognitive behavioral therapy and antidepressant medications.
    B. Antidepressant medications and behavior modification.
    C. Behavior modification and antipsychotic medications.

D. Antipsychotic medication and group psychotherapy.

12. What are the most appropriate referrals the pediatric nurse practitioner should make on all teens diagnosed with anorexia nervosa?
    A. Registered dietitian and sociologist.
    B. Registered dietitian, psychologist, medical provider, and social worker.
    C. Psychologist, medical provider, and hospitalist.
    D. Social worker and physiologist.

13. Which of the following is the best action the pediatric nurse practitioner should take for a 13-year-old female patient with amenorrhea and osteopenia?
    A. Start Fosamax to increase bone growth.
    B. Order a repeat DEXA scan to verify findings.
    C. Provide nutritional counseling to promote weight restoration, which should result in the onset of menses.
    D. Order two Tums tablets per day to increase calcium.

14. Which statement is true about the prevalence of anorexia in the United States?
    A. 10% of all adolescent females are affected.
    B. 5% of all male adolescents are affected.
    C. 0.5% to 1% of females have anorexia nervosa.
    D. 0.5% to 1% of males have anorexia nervosa.

15. What patient's presentation would be most indicative of bulimia nervosa?
    A. 14-year-old female with lanugo, cold hands and feet, and secondary amenorrhea.
    B. 13-year-old male with loss of wet dreams, calluses on fingers, no gag reflex, and cheilosis.
    C. 16-year-old female with a BMI of 16 and poor self-esteem.
    D. 10-year-old male with no onset of pubertal changes and BMI of 5.

16. The pediatric nurse practitioner sees the following four patients one afternoon.

Which patient shows signs of anorexia nervosa?
A. 14-year-old female with BMI of 14, lanugo, pedal edema, and hypothermia.
B. 16-year-old male with loss of wet dreams, enlarged thyroid, and acute weight loss.
C. 13-year-old female with stunted growth, BMI of 25, and amenorrhea.
D. 10-year-old male with acanthosis nigricans, BMI of 12, and blood pressure of 80/50 mm Hg.

17. Which of the following statements is true regarding females/males from other countries with eating disorders?
A. Third-world countries do not recognize eating disorders.
B. Foreign citizens who live in the United States are more at risk for eating disorders.
C. Spain and Italy have more eating disorders than other countries.
D. Males are more likely than females to have eating disorders in foreign countries.

18. You saw a 16-year-old female, a known anorexic, 5 days ago. At that time, she had been eating only about 500 calories per day for 3 months. Today, she presents for her follow-up visit with you and mom states she has been eating all of her meals and three snacks per day (about 2000 calories/24 hours) since she was last in your office. What is the best action to take today?
A. Provide positive encouragement and schedule a weight check in 7 days.
B. Counsel on obesity prevention.
C. Admit to the hospital.
D. Order and evaluate serum electrolytes.

19. What lab value is most diagnostic of refeeding syndrome?
A. Hypophosphatemia
B. Hyponatremia
C. Hypermagnesemia
D. Hypokalemia

20. What is a serious complication of refeeding syndrome?

A. Hypoglycemia.
B. Metabolic syndrome.
C. Congestive heart failure.
D. Hypertensive crisis.

21. What patient is most likely to be at risk once hospitalized for refeeding syndrome?
A. 16-year-old male with morbid obesity and 12-pound weight loss in last 2 months.
B. 12-year-old male with anorexia with steady weight gain.
C. 15-year-old female with unstable diabetes and stable weight gain.
D. 15-year-old female with morbid obesity and a 36-pound weight loss in 1 month.

22. Which scenario is most likely diagnostic for EDNOS?
A. Use of daily laxatives and binging episodes with subsequent vomiting for 6 months.
B. Eating uncontrollably and developmental delay.
C. Normal menstruation, use of laxatives for 1 month, and at 80% of ideal body weight.
D. Loss of menses for 2 years, weight at 75% of ideal body weight, spitting out food.

23. Patients with anorexia will demonstrate:
A. An intense fear of gaining weight.
B. A refusal to maintain body weight above 90% of ideal body weight.
C. A positive body image.
D. A sense of lack of control of eating.

24. What are the most likely comorbid disorders that can accompany eating disorders?
A. Depression and psychosis.
B. Depression and anxiety.
C. Obsessive compulsive disorder and anxiety.
D. Anxiety and phobias.

25. The most dangerous outcome for disordered eating behavior is:
A. Hyperglycemia.
B. Hypothermia.
C. Liver disease.
D. Cardiac arrest.

ANSWERS

1. *Answer:* A
   Rationale: Mortality rates for both anorexia and bulimia range from 5% to 10%.

2. *Answer:* A
   Rationale: The presentation of this 12-year-old anorexia patient is adequate for admission based on AAP guidelines for hospitalization. Criteria are: pulse less than 50 beats per minute during the day and temperatures less than or equal to 36.0° C. Although the blood pressure does not meet criteria, the pulse and the temperature indicate systemic impacts of disordered eating behaviors. Although there is an association with anorexia and the development of mitral valve prolapse, unless a diastolic clink is heard, an echocardiogram is not an appropriate test at this time. An electrocardiogram might be better if you are concerned about prolonged QT interval, or changes in the T-waves based on electrolyte abnormalities. She is only 14, there has not been enough time to develop the so called "athletic heart." It would be prudent at this time to investigate eating behaviors as well as compensatory behaviors like vomiting and laxative use in this patient. Lastly, once this patient achieves acute medical stabilization, the body will need time to recover and the introduction of physical activity should be slow and well-monitored.

3. *Answer:* B
   Rationale: If the patient's vital signs are significant enough to merit acute medical stabilization and hospitalization, it will require at least 10 days of nutrition for reversing cardiac instability. Along those lines, the possibility of the patient suffering from refeeding syndrome is high (usually around 3 to 7 days postinitiation of refeeding), and will also need to be monitored in the hospital. Increase the feeds slowly, about 200-400 calories a day is the average; rapid refeeding can cause multisystem failure. Residential treatment is not the first-line treatment and is usually used once outpatient treatment has failed. Most inpatient facilities require that patients who need residential treatment are medically stable.

4. *Answer:* C
   Rationale: There is a paucity of information about young men with eating disorders. Although homosexuality can be one of the factors that affect young men with eating disorders, it is not thought to be the primary factor. It is also thought that men are affected by body image, but no association with depression and body dysmorphic disorder have been made to date. It is estimated that the female-to-male ratio is about 10-20:1 (or about 10%). There is no data showing that more men have bulimia than anorexia.

5. *Answer:* A
   Rationale: Anorexia is, in summary, the starvation of one's own body. There is a decreased level of vitamin D, zinc, calcium, folate, vitamin B$_{12}$, magnesium, copper, riboflavin, thiamine, and essential fatty acids (mostly omega 3 and 6). These can be supplemented in the diet with both food and oral supplements. Suggestions for supplementation vary. Refer to article and position paper by American Dietetic Association for suggestions. Studies are currently looking at essential fatty acids and their impact on the body.

6. *Answer:* D
   Rationale: There are several factors that have been identified and linked to the initiation of disordered eating behaviors. The most important factors are the desire to lose weight and the initiation of dieting behavior. They may be normal weight or even slightly lower weight at the onset of dieting. Although vomiting and diuretic use are behaviors that might also be practiced, the initial desire is to lose weight. Family history includes primary or secondary relatives with eating disorders.

7. *Answer:* C
   Rationale: It is estimated that 50% of children and adolescents who are discovered in pediatric settings do not meet official criteria for anorexia nervosa or bulimia nervosa. It is thought, however, that about 50% of those patients initially diagnosed with ED-NOS will go on to meet criteria for anorexia nervosa or bulimia nervosa. They may have similar medical signs and symptoms and will require the same types of treatment as the officially diagnosed patients. It is purported

that EDNOS should be treated as aggressively anorexia nervosa or bulimia nervosa.

8. *Answer:* A

Rationale: Medical complications include significant metabolic abnormalities, such as hypophosphatemia, hypomagnesemia, hypokalemia, hypoglycemia, normal or low albumin, hypocalcemia, and hyponatremia. Not only can these electrolyte abnormalities be caused by anorexia or bulimia, but can also recur in the refeeding phase of nutritional therapy.

9. *Answer:* B

Rationale: There are several disease processes that can present with the initial signs and symptoms of eating disorders in addition to other illnesses. Children and adolescents with eating disorders can also present with other disease processes. This patient has a known eating disorder and has stable vital signs which indicate metabolic stability. An elevated erythrocyte sedimentation rate is not typical for patients with eating disorders; usually they are normal to low. Although a C-reactive protein may help you rule out an acute infection, the sedimentation rate merits further investigation at this point. The differential diagnosis includes inflammatory bowel disease, tuberculosis, hypo/hyperthyroidism, diabetes, malignancies, rheumatologic disease, and problems with the pituitary gland.

10. *Answer:* A

Rationale: This patient presents with a dangerous electrolyte imbalance and should be immediately hospitalized for stabilization.

11. *Answer:* A

Rationale: There are many treatment methods available for the various psychiatric diseases. All patients who might need psychiatric consultation should be seen by a professional specializing in the psychiatric needs of children and adolescents. According to the Cochrane Database examination of data from 2003, cognitive behavior therapy is the most effective treatment for bulimia nervosa. Some studies purport that cognitive behavioral therapy (CBT) and SSRIs are the most effective treatment, but most studies show that CBT is extremely effective in decreasing the purging/binging desires. Individual therapy and psychoanalysis might be helpful; however, it is not the first-line treatment. Antipsychotic medications are not first-line at this time.

12. *Answer:* B

Rationale: A formal outpatient treatment center that houses nutrition, psychiatry, adolescent medicine, or primary care and social work would be an ideal environment for children and adolescents with eating disorders. However, a primary care provider who is willing to investigate resources in the area, arrange psychiatric care through insurance and communicate with eating disorder specialists can also achieve a good outpatient environment. If the team is spread throughout the community, constant communication with the various providers is imperative. It is important to recognize it is not just a psychiatric disease and nutrition is only a part of the total treatment process. It is also a process that ebbs and flows, with acute hospitalization being a possibility. Once the patient is medically stable, returning to the outpatient team is important for long-term care and outcome.

13. *Answer:* C

Rationale: Approximately 40% to 60% of bone mass is deposited during puberty and peak mass is usually achieved by late adolescence or early adulthood. Although this area of research is very controversial, it appears that nutritional health, weight gain, and return of menses are the markers used to evaluate improved health. The biphosphanates are being investigated but are not first-line treatment. Estrogen replacement may be good for patients with very low percent body fat, but are also not first-line treatment. It is thought that weight restoration, estrogen (from menses), and nutrition appear to have the best result.

14. *Answer:* C

Rationale: The prevalence of anorexia in adolescent females is 0.5% and 1% to 5% of girls ages 15 to 19 have bulimia. Anorexia is thought to occur more in the adolescent age group while bulimia occurs more in the young adult population.

15. *Answer:* B

Rationale: The symptoms of bulimia include changes in the hormonal gonadal axis (loss of menses or loss of wet dreams), calluses on fingers indicating possibility of vomiting (Russells' signs), loss of gag reflex from persistent vomiting, and cheilosis from vomiting or vitamin deficiency. Additionally, these patients have parotid enlargement, are of normal weight or overweight, and have dental enamel erosion secondary to acid effects of vomiting.

16. *Answer:* A

Rationale: Signs of anorexia include cold hands and feet, edema (secondary to changes in protein), lanugo (hair growth with attempt to keep body warm), hypothermia, low BMI, amenorrhea, and mitral valve prolapse from decreased heart size. Answer C presents symptoms of bulimia while answers B and D should be evaluated for other medical disease processes.

17. *Answer:* B

Rationale: It is not known that Spain and Italy have greater or fewer eating disorders than other countries. Foreign citizens who have exposure to western culture are more at risk for developing eating disorders.

18. *Answer:* D

Rationale: Someone who is taking in a small amount of calories over a set period of time will slow his or her metabolic systems down and decrease weight. The body learns to operate at the low calorie intake and conserves energy. If there is a large increase in caloric intake suddenly, the body often cannot recover fast enough. A large amount of energy is necessary and a large amount of phosphorus is consumed as the body adapts to the increase in energy consumption. It may take 3 to 7 days for the effects of refeeding to show up and providers should monitor their patients carefully. Although referral to a therapist is a good idea, it is not the priority at this visit. Encouraging the family is also important, but again, most importantly lab tests should be obtained to evaluate for refeeding syndrome.

19. *Answer:* A

Rationale: The most common sequelae in refeeding is hypophosphatemia. There can also be decreases in magnesium, potassium, and glucose.

20. *Answer:* C

Rationale: Refeeding syndrome can impact various systems in the body secondary to losing phosphorus, including cardiac, neurologic, hepatic, and hematologic changes. The liver is usually overwhelmed with the increase in calories after a long period of starvation and liver function test results can dramatically increase with refeeding. The most important effect is the cardiac changes that can result, including congestive heart failure and myocardial infarction due to electrolyte depletion.

21. *Answer:* D

Rationale: Patients at most risk for refeeding syndrome include those with anorexia, classic kwashiorkor, classic marasmus, chronic malnutrition and underfeeding, chronic alcoholism, morbid obesity with acute and massive weight loss, prolonged fasting, prolonged intravenous starvation, and prolonged intravenous hydration. Although patient B has anorexia, she has had steady and slow refeeding for several months, which is safe. There is no indication that adolescents with diabetes are at risk for refeeding syndrome.

22. *Answer:* C

Rationale: Patient C is the only one who doesn't meet criteria for anorexia nervosa or bulimia nervosa because he or she has not had the behavior long enough and does not meet the weight criteria. Patient A meets criteria for bulimia, patient B most likely has Prader Willi syndrome, and patient D meets criteria for anorexia nervosa.

23. *Answer:* A

Rationale: Patients with anorexia will have an intense fear of weight gain; usually they have poor body image, and demonstrate very high control over their eating behaviors.

24. *Answer:* B

Rationale: Depression, OCD, and anxiety all can be found in eating disorders, but the most common disorders that occur are both anxiety and depression. Patients who are profoundly malnourished can have changes in their mood that may mimic depression.

25. *Answer:* D

Rationale: Prolonged QT interval corrected for heart rate (QTc) has been found in patients with both anorexia and bulimia which can cause changes in heart rhythm and possibly cardiac arrest.

BIBLIOGRAPHY

American Academy of Pediatrics (AAP) (2003). Identifying and treating eating disorders. *Pediatrics, 111*(1), 204-211.

American Dietetic Association Reports. (2001). Position of the American Dietetic Association: Nutrition intervention in the treatment of anorexia nervosa, bulimia nervosa, and eating disorders not otherwise specified (EDNOS). *J Am Diet Soc, 101*(7), 810-819.

American Psychiatric Association. (1994). *Diagnostic and statistical manual of mental disorders* (4th ed.). Washington DC: Author.

Bacaltchuk, J., Hay, P., Trefiglio, R. (2001). Antidepressants versus psychological treatments and their combination for bulimia nervosa. The Cochrane Database of Systematic Reviews, Issue 4. Art. No.: CD003385. DOI: 10.1002/14651858. CD003385.

Bottas, A. & Richter, M. (2002), Pediatric autoimmune neuropsychiatric disorders associated with streptococcal infections (PANDAS). *Pediatr Infect Dis, 21*(1), 67-71.

Carter, F., McIntosh, V., Joyce, P., et al. (2003). Role of exposure with response prevention in cognitive behavioral treatment for bulimia nervosa: Three year follow-up results. *Int J Eat Disord, 33*(2), 127-135.

Centers for Disease Control and Prevention (CDC). (2003). Report from the National Youth Risk Behavior Survey. Retrieved May 21, 2006, from www.cdc.gov/mmwr/preview/mmwrhtml/ss5302a1.htm.

Cobb, K., Bachrach, L., Greendale, G., et al. (2003). Disordered eating, menstrual irregularity and bone mineral density in female runners. *Med Sci Sports Exer, 35*(5), 711-719.

Connan, F., Lightman, S., & Treasure, J. (2000). Biochemical and endocrine complications. *Eur Eat Disord Rev, 8*, 144-157.

Diamond-Raab, L., & Orrell-Valente, J.K. (2002). Art therapy, psychodrama, and verbal therapy. An integrative model of group therapy in the treatment of adolescents with anorexia nervosa and bulimia nervosa. *Child Adolesc Psychiatric Clin North Am, 11*(2), 343-364.

Fairburn, C., & Harrison, P. (2003). Eating disorders. *Lancet, 317*(9355), 407-416.

Fisher, M. (2006) Treatment of eating disorders in children, adolescents and young adults. *Fed Review, 27*(1), 5-15.

Fisher, M., Simpser, E., & Schneider, M. (2000). Hypophosphatemia secondary to oral refeeding in anorexia nervosa. *Int J Eat Dis, 28*(2), 181-187.

Frisch, M., Herzog, D., Franco, D. (2006). Residential treatment for eating disorders. *Intl J Eating Dis, 39*(3), 1-9.

Golden, N. (2003). Osteopenia and osteoporosis in anorexia nervosa. *Adolesc Med, 14*(1), 97-108.

Golden, N.H., Katzman, D. K., Kreipe R. E., et al. (2003). Eating disorders in adolescents: Position paper of the Society of Adolescent Medicine. *J Adol Health, 33*(6), 496-503.

Gordon, C. (2003). Normal bone accretion and effects of nutritional disorders in childhood. *J Women's Health, 12*(2), 137-143.

Hay, P., Bacaltchuk, J., & Stefano, S. (2004). Psychotherapy for bulimia nervosa and binging. The Cochrane Database of Systematic Reviews, Issue 3, Art No.: CD000562. DOI: 10.1002/14651858.CD000562.pub2.

Katzman, D. (2003). Osteoporosis in anorexia nervosa. A brittle future-current drug targets. *Curr Drug Targets CNS Neurol Disord, 2*(1), 11-15.

Katzman, D. (2005). Medical complications in adolescents with anorexia nervosa: A review of the literature. *Int J Eat Disord, 37*(Suppl), s52-s59.

Kazis, K., & Iglesias, E. (2003). The female athletic triad. *Adolesc Med, 14*(1), 87-95.

Keel, P. Dorer, D., Franco, D., et al. (2005). Postremission predictors of relapse in women with eating disorders. *Am J Psychiatry, 162*(12), 2263-2268.

Kotler, L., & Walsh, T. (2000). Eating disorders in children and adolescents: Pharmacological therapies. *Eur Child Adolesc Psychiatry, 9*(1), I 108-I 116.

Kreipe, R., & Birndorf, S. (2000). Eating disorders in adolescents and young adults. *Med Clin North Am, 84*(4), 1027-1049.

Levine, R. (2002). Endocrine aspects of eating disorders in adolescents. *Adolesc Med, 13*(1), 129-143.

Lock, J. (2002). Treating adolescents with eating disorders in the family context: Empirical and theoretical considerations. *Child Adolesc Psychiatry Clin North Am, 11*(2), 331-342.

Marinella, M. (2004). Refeeding syndrome. Implications for the impatient rehabilitation unit. *Am J Physical Med Rehab, 83*(1), 65-68.

Martin, H., & Ammerman, S. (2002). Adolescents with eating disorders. Primary care screening, identification, and early intervention. *Nurs Clin North Am, 37*(3), 537-551.

McLean, N., Griffin, S., Toney, K., & Hardeman, W. (2003). Family involvement in weight control, weight maintenance and weight-loss interventions: A systematic review of randomized trials. *Int J Obes Relat Metab Disord, 27*(9), 987-1005.

Mehler, P. (2003). Osteoporosis in anorexia nervosa: Prevention and treatment. *Int J Eat Disord, 33*(2), 113-126.

Metzl, J. (1999). Caring for the young dancer (*gymnast, figure skater). Contemp* Pediatr, 16(9), 138-164.

Milos, G., Spindler, A., & Schnyder, V. (2004). Psychiatric comorbidity and eating disorder inventory (EDI) profiles in eating disorder patients. *Canadian J Psychiatry, 49*(3), 179-184.

Mitchell, J., & Crow, S. (2006). Medical complications of anorexia nervosa and bulimia nervosa. *Curr Opinion Psych, 19*, 438-443.

Mont, L., Castro, J., Herreros, B., et al. (2003). Reversibility of cardiac abnormalities in adolescents with anorexia nervosa after weight recovery. *J Am Acad Child Adolesc Psychiatry, 42*(7), 808-813.

Muise, A., Stein, D., & Arbess, G. (2003), Eating disorders in adolescent boys: A review of the adolescent and young adult literature. *J Adolesc Health, 33*(6), 427-435.

Nicholls, D., & Stanhope, R. (2000). Medical complications of anorexia nervosa in children and young adolescents. *Eur Eat Disord Rev, 8*, 170-180.

Palla, B., & Litt, I. (1988). Medical complications of eating disorders in adolescents. *Pediatrics, 81*(5), 613-623.

Patrick, L. (2001). Eating disorders: A review of the literature with emphasis on medical complications and clinical nutrition. *Alt Med Rev, 7*(3), 184-202.

Phillips, E, & Pratt, H. (2005). Eating disorders in college. *Ped Clinics N Am, 52*(1), 85-96.

Robb, A. & Dadson, M. (2002). Eating disorders in males. *Child Adolesc Psychiatr Clin N Am, 11*(2), 399-418.

Rome, E. (2003). Eating disorders. *Obstet Gynecol Clin, 30*(2), 353-377.

Rome, E., & Ammerman, S. (2003). Medical complications of eating disorders: An update. *J Adol Health, 33*(6), 418-426.

Rome, E., Ammerman, S., Rosen, D., et al. (2003). Children and adolescents with eating disorders: The state of the art. *Pediatrics, 111*(1), e98-e108.

Rosenblum, J., & Foreman, S. (2002). Evidence based treatment of eating disorders. *Curr Opin Pediatr, 14*(4), 379-383.

Schapman-Williams, A., Lock J., & Couturier, J. (2006). Cognitive-behavioral therapy for adolescents with binge-eating syndromes. *Intl J Eating Disorders, 39*(3), 252-255.

Seibel, M. (2002). Nutrition and molecular markers of bone remodeling. *Curr Opin Clin Nutr Metab Care, 5*(5), 525-531.

Simopoulous, A.P. (2000). Human requirement for N-3 poly-unsaturated fatty acids. *Poult Sci, 79*(7), 968-970.

Solomon, S. & Kirby, D. (1990) The refeeding syndrome. *JPEN J Parenter Enteral Nutr, 14*, 90-97.

Sundaran, G., & Bartlett, D. (2001). Preventive measures for bulimic patients with dental erosion. *Eur J Prosthodontic Restorative Dentistry, 8*, 25-29.

Swenne, I., & Engstrom, I. (2005). Medical assessment of adolescent girls with eating disorders. An evaluation of symptoms and signs of starvation. *Acta Paediatr, 94*(10), 1363-1371.

Treasure, J., & Schmidt, U. (June 2004). Anorexia nervosa. *In Clin Evid, 11*, 1192--1203.

Walsh, J., Wheat, M., & Freund, K. (2000). Detection, evaluation, and treatment of eating disorders: The role of the primary care physician. *J Gen Intern Med, 15*(8), 577-590.

Winston, A.P., & Stafford, P.J. (2000). Cardiovascular effects of anorexia nervosa. *Eur Eat Disord Rev, 8*(2), 117-125.

46 Epilepsy

MARIA S. CHICO

Select the best answer for each of the following questions:

1. The antiepileptic medication most likely to cause oral contraception failure is:
   A. Lamotrigine.
   B. Carbamazepine.
   C. Levetiracetam.
   D. Valproate.

2. The best treatment for total cure of partial epilepsy in a child is:
   A. Cortical resection.
   B. Phenytoin.
   C. Vagus nerve stimulator (VNS).
   D. Ketogenic diet.

3. Children with epilepsy should be restricted from which of the following activities?
   A. School field trips.
   B. Swimming alone.
   C. Soccer.
   D. Airline travel.

4. A seizure with focal origin involving one hemisphere is classified as:
   A. Generalized.
   B. Partial.
   C. Mixed.
   D. Atonic.

5. Initial diagnostic testing conducted in the primary care setting to evaluate the etiology of seizures includes:
   A. EEG.
   B. Muscle/skin biopsy.
   C. CBC, serum glucose, electrolytes, chemistry, urine ketones.
   D. Cranial ultrasound.

6. A 14-year-old patient presents with the following history: brief sudden generalized muscle contractions affecting the extremities—mainly upon awakening, duration of less than 2 minutes, no loss of consciousness is involved. Otherwise healthy without change in body habitus or evidence of cognitive decline. The most likely seizure type is:
   A. Generalized tonic/clonic.
   B. Complex partial.
   C. Juvenile myoclonic epilepsy.
   D. Atonic.

7. A 3-year-old child presents to clinic with history of a single seizure, duration of 2 minutes that occurred this past week. The child's immunizations are up to date and his BMI is at the 50th percentile. The pediatric nurse practitioner would first obtain:
   A. Chemistry profile, electrolytes, CBC.
   B. Detailed history of the event.
   C. Brain CT scan.
   D. CSF for cell count and culture.

8. The most appropriate treatment for this patient is:
   A. Carbamazepine.
   B. Valproate.
   C. Phenytoin.
   D. No treatment is indicated at this time.

9. Children with uncontrolled nocturnal, generalized, tonic/clonic seizures are at high risk for:
   A. JME (juvenile myoclonic epilepsy).
   B. SUDEP (sudden unexpected death from epilepsy).

C. BRE (benign rolandic epilepsy).
D. LTM (long-term video EEG monitoring).

10. Ketogenic diet for the treatment of epilepsy involves:
A. High carbohydrate to low fat ratio.
B. High fatty acids and carbohydrates and low protein.
C. High fat to low carbohydrate/protein ratio.
D. High protein and low fatty acids.

11. Surgical intervention for intractable epilepsy is most appropriate for which seizure type?
A. Atonic.
B. Myoclonic.
C. Clonic.
D. Complex partial.

12. Children with epilepsy most at risk for cognitive decline include those:
A. With high-severity seizures.
B. In remission without therapy.
C. With brief, infrequent seizures.
D. In supportive home environments.

13. The antiepileptic medication known to cause anorexia and concomitant weight loss is:
A. Valproate.
B. Phenytoin.
C. Topiramate.
D. Lamotrigine.

14. The antiepileptic medication known to cause increased appetite and subsequent weight gain is:
A. Valproate.
B. Phenytoin.
C. Topiramate.
D. Lamotrigine.

15. A factor which indicates a poor prognosis of epilepsy is:
A. Normal neuroimaging studies.
B. Control of seizures with dual antiepileptic medications.
C. Presence of postictal phase.
D. High initial seizure density.

16. Median age of onset in pediatric epilepsy is:
A. 15 to 18 years.
B. First 6 months of life.
C. 5 to 6 years.
D. Second decade of life.

17. A 3-year-old child comes in to the clinic for a well child visit. The child was diagnosed with juvenile myoclonic epilepsy about 12 months ago. The mother expresses her concern that she caused this condition by traveling to Thailand while pregnant. The best response for the pediatric nurse practitioner would be:
A. I'll put in a referral to the air travel medicine department.
B. The cause of juvenile myoclonic epilepsy has been linked to genetics.
C. This disorder is caused by exposure to environmental toxins during your pregnancy.
D. Did you visit any other countries while pregnant with this child?

18. The pediatric nurse practitioner should consider referral to a pediatric neurologist when the patient exhibits:
A. Subtherapeutic antiepileptic levels.
B. Regression of cognitive function.
C. Noncompliance with antiepileptic medication.
D. A growth spurt on antiepileptic medications.

19. Which of the following seizure type causes impairment of consciousness?
A. Psychogenic.
B. Complex partial.
C. Tonic-clonic.
D. Simple partial.

20. The antiepileptic medication utilized for the treatment of both partial and generalized seizures is:
A. Lamotrigine.
B. Valproate.
C. Carbamazepine.
D. Topiramate.

21. The best time to obtain antiepileptic medicine levels is:

A. Two hours after the dose is given.
B. Random afternoon level.
C. Morning trough (prior to morning dose).
D. Postprandial (after meals).

22. Tapering off anticonvulsant medication can be considered after:
A. 1 year of treatment.
B. 4 seizure-free years.
C. 6 months of treatment.
D. 2 seizure-free years.

23. Epilepsy is characterized by:
A. Recurrent, unprovoked seizures.
B. A single febrile seizure.
C. Mental retardation.
D. Cerebral palsy.

24. After vagus nerve stimulator (VNS) therapy, what percentage of patients with epilepsy will have greater than a 50% reduction in the number of seizures?
A. 5%
B. 10%
C. 33%
D. 50%

NOTES

ANSWERS

1. *Answer:* B
    Rationale: Carbamazepine causes contraception failure; the others do not.

2. *Answer:* A
    Rationale: Cortical resection provides a cure and complete remission of seizures. The other choices do not cure partial epilepsy.

3. *Answer:* B
    Rationale: Seizure while swimming alone may cause drowning.

4. *Answer:* B
    Rationale: Partial seizure involves one hemisphere of the brain.

5. *Answer:* C
    Rationale: CBC, serum glucose, electrolytes, chemistry, and urine ketones are routine laboratory diagnostics; the other diagnostic tests are obtained at tertiary centers.

6. *Answer:* C
    Rationale: Juvenile myoclonic epilepsy is a common seizure type that occurs in adolescence, mainly upon awakening; the other seizures occur randomly across all ages.

7. *Answer:* B
    Rationale: The chief complaint does not always reveal the detailed history needed to formulate an accurate differential diagnosis. The history will then guide any diagnostics to be performed.

8. *Answer:* D
    Rationale: No treatment is usually indicated for first single seizure.

9. *Answer:* B
    Rationale: The risk factors for sudden, unexpected death from epilepsy are uncontrolled nocturnal, generalized tonic/clonic seizures; JME and BRE are seizure types and LTM is a neurophysiology study.

10. *Answer:* C
    Rationale: The ketogenic diet is high in fat and low in carbohydrate/protein. Management should be done by qualified registered dietitian.

11. *Answer:* D
    Rationale: Surgery is indicated for partial seizures; the others listed are generalized seizures.

12. *Answer:* A
    Rationale: Uncontrolled seizures are the single highest risk factor for cognitive decline. Polytherapy with antiepileptic medication can have a negative effect on a child's cognitive functioning, especially if the side effect profile of the drug alters cognition. Children with low-severity seizures usually maintain average school performance. Supportive family environments can positively affect cognitive functioning.

13. *Answer:* C
    Rationale: All the other medications, except topiramate, either cause weight gain or no change in weight.

14. *Answer:* A
    Rationale: All the other medications, except valproate, either cause weight loss or no change in weight.

15. *Answer:* D
    Rationale: Poor prognostic factors in children with epilepsy include high initial seizure density, presence of a metabolic disorder, and cerebral structural abnormalities.

16. *Answer:* C
    Rationale: The median age of onset of pediatric epilepsy is 5 to 6 years old.

17. *Answer:* B
    Rationale: Juvenile myoclonic epilepsy is a genetic disorder located on the chromosome 6p15q14. The gene has not been identified yet. It has not been linked to infections, diseases, or fever.

18. *Answer:* B
    Rationale: The other choices, suboptimal medication levels, noncompliance, and growth issues, are situations that the pediatric nurse practitioner can manage.

19. *Answer:* C

Rationale: In tonic-clonic seizures, consciousness is completely lost. In simple partial seizures and and complex partial seizures there is no loss of consciousness. Psychogenic is not a type of seizure.

20. *Answer:* B

Rationale: Valproate is used for both partial and generalized seizures. All the others are used for partial seizures.

21. *Answer:* C

Rationale: The best time to obtain antiepileptic levels is just prior to the morning scheduled dose (trough level.)

22. *Answer:* D

Rationale: After 2 years without seizures, a normal EEG and unchanged physical examination anticonvulsant medications can be tapered off over a 3- to 6-month period of time.

23. *Answer:* A

Rationale: Recurrent, unprovoked seizures define epilepsy; the other choices define brain dysfunction.

24. *Answer:* C

Rationale: Vagus nerve stimulator therapy is most effective with generalized epilepsy. One-third of the patients will have greater than 50% reduction in seizures, one-third will have less than 50% reduction in seizures, and one-third will have no changes in their seizure frequency.

BIBLIOGRAPHY

American Academy of Pediatrics, Provisional Committee on Quality Improvement and Subcommittee on Febrile Seizures. (1996). Practice Parameter: The neurodiagnostic evaluation of the child with a first simple febrile seizure. *Pediatrics, 97*(5), 769-772.

American Epilepsy Society. (2004). Basic mechanisms underlying seizures and epilepsy. Retrieved on May 21, 2006, from http://www.aesnet.org/Visitors/ProfessionalDevelopment/MedEd/ppt/ppts03/BASICORE.PDF.

Austin, J., Huberty, T., Huster, G., & Dunn, D. (1999). Does academic achievement in children with epilepsy change over time? *Dev Med Child Neurol, 41*(7), 473-479.

Austin, J.K., Dunn, D.W., Johnson, C.S., & Perkins, S.M. (2004). Behavioral issues involving children and adolescents with epilepsy and the impact of their families: Recent research data. *Epilepsy Behav, 5*(Suppl. 3), S10-S17.

Blair, J., & Selekman, J. (2004). Epilepsy. In P.L. Jackson & J.A. Vessey (Eds.). *Primary care of the child with a chronic condition* (4th ed.). St. Louis: Mosby.

Fastenau, P.S., Shen, J., Dunn, D.W., et al. (2004). Neuropsychological predictors of academic underachievement in pediatric epilepsy: Moderating roles of demographic, seizure and psychosocial variables. *Epilepsia, 45*(10), 1261-1272.

French, J.A., Kanner, A.M., Bautista, J., et al. (2004). Efficacy and tolerability of the new antiepileptic drugs I: treatment of new onset epilepsy: report of the Therapeutics and Technology Assessment Subcommittee and Quality Standards Subcommittee of the American Academy of Neurology and the American Epilepsy Society.. *Neurology, 62*(8), 1252-1260.

Johnston, M.V. (2004). Seizures in childhood. In R.E. Behrman, R.M. Kliegman, & H.B. Jenson (Eds.). *Nelson textbook of pediatrics* (17th ed.). Philadelphia: Saunders.

Kwan, P., & Sander, J.W. (2004). The natural history of epilepsy: An epidemiological view. *J Neurol Neurosurg Psychiatry, 75*(10), 1376-1381.

Loring, D.W., & Meador, K.J. (2004). Cognitive side effects of antiepileptic drugs in children. *Neurology, 62*(6), 872-877.

Marsh, L., & Rao, V. (2002). Psychiatric complications in patients with epilepsy: A review. *Epilepsy Res, 49*(1), 11-33.

Ojemann, J.G., Park, T.S. (2001). Surgical treatment: Surgery and outcome. In J. Pellock, W.E. Dodson, B. Bourgeois (Eds). *Pediatric epilepsy diagnosis and therapy* (2nd ed.). New York: Demos.

Ottman, R. (2001). Genetic influences on risk for epilepsy. In J. Pellock, W.E. Dodson, B. Bourgeois (Eds). *Pediatric epilepsy diagnosis and therapy* (2nd ed.). New York: Demos.

Shinnar, S., Berg, A.T., O'Dell, C., et al. (2000). Predictors of multiple seizures in a cohort of children prospectively followed from the time of their first unprovoked seizure. *Ann Neurol, 48*(2), 140-147.

47 Hemoglobinopathies

MIRELLA VASQUEZ BROOKS

Select the best answer for each of the following questions:

1. Which of the following is NOT considered a common hemoglobinopathy?
   A. Sickle-cell anemia.
   B. Iron deficiency anemia.
   C. Hemoglobin E.
   D. α-thalassemia.

2. Michael, age 7, is brought into the office by his parents. Mr. Smith asks the pediatric nurse practitioner "How is α-thalassemia transmitted?" The most appropriate response by the pediatric nurse practitioner is that it is a(n):
   A. X-lined inheritance.
   B. Dominant inheritance.
   C. Autosomal recessive inheritance.
   D. Split-gene inheritance.

3. Dan, age 17, is an African American male who is being tested for α-thalassemia. Which tests should be ordered today?
   A. Hemoglobin electrophoresis, CBC, and iron studies.
   B. Hemoglobin C, hematocrit, and iron studies.
   C. Hemoglobin AIC, multimeric, and iron studies.
   D. Hemoglobin electrophoresis, platelet aggregation, and iron studies.

4. Which of the following is an X-linked recessive disorder that is commonly seen in African American children?
   A. α-thalassemia.
   B. Sickle-cell anemia.
   C. Hemophilia.

   D. von Willebrand's disease.

5. Which of the following test is the most definitive to use in the diagnosis of sickle cell anemia?
   A. Bleeding time.
   B. Genetic testing.
   C. Hemoglobin electrophoresis.
   D. Multimeric analysis.

6. Which of the following conditions is NOT caused by a genetic mutation of chromosome 11?
   A. Hemoglobin C.
   B. Hemoglobin E.
   C. Hemoglobin S.
   D. α-thalassemia.

7. Treatment of thalassemia trait should include:
   A. Transfusions.
   B. Bone marrow transplant.
   C. Iron chelation therapy.
   D. No treatment is needed.

8. Treatment for thalassemia intermedia should include:
   A. Transfusions.
   B. Bone marrow transplant.
   C. Iron chelation therapy.
   D. No treatment needed.

9. During a clinic visit, the pediatric nurse practitioner knows that Brian, a 6-year-old child receiving transfusions for thalassemia major, should have:
   A. Monitoring of fluid overload.
   B. Regular evaluation of liver and kidney function.

C. Monitoring for iron deficiency.
D. Genetic counseling.

10. Which type of thalassemia condition causes a shortened life span and impaired fertility in patients?
A. Thalassemia major.
B. Thalassemia minor.
C. Thalassemia intermedia.
D. Thalassemia globulin.

11. It is appropriate to consider genotyping in children with α-thalassemia at high risk for loss of:
A. 1 or 2 genes.
B. 2 or 3 genes.
C. 3 or 4 genes.
D. 5 or 6 genes.

12. Which of the following is the most severe of the phenotype notations for α-thalassemia?
A. Minor.
B. Major.
C. Hemoglobin H disease.
D. Bart's hydrops fetalis.

13. Which of the following is FALSE regarding surviving infants with four gene deletions?
A. Require transfusion therapy.
B. Life expectancy is normal.
C. Primary care should be managed collaboratively with a pediatric hematologist.
D. May be a candidate for hematopietic stem cell transplantation.

14. Which of the following cardiovascular effects is NOT a long-term effect in a child with sickle-cell anemia?
A. Compensatory increased cardiac output.
B. Left ventricular hypertrophy as a result of chronic anemia.
C. Right ventricular hypertrophy as a result of immature RBC.
D. Pulmonary hypertension is rare except in those with acute or chronic pulmonary disease.

15. What is the life span of a red blood cell (RBC) in individuals with hemoglobin C disease?

A. 100 days.
B. 70 days.
C. 40 days.
D. 20 days.

16. Which of the following is NOT considered a standard of care for a child with hemoglobin C disease?
A. Annual complete blood cell count (CBC).
B. Collaboration with a pediatric hematologist.
C. Routine preventive care visits.
D. Bimonthly evaluation of liver and kidney function.

17. Which of the following statements regarding hemoglobinopathies is true?
A. Abnormal structure of one of the globin chains of the hemoglobin molecule.
B. Abnormal structure of one the clotting factors.
C. Abnormal structure of the platelets.
D. Abnormal structure of one of the beta chains of the hematocrit molecule.

18. Which ethnic group has the highest overall hemoglobin E incidence rate?
A. Mediterranean and Middle Easterners.
B. Southeast Asians and Native Americans.
C. Western Europeans.
D. South American.

19. The lab results come back on Baby Presley. Which of the following labs are indicative of a definitive diagnosis of α-thalassemia?
A. FA+ hemoglobin Bart's.
B. FA+ hemoglobin S.
C. FA+ hemoglobin B.
D. FA+ hemoglobin H.

20. Which of the following instructions should NOT be included in the teaching plan for the parents of a child with anemia associated with hemoglobin S disease?
A. Parents need to know the child's baseline hemoglobin level.
B. Parents should be able to identify signs of worsening anemia that require evaluation.

C. Parents need to understand the cause of the anemia.

D. Parents need to get tested for hemoglobin S disease.

21. Three signs and symptoms of β-thalassemia minor (trait) are:

A. Microcytic anemia, abnormal red blood cell count, and asymptomatic.

B. Macrocytic anemia, normal red blood cell count, and symptomatic.

C. Microcytic anemia, normal red blood cell count, and asymptomatic.

D. Macrocytic anemia, abnormal red blood cell count, and symptomatic.

22. Sickle-cell anemia is caused by:

A. Exposure to radiation.

B. A genetically induced production of abnormal hemoglobin S.

C. A deficiency of dietary folic acid.

D. Long-term use of steroids.

23. When should Larry, a 1-week-old infant diagnosed with α-thalassemia, have a follow-up visit?

A. In 1 week.

B. By 1 month of age.

C. By 1 year of age.

D. No follow-up is needed.

NOTES

ANSWERS

1. **Answer:** B
   Rationale: Hemoglobinopathies are genetic defects; iron deficiency is not genetic in orgin. The most common hemoglobinopathies are α-thalassemia, β-thalassemia, hemoglobin C, hemoglobin E, and sickle cell anemia.

2. **Answer:** C
   Rationale: Thalassemia is a genetic disorder transmitted in an autosomal recessive inheritance. A person can only be affected with thalassemia if they inherit the trait from their parents.

3. **Answer:** A
   Rationale: Testing in older children should include hemoglobin electrophoresis, CBC, and iron studies.

4. **Answer:** B
   Rationale: The prevalence of sickle cell trait is 8% to 10% in the black population. One in 500 or 15% of the black population has sickle cell disease.

5. **Answer:** C
   Rationale: Hemoglobin electrophoresis is a test that determines the presence of hemoglobin S.

6. **Answer:** D
   Rationale: α-thalassemia is a genetic mutation of chromosome 16.

7. **Answer:** D
   Rationale: No treatment is needed for patients with thalassemia trait.

8. **Answer:** A
   Rationale: Treatment for thalassemia intermedia often requires transfusions and should be managed collaboratively with a pediatric hematologist.

9. **Answer:** B
   Rationale: Children receiving transfusions should also have regular evaluation of liver and kidney function, monitoring of iron overload, and testing for blood-borne infectious diseases (hepatitis B and C, HIV). Genetic testing should occur when the child reaches adolescence.

10. **Answer:** A
    Rationale: Individuals with thalassemia major may have a shortened life span and may also have impaired fertility.

11. **Answer:** C
    Rationale: Consider genotyping in populations at high risk for loss of three or four genes.

12. **Answer:** D
    Rationale: Examples of phenotype notation in order of severity: carrier, minor, hemoglobin H disease, and Bart's hydrops fetalis.

13. **Answer:** B
    Rationale: Surviving infants with four gene deletions require chronic transfusion therapy, may be candidates for hematopoietic stem cell transplantation, and primary care should be managed in collaboration with a pediatric hematologist.

14. **Answer:** C
    Rationale: Individuals with sickle cell disease will develop chronic organ damage. Cardiovascular effects are left ventricular hypertrophy as a result of chronic anemia, compensatory increased cardiac output, and pulmonary hypertension (which is rare except in those with acute or chronic pulmonary disease).

15. **Answer:** C
    Rationale: A hemoglobin C RBC life span is about 40 days compared with a normal life span of 120 days.

16. **Answer:** D
    Rationale: Standard care for a child with hemoglobin C disease includes seeing child according to routine preventive care schedule, annual CBC, and consultation with a pediatric hematologist.

17. **Answer:** A
    Rationale: Genetic defects that involve changes in the amino acid sequence of either

the α-or β-globin chains of hemoglobin are termed *hemoglobinopathies*. Hundreds of these defects have been described.

18. *Answer:* B
Rationale: Hemoglobin E is most common in Southeast Asians and Native Americans.

19. *Answer:* A
Rationale: Diagnostic newborn screening indicative of α-thalassemia are FA+ Bart's. FA means that amount of fetal hemoglobin is greater than adult hemoglobin (normal for a newborn). Bart's hemoglobin is indicative of one to four missing or dysfunctional genes.

20. *Answer:* D
Rationale: Teaching parents to understand the importance of knowing the cause of anemia, signs of worsening anemia that require evaluation (pallor, significantly increased fatigue), and knowing the child's baseline hemoglobin should all be included in the teaching plan. Hemoglobin S is an autosomal recessive inheritance. Both parents have the sickle cell trait.

21. *Answer:* C
Rationale: The signs and symptoms of β-thalassemia are mild to moderate microcytic anemia, target cells are seen on the peripheral blood smear, normal red blood cell count, and patients are likely asymptomatic.

22. *Answer:* B
Rationale: In patients with sickle cell anemia, their RBCs contain hemoglobin S.

23. *Answer:* B
Rationale: Follow-up testing should be done by 1 month of age.

BIBLIOGRAPHY

Brigham & Women's Hospital (BWH). (2002). Hemoglobin synthesis. Retrieved June 26, 2006, from http://sickle.bwh.harvard.edu/hbsynthesis.html.

Carter, S.M., & Gross, S.J. (2005). Hemoglobin C disease. Retrieved May 21, 2006, from www.emedicine.com/med/topic976.htm.

Cohen, A.R., Galanello, R., Pennell, D.J., et al. (2004). Thalassemia. *Hematology Am Soc Hematol Educ Program*, 14-34.

Dodds, N., & Shahidi, H. (2005). Pediatrics, sickle cell disease. Retrieved February 20, 2005, from www.emedicine.com/emerg/topic406.htm.

Dover, G.J., & Platt, O. (2003). Sickle cell disease. In D.G. Nathan, S.H. Orkin, A.T. Look, & D. Ginsburg (Eds.). *Nathan and Oski's hematology of infancy and childhood* (6th ed.). Philadelphia: Saunders.

Lisak, M.E. (2004). Sickle cell disease. In P.J. Allen & J. Vessey (Eds.). *Primary care of the child with a chronic condition* (4th ed.). St. Louis: Mosby.

Nagel, R. (2003). Human hemoglobins: Normal and abnormal. In D.G. Nathan, S.H. Orkin, A.T. Look, & D. Ginsburg (Eds.). *Nathan and Oski's hematology of infancy and childhood* (6th ed.). Philadelphia: Saunders.

Orkin, S.H., & Nathan, D.G. (2003). The thalassemias. In D.G. Nathan, S.H. Orkin, A.T. Look, & D. Ginsburg (Eds.). *Nathan and Oski's hematology of infancy and childhood* (6th ed.). Philadelphia: Saunders.

Schatz, J., Finke, R., & Roberts, C.W. (2004). Interactions of biomedical and environmental risk factors for cognitive development: A preliminary study of sickle cell disease. *J Dev Behav Pediatr, 25*(5), 303-310.

Segel, G.B., Hirsh, M.G., & Feig, S.A. (2002a). Managing anemia in pediatric office practice: Part 1. *Pediatr Rev, 23*(3), 75-83.

Segel, G.B., Hirsh, M.G., & Feig, S.A. (2002b). Managing anemia in pediatric office practice: Part 2. *Pediatr Rev, 23*(4), 111-121.

Viprakasit, V., Tamphaichitr, V.S., Mahasandana, C., et al. (2001). Linear growth in homozygous beta-thalassemia and beta-thalassemia/hemoglobin E patients under different treatment regimens. *J Med Assoc Thai, 84*(7), 929-941.

Walters, M.C., Storb, R., Patience, M., et al. (2000). Impact of bone marrow transplantation for symptomatic sickle cell disease: An interim report. Multicenter investigation of bone marrow transplantation for sickle cell disease. *Blood, 95*(6), 1918-1924.

Zimmerman, S.A., Schultz, W.H., Davis, J.S., et al. (2004). Sustained long-term hematologic efficacy of hydroxyurea at maximum tolerated dose in children with sickle cell disease. *Blood, 103*(6), 2039-2045.

RICHELLE T. MAGDAY ASSELSTINE

Select the best answer for each of the following questions:

1. A diagnosis of juvenile rheumatoid arthritis (JRA) would be suspected if a child presents with which set of symptoms?
   A. Erythematous joints, joint pain, fever, rash.
   B. Morning stiffness, altered mobility, joint pain, fever, rash.
   C. Nausea, one-sided weakness, irritability, intolerance to heat or cold.
   D. Change in daily activities, photosensitivity, anemia, loss of appetite.

2. Macrophage activation syndrome (MAS), reactive hematophagocytic lymphohistiocytosis, and cricoarytenoid arthritis are complications in systemic JRA that require what type of action by the pediatric nurse practitioner?
   A. Prescription of high dose nonsteroidal antiinflammatory medications (NSAIDs).
   B. Careful monitoring without immediate treatment.
   C. Referral to the emergency department for high-dose intravenous steroids and consultation with a rheumatoid specialist.
   D. Oral steroids and physical therapy three to four times per week.

3. Which one of the following diagnoses would you suspect in a 13-year-old male who presents with inflammation in his right ankle and knees, no pain, rheumatoid factor negative, and ANA positive?
   A. Oligoarthritis.

B. Polyarthritis.
C. Systemic JRA.
D. Osteoarthritis.

4. Christina is a 12-year-old with oligoarthritis who is currently taking naproxen for her JRA. She comes to clinic to have a preoperative clearance for arthroscopic surgery on her ankle in 5 days. What instructions should she receive regarding her naproxen?
   A. Double-dosing of the naproxen after the surgery to help postoperative pain.
   B. Continue taking the medication until the day of the surgery, then discontinue until 2 weeks postoperative.
   C. Continue daily doses of naproxen pre- and postoperatively.
   D. Discontinue the naproxen immediately and resume only when instructed by a health care provider.

5. Progressive joint involvement occurs in approximately what percentage of children with systemic JRA?
   A. 30%
   B. 75%
   C. 50%
   D. 90%

The following six questions pertain to this scenario:

Melissa is a 10-year-old who has been diagnosed with systemic JRA. Her BMI is at the 10th percentile for her age. Her parents only speak Spanish and Melissa has to translate to the health care team. She is currently taking methotrexate subcutaneous once a week, folic acid orally every day except for days she receives methotrexate, etanercept subcutaneously once a week, naproxen orally twice a day, and a multivitamin daily. After 3 years of corticosteroid therapy, Melissa was weaned off about 3 months ago. They only have one car which dad must use to go to work. Mom uses public transportation to bring Melissa to clinic for her weekly methotrexate and etanercept shots. Melissa is the oldest of three children. Melissa tries as much as possible to be active at school and knows her limitations on physical activity.

6. Mom has some concerns about Melissa's health status in the days after receiving her shots. Melissa gets very fatigued and sometimes is too tired to get out of bed. Overall, both medications help with pain management and JRA symptoms, but she worries about the fatigue. As her pediatric nurse practitioner, you explain that:

A. Methotrexate and etanercept's side effects include fatigue, suppressing the body's immune system and lowering the white blood cell count, making Melissa feel weak at times and harder for her body to fight infection.

B. Melissa doesn't get enough exercise and a more rigorous regimen will help Melissa be more active and feel less fatigued.

C. The dose of medication is too low based on Melissa's age and increasing the dose will decrease fatigue.

D. Melissa's fatigue is not related to her medications and perhaps she is not getting proper rest at night.

7. During the appointment, Melissa translates for her mother. You are discussing important issues regarding Melissa's medication. The next best course of action is to:

A. Ask Melissa if there is an adult family member who can translate.

B. Find medical staff in your office who can translate or contact a medical interpreter for accurate translation.

C. Have Melissa call her father at work to help translate to mom.

D. Continue to have Melissa translate to her mom.

8. Melissa and her mother are constantly late to medication administration appointments because of their reliance on public transportation. They often arrive to the clinic after it has already closed or at times do not come at all because it takes up too much of their time to get to the clinic. What is the BEST course of action for the pediatric nurse practitioner?

A. Schedule Melissa for appointments every 2 weeks for medication.

B. Counsel the family on the importance of the medication and discuss the possibility of home administration to assure that Melissa gets her medications weekly.

C. Stress the importance of receiving the medication consistently and tell mom that she must make sure to get on the bus earlier than usual on the days that Melissa needs the shot.

D. Work with Melissa's father regarding taking off work and driving Melissa in for her shots.

9. Melissa has been noticing that her friends at school are much taller than her. When asked why, you explain:

A. Some people just grow faster than others, you will catch up eventually.

B. The methotrexate and etanercept you are taking causes slow growth.

C. The folic acid is causing a delay in growth.

D. The long-term corticosteroids you used to take interfered with your normal growth.

10. Melissa's school nurse has called and she reports that at times Melissa has great difficulty getting up and down the stairs to her classes. Because Melissa's condition is chronic, for best outcomes at school, the pediatric nurse practitioner's should:

A. Encourage Melissa's mother to switch her to a school that has only one floor.

B. Initiate a case conference with Melissa's family, health care providers, and the school in order to make special accommodations at school.

C. Encourage Melissa to be home-schooled.

D. This matter should be deferred to the school to handle.

11. Routine labs to be monitored for Melissa should include the following:
    A. ESR, LFTs.
    B. Urinalysis, CBC.
    C. CMP, ESR, urinalysis, CBC, CRP.
    D. CBC, CRP, and ESR.

12. Poorest prognosis exists for the children with JRA who have the following characteristics:
    A. Seronegative rheumatoid factor, ANA negative, vision involvement.
    B. Bracing requirements, hyperlaxity in joints.
    C. Positive rheumatoid factor, 5+ joint involvement, hip disease, hand and vision involvement.
    D. Bilateral joint involvement of the ankles and knees, ANA positive.

13. Family factors which can potentially limit a child's ability to cope with JRA include:
    A. Emphasis on self-mastery.
    B. Highly cohesive family.
    C. Environment of flexibility.
    D. Codependency.

14. You discover that Emily constantly complains of joint pain in her fingers, especially after school. You provide a letter to mother for school explaining what JRA is and encourage mother to discuss with her teachers to:
    A. Help with pain issues, joint preservation, and alternative ways to complete homework assignments and note-taking while still fulfilling requirements.
    B. Excuse Emily from homework on the days that she has pain.
    C. Get funding for a laptop computer so that all homework and notes can be typed instead of written.
    D. Make special exceptions for Emily for mom to write her homework assignments for her.

15. Which of the following statements is FALSE?

A. Daily fever over at least 2 weeks, with daily high-spiking fevers of greater than or equal to 39° C followed by normal or subnormal temperatures helps to classify systemic JRA.
B. Despite the type of JRA at onset, JRA can potentially become systemic.
C. The Rehabilitation Act 504 is a federal law for nondiscrimination against disabilities and requires special provisions to be made in schools.
D. Mouth sores are a symptom of JRA, not a side effect from medications such as methotrexate.

16. Nonpharmacologic approaches to JRA pain in children include all of the following EXCEPT:
    A. Distraction.
    B. Cognitive behavioral therapy.
    C. Exercise.
    D. Joint splinting.

17. Kristen is a 4-year-old who is newly diagnosed with JRA. Which of the following referrals should the pediatric nurse practitioner make for Kristen?
    A. Ophthalmologist
    B. Cardiologist
    C. Urologist
    D. Pulmonologist

18. What anticipatory guidance should be provided to an adolescent female with JRA?
    A. Puberty and secondary sex characteristics may occur earlier than normal.
    B. Mean height in teens with JRA is often greater than the average teen.
    C. Puberty and secondary sex characteristics may be delayed.
    D. Mean weight in teens with JRA is often greater than the average teen.

19. What anticipatory guidance will you give to Elijah, a 10-year-old with JRA, and his family about taking the oral form of methotrexate?
    A. This medication may cause constipation; eat a high-fiber diet.
    B. The taste of oral methotrexate is unpalatable and taking the medication with root beer or a carbonated beverage may improve the taste.

C. Elijah will be less susceptible to infection with this medication.
D. The medication may cause insomnia; monitor sleep patterns.

20. Eric, a 14-year-old with JRA, is currently on systemic corticosteroids to reduce inflammation. Which of the following routine adolescent immunizations is contraindicated for Eric?
   A. Inactive polio.
   B. Hepatitis B.
   C. Tdap.
   D. Varicella.

21. The primary goals of vocational counselor referral for an adolescent with JRA are:
   A. Assistance with job or career choices, college issues, and transition to independence.
   B. Gaining understanding in coping, sexuality, and intimacy issues.
   C. Long-term medication and nutritional counseling.
   D. Assistance with government financial issues, disability assistance, and advocacy.

22. Daily calcium and vitamin D supplementation should be emphasized for all children with JRA to:
   A. Enhance T-cell formation.
   B. Reduce joint swelling.
   C. Prevent bone loss.
   D. Decrease the risk of gastrointestinal bleeding.

23. Which of the following statement is NOT true regarding Koebner's phenomenon?
   A. Trauma to uninvolved skin can trigger the onset of a skin disease.
   B. It is associated with oligoarthritis form of JRA.

C. Lesions may mark the initial onset of psoriasis, or may be a new lesion in an existing case of psoriasis.
D. This phenomenon can be seen in various skin diseases.

24. Liza, a 14-year-old teenage girl with oligoarthritis in her left knee, presents to the clinic with left knee joint pain. She is currently on the maximum dose of naproxen for her age, weight, and height. On exam, her left knee is swollen with effusion. The x-rays of her knee are inconclusive. The BEST course of action is to:
   A. Order an MRI of the knee and refer Liza to an orthopedic surgeon for consultation.
   B. Prepare to tap fluid from the knee and send a culture of the aspirate.
   C. Prescribe an additional NSAID to help with the swelling and pain.
   D. Refer to physical therapy three to four times per week.

25. Which of the following is a FALSE statement?
   A. Immunosusceptability and external environmental triggers are necessary for the development of JRA.
   B. B-cell activation, complement consumption, release of interleukin-6 (IL-6), IL-13, tumor necrosis factor (TNF), and other proinflammatory cytokines lead to joint damage.
   C. Siblings tend to develop the same type of JRA.
   D. The United States and Canada currently adopt the JRA classification from the International League of Associations for Rheumatology (ILAR).

ANSWERS

1. *Answer:* B
   Rationale: A, C, and D are incorrect as signs and symptoms for JRA. Children with JRA do NOT have the following symptoms: erythematous joints, nausea, one-sided weakness, intolerance to heat or cold, or photosensitivity.

2. *Answer:* C
   Rationale: Although rare, MAS, reactive hematophagocytic lymphohistiocytosis, and cricoarytenoid arthritis are serious complications of systemic JRA that require immediate intervention by the pediatric nurse practitioner, emergency department, and pediatric rheumatologist. The treatment includes high-dose intravenous steroids.

3. *Answer:* A
   Rationale: Unlike the other classifications of JRA, oligoarthritis JRA is often asymmetric and the most commonly affected joints are the knees and ankles. Up to four joints can be affected. Although inflammation is present, pain is not always reported. Late-onset oligoarthritis tends to occur in males older than age 10.

4. *Answer:* D
   Rationale: Naproxen and other NSAIDs will thin the blood and may cause intraoperative and postoperative bleeding. To reduce the risk of bleeding during surgery, these medications should be stopped preoperatively.

5. *Answer:* C
   Rationale: 50% of the children with systemic JRA have progressive joint involvement as well as complications such as pericarditis and infection. The other 50% may have complete resolution of their symptoms by adulthood.

6. *Answer:* A
   Rationale: Side effects from both etanercept and methotrexate affect the body's immune system and can cause fatigue, low white blood cell counts, and increase the risk of infection. These two medications are classified as DMARDs, or disease modifying antirheumatic drugs.

7. *Answer:* B
   Rationale: Melissa should not be depended on to translate nor should another family member translate. Medical staff within the office who can translate should be utilized or obtain medical translation services from an outside company.

8. *Answer:* B
   Rationale: With systemic JRA, DMARDs and other medications are for maintenance and are taken long-term. Methotrexate and etanercept, given just like insulin shots, can be given at home if taught properly. This can be done with the least interruption to the dynamics of the family. Education and support are needed for proper administration.

9. *Answer:* D
   Rationale: Anticipatory guidance is important for those who are on long-term corticosteroid therapy during childhood, as it will interfere with normal growth patterns, causing short stature. Other characteristics include a rounded face and weakened bones.

10. *Answer:* B
    Rationale: By law, schools are to provide special accommodations for students with physical disabilities and still include them in their normal classes. It is important to keep Melissa in regular classes as much as possible and still be sensitive to her physical challenges. Bringing together the family, health care providers, and school officials will create best outcomes.

11. *Answer:* C
    Rationale: CMP, ESR, urinalysis, CBC, and CRP must all be monitored routinely to determine if there are any adverse effects from medication and to also monitor the disease process. Although not all are monitored in the same frequency, if any of these labs are not routinely checked, vital information could be missed.

12. *Answer:* C
    Rationale: A positive rheumatoid factor, 5+ joint involvement, hip disease, and hand and vision involvement are good indicators of long-term disability and poor prognosis.

13. *Answer:* D

Rationale: All the choices except for D can enhance the child's ability to cope with a chronic disease. Assuring independence as a child grows will help quality of life, coping, and functionality.

14. *Answer:* A

Rationale: Encourage mom to openly discuss these issues and challenges with her teachers. A letter from the pediatric nurse practitioner describing her ailments may aid in the discussion to help alleviate some pain, while preserving joint function and still make sure she properly fulfills her education requirements.

15. *Answer:* D

Rationale: Mouth sores are a side effect of methotrexate and other DMARDs; they are not a symptom of JRA.

16. *Answer:* D

Rationale: Splinting of the joints is used to maintain alignment, reduce flexion contractures, and provide support during functional activities. It is not necessarily done to control pain.

17. *Answer:* A

Rationale: Children with JRA are at risk for developing uveitis; all children diagnosed with JRA should be evaluated by an ophthalmologist.

18. *Answer:* C

Rationale: Adolescents with JRA may have delayed puberty with delayed development of secondary sexual characteristics. Almost half of teens with JRA have linear growth retardation and in certain types of JRA, mean height and weight are lower than the average adolescent.

19. *Answer:* B

Rationale: Compliance with the oral form is difficult for children because the taste is not favorable. Providing suggestions to mask the flavor will increase compliance.

20. *Answer:* D

Rationale: Corticosteroid medications suppress the immune system, therefore all live vaccinations should be withheld until these medications are discontinued and the recommended wait time has lapsed. The pediatric nurse practitioner can obtain accurate and up to date information about the wait time for live attenuated immunizations after steroid medications from the Centers for Disease Control website (www.CDC.gov).

21. *Answer:* A

Rationale: B, C, and D are not issues that a vocational counselor is able to address for adolescents with JRA.

22. *Answer:* C

Rationale: Children with JRA are especially prone to bone loss because of lack of activity secondary to pain, and/or effects from medication. Because of bone and joint challenges, this population needs optimal bone growth for best outcomes.

23. *Answer:* B

Rationale: Koebner's phenomenon is indicative of systemic JRA, and not the other two types of JRA. However, it is not exclusive to systemic JRA; it can be seen in certain other skin diseases.

24. *Answer:* A

Rationale: MRI will assist in the accurate diagnosis of this condition.

25. *Answer:* D

Rationale: Historically, the U.S. and Canada classify JRA using the American College of Rheumatology classifications. ILAR may be used in the future, but this has not been established yet.

BIBLIOGRAPHY

American Academy of Pediatrics (AAP) (1993). Guidelines for ophthalmologic examinations in children with juvenile rheumatoid arthritis. *Pediatrics, 92*(2) part 1 of 2, 295-296. See http://aappolicy.aappublications.org/cgi/content/abstract/pediatrics;92/2/295.

Bowyer, S.L., Roetcher, P.A., Higgins, G.C., et al. (2003). Health status of patients with juvenile rheumatoid arthritis at 1 and 5 years after diagnosis. *J Rheumatol, 30*(2), 394-400.

Cassidy, J.T., Levinson, J.E., Bass, J.C., et al. (1986). A study of classification criteria for a diagnosis of juvenile rheumatoid arthritis. *Arthritis Rheumatol, 29*(2), 274-281

Cassidy, J.T., & Petty, R.E. (2001). Juvenile rheumatoid arthritis. In J.T. Cassidy, & R.E. Petty (Eds.). *Textbook of pediatric rheumatology* (4th ed.). Philadelphia: Saunders.

Cimaz, R., & Simonini, G. (2003). Review for the primary care physician: Differential diagnosis of arthritis in children. *Pediatric* rheumatology online journal, retrieved June 1, 2005, from www.pedrheumonlinejournal.org/issues1/DIFFERENTIAL%20PROJ.htm.

Duffy, C.M. (2004). Health outcomes in pediatric rheumatic diseases. *Curr Opin Rheumatol, 16*(2), 102-108.

Duffy, C., Tucker, L., Burgos-Vargas, R. (2000). Update on functional assessment tools. *J Rheumatol, 27*(Suppl. 58), 11-14.

Gerhardt, C.A., Vannatta, K., McKellop, J.M., et al. (2003). Brief report: Childrearing practices of caregivers with and without a child with juvenile rheumatoid arthritis: Perspectives of caregivers and professionals. *J Pediatr Psychol, 28*(4), 275-279.

Giannini, E.H., & Petty, R.E. (2001). Treatment of juvenile rheumatoid arthritis. In J.W. Koopman (Ed.). *Arthritis and allied conditions: A textbook of rheumatology* (14th ed.). New York: Lippincott Williams & Wilkins.

Giannini, E.H., Ruperto, N., Ravelli, A., et al. (1997). Preliminary definition of improvement in juvenile arthritis. *Arthritis Rheum, 40*(7), 1202-1209.

Howe, S., Levinson, J., Shear, E., et al. (1991). Development of a disability measurement tool for juvenile rheumatoid arthritis: The juvenile arthritis functional assessment report for children and their parents. *Arthritis Rheum, 34*(7), 873-880.

Huygen, A.C., Kuis, W., & Sinnema, G. (2000). Psychological, behavioural, and social adjustment in children and adolescents with juvenile chronic arthritis. *Ann Rheum Dis, 59*(4), 276-282.

LeBovidge, J.S., Lavigne, J.V., Donenberg, G.R., & Miller, M.L. (2003). Psychological adjustment of children and adolescents with chronic arthritis: A meta-analytic review. *J Pediatr Psychol, 28*(1), 29-39.

Lotlto, A.P.N., Muscara, M.N., Kiss, M.H.B., et al. (2004). Nitric oxide-derived species in synovial fluid from patients with juvenile idiopathic arthritis. *J Rheumatol, 31*(5), 998-1000.

Lovell, D.J., Howe, S., Shear, E., et al. (1989). Development of a disability measurement tool for juvenile rheumatoid arthritis: The Juvenile Arthritis Functional Assessment Scale. *Arthritis Rheuml, 32*(11), 1390-1395.

Marin, C., Sanchez-Alegre, M.L., Gallego, C., et al. (2004). Magnetic resonance imaging of osteoarticular infections in children. *Curr Prob Diag Radiol, 33*(2), 43-59.

Miller, M., & Cassidy, J.T. (2004). Juvenile rheumatoid arthritis. In R.E. Behrman, R.M. Kliegman, & H.B. Jenson (Eds.). *Nelson textbook of pediatrics* (17th ed.). Philadelphia: Saunders.

Miller, M.L., LeBovidge, J., & Feldman, B. (2002). Health-related quality of life in children with arthritis. *Rheum Dis Clin North Am, 28*(3), 493-501, vi.

Prahalad, S., Bove, K.E., Dickens, D., et al. (2001). Etanercept in the treatment of macrophage activation syndrome. *J Rheumatol, 28*(9), 2120-2124.

Ravelli, A. (2004). Toward an understanding of the long-term outcome of juvenile idiopathic arthritis. *Clin Exper Rheumatol, 22*(3), 271-275.

Reece, G. (2004). A 41/2 year old with a swollen knee. *J Pediatr Health Care, 18*(3), 153, 161-162.

Reiter-Purtill, J., Gerhardt, C.A., Vannatta, K., et al. (2003). A controlled longitudinal study of the social functioning of children with juvenile rheumatoid arthritis. *J Pediatr Psychol, 28*(1), 17-28.

Rettig, P.A., Merhar, S.L., & Cron, R.Q. (2004). Juvenile rheumatoid arthritis and juvenile spondyloarthropathy. In P.L. Jackson & J.A. Vessey (Eds.). *Primary care of the child with a chronic condition* (4th ed.). St. Louis: Mosby.

Rosen, P., Hopkin, R.J., Glass, D.N., & Graham, T.B. (2004). Another patient with chromosome 18 deletion syndrome and juvenile rheumatoid arthritis. *J Rheumatol, 31*(5), 992-997.

Rosenberg, A.M. (2002). Uveitis associated with childhood rheumatic diseases. *Curr Opin Rheumatol, 14*(5), 542-547.

Sandborg, C.I., & Wallace, C.A. (1999). Position statement of the American College of Rheumatology regarding referral of children and adolescents to pediatric rheumatologists. *Arthritis Care Res, 12*(1), 48-51.

Shaw, K.L., Southwood, T.R., & McDonagh, J.E. (2004). User perspectives of transitional care for adolescents with juvenile idiopathic arthritis. *Rheumatology, 43*(6), 770-778.

Simon, D., Lipman, A., Jacox, A., et al. (2002). *Guidelines for the management of pain in osteoarthritis, rheumatoid arthritis, and juvenile chronic arthritis* (2nd ed.). Glenview, IL: American Pain Society.

Spencer, C.H., & Bernstein, B.H. (2002). Hip disease in juvenile rheumatoid arthritis. *Curr Opin Rheumatol, 14*(5), 536-541.

Taylor, J., & Erlandson, D.M. (2001). Pediatric rheumatic diseases. In L. Robbins (Ed.). *Clinical care in the rheumatic diseases* (2nd ed.). Atlanta: American College of Rheumatology.

White, P.H. (1999). Transition to adulthood. *Curr Opin Rheumatol, 11*(5), 408-411.

White, P. Silman, A.J., Smolen, J.S., (2003). Clinical features of juvenile rheumatoid arthritis. In M.C. Hochberg, et al. (Eds.). *Rheumatology* (3rd ed., Vol. 1.). St. Louis: Mosby.

49 Learning Disorders and Attention Deficit Hyperactivity Disorder

DEBORAH SHELTON

Select the best answer for each of the following questions:

1. The most recent educational federal guidelines for determining whether a student in a public school is eligible for special programs for learning disabilities include:
   A. The child is immature for his age.
   B. The family refuses to participate in directing the education of their child.
   C. The learning problem is associated with cultural differences.
   D. A central nervous system processing deficit.

The next five questions relate to the following scenario:

Beth, age 13, has a long history of school problems. She failed second grade and was removed from a special classroom after she kept getting into fights with the other children. Now in a normal sixth-grade class, she is failing reading and English, is barely passing in math and spelling, but doing well in art and sports. She is described as a slow learner with a poor memory, and in need of much individual attention. Her medical history is unremarkable. Upon examination, she is found to be an open and friendly girl, but very sensitive about her academic problems. She has an IQ of 97 and scores 4.8 for reading, 5.3 for spelling and 6.3 for math on her achievement tests.

2. The differential diagnosis for academic problems in children and adolescents are:
   A. Attention deficit/hyperactivity disorder (ADHD), conduct disorder, learning disorder.
   B. Oppositional defiant disorder, depression, eating disorder.
   C. Poor schooling, depression, and mental retardation.
   D. Bipolar disorder, depression, dysthymia.

3. Based on the description above, what is Beth's most likely primary diagnosis?
   A. ADHD.
   B. Conduct disorder.
   C. Learning disorder.
   D. Mental retardation.

4. Which criteria of your diagnosis do you suspect Beth meets?
   A. Motor skills disorder.
   B. Reading disorder.
   C. Disorder of written expression.
   D. Mathematics disorder.

5. To confirm the proposed diagnosis, what screening questions you might ask Beth?
   A. When the teacher is speaking in class, do you have trouble understanding or keeping up?
   B. Do you feel you can run, jump, and climb as well as your friends can?
   C. Do you understand jokes when your friends tell them?
   D. Can you sound out words as well as your classmates can?

6. A treatment plan for Beth would include:
   A. Family therapy and a youth group.
   B. Remedial reading and social skills training.

C. Individual therapy and medication.
D. Special education services and physical training.

7. When the presenting problem is academic difficulty, the differential diagnostic process must clarify the reason for the academic difficulty. The areas of inquiry into factors contributing to the student's learning difficulties include:
A. The child's psychoeducational status, family functioning, and cultural context.
B. The quality of the school, its teachers, and its scorecard on standardized testing.
C. Parenting issues, couples issues, and family issues.
D. The value systems of peers and the community at large.

8. Studies show that approximately 30% of youth diagnosed as having a learning disability have which comorbid condition?
A. Depression.
B. Childhood schizophrenia.
C. Eating disorder.
D. Conduct disorder.

9. Genetic studies of learning disorders have shown a familial pattern in:
A. 70% of children with learning disabilities.
B. 40% to 50% of children with learning disabilities.
C. 22% of children with learning disabilities.
D. 5% of children with learning disabilities.

10. The neurobiological basis of learning is located in which parts of the brain?
A. Olfactory nerve and hippocampus.
B. Hippocampus, cortex, and cerebellum.
C. Cerebellum and cortex.
D. Neurons that layer the hippocampus.

11. The most widely studied drugs in the treatment of ADHD, the stimulants, affect:
A. Dopamine and norepinephrine.
B. 3-methoxyl-4-hydroxyphenyglycol (MHPG), a metabolite of norepinephrine.
C. Norepinephrine.
D. Dopamine.

12. Diagnostic features of ADHD includes:
A. Symptoms that cause impairment must have been present before age 7 years.
B. Children who present with inattention and have behavioral patterns marked by sluggishness, daydreaming, and hypoactivity.
C. Disruptive behavior that violates age-appropriate societal norms.
D. Extreme irritability.

13. Failure to complete tasks should be considered in making a diagnosis of ADHD only if:
A. Marked impairment in the use of nonverbal behaviors exists.
B. Nonaggressive behavior causes property loss or damage.
C. Associated symptoms include lying, truancy, and staying out after dark without permission.
D. It is due to inattention as opposed to other possible reasons (e.g., defiance).

14. Hyperactivity, a primary concern to the diagnosis of ADHD may vary with the individual's age and developmental level. A toddler or preschooler with this disorder would be different from normally active young children by:
A. Being constantly on the go and into everything; unable to sit and listen to a story.
B. Being impatient, blurting out answers to questions before the questions are asked.
C. Being increasingly aggressive in nature.
D. Being preoccupied for the majority of time.

15. Many individuals present with symptoms of both inattention and hyperactivity-impulsivity, however there are individuals in whom one or the other pattern is predomi-

nant. Criteria for ADHD, predominantly hyperactive-impulsive type, include:

A. Six or more symptoms of inattention and six or more symptoms of hyperactivity-impulsivity that have persisted for more than 6 months.
B. Six or more symptoms of inattention, but fewer than six symptoms of hyperactivity-impulsivity that have persisted for more than 6 months.
C. Six or more symptoms of hyperactivity-impulsivity and six or more symptoms of inattention that have persisted for more than 6 months.
D. Six or more symptoms of hyperactivity-impulsivity, but fewer than six symptoms of inattention that have persisted for more than 6 months.

The next four questions relate to the following scenario:

Mark is an 11-year-old boy who is brought to you for a psychiatric consultation by his parents for problems he has "had since he was born." He is described as socially immature and has had trouble making friends. His mother sees him as unhappy and his father as unfocused and lazy. Mark has trouble waiting in line at school, and has had difficulty with change and transitions. He was an average student in elementary school, but his grades dropped in seventh grade. When doing homework, Mark's father thinks he wastes time daydreaming instead of focusing on his homework. His father also thinks he is absent-minded, has poor eye contact, and lacks social skills. His mother notes that Mark usually starts school off on a positive note, but as the work gets more difficult and complex, he becomes disorganized.

16. Mark meets the criteria for ADHD, but you note that there is an absence of symptoms of hyperactivity. You would further refine the diagnosis as:

A. ADHD, predominantly hyperactive-impulsive type.
B. ADHD, predominantly inattentive type.
C. ADHD, combined type.
D. ADHD, predominantly depressed type.

17. Mark is unable to tolerate the prescribed stimulant medication. You decide to use desipramine 4.6 mg/kg/day, a nonstimulant medication, for Mark. You advise his parents that:

A. Periodic monitoring every 6 months will be required.
B. He may lose weight due to lack of appetite.
C. You will have to monitor for cardiovascular side effects (EKG).
D. He is likely to develop tics.

18. As you meet with Mark's teacher and parents to determine a plan of treatment for Mark, you suggest:

A. Brief group therapy (four sessions) for social skill development.
B. Developing behavioral interventions with positive reinforcements.
C. Retaining Mark in regular classrooms because he prefers it.
D. That use of medication will be enough without psychosocial intervention.

19. You decide to provide parent education to reduce some of the feelings that Mark's father, in particular, has about his son. Your education includes:

A. While symptoms are not "voluntary," Mark can be held responsible for reasonable expectations.
B. Suggestions for relaxation exercises for Mark's parents to practice in the evening.
C. Suggestions for Mark's parents to be more lenient with Mark around his homework.
D. That individual therapy is the only treatment that will help Mark.

20. The prevalence of ADHD in school-aged children is estimated at:

A. 3 to 7%.
B. 20 to 25%.
C. 30%.
D. 75%.

21. A first-line medication in treatment of ADHD for youth with comorbid tic disorders is:

A. Wellbutrin.
B. Clonidine.

C. Ritalin.

D. Concerta.

22. The most recent American Academy of Child and Adolescent Psychiatry (AACAP) practice parameters recommend the following monitoring for children treated with stimulant medications:

A. Height, weight, blood pressure, and pulse checked annually with a physical exam.

B. Height, weight, and eating patterns monitored weekly with a physical exam annually.

C. Height, weight, blood pressure, and pulse checked quarterly with a physical exam annually.

D. Height and weight monitored by the parents monthly with a physical exam annually.

23. Essential components of parent training programs for behavior management of their children with ADHD include:

A. To be nonresponsive to all behaviors, positive or negative.

B. Punishment of misbehavior at the end of the day.

C. Interrupting coercive interchange between parents and child.

D. To overly praise the behaviors of the child.

24. Contingency management skills learned by parents are useful in handling the misbehavior of their children with ADHD. These skills entail clear and frequent feedback to the child about his or her behavior, sometimes taking the form of point or token systems. For adolescents, which strategy would be more developmentally appropriate?

A. Bigger rewards for bigger kids.

B. Less frequent feedback is necessary for older kids.

C. Negotiations with parents around negotiable topics.

D. Peer-driven strategies.

25. Confidentiality is particularly challenging when working with a rural family and child with ADHD because the communities are small and you are likely to encounter this family in a social setting. A strategy to deal with this is:

A. Pretend you don't know them "professionally."

B. Avoid participating in any community activities they might attend.

C. Discuss with parents directly what you have heard about them.

D. There is no need for additional concerns about boundaries.

ANSWERS

1. *Answer:* D
   Rationale: Four criteria defined in the federal guidelines determine a student's eligibility for special programs for learning disabilities in a public school system: documented evidence that a general education has been found ineffective, evidence of a disorder in one or more of the psychological processes required for learning, evidence of academic achievement below the student's level of intellectual functioning, evidence that learning problems are not due primarily to other handicapping conditions (visual, auditory, retardation, cultural differences, or environmental deprivation).

2. *Answer:* A
   Rationale: The differential diagnosis of academic problems includes consideration of poor schooling, mental retardation, ADHD, oppositional defiant disorder, conduct disorder, and learning disorder.

3. *Answer:* C
   Rationale: Beth's average intelligence rules out mental retardation. Despite her fighting in class, there is no description of other behaviors that would justify a diagnosis of ADHD or conduct disorder. There is positive evidence suggesting a learning disorder.

4. *Answer:* B
   Rationale: She seems to have difficulty with reading and performs significantly below her expected level on the reading achievement exam. The criteria for a reading disorder include reading achievement as measured by a standardized test of accuracy and comprehension is substantially below what is expected given the person's age, measured intelligence, and age-appropriate education. The disturbance in criterion A significantly interferes with academic achievement or activities of daily living that require reading skills. Given this diagnosis, it is reasonable to regard her fighting as an associated feature of the learning disorder.

5. *Answer:* D

Rationale: Screening questions for a reading disorder address reading accuracy and comprehension given what would be expected for age, intelligence, and education. This can be assessed by asking the child to compare him- or herself with peers.

6. *Answer:* B
   Rationale: Treatment directed at the underlying disability consists of educational interventions. Psychologic interventions are directed at any emotional, social, or family difficulty. Beth has difficulty reading, so targeted assistance with this would be appropriate. There is no evidence of family discord, but Beth's fighting behaviors may indicate some need for social skills training to build self-esteem among her peer group.

7. *Answer:* A
   Rationale: Three principal areas of inquiry into the factors contributing to the student's learning difficulties include the child's psychiatric, medical, or psychoeducational status; the family's functioning; and the environment or cultural context in which the student functions.

8. *Answer:* D
   Rationale: Studies of youth diagnosed as having conduct disorder or young adults diagnosed as having a personality disorder show that one-third have unrecognized, or recognized and poorly treated, learning disabilities.

9. *Answer:* B
   Rationale: Several studies have shown a familial pattern in approximately 40% to 50% of children with learning disabilities. In longitudinal studies of twins, identical pairs are more likely than fraternal pairs to be concordant for academic difficulties.

10. *Answer:* B
    Rationale: The neurologic basis of learning is located in the structures of the brain involved in forming and storing information. These include the hippocampus, cortex, and the cerebellum.

11. *Answer:* A

Rationale: In part, hypotheses about the neurochemistry of the disorder have arisen from the impact of many medications that exert a positive effect. The most widely studied, the stimulants, affect both dopamine and norepinephrine, leading to a neurotransmitter hypothesis that include possible dysfunction in both the adrenergic and dopaminergic systems.

12. *Answer:* A
Rationale: Although children with ADHD often exhibit hyperactive and impulsive behavior that may be disruptive, this behavior does not by itself violate age-appropriate social norms. Some hyperactive-impulsive or inattentive symptoms that cause impairment must have been present before age 7 years, although many individuals are diagnosed after the symptoms present for several years.

13. *Answer:* D
Rationale: Youth with ADHD may have difficulty completing a task and following through on requests or instructions. Failure to complete tasks should be considered in making this diagnosis only if it is due to inattention as opposed to other possible reasons (Criterion A1d).

14. *Answer:* A
Rationale: Toddlers and preschoolers with this disorder differ from normally active young children by being constantly on the go and into everything; they dart back and forth, are "out the door before their coat is on," jump or climb on furniture, run through the house, and have difficulty participating in sedentary group activities in preschool classes, such as listening to a story.

15. *Answer:* D
Rationale: ADHD, predominantly hyperactive-impulsive type should be used if six or more symptoms of hyperactivity-impulsivity, but fewer than six symptoms of inattention, have persisted for more than 6 months. Inattention may often still be a significant clinical feature in such cases.

16. *Answer:* B

Rationale: Mark meets the diagnosis of ADHD. This disorder usually involves symptoms of hyperactivity and impulsivity. Mark has few, if any, of these symptoms; hence the diagnosis would be further specified as predominantly inattentive type.

17. *Answer:* C
Rationale: Tricyclic antidepressants such as desipramine are effective in the treatment of ADHD. However, their use has been largely supplanted by the use of stimulants such as atomoxetine (Straterra) because of their low risk for cardiovascular toxicity, reduced need to monitor serum levels, and unlikelihood of exacerbating tics.

18. *Answer:* B
Rationale: Medication alone is not enough to satisfy the therapeutic needs of children with ADHD. Social skills groups, training for parents, and behavioral interventions that can be used consistently between home and school are often efficacious in the overall management of children with ADHD. Brief group interventions are not reasonable for the child with attention problems.

19. *Answer:* A
Rationale: A common goal of therapy is to help parents of children with ADHD recognize that while the child does not "voluntarily" exhibit symptoms of ADHD, he is still capable of being responsible for meeting reasonable expectations. Parents should be helped to realize that in spite of their child's difficulties, all children face normal tasks of maturation, including building self-esteem when he develops a sense of mastery.

20. *Answer:* A
Rationale: The prevalence of ADHD has been estimated at 3% to 7% of school-aged children. Data on adolescents and adults are limited.

21. *Answer:* B
Rationale: Originally used as antihypertensive medication for adults, clonidine (Catapres) has been considered a first-line therapy for children with ADHD with tic disorders and Tourette's syndrome. Other first-

line medications recommended include atomoxetine (Straterra) and guanfacine (Tenex).

22. *Answer:* C

Rationale: It is recommended that children and adolescents being treated with stimulants have their height, weight, blood pressure, and pulse checked on a quarterly basis and have a physical exam annually.

23. *Answer:* C

Rationale: The essential components of parent training for behavior management include: interrupting the pattern of coercive and often escalating interchange between parent and child; systematic implementation of positive parent-child exchanges that are noncontingent, which strengthens the parent-child bond; praising appropriate behaviors, while as often as possible ignoring misbehavior; implementation of disciplinary strategies such as time-out when the child's misbehavior cannot be safely ignored.

24. *Answer:* C

Rationale: Contingency management skills with adolescents are more successful when the teen takes a more active role in shaping the program and by negotiating with parents around those problems that are negotiable.

25. *Answer:* C

Rationale: Boundaries, confidentiality, and conflicts of interest are particularly challenging in rural practice. It is important to keep an open mind, but to discuss with parents directly what you have heard about them, and clearly define boundaries between you and your patients, but also with the community.

BIBLIOGRAPHY

American Academy of Pediatrics. (2000). Clinical practice guidelines: Diagnosis and evaluation of the child with attention-deficit/hyperactivity disorder. *Pediatrics, 105*(5), 1158-1170.

American Academy of Pediatrics. (2001). Clinical practice guideline: Treatment of the school-aged child with attention-deficit/hyperactivity disorder. *Pediatrics, 108*(4), 1033-1044.

American Psychiatric Association. (2000). *Diagnostic and statistical manual of mental disorders* (4th ed.). Text revision. Washington, DC: Author.

Anastopoulos, A. & Shelton, T. (2001). *Assessing attention-deficit/hyperactivity disorder*. New York: Kluwer Academic/Plenum Publishers.

Institute for Clinical Systems Improvement (ICSI) (2003). *Diagnosis and management of ADHD* (5th ed.). Bloomington, MN: Author.

Jellinek, M., Patel, B.P., & Froehle, M.C. (Eds.). (2002). *Bright futures in practice: Mental health— volume 1. Practice guide*. Arlington, VA: National Center for Education in Maternal and Child Health.

Jensen, P. (2000). Current concepts on etiology, pathophysiology and neurobiology. *J Am Acad Child Adolesc Psychiatry, 9*(3), 557-572.

Pliszka, S. (2000). Patterns of psychiatric comorbidity of attention-deficit/hyperactivity disorder. *Child Adolesc Psychiatric Clin North Am, 9*(3), 525-540.

Selekman, J., & Moore, C. (2004). Attention deficit hyperactivity disorder. In P. Jackson & J. Vessey (Eds.). *Primary care of the child with a chronic condition*. St. Louis: Mosby.

Solanto, M. (2001). Attention-deficit/hyperactivity disorder: Clinical features. In M. Solanto, A. Arnsten, & F.X. Xastellanos (Eds.). *Stimulant drugs and ADHD: Basic and clinical neuroscience*. New York: Oxford University Press.

Stubbe, D. (2000). Attention-deficit/hyperactivity disorder overview: Historical perspective, current controversies, and future directions. *Child Adolesc Psychiatric Clin North Am, 9*(3), 469-479.

50 Renal Failure

MELANIE KLEIN

Select the best answer for each of the following questions:

Please use the following scenario to answer questions 1 through 6:

Matt is a previously healthy 16-year-old African American boy who comes to you with complaints of fatigue and weight loss. He is 155 cm tall and weighs 41 kg. He is afebrile and has a blood pressure of 142/82 mm Hg. In getting a history from Matt and his mother, you find that Matt has not seen a health care provider in more than 8 years. When you question his mother about his short stature, she tells you "He's always been the runt of the litter. He's a very picky eater." She also tells you, "He can't keep up with his brothers and is failing school because he keeps falling asleep." You order chemistries on Matt and find his creatinine is 2.8 mg/dl. All other labs are within normal limits.

1. Using the Schwartz formula for estimating creatinine clearance, what is Matt's glomerular filtration rate (GFR)?
   A. 38.7 ml/min/1.73 m².
   B. 94.5 ml/min/1.73 m².
   C. 60.5 ml/min/1.73 m².
   D. 46.2 ml/min/1.73 m².

2. According to his estimated GFR, Matt's kidney failure can be classified as what stage?
   A. Stage 1.
   B. Stage 2.
   C. Stage 3.
   D. Stage 4.

3. The likely cause of Matt's chronic kidney disease is:
   A. Wilms' tumor.
   B. Potter's syndrome.
   C. Autosomal dominant polycystic kidney disease.
   D. Glomerulonephritis.

4. What other signs and symptoms are associated with Matt's stage of chronic kidney disease (CKD)?
   A. Hypercalcemia, hypophosphatemia, and hyperactivity.
   B. Change in urine output, anemia, and hyperparathyroidism.
   C. Metabolic alkalosis and hyperalbuminemia.
   D. Seizures, rash, and fine tremors.

5. The next step would be to:
   A. Arrange for an urgent appointment with the local nephrologist.
   B. Ask the patient to check his blood pressures intermittently at the local pharmacy and follow up with you in 6 months.
   C. Send him to the emergency department.
   D. Start Matt on antihypertensive medication and see him back in 1 month.

6. Indications for sending Matt to the emergency department would include:
   A. Potassium of 3.8 mmol/L, calcium of 9.7 mg/dl, and BP of 100/60.
   B. Potassium of 4.9 mmol/L, phosphorus of 5.2 mg/dl, and BP of 115/70.
   C. Potassium of 7.0 mmol/L, calcium of 5.1 mg/dl, and BP of 190/110.

D. Sodium 145 mmol/L, PTH 300 pg/mL, and hemoglobin of 11 g/dl.

7. In children under the age of 5 years, the most common cause of chronic renal failure is:
   A. Systemic lupus erythematosus.
   B. Congenital malformations or obstruction.
   C. Drug-induced interstitial nephritis.
   D. Poststreptococcal glomerulonephritis.

8. You are seeing a 4-year-old white girl for her well child visit. Upon palpation of her abdomen, you note a large mass in the right upper quadrant. The likely diagnosis is:
   A. Renal dysplasia.
   B. Focal segmental glomerulosclerosis.
   C. Wilms' tumor.
   D. Sickle cell nephropathy.

9. The most practical way to estimate the creatinine clearance of a 18-month-old child is:
   A. Kidney biopsy.
   B. Schwartz formula.
   C. 24-hour urine collection.
   D. Insulin urinary clearance.

10. Treatment of hyperkalemia includes:
   A. ACE inhibitors.
   B. Spironolactone.
   C. Kayexalate.
   D. Calcium carbonate.

11. Nikki is a 7-year-old girl who is 128.8 cm tall and has a serum creatinine of 1.9. Using the Schwartz formula for estimating creatinine clearance, what is Nikki's GFR?
   A. 37.3 ml/min/1.73 m².
   B. 47.4 ml/min/1.73 m².
   C. 30.5 ml/min/1.73 m².
   D. 68.7 ml/min/1.73 m².

12. Normal renal function at birth is:
   A. 80-120 ml/min/1.73 m².
   B. 60-80 ml/min/1.73 m².
   C. 30-60 ml/min/1.73 m².
   D. 10-30 ml/min/1.73 m².

13. Abnormal development of nephrons with undifferentiated cells is indicative of:

A. Renal dysplasia.
B. Renal hypoplasia.
C. Cloacal abnormalities.
D. Ureteropelvic junction (UPJ) obstruction.

14. Optimal treatment for children with CKD is provided by:
   A. Pediatric nurse practitioner and primary care MD.
   B. Primary care provider and gastroenterologist.
   C. Pediatric nephrologist, primary care provider, and interdisciplinary team.
   D. Internal medicine, urologist, and primary care provider.

15. Common sequelae of late-stage CKD are:
   A. Obesity and hyperglycemia.
   B. Reactive airway disease and allergies.
   C. Excessive growth and premature bone aging.
   D. Poor school performance and increased fatigue.

16. Signs of Alport's syndrome include:
   A. Malar rash, edema, and proteinuria.
   B. High-frequency sensiorneural hearing loss and hematuria.
   C. Lack of abdominal musculature, cryptorchidism, and dilated urinary tract.
   D. Multiple cystic lesions and congenital hepatic fibrosis.

17. The correct equation for the Schwartz formula for estimating GFR in a pediatric patient is:
   A. $\dfrac{(U \times V/P)1.73}{BSA}$
   B. $\dfrac{k \times L}{P_{cr}}$
   C. $\dfrac{P_{cr} \times L}{k}$
   D. $\dfrac{U \times BSA}{V/P}$

18. Short stature related to kidney failure is:
   A. Equally distributed between boys and girls and throughout all ages.

B. More common in boys and younger children.
C. More common girls and older children.
D. Equally distributed between boys and girls in the older age groups.

19. Routine monitoring of children with CKD includes:
   A. Serum electrolytes and CBC.
   B. Thyroid function tests and antinuclear antibodies.
   C. Immunoglobulins.
   D. Urine cultures and urine catecholamines.

20. The most common symptom(s) of stage 3 CKD is (are):
   A. Hypocalcemia.
   B. Hypertension and metabolic acidosis.
   C. Uremia.
   D. Hyperkalemia.

21. Goals of CKD management include:
   A. Reversal of all kidney damage.
   B. Minimizing medications by treating only the urgent symptoms.
   C. Increasing the progression of disease in order to treat with a kidney transplant as soon as possible.
   D. Slowing the progressive loss of kidney function.

22. The preferred treatment for stage 5 CKD is:
   A. Hemodialysis.
   B. Peritoneal dialysis.
   C. Kidney transplant.
   D. Immunosuppressive therapy.

23. A role of the primary care pediatric nurse practitioner when caring for a child with CKD is to:
   A. Manage all aspects of the child's care.
   B. Consolidate and reinforce education and information with the patient and family.
   C. Hand over primary care responsibilities to the nephrology team.
   D. Independently prescribe medications to manage the symptoms of CKD.

24. Which statement is NOT true regarding primary preventive services for a child with chronic renal failure?
   A. Yearly attenuated virus vaccines are contraindicated.
   B. Live attenuated virus vaccines are contraindicated.
   C. Growth assessment should be done annually.
   D. Evaluate blood pressure at each well child visit.

25. Ralph, a 5-year-old who has chronic renal failure, is scheduled to undergo a kidney transplant. Prior to surgery, it is very important to:
   A. Assess his immunization status and give all necessary live virus vaccines if he is not immunosuppressed.
   B. Withhold his annual influenza vaccine.
   C. Send a urine culture and if positive, treat with appropriate antibiotics.
   D. Discontinue dialysis 1 month prior to surgery.

ANSWERS

1. *Answer:* A
   Rationale: Using the Schwartz formula of $k \times L/P_{cr}$ where $k = 0.7$ for an adolescent boy, the estimated GFR is 38.7 ml/min/1.73 m².

2. *Answer:* C
   Rationale: Matt's estimated GFR is 38.7 ml/min/1.73 m², which corresponds to CKD stage 3 (30-59 ml/min/1.73 m²).

3. *Answer:* D
   Rationale: Glomerulonephritis is the most common cause of chronic kidney disease in adolescent African American boys. Potter's syndrome is bilateral renal agenesis, which is diagnosed in infancy; Wilms' tumor is more common in preschool-age children; and autosomal dominant polycystic kidney disease is most commonly diagnosed in the sixth to seventh decade of life.

4. *Answer:* B
   Rationale: CKD can cause an increase or decrease in urine output. As CKD progresses, the kidneys decrease production of erythropoetin, causing anemia, and the progressive inability to excrete phosphorus through the kidney and absorb calcium in the GI system causes an imbalance of calcium (hypocalcemia) and phosphorus (hyperphosphatemia), triggering the parathyroid gland to increase production of parathyroid hormone. Progressive CKS also presents with increased fatigue, metabolic acidosis, and occasionally hypoalbuminemia.

5. *Answer:* A
   Rationale: Matt should be seen by the local pediatric nephrologist within the next few days. He has significant CKD and though nothing on his physical exam or lab findings warrant immediate transport to the emergency department, he should be seen as soon as possible.

6. *Answer:* C
   Rationale: Matt has severe hypertension and is at risk for neurologic complications such as seizures. The hyperkalemia and hy-pocalcemia place him at high risk for a cardiac arrhythmia. None of the findings in the remaining choices are of imminent danger to the patient.

7. *Answer:* B
   Rationale: Congenital malformations or obstructions are the most common cause of chronic kidney disease in children under the age of 5 years.

8. *Answer:* C
   Rationale: Wilms' tumor presents in preschool-age children and often a mass is palpable either unilaterally or bilaterally. The remaining choices do not present with abdominal masses.

9. *Answer:* B
   Rationale: The Schwartz formula is the most practical way to estimate GFR. Insulin clearance involves continuous infusion of medication and repeated blood sampling that is impractical in pediatrics. A 24-hour urine collection is extremely difficult to perform in an 18-month-old, unless the child is catheterized with a Foley catheter during the collection period. Kidney biopsies do not provide any estimate of GFR.

10. *Answer:* C
    Rationale: Kayexalate is sodium polystyrene sulfonate and exchanges sodium for potassium in the serum and excretes it through the feces. ACE inhibitors and spironolactone can increase potassium. Calcium carbonate has no effect on serum potassium.

11. *Answer:* A
    Rationale: Using the Schwartz formula of $k \times L/P_{cr}$ where $k = 0.55$ for a child, the estimated GFR is 37.3 ml/min/1.73 m².

12. *Answer:* C
    Rationale: Normal renal function at birth is 30 to 60 ml/min/1.73 m². GFR increases postnatally and achieves adult norms by the age of 2. This progressive increase in GFR is thought to be related to increasing glomerular perfusion pressure, increases in renal blood flow, and maturation of cortical nephrons.

13. *Answer:* A

Rationale: Renal dysplasia is defined as the abnormal development of nephrons with undifferentiated cells. Hypoplasia is defined as the compromised growth and development of nephrons leading to a small kidney with fewer nephrons, cloacal abnormalities occur during the 4th and 6th weeks of fetal development when the cloaca fails to divide into an anterior urogenital sinus and a posterior anorectal canal. UPJ obstruction is a narrowing or complete obstruction of the ureteropelvic junction.

14. *Answer:* C

Rationale: Optimal treatment of children with CKD is not provided by one health care provider alone. Care of the child with CKD involves providers from a variety of specialties, including nephrologists, nurses, social workers, nutritionists, mental health professionals, and primary care providers.

15. *Answer:* D

Rationale: Significant CKD is associated with increased fatigue and decreased endurance with physical activity. Cognitive development is affected as well, as this is thought to be related to uremia and the build-up of immeasurable toxins in the body.

16. *Answer:* B

Rationale: Hearing loss and hematuria are classic symptoms of Alport's syndrome. A macular rash, edema, and proteinuria are seen with systemic lupus erythematosus. A lack of abdominal musculature, cryptorchidism, and dilated urinary tract are associated with Eagle-Barrett (prune belly) syndrome. Multiple renal cysts and congenital hepatic fibrosis are associated with autosomal recessive polycystic kidney disease.

17. *Answer:* B

Rationale: The correct equation for the Schwartz formula is $k \times L/P_{cr}$ where k equals a constant dependent on age, L equals length or height and P_{cr} equals plasma creatinine.

18. *Answer:* B

Rationale: Short stature secondary to CKD is seen most often in boys and younger children. Younger children also show the most catch-up growth once they are started on growth hormone therapy or they receive a kidney transplant.

19. *Answer:* A

Rationale: It is essential to routinely monitor for imbalances in serum electrolytes, including BUN, creatinine, potassium, calcium, phosphorus, bicarbonate, and albumin. Complete blood counts are used to monitor for development or progression of anemia.

20. *Answer:* B

Rationale: The most common symptoms of stage 3 CKD are hypertension and metabolic acidosis. Electrolyte imbalances such as hyperkalemia, hypocalcemia, and uremia are not seen until late stage 4 or stage 5 CKD.

21. *Answer:* D

Rationale: Significant effort is made to slow the progression of CKD by treating symptoms and lab abnormalities as soon as they appear. Appropriate treatment of blood pressure, proteinuria, calcium, phosphorus imbalances, and metabolic acidosis can retard the progression of CKD and lengthen the time the child has before starting any type of renal replacement therapy.

22. *Answer:* C

Rationale: Kidney transplantation is the preferred treatment for CKD as it provides improved growth, cognitive function, and school attendance and achievement, a higher quality of life and significantly higher renal function when compared to dialysis.

23. *Answer:* B

Rationale: A central role for pediatric nurse practitioners in the care of children with CKD is to consolidate and reinforce the information and education provided by the nephrology team. Optimal care of the child with CKD involves the nephrology team and the primary care provider.

24. *Answer:* B

Rationale: Live attenuated virus vaccines are only withheld in immunosuppressed children with chronic renal failure. Yearly influenza vaccines and monitoring of BP and growth are all important primary preventive care practices.

25. *Answer:* A

Rationale: Live vaccines should be given before a kidney transplant because the child will be on life-long immunosuppressive therapy. Most children with chronic renal failure will have bacteriuria and should not be treated with antibiotics unless they have associated symptoms of a UTI such as fever, nausea, vomiting, and pain. Children with chronic renal failure should receive annual influenza immunizations. Dialysis-dependent children could not tolerate a month without treatment.

BIBLIOGRAPHY

Avner, E.D. (2004). Chronic renal failure. In E.D. Avner, W.E. Harmon, & P. Niaudet (Eds.). *Pediatric nephrology* (5th ed.). Philadelphia: Lippincott Williams & Wilkins.

DeFoor, W., Minevich, E., McEnery, P., et al. (2003). Lower urinary tract reconstruction is safe and effective in children with end stage renal disease. *J Urol, 170*(4), 1497-1500.

Harris, M., Hofman, P.L., & Cutfield, W.S. (2004). Growth hormone treatment in children: Review of safety and efficacy. *Paediatr Drugs, 6*(2), 93-106.

Hogg, R.J., Furth, S., Lemley, K.V., et al. (2003). National Kidney Foundation's Kidney Disease Outcomes Quality Initiative clinical practice guidelines for chronic kidney disease in children and adolescents: Evaluation, classification, and stratification. *Pediatrics, 111*(6, Pt. 1), 1416-1421.

Klein, M., & Namrow, A. (2004). Chronic renal failure. In P.J. Allen & J.A. Vessey (Eds.). *Primary care of the child with a chronic condition* (4th ed.). St. Louis: Mosby.

Reilly, N.J. (2001). *Urologic nursing: A study guide* (2nd ed.). Pitman, NJ: Anthony J. Jannetti.

Roth, K.S., Koo, H.P., Spottswood, S.E., & Chan, J.C.M. (2002). Obstructive uropathy: An important cause of chronic renal failure in children. *Clin Pediatr, 41*(5), 309-314.

Salusky, I.B., Kuizon, B.G., & Juppner, H. (2004). Special aspects of renal osteodystrophy in children. *Semin Nephrol, 24*(1), 69-77.

Vogt, B.A., & Avner, E.D. (2004). Renal failure. In R.E. Behrman, R.M. Kliegman, & H.B. Jenson (Eds.). *Nelson textbook of pediatrics* (17th ed.). Philadelphia: Saunders.

CHAPTER 51

Spina Bifida and Other Myelodysplasias

MICHELE A. THOLCKEN

Select the best answer for each of the following questions:

1. Folic acid supplementation is important for women of childbearing age to prevent neural tube defects. The recommended dosage for women who have had one child with myelomeningocele is:
   A. 0.8 mg.
   B. 0.4 mg.
   C. 4.0 mg.
   D. 2.0 mg.

2. The pediatric nurse practitioner understands that neural tube defects occur in the:
   A. First 30 days of gestation.
   B. Fourth month of gestation.
   C. Third trimester
   D. Latter part of the first trimester.

3. The incidence of scoliosis in the child with a myelomeningocele is:
   A. 50%.
   B. 90%.
   C. 10%.
   D. 30%.

4. The pediatric nurse practitioner recognizes that the diagnosis of myelomeningocele describes a:
   A. Herniated meningeal sac that protrudes through a vertebral arch.
   B. Tube or hollow cavity with spinal fluid that connects the central canal of the cord and is enclosed in a membrane.
   C. Condition in which the brain and spinal cord are exposed.

   D. Cystic swelling of the meningeal sac that protrudes beyond the vertebral bodies and contains portions of the spinal cord and nerve roots.

5. You are reading the history of a new patient, a 3-year-old girl with repaired myelomeningocele, and note that the child has a ventriculoperitoneal shunt which was placed soon after the closure of the myelomeningocele. You understand that the most likely reason for the placement of this shunt was to:
   A. Create a space for the cerebrospinal fluid in the spinal canal.
   B. Drain an accumulation of pus from the brain caused by meningitis.
   C. Drain cerebrospinal fluid entrapped in the fourth ventricle of the brain.
   D. Drain an overproduction of cerebrospinal fluid.

6. When assessing the condition of a child's ventriculoperitoneal shunt, the pediatric nurse practitioner will assess the child's:
   A. Head, neck, and abdominal area.
   B. Head, neck, and chest.
   C. Lumbar area of the spine and abdomen.
   D. Chest and lumbar spine area.

7. You are seeing 4-year-old Millie in clinic today. She is complaining of feeling sick to her stomach, has vomited three times in the last 5 hours, axillary temperature is 38.4° C, and other vitals are in normal range. Millie's past medical history includes a repaired myelomeningocele at L2-L5 with a ventriculoperitoneal (VP) shunt. Based on

the above presentation of symptoms and her history, which differential diagnoses would you suspect?

A. Gastrointestinal virus, shunt malfunction, or urinary tract infection.
B. Infected shunt or gastrointestinal virus.
C. Infected shunt, urinary tract infection, or gastrointestinal virus.
D. Shunt malfunction or gastrointestinal virus.

8. You are conducting a history of 6-year-old Isabel who was born with a myelomeningocele at L4-L5 area of the spine. The mother and child report that Isabel usually has problems with constipation but a couple of teaspoons of lactulose every day has helped her have normal soft stools every other day. She has been having problems with 2 or 3 episodes of liquid stool for the last 2 days and no formed stool. After physical examination, your first action is to:

A. Instruct Isabel's mom to give the child a dose of Imodium appropriate for Isabel's age and weight if she has another liquid stool.
B. Order a kidney, urine, bladder (KUB) or abdominal x-ray of Isabel.
C. Prescribe a clear liquid diet for 24 hours and have Isabel's mother call the clinic the next day with a report.
D. Alleviate mom's concerns by explaining that Isabel is having a problem common to children, continue with regular routine and this problem will go away in a few days.

9. You are reviewing the chart of a new 4-year-old patient who is in need of immunizations. The child was born with a meningocele defect at T10-L1. You would expect this child to:

A. Be sitting in a wheelchair.
B. Have crutches as an assistive device for walking.
C. Have ambulatory skills of a normal 4-year-old.
D. Be wearing ankle-foot orthoses (AFOs) to ambulate.

10. The pediatric nurse practitioner recognizes that the Arnold-Chiari II malformation describes:

A. Stenosis of the third ventricle of the brain.
B. Cystic formations throughout the cerebrum.
C. A fluid-filled canal in the cervical area of the spinal cord.
D. Elongation of the posterior cerebellum and brainstem into the foramen magnum.

11. Urinary dysfunction with myelomeningocele is best monitored with the use of:

A. Serum evaluations of the child's BUN and MRIs of the kidneys.
B. Serum creatinine and ultrasound of the urinary tract.
C. Intravenous pyelograms on an annual basis.
D. CBC with differential and KUB every 6 months.

12. The best management for urinary incontinence associated with neurogenic bladder is:

A. Sterile intermittent catheterization.
B. A urologic surgical intervention that results in a vesicostomy.
C. Clean intermittent catheterization.
D. An indwelling Foley catheter and prophylactic antibiotics.

13. Jill is a 12-year-old girl with myelomeningocele and neurogenic bladder who presents at your office today. She has just returned from summer camp where she experienced several episodes of increased body temperature, shortness of breath, and feeling very tired. Your history will take a special focus on:

A. Use of prophylactic antibiotics to prevent urinary tract infection.
B. Symptoms of urinary tract infection over the past few weeks.
C. Menstrual history, especially while she was at camp.
D. Use of anticholinergics for managing urinary continence.

14. When treating children with myelomeningocele and Arnold-Chiari II malforma-

tion, the pediatric nurse practitioner understands that these children are at high risk for the dangerous complication of:

A. Hip dislocation.
B. Respiratory arrest.
C. Urinary tract infection.
D. Decubitus ulcer.

15. The accepted standard for managing urinary tract infections in children with myelomeningocele and neurogenic bladder is to:

A. Treat every urine culture that is positive for bacteria.
B. Keep the children on a prophylactic antibiotic throughout life.
C. Treat urine cultures when they are accompanied by symptoms and/or reflux.
D. Treat based on the results of the urinalysis and forgo the expense of culture and sensitivity.

16. The least invasive intervention that can reverse upper tract renal problems such as vesicoureteral reflux and/or hydronephrosis in the child with a neurogenic bladder is:

A. Bladder augmentation accompanied with an appendicovesicostomy.
B. The Malone ACE procedure.
C. Placement of an indwelling Foley catheter.
D. Following a schedule of clean intermittent catheterization.

17. The mother of 16-year-old Manuel brings him to your office because he has been asking her many questions about whether "he can have a woman" and other sexual questions that she does not want to hear. His mother thinks that since Manuel is paralyzed and uses a wheelchair everywhere he goes, he should not be thinking about sex. She is sure he cannot have sex. Manuel is angry and thinks differently. The best way to start this session is by telling them both:

A. Manuel's mother is right and Manuel is not thinking correctly for a person who is paralyzed.
B. People who are paralyzed have sexual desires like those of people who can walk, but they are unable to have sexual intercourse.

C. That people like Manuel are interested in sexual activity but never derive any pleasure from engaging in it.
D. It is normal for Manuel to have these thoughts and desires and there are strategies for safely engaging in pleasurable sexual activity.

18. Suzie is a healthy 4-year-old with repaired myelomeningocele at T10-L2. She is a household ambulator with the assistance of bilateral AFOs and forearm crutches. She arrives in your clinic for an update on immunizations. She is seated in a wheelchair wearing her AFOs. In addition to your general physical exam of Suzie, you will:

A. Order a urine specimen to be collected and sent for culture and sensitivity.
B. Assess the condition of her skin on her gluteus and under her AFOs.
C. Have a urine specimen collected for dipstick and urinalysis.
D. Order a KUB.

19. Eighteen-month-old Joey who was born with a large myelomeningocele at L1-L5 has been brought to clinic by his mother for his immunizations. He has an axillary temperature of 38.4° C, other vitals are in the normal range. His mom says she has been catheterizing him four times a day, his urine is clear and yellow with no foul odor. He does not have a cough, has been eating well, scooting himself around the house and even tries to pull himself up to stand with his flaccid legs. On examination you note a red, warm to the touch area on his left thigh, there are no other remarkable findings in the physical exam. The differential diagnosis highest on your list is:

A. Fractured left femur.
B. Urinary tract infection.
C. Deep vein thrombosis.
D. Phlebitis.

20. The care of children with myelodysplasia and the accompanying disorders is best managed by:

A. The child's pediatrician.
B. A pediatric urologist.
C. A competent pediatric nurse practitioner.

D. A multidisciplinary team.

21. Parents of children with myelodysplasias experience denial, anger, and sadness with the birth and subsequent long-term care of child with multiple disabilities. The pediatric nurse practitioner understands that this:
   A. Is a normal reaction described as chronic sorrow.
   B. Is an example of abnormal coping on the part of the parents.
   C. Indicates the parents are in need of more education in the care of the child.
   D. Is probably a type of depressive reaction and parents need to be referred to a psychiatrist for prompt treatment.

22. The physician specialists most commonly needed by the child with diagnosis of myelomeningocele, Arnold-Chiari II malformation, and neurogenic bladder are:
   A. Urologist, cardiologist, neurosurgeon, and neurologist.
   B. Orthopedic surgeon and urologist.
   C. Neurosurgeon, orthopedic surgeon, and gastroenterologist.
   D. Gastroenterologist, urologist, neurosurgeon, orthopedic surgeon, and neurologist.

23. Cognitive deficits in children with myelodysplasias are common. A decrease in cognitive functioning in this population is directly related to the:
   A. Type of myelodysplasia.
   B. Level of the lesion.

C. Number of insertions of ventriculoperitoneal shunts.
   D. Number of surgeries the child must have in the first 3 years of life.

24. The current surgical management of the neurogenic bowel in children with myelomeningocele is commonly called:
   A. Colostomy.
   B. Ileostomy.
   C. Decompression of the bowel.
   D. MACE procedure.

25. Jenny, a 16-year-old with myelomeningocele and neurogenic bladder, has come to your office today because she thinks she has another urinary tract infection. She is excited about a new surgery that will fix her bladder. She goes on to tell you that she will not leak urine or have to catheterize herself. You have known Jenny for several years and know she has trouble sticking to her catheterization schedule. You explain to Jenny that:
   A. She will need to continue to catheterize herself the same way.
   B. The surgery will allow her to catheterize an opening in her abdomen called a stoma.
   C. The surgery results is an opening in her abdomen that drains urine continuously and she will have to wear a covering over the area to keep herself dry.
   D. She has misunderstood and there are no surgeries to help people with neurogenic bladders stay dry.

ANSWERS

1. *Answer:* C
   Rationale: The present standard for folic acid supplementation for all women of child-bearing age is 0.4 mg. The dose is 10 times that amount for women who have had one child with myelomeningocele (4.0 mg).

2. *Answer:* A
   Rationale: Neural tube defects occur between the 17th and 30th day of gestation.

3. *Answer:* B
   Rationale: Scoliosis is an extremely common disorder in children with myelomeningocele due to the abnormal muscle pull below the level of the lesion.

4. *Answer:* D
   Rationale: Myelomeningocele is the protrusion of the meningeal sac on the back of the infant, it protrudes beyond the vertebral bodies and is the only defect that also contains a portion of the spinal cord and nerve roots. Answer A is the description of the meningocele. Answer B is the description of syringomeningocele, and answer C is the description of craniorachischisis or total dysraphism.

5. *Answer:* C
   Rationale: The ventriculoperitoneal shunt placed after closure of the myelomeningocele drains cerebrospinal fluid that is entrapped in the brain due to an obstruction. That obstruction is usually a brain malformation that accompanies myelomeningocele, such as the Arnold Chiari malformation. Answer A is incorrect because a ventriculoperitoneal shunt is not placed in the spinal canal and does not drain CSF from that area. Answer B is incorrect because meningitis and accumulation of pus does not occur in the 24- to 48-hour-old neonate with myelomeningocele and hydrocephalus. Answer D is incorrect because the overaccumulation of cerebrospinal fluid in the brain following closure of the myelomeningocele is rarely caused by overproduction of CSF and the stem states, "the most likely reason."

6. *Answer:* A

Rationale: The ventriculoperitoneal shunt is inserted into the brain and is threaded under the skin down the neck into the peritoneum of the abdomen. Answers B, C, and D assess areas where the ventriculoperitoneal shunt would not be found.

7. *Answer:* C
   Rationale: Elevated temperature in the child with myelomeningocele with a ventriculoperitoneal shunt can be an indicator of infection in the shunt or the urinary tract as most children with myelomeningocele have neurogenic bladders and all children are susceptible to childhood disorders. Answer A and D are incorrect because shunt malfunction is not associated with an elevated temperature. Answer B is incorrect because it does not include urinary tract infection which always needs to be ruled out as a source of elevated body temperature in these children.

8. *Answer:* B
   Rationale: Diarrhea in a child with myelomeningocele who also has problems with constipation must first be suspected as liquid stool passing by an impaction. Answers A, C, and D do not include additional assessment before proceeding to treatment.

9. *Answer:* C
   Rationale: The diagnosis of meningocele indicates that the cord and nerve roots are not part of the birth defect; thus, innervation to all muscle groups below the lesion are not affected.

10. *Answer:* D
    Rationale: Arnold-Chiari II is the elongation of the posterior portion of the cerebellum and the brainstem into the foramen magnum.

11. *Answer:* B
    Rationale: Serum creatinine is the most sensitive serum indicator of renal function and ultrasound of the urinary tract is the least invasive technique for assessing the condition of the kidneys, ureters, and bladder. Answer A is incorrect because the BUN results are not as sensitive as serum creatinine and an MRI is not accepted practice for

routine assessments of the urinary tract because a child usually must be sedated and the MRI is costly. Answer C and D are incorrect because of the exposure of the child to dangerous radioactivity associated with the IVP and KUB.

12. *Answer:* C
     Rationale: Clean intermittent catheterization has been proven over three decades to be the simplest and most cost-effective method for managing the neurogenic bladder.

13. *Answer:* D
     Rationale: Oxybutynin chloride can cause heat prostration because it limits the person's ability to sweat. Patients who are taking oxybutynin and are involved in outside activities during the summer complain of feeling very tired and unable to catch their breath at the same time or soon before their body temperature rises. Answer B is incorrect because shortness of breath is not associated with symptomatic urinary tract infections.

14. *Answer:* B
     Rationale: Children with Arnold-Chiari II malformation develop sleep apnea and can experience sudden respiratory arrest. This is caused by the compression of the brainstem which has the potential to worsen with the complication of tethered cord. The other three options are not associated with Arnold-Chiari II malformation.

15. *Answer:* C
     Rationale: The standard for treating urinary tract infections in patients with myelomeningocele is to treat only when signs and/or symptoms of urinary tract infection accompany culture reports. Long-term clean intermittent catheterization leads to colonization of the bladder. Answer B is incorrect because the long-term use of prophylactic antibiotics is discouraged because of the risk of developing organisms that are resistant to all antibiotics. Answer A is incorrect because treating every urine culture leads to the same problem as the use of prophylactic antibiotics. Answer D is incorrect because the urinalysis is nonspecific and does not guide the

pediatric nurse practitioner in treating the child appropriately.

16. *Answer:* D
     Rationale: Clean intermittent catheterization is the least expensive method of reversing upper urinary tract damage. Answer A involves extensive bladder and colon and/or gastric surgery. Answer B is not a procedure to manage the neurogenic bladder. Instead it is a surgical intervention to manage the neurogenic bowel. Answer C is inexpensive but is bothersome, and is not considered an acceptable method to reverse upper urinary tract damage because of the high risk of infection and bladder stones.

17. *Answer:* D
     Rationale: Sexual development, interest, and desires are a normal part of development for the person disabled by a paralyzing defect. Sexual intercourse is possible and has pleasurable aspects for the paralyzed person as most of sexuality is in the mind and there are other areas of the body that a person can feel and experience pleasure through touching, caressing, and kissing.

18. *Answer:* B
     Rationale: This is a healthy child whose greatest risk at this time is skin breakdown due to the wearing of hard plastic orthotics on insensate skin and sitting for long periods on another area of insensate skin.

19. *Answer:* A
     Rationale: Children who do not have normal muscle innervation to provide the ability to bear weight develop osteopenia and as early as their teens, osteoporosis. The child who has no sensation is often unaware of his or her legs and falls and/or bends the extremity to the point of fracturing a bone. They do not experience pain in the affected extremity. B is incorrect because his urine is clear. Answers C and D are incorrect as children with myelomeningocele do not develop deep vein thrombosis or phlebitis when they are otherwise healthy.

20. *Answer:* D
     Rationale: Children with myelodysplastic disorders have multiple, complicated

needs and require a team of specially trained providers to coordinate and provide comprehensive care.

21. *Answer:* A
Rationale: Parents of children with chronic disorders experience a type of grief and sorrow, known as chronic sorrow. They are grieving the loss of the expected child and expected accomplishments.

22. *Answer:* D
Rationale: Children with the complicated disorders of myelomeningocele, Arnold-Chiari II malformation, and neurogenic bladder need the full complement of physician specialists. Children with these disorders do not usually have cardiac disorders.

23. *Answer:* C
Rationale: Research demonstrates that the number of times a child experiences increased intracranial pressure with resulting placement of shunts has a significant effect on the child's cognition.

24. *Answer:* D
Rationale: Colostomy and ileostomy were gold standards for managing bowel incontinence associated with neurogenic bowel. They were replaced in the 1990s with the surgical intervention called the Malone antegrade continent enema. There is not a procedure called decompression of the bowel to manage bowel incontinence.

25. *Answer:* B
Rationale: The newest most helpful surgery for managing urinary incontinence in the paralyzed person is the continent appendicovesicostomy. This is a surgical intervention resulting in a continent stoma located on the abdomen which the person catheterizes on the same schedule followed prior to surgery. Surgeons usually insist that the candidate for the surgery demonstrate motivation and ability to follow a self-catheterization schedule before performing the surgery.

BIBLIOGRAPHY

American Academy of Pediatrics (AAP) Committee on Bioethics. (1999). Fetal therapy—Ethical considerations. *Pediatrics, 103*(5 Pt 1), 1061-1063.

Benasich, A.A. (2004). Foundations—Early brain development. Retrieved June 1, 2005, from http://babylab.rutgers.edu/foundations/outlines/Brain%20Devoutline04.doc.

Biggio, J.R. Jr., Owen, J., Wenstrom, K.D., & Oakes, W.J. (2001). Can prenatal ultrasound findings predict ambulatory status in fetus with open spina bifida? *Am J Obstet Gynecol, 185*(5), 1016-1020.

Bureau for Children with Medical Handicaps (BCMH), Myelodysplasia Standards Committee. *Standards of care and outcome measures for children with myelodysplasia.* Columbus, OH: Ohio Department of Health. Retrieved June 26, 2006, from www.odh.state.oh.us/ODHPrograms/CMH/bifida.pdf.

Chervenak, F.A., McCullough, L.B., & Birnbach, D.J. (2004). Ethical issues in fetal surgery research. *Best Pract Res Clin Anaesthesiol, 18*(2), 221-230.

Churchill, B.M., Abramson, R.P., & Wahl, E.F. (2001). Dysfunction of the lower urinary and distal gastrointestinal tracts in pediatric patients with known spinal cord problems. *Pediatr Clin North Am, 48*(6), 1587-1630.

Drolet, B.A. (2000). Cutaneous signs of neural tube dysraphism. *Pediatr Clin North Am, 47*(4), 813-823.

Elder, J.S. (2004). Neuropathic bladder. In R.E. Behrman, R.M. Kliegman, & H.B. Jenson (Eds.). *Nelson textbook of pediatrics* (17th ed.). Philadelphia: Saunders.

Foster, M.R. (2004). Spina bifida. Retrieved June 2, 2005, from www.emedicine.com/orthoped/topic557.htm.

Green, N. (2002). Folic acid supplementation and prevention of birth defects. *J Nutr, 132*(8 Suppl), 2356S-2360S.

Greenlee, J.D.W., Donovan, K.A., Hasan, D.M., & Menezes, A.H. (2002). Chiari malformation in the very young child: The spectrum of presentations and experience in 31 children under age 6 years. *Pediatrics, 110*(6), 1212-1219.

Haslam, R.H.A. (2004). Neurologic evaluation. In R.E. Behrman, R.M. Kliegman, & H.B. Jenson (Eds.). *Nelson textbook of pediatrics* (17th ed.). Philadelphia: Saunders.

Hirose, S., Meuli-Simmen, C., & Meuli, M. (2003). Fetal surgery for myelomeningocele: Panacea or peril? *World J Surg, 27*(1), 87-94.

Johnson, M.P., Sutton, L.N., Rintoul, N., et al., (2003). Fetal myelomeningocele repair: Short-term clinical outcomes. *Am J Obstet Gynecol, 189*(2), 482-487.

Johnston, M.V., & Kinsman, S. (2004). Congenital anomalies of the central nervous system. In R.E. Behrman, R.M. Kliegman, & H.B. Jenson (Eds.). *Nelson textbook of pediatrics* (17th ed.). Philadelphia: Saunders.

Lazzaretti, C.C., & Pearson, C. (2004). Myelodysplasia. In P.L. Jackson & J.A. Vessey (Eds.). *Primary care of the child with a chronic condition* (4th ed.). St. Louis: Mosby.

Mazzola, C.A., Albright, A.L., Sutton, L.N., et al. (2002). Dermoid inclusion cysts and early spinal cord tethering after fetal surgery for myelomeningocele. *N Engl J Med, 347*(4), 256-259.

Merropol, E. (2001). Latex (natural rubber) allergy in spina bifida. Spina Bifida Association of America fact sheet. Washington, DC: Spina Bifida Association of America.

Mingin, G.C., Nguyen, H.T., Mathias, R.S., et al. (2002). Growth and metabolic consequences of bladder augmentation in children with myelomeningocele and bladder exstrophy. *Pediatrics, 110*(6), 1193-1198.

Nieto, A., Mazon, A., Pamies, R., et al. (2002). Efficacy of latex avoidance for primary prevention of latex sensitization in children with spina bifida. *J Pediatr, 140*(3), 370-372.

NINDS—National Institute of Neurological Disorders and Stroke (2006). NINDS Chiari malformation information page. Updated June 19, 2006. Retrieved June 26, 2006, from www.ninds.nih.gov/disorders/chiari/chiari.htm.

Rintoul, N.E., Sutton, L.N., Hubbard, A.M., et al. (2002). A new look at myelomeningoceles: Functional level, vertebral level, shunting, and the implications of fetal intervention. *Pediatrics, 109*(3), 409-413.

Schneider, J.W., & Krosschell, K.J. (2001). Congenital spinal cord injury. In D.A. Umphred (Ed.). *Neurological rehabilitation* (4th ed.). St. Louis: Mosby.

Strayer, A. (2001). Chiari I malformation: Clinical presentation and management. *J Neurosci Nurs, 33*(2), 90-96, 104.

NOTES

6

DIAGNOSTIC, MEDICATION, AND TREATMENT GUIDES FOR CHILDREN AND ADOLESCENTS

CHAPTER 52

Readiness for Handling Pediatric Emergencies in the Primary Care Office

LISA MARIE BERNARDO

Select the best answer for each of the following questions:

1. The pediatric nurse practitioner's role in office emergency preparedness planning includes all of the following EXCEPT:
   A. Having access to the proper emergency equipment per sample emergency drug and equipment lists in AAP *Blue Book*.
   B. Receiving ongoing education and training in identification and treatment of selected emergencies.
   C. Knowing the community resources for referral and to confidently render care under such circumstances.
   D. Pediatric nurse practitioners are required to complete pediatric advanced life support (PALS) certification prior to practicing in a clinic or outpatient setting.

2. While pediatric emergencies in the office setting are an infrequent event, the type of emergency that is most frequently reported is:
   A. Poisoning.
   B. Respiratory.
   C. Major trauma.
   D. Orthopedic.

3. A mother presents to the receptionist at the clinic with her 5-year-old child who reportedly fell from a two-story window 20 minutes ago. The child is unconscious and limp with shallow breathing and pale skin. The BEST action for the receptionist would be to:

   A. Immediately call the pediatric nurse practitioner to the front desk.
   B. Ask the mother take a seat and complete the intake form.
   C. Escort the mother and child to the designated emergency treatment room and call for help.
   D. Tell the mother to call 911 from the lobby payphone.

4. When enacting the response plan, the pediatric nurse practitioner gives all of the following information to the EMS dispatcher EXCEPT:
   A. Patient name.
   B. Location of the office (street address, building number, room number).
   C. Nature of the emergency (e.g., 3-year-old child with severe respiratory distress).
   D. Child's health insurance number.

5. In an emergency, the pediatric nurse practitioner trained in pediatric advanced life support should be prepared to:
   A. Maintain and stabilize the child's airway, with or without airway adjuncts.
   B. Perform a venous cut-down.
   C. Perform chest decompression.
   D. Administer intracardiac epinephrine.

6. What system allows for quick reference to determine appropriate equipment size, fluid volumes, and medication doses?
   A. Pediatric advanced life support (PALS).
   B. Emergency medical system (EMS).
   C. Basic life support (BLS).
   D. Broselow-Luten system.

7. Many times parents cannot accompany their child in the air or ground ambulance to the hospital. Under such circumstances, the pediatric nurse practitioner could do all of the following EXCEPT:
   A. Contact a family friend or relative to drive the parents to the hospital.
   B. Provide written explanations of illness, treatment, and where the child is being transported with address, directions, and telephone numbers.
   C. Drive the parents to the hospital in his or her own car.
   D. Ask the secretary or receptionist to escort EMS and the parents from the building.

8. Because the treatment and transport of an emergently ill child is very stressful for the office staff, the pediatric nurse practitioner or pediatrician in charge of the emergency should gather the office staff and reflect on the day's events at the end of the day. At this time:
   A. The office's malpractice insurer should be contacted.

B. Words of encouragement ("We did the best we could") should be expressed.
C. The emergency preparedness plan should be completely rewritten.
D. Blame should be placed on the staff for not doing their best.

9. Pediatric nurse practitioners should collaborate with EMS to accomplish all of the following EXCEPT:
   A. Improve their response time to their office.
   B. Enhance professional communications.
   C. Teach them about pediatric care.
   D. Participate in their mock codes.

10. Mock codes are mechanisms used to allow health care providers and staff to:
   A. Practice emergency skills that are not often used.
   B. Provide patient's information to the emergency department.
   C. Gain certification in emergency care.
   D. Check emergency equipment daily.

NOTES

ANSWERS

1. *Answer:* D
   Rationale: PALS certification is not a standard requirement for pediatric nurse practitioner practice in outpatient settings.

2. *Answer:* B
   Rationale: Respiratory-related conditions are the most frequently reported emergencies in the pediatric office setting. This finding coincides with respiratory emergencies being the most common medical emergency, overall, in pediatric emergency care.

3. *Answer:* C
   Rationale: The receptionist has the lowest level of training, yet is the first one to come in contact with a seriously ill or injured child. The receptionist's actions show that an emergency is recognized, the prepared room will be used, and help is needed.

4. *Answer:* D
   Rationale: Health insurance information is not critical information at this time.

5. *Answer:* A
   Rationale: The pediatric nurse practitioner should be prepared to assume airway control in an emergency situation; the remaining procedures are unlikely to be performed in an office setting.

6. *Answer:* D
   PALS is training in pediatric advanced life support and includes CPR, entotracheal tube intubation, intraosseous access, and medication calculation. BLS is basic life support training which includes adult, child, and infant CPR. EMS is activated in the event of an emergency. The Broselow-Luten system is a color coded measuring tape that offers quick reference for equipment size, supplies, and medication doses based on the child's height.

7. *Answer:* C
   Rationale: The pediatric nurse practitioner should never transport a child or family in his or her personal vehicle due to liability issues as well as potential abandonment of patients waiting in the office for treatment.

8. *Answer:* B
   Rationale: Because office staff should be well-prepared for emergencies, everyone's actions should be acknowledged in a positive light to promote confidence. Problems identified in the emergency response/treatment, plus revisions to protocols and procedures can be addressed at a future meeting.

9. *Answer:* A
   Rationale: EMS may not have control in their response times to the primary care office due to its location, availability of the EMS crew, and other factors that pediatric nurse practitioners are unable to control.

10. *Answer:* A
    Rationale: Mock codes are practice scenarios that allow health care providers and staff the opportunity to practice emergency skills. Mock codes do not result in emergency certification nor do they provide patient data to the emergency department. Although checking emergency equipment is important, the purpose of a mock code is not to check equipment daily.

BIBLIOGRAPHY

American Association of Colleges of Nursing (1996). *The essentials of master's education for advanced practice nursing.* Washington DC: American Association of Colleges of Nursing Publishing.

Association of Faculties of Pediatric Nurse Practitioner Programs (AFPNP). (1996). *Philosophy, conceptual model, terminal competencies for the education of pediatric nurse practitioners.* Cherry Hill, NJ: AFPNP/NAPNAP.

Bernardo, L.M. (2001). Pediatric implications in bioterrorism, Part I: Physiologic and psychosocial differences. *Int J Trauma Nurs, 7*(1), 14-16.

Bernardo, L.M., & Kapsar, P. (2003). Pediatric implications in bioterrorism: Education for health care providers. *Disaster Manag Response, 1*(2), 52-53.

Bordley, W.C., Travers, D., Scanlon, P., et al. (2003). Office preparedness for pediatric emergencies: A randomized, controlled trial of an office-based training program. *Pediatrics, 112*(2), 291-295.

Davis, C.O., & Rodewald, L. (1999). Use of EMS for seriously ill children in the office: A survey of primary care physicians. *Prehospital Emerg Care, 3*(2), 102-106.

Flores, G., & Weinstock, D. (1996). The preparedness of pediatricians for emergencies in the office: What is broken, should we care, and how can we fix it? *Arch Pediatr Adolesc Med, 150*(3), 249-256.

Frush, K., Cinoman, M., Bailey, B., & Hohenhaus, S. (2001). *Office preparedness for pediatric emergencies: Provider manual*. Washington, DC: Department of Health and Human Services, Health Resources and Services Administration, Emergency Medical Services for Children Program.

Heath, B., Coffey, J., Malone, P., & Courtney, J. (2000). Pediatric office emergencies and emergency preparedness in a small rural state. *Pediatrics, 106*(6), 1391-1396.

Knapp, J.F. (2000). Commentary: Pediatric emergencies in the office, hospital, and community: Organizing systems of care. *Pediatrics, 106*(2), 337-338.

Mansfield, C., Price, J., Frush, K., & Dallara, J. (2001). Pediatric emergencies in the office: Are family physicians as prepared as pediatricians? *J Fam Pract, 50*(9), 757-761.

National Organization of Nurse Practitioner Faculties. (2002). *Nurse practitioner primary care competencies in specialty areas: Pediatrics*. Washington, DC: U.S. Department of Health and Human Services, Health Resources and Services Administration, Bureau of Health Professions, Division of Nursing.

Primm, P., Hodge, D., Ringwood, J., et al. (Eds). (2002). *Office PERC: Preparedness for emergency response to children* (CD-ROM). Washington, DC: U.S. Department of Health and Human Services, Division of Maternal Child Health.

Rosenfield, R.L., & Bernardo, L.M. (2001). Pediatric implications in bioterrorism, Part II: Post-exposure diagnosis and treatment. *Int J Trauma Nurs, 7*(4), 133-136.

Samson, R.A., Berg, R.A., & Bingham, R. (2003). Use of automated external defibrillators for children: An update: An advisory statement from the Pediatric Advanced Life Support Task Force, International Liaison Committee on Resuscitation. *Pediatrics, 112*(1 Pt 1), 163-168.

Seidel, J., & Knapp, J. (Eds.). (2000). *Childhood emergencies in the office, hospital, and community: Organizing systems of care* (2nd ed.). Elk Grove Village, IL: American Academy of Pediatrics.

Stokes, E., Gilbert Palmer, D., Skorga, P., et al. (2004). Chemical agents of terrorism: Preparing nurse practitioners. *Nurse Pract, 29*(5), 30-41.

Toback, S. (2002). Prepare your office for a medical emergency. *Contemp Pediatr, 4*, 107.

Veenema, T.G. (2003). Chemical and biological terrorism preparedness for staff development specialists. *J Nurse Staff Dev, 19*(5), 218-227.

Zonia, C.L., and Moore, D.S. (2004). Review of guidelines for pediatric advanced life support. *J Am Osteopath Assoc, 104*(1), 22-23.

NOTES

53 Diagnostic Tests for Pediatric Clinical Decision Making

AMY HOWELLS

Select the best answer for each of the following questions:

1. What is the best way to determine the practical value of a diagnostic test?
   A. Ordering the test will appease the parents of the child.
   B. The subsequent health outcomes of the child have been considered.
   C. The test will narrow the differential diagnosis, but not guide treatment.
   D. The test will confirm a diagnosis that will be treated regardless of the results.

2. You have a patient who lives in an area where a certain disease that can be easily treated in the early stages has a high prevalence. Your patient has not yet shown symptoms of any illness. You want to determine whether your patient is at risk for this disease. Your first step is to order a:
   A. Diagnostic test.
   B. Specific test.
   C. Screening test.
   D. Sensitive test.

3. What are some commonly used point-of-care diagnostic tests?
   A. Hemoglobin, pregnancy tests, blood culture.
   B. "Rapid strep," stool occult blood, microscopy of vaginal fluids.
   C. pH of gastric fluid, whiff test of vaginal fluid, urine culture.
   D. Urine microscopy, hematocrit, serum potassium.

4. What are defining characteristics of point-of-care diagnostic tests?
   A. Specific, simple to conduct, inexpensive.
   B. Accurate, simple to conduct, disposable.
   C. Specific, disposable, inexpensive.
   D. Simple to conduct, specific, difficult to interpret.

5. It is important to use the proper collection tubes for venous blood specimens because:
   A. All tubes have additives.
   B. All samples are collected in the same manner.
   C. The tubes are all the same size.
   D. The samples may be whole blood, serum, or plasma.

6. Common sites for a capillary blood specimen in infants and children include:
   A. Abdomen, heels, earlobes.
   B. Fingertips, toes, heels.
   C. Heels, elbows, earlobes.
   D. Fingertips, heels, earlobes.

7. You ordered a chemistry panel for your patient that includes a sodium, potassium, chloride, bicarbonate, BUN, creatinine, and glucose. The results are sodium 138, potassium 6.1, chloride 99, bicarbonate 22, BUN 36, creatinine 0.4, and glucose 102. You learn the specimen was a capillary blood sample. What is a possible explanation for this result?
   A. The lab has a new technician.
   B. The sample was hemolyzed during the collection process.

C. The specimen was labeled incorrectly.
D. The specimen was not sent on ice.

8. When collecting a urine sample, why is the first morning specimen preferred?
   A. It is the most concentrated.
   B. It is sterile.
   C. It has more volume.
   D. It is the easiest to obtain.

9. What urine specimens can be sent for culture?
   A. Clean-catch specimens, catheter specimens, urinary bag specimens.
   B. Urinary bag specimens, suprapubic aspiration specimens, catheter specimens.
   C. Catheter specimens, clean-catch specimens, suprapubic specimens.
   D. Catheter specimens, diaper specimens, clean-catch specimens.

10. Under what circumstances is the pediatric nurse practitioner able to obtain a suprapubic specimen?
    A. In the case of an emergency.
    B. When the pediatric nurse practitioner has undergone special training.
    C. When the parent gives consent.
    D. When the child cannot void spontaneously.

11. A 12-year-old female presents to the clinic with frequency and pain when urinating. She has had the symptoms for several days and reports the use of a medicine "to help the pain" that her mother bought over the counter. A clean-catch specimen is obtained for urinalysis and culture. The color of the urine is noted to be dark orange. What is the most likely reason for the color of the urine?
    A. Blood
    B. Lotrimin
    C. Pyridium
    D. Melanin

12. A 3-year-old female presents to the clinic with fever, irritability, and mom reports that she is "having frequent accidents" even though she has been potty trained for a year. You obtain a urine sample via a disposable

urinary bag for urinalysis. The results show cloudy color, negative glucose, negative ketones, positive leukocytes, and positive nitrites. What is your next step?
    A. Nothing, this is normal.
    B. Send bag specimen for culture.
    C. Diagnose a urinary tract infection.
    D. Obtain a catheter specimen for culture.

13. You are obtaining a history from a patient who has had diarrhea for 3 days. The patient just returned from a trip to Guatemala, where he was visiting family. The mother reports that the stools have been particularly foul-smelling, so she was starting to worry. The patient has also been running a low-grade fever, for which the mother has given him Ibuprofen. You decide to order a stool sample. What information gathered in the history could affect the results of the stool sample?
    A. The patient has diarrhea.
    B. The patient has taken Ibuprofen.
    C. The patient has traveled outside the country.
    D. The patient has foul-smelling stools.

14. What diagnostic tests require a larger than normal stool sample?
    A. Microscopy for ova and parasites, fat content.
    B. Occult blood, microscopy for ova and parasites.
    C. Fat content, gram stain.
    D. Trypsin, rotavirus antigen.

15. A sputum specimen can be obtained by the following method:
    A. Having the patient spit into a cup.
    B. Having the patient suck on a cotton pledget.
    C. Suctioning the patient's trachea.
    D. Swabbing the tonsillar area.

16. You obtain a sputum culture from a 13-year-old boy who presents with a 7-day history of cough that is not improving. You ask for a sputum culture and sensitivity to be performed on the specimen. What information can this test give you?
    A. Detect the presence of *Mycobacterium tuberculosis*.

B. Identify a specific microorganism and the medication to which it is sensitive.
C. Detect a virus.
D. Identify the presence of cancerous cells.

17. A 6-year-old boy presents to the clinic with a 1-day history of sore throat. A rapid strep test is performed and the results are negative. Your next step would be:
    A. Nothing, the test is highly sensitive.
    B. Ask for the patient to repeat the test the next day.
    C. Start antibiotics anyway, drug resistance is not a problem in your region.
    D. Send a back-up throat culture.

18. Vaginal fluids are obtained by swabbing the walls of the vagina when performing a pelvic examination. What information CANNOT be obtained with this type of vaginal specimen?
    A. Papanicolaou tests.
    B. Vaginal pH.
    C. Whiff test.
    D. Wet mount microscopy.

19. A wet mount microscopy is performed on vaginal fluids obtained during a pelvic examination. The presence of pseudohyphae is noted. What does this finding suggest?
    A. This finding is normal.
    B. Bacterial vaginosis.
    C. *Candida* infection.
    D. Precancerous cells.

20. When using a Wood's lamp to observe fluorescence on the skin of a patient, you note the color to be pale yellow. What is this most likely indicative of?

A. Tinea capitis.
B. Pityriasis versicolor.
C. Candida.
D. *Corynebacterium minutissimum.*

21. Which dermatophyte has a characteristic "spaghetti-and-meatballs" appearance under the microscope?
    A. Candida.
    B. Pityriasis versicolor.
    C. Tinea cruris.
    D. Tinea versicolor.

22. A skin culture can be considered negative after how many days?
    A. 5
    B. 7
    C. 10
    D. 21

23. A pregnant woman in the emergency department who has twisted her ankle is told that an x-ray will not be performed. When the woman asks why the 6-year-old child next to her will undergo an x-ray for an ankle injury but she will not, you reply:
    A. Because the child is more likely to have a broken bone.
    B. Children are still growing.
    C. Your unborn child could be harmed by an x-ray.
    D. X-rays are not indicated for adults.

24. When using contrast dyes for radiographic procedures, what potential risk exists?
    A. Allergic reactions.
    B. Increase in radiation exposure.
    C. Poor study results due to the contrast.
    D. There is no risk involved.

ANSWERS

1. *Answer:* B
    Rationale: The practical value of a test can only be assessed by taking into account the subsequent health outcomes. Testing should not be done if the intention is to treat regardless of the results.

2. *Answer:* C
    Rationale: A screening test is used for individuals without current symptoms of a specific disease to detect presymptomatic disease or risk for disease. A diagnostic test is a method of distinguishing individuals with a disease from individuals without the disease. Sensitivity and specificity refer to characteristics of both screening and diagnostic tests.

3. *Answer:* B
    Rationale: Point-of-care tests must be sensitive, specific, simple to conduct, and inexpensive. Tests that are performed in a lab, such as cultures and serum tests, would not fit these criteria.

4. *Answer:* A
    Rationale: Point-of-care tests are not required to be disposable and they should not be difficult to interpret.

5. *Answer:* D
    Rationale: Not all tubes have additives or are the same size. Samples may be collected by various methods, such as a heel stick or venipuncture.

6. *Answer:* D
    Rationale: Fingertips, heels, and earlobes are often used for capillary samples because these sites are accessible, and they have capillary beds close to the skin's surface.

7. *Answer:* B
    Rationale: The value that is not in the normal range is potassium of 6.1. This value may have occurred because of hemolysis. Hemolysis can occur if the technician drawing the sample had to squeeze the site to obtain blood or used a scraping motion to collect the blood in the tube.

8. *Answer:* A

Rationale: The first void in the morning is usually the most concentrated, but may not be sterile, depending on the mode of collection.

9. *Answer:* C
    Rationale: Culture specimens must be sterile. Specimens obtained with a urinary bag or from a diaper are not sterile.

10. *Answer:* B
    Rationale: A pediatric nurse practitioner must have special training to perform any procedure that is not taught in the program from which he or she graduated.

11. *Answer:* C
    Rationale: Blood usually presents as red urine, while melanin would present as black urine. Pyridium can cause urine to be dark orange or brown.

12. *Answer:* D
    Rationale: Positive leukocytes and nitrites may be an indicator of a urinary tract infection. A catheter specimen is necessary because a 3-year-old is unlikely to be able to perform a clean-catch technique, and a sterile specimen should be sent for culture and sensitivity.

13. *Answer:* B
    Rationale: The anticlotting mechanism of NSAIDs may result in trace amounts of blood in the stool. While the other components of the history are important, they are unlikely to affect the results of the test.

14. *Answer:* A
    Rationale: Microscopy for ova and parasites usually requires three specimens to identify the organism. To determine the fat content of stool, a 72-hour sample is required. Other tests only require a small amount of stool.

15. *Answer:* C
    Rationale: Asking a patient to spit in a cup, suck on a cotton pledget, or swabbing the tonsillar area will provide a sample of saliva. A patient may be able to cough up a specimen, or the trachea can be suctioned to obtain sputum.

16. *Answer:* B

Rationale: A sputum acid-fast bacilli must be checked to detect *Mycobacterium tuberculosis*. Sputum cytology would identify the presence of cancerous cells. A culture and sensitivity would identify the microorganism and the medication to which it is most sensitive.

17. *Answer:* D

Rationale: A back-up throat culture should be sent in this instance, because there are dangerous sequelae (rheumatic fever, poststreptococcal glomerulonephritis) that can occur if a group A B-hemolytic streptococcus infection (GABHS) infection goes untreated . The rapid strep test may not indicate an infection if the symptoms have a recent onset. Because of drug resistance, it is preferable to treat documented infections rather than start empiric therapy.

18. *Answer:* A

Rationale: Papanicolaou tests are performed on specimens obtained with a specially designed spatula that scrapes the cervical canal and the squamocolumnar junction.

19. *Answer:* C

Rationale: The presence of pseudohyphae or yeast buds suggests a Candida infection. Clue cells that look like ground black pepper would suggest a bacterial vaginosis.

20. *Answer:* B

Rationale: Tinea capitis fluoresces a blue-green, *Corynebacterium minutissimum* shows a coral red color, and Candida does not fluoresce.

21. *Answer:* D

Rationale: Candida cells are round or oval. The dermatophyte that causes tinea versicolor has a characteristic appearance which is described as "spaghetti and meatballs."

22. *Answer:* D

Rationale: While a skin culture can be positive after 7 to 10 days, a full 21 days must past before the culture is determined to be negative.

23. *Answer:* C

Rationale: An x-ray is only indicated for pregnant women when it is medically required for treatment because the radiation, although minimal, may negatively affect fetal development.

24. *Answer:* A

Rationale: The contrast will enhance the study and no more radiation than normal would be used. The risk for allergic reaction exists with any medication given to a patient.

BIBLIOGRAPHY

French, L., Horton, J., & Matousek, M. (2004). Abnormal vaginal discharge: Using office diagnostic testing more effectively. *J Fam Pract, 53*(10), 805-814.

Hainer, B.L. (2003). Dermatophyte infections: Practical therapeutics. *Am Fam Phys, 67*(1), 101-108.

Higgins, J.C.C. (2000). The status of physician office labs since CLIA '88. *J Med Pract Manage, 16*(2), 99-102.

Kee, J.L. (2005). *Laboratory and diagnostic tests with nursing implications* (7th ed.). Upper Saddle River, NJ: Pearson.

MDS Metro Laboratory Services. (2005a). Urinalysis. Retrieved May 21, 2006, from www.mdsdx.com/MDS_Metro_Laboratories/Patients/MedicalConditions/Urinalysis.asp.

MDS Metro Laboratory Services. (2005b). Stool sample for occult blood. Retrieved May 21, 2006, from www.mdsdx.com/mds_metro_laboratories/patients/instructions/stool_sample_for_occult_blood.asp.

Mol, B.W., Lijmer, J.G., Evers, J.L.H., & Bossuyt, P.M.M. (2003). Characteristics of good diagnostic studies. *Sem Reprod Med, 21*(1), 17-25.

National Library of Medicine. (2005). Stools: floating. Medical encyclopedia. Retrieved November 17, 2005, from www.nlm.nih.gov/medlineplus/print/ency/article/003128.htm.

Nicholson, J.F., & Pesce, M.A. (2004). Laboratory testing in infants and children. In R.E. Behrman, R.M. Kliegman, & H.B. Jenson (Eds.). *Nelson textbook of pediatrics* (17th ed.). Philadelphia: Saunders.

Pagana, K.D., & Pagana, T.J. (2005). *Mosby's diagnostic and laboratory test reference* (7th ed.). St. Louis: Mosby.

Riegelman, R.K. (2004). *Studying a study and testing a test: How to read the medical evidence* (5th ed.). Philadelphia: Lippincott Williams & Wilkins.

54 Pharmacodynamic Considerations Unique to Neonates, Infants, Children, and Adolescents

IRMA LARA AND ROSE A. SALDIVAR

Select the best answer for each of the following questions:

1. When preparing an intravenous infusion for an infant, it would be important to:
   A. Use a short needle to prevent plugging.
   B. Hang the intravenous fluid no higher than 4 feet above the infant's head.
   C. Use a calibrated fluid pump for the intravenous infusion.
   D. Use minimal adhesive tape; this reduces allergic reaction to the tape.

2. The danger of fluid overload developing is a potential problem in the infant receiving an intravenous infusion. For which of the following would you observe?
   A. Increased pulse rate and decreased blood pressure.
   B. Increased pulse rate and increased blood pressure.
   C. Decreased pulse rate and decreased blood pressure.
   D. Decreased blood pressure and swelling of the feet.

3. Adult body water accounts for approximately 60% of total weight. A full-term neonate's body water is approximately what percentage of total weight?
   A. 45% to 55%.
   B. 55% to 60%.
   C. 70% to 75%.
   D. 75% to 80%.

4. In the neonate, the proportion of body water varies from the adult in which of the following ways?
   A. The proportion of intracellular fluid increases as the infant matures.
   B. The neonate exchanges extracellular fluid more rapidly than an adult.
   C. A larger milligram per kilogram dosage of water-soluble drug is needed.
   D. A smaller milligram per kilogram dosage of water-soluble drug is needed.

5. As the pediatric nurse practitioner, you prescribed penicillin V (Veetids) 250 mg by mouth every 12 hours for a child with a respiratory infection. The child's weight is 50 pounds. The safe pediatric dose is 25 to 50mg/kg/day. You have determined this dose to be:
   A. Too high.
   B. Too low.
   C. Within the safe range.
   D. There is not enough information to determine safe dose.

6. A 2-month-old is recovering from pneumonia. Her medications include oral penicillin. The infant develops gastritis with regurgitation. As the pediatric nurse practitioner, you are aware that the administration of oral medication at this time may result in:
   A. Increased therapeutic response.
   B. Prolonged therapeutic response.
   C. Altered timing of the therapeutic effect.
   D. No effect in penicillin absorption.

7. A 1-month-old is given medication which is dependent on protein binding for drug distribution. As the pediatric nurse practitioner, you are aware that it may be necessary to:
A. Decrease the amount of drug and shorten the dosage interval.
B. Increase the amount of drug and give at longer intervals.
C. Decrease the amount of drug and give at longer intervals.
D. Increase the amount of drug and shorten the dosage intervals.

8. Medication absorption via the intestine in the neonate is limited by the following characteristic:
A. The length of the intestinal lumen is short compared to the adult.
B. These is a relatively small surface area for drug absorption.
C. Due to neuromuscular immaturity, peristalsis is slow.
D. Intestinal peristalsis is rapid and unpredictable.

9. Which statement regarding pediatric percutaneous absorption and medication administration is correct?
A. Due to alkalinity of the skin, infants require topical medication for frequent infections.
B. Natural skin barriers are present in the skin of infants which prevent the absorption of topical medications.
C. Infants absorb greater amounts of topical medications, causing potential side effects.
D. Body surface area is smaller for an infant than an adult.

10. Knowledge of the metabolism of medications is essential for drug administration in the neonate. During the first month of life, you will observe for which response to medication administration?
A. Reduced drug half-life.
B. Prolonged therapeutic effect.
C. Increased elimination half-life.
D. Slow clearance rate.

11. To give eardrops to a 4-year-old, which of the following would be the best technique to use?
A. Pull the pinna of the ear downward.
B. Lift the pinna of the ear down and back.
C. Pull the pinna of the ear upward.
D. Pull the pinna of the ear up and back.

12. The pediatric nurse practitioner prescribed penicillin G procaine (Wycillin), 1,000,000 Units IM for a strep throat infection. The child's weight is 62 pounds. The safe pediatric dose reads "greater than 60 pounds: 600,000 to 1,200,000 Units daily." You have determined that:
A. The dose is too high.
B. The dose is too low.
C. The dose is within the safe range.
D. There is not enough information to determine safe dose.

13. As a pediatric nurse practitioner, you plan to apply EMLA cream to decrease the pain of a procedure. Which of the following would be the best application technique?
A. Wipe the cream off at least 15 minutes before the procedure.
B. Apply it immediately prior to the procedure.
C. Avoid covering the site after application to prevent it from discoloring.
D. Apply it at least 1 hour before the procedure.

14. The mother of a 6-year-old child states that her child was diagnosed with thrombocytopenia after having a viral illness. Which medication should be avoided in children with thrombocytopenia?
A. Amoxicillin (Amoxil).
B. Cefaclor (Ceclor).
C. Acetaminophen (Tylenol).
D. Acetylsalicylic acid (Aspirin).

15. The pediatric nurse practitioner is providing medication administration instructions to the parents of a child on the use of erythromycin. What instructions would you give the parents about how to take this medication?
A. Medication should be administered with meals.

B. Medication should be administered on an empty stomach.
C. Medication should be administered with fruit juice.
D. Medication should be crushed and administered with apple sauce.

16. The pediatric nurse practitioner is instructing the parents of a 6-month-old child on how to properly administer eye drops. Which medication administration instructions are correct?
   A. Lay child on her right side for eye drop instillation.
   B. Lay child on her left side for eye drop instillation.
   C. Lay child prone for eye drop instillation.
   D. Lay child supine for eye drop instillation.

17. What statement best reflects a strategy the pediatric nurse practitioner can implement to improve compliance of medication administration among children attending school or daycares?
   A. Prescribing medications with once a day administration.
   B. Prescribing medications with four times a day administration
   C. Prescribing medications that have a pleasant taste.
   D. Prescribing medications that are affordable.

18. Which of the following medications has a narrow therapeutic window and will be an essential candidate for therapeutic monitoring?
   A. Acetaminophen.
   B. Trimethoprim-sulfamethoxazole (Septra).
   C. Vancomycin.
   D. Tetracycline.

19. Which of the following is the most appropriate first-line antibiotic to be used in the treatment of acute otitis media?
   A. Azithromycin (Zithromax).
   B. Amoxicillin/clavulanate (Augmentin).
   C. Amoxicillin (Amoxil).
   D. Cefaclor (Ceclor).

20. The mother of a newborn infant states that her baby has white plaques on the buccal mucosa, tongue, and pharynx. These plaques do not scrape off easily and bleed when they are removed. You diagnose the infant with thrush (oral candidiasis) and your treatment of choice is:
   A. Amoxicillin oral suspension applied to oral mucosa four times a day for 10 days.
   B. Erythromycin 50/kg/day for 10 days.
   C. Nystatin oral suspension 2 ml four times daily applied to oral mucosa for 10 days.
   D. Omnicef suspension 7mg/kg every 12 hours for 10 days.

21. What is the treatment of choice for gonococcal conjunctivitis in the newborn?
   A. Ceftriaxone 25 to 50 mg/kg/day and immediate referral to an ophthalmologist.
   B. Erythromycin 50 mg/kg/day for 10 days and subsequent referral to an ophthalmologist.
   C. Sodium sulfacetamide 10% ophthalmic solution four times a day and does not need a referral to an ophthalmologist.
   D. Topical penicillin G 50,000 U/kg for 10 days and referral to an optometrist.

22. You are assessing a 14-month-old toddler and find a scaly papulovesicular rash between his fingers and on his thighs and ankles. Excoriations in a linear pattern are also present on his thighs and ankles. The mother reports that the child scratches primarily during the night. As the pediatric nurse practitioner you diagnose scabies. What would be the treatment of choice?
   A. Bacitracin ointment.
   B. Elidel 30 % cream.
   C. Elimite cream.
   D. Lindane cream or lotion.

23. When administering intramuscular injections on a child under 4 years of age, what muscle must you avoid?
   A. The posterior gluteal muscle.
   B. The deltoid muscle.
   C. The lateralis lateral aspect.
   D. The rectus femoris anterior aspect.

24. You are evaluating a sexually active 15-year-old female who was diagnosed with a Chlamydia infection and needs to undergo treatment. The recommended regimen for Chlamydia is:
    A. Doxycyline 100 mg orally daily for 3 days.
    B. Levofloxacin 300 mg orally daily for 5 days.
    C. Clotrimazole vaginal cream for 5 days.
    D. Azithromycin 1 g orally in a single dose.

25. What is the recommended treatment for bacterial vaginosis in a sexually active nonpregnant female?
    A. Metronidazole gel 0.35% one applicatorful intravaginally once a day for 3 days.
    B. Clindamycin ovules 100 mg intravaginally once at bedtime.
    C. Metronidazole 500 mg orally twice a day for 7 days.
    D. Clindamycin 300 mg orally twice a day for 5 days.

NOTES

ANSWERS

1. *Answer:* C
   Rationale: All children should be placed on a calibrated fluid pump because of the danger of fluid overload. Selection of the catheter length and gauge depends on the prescribed therapy and IV placement site. Typically 22 to 24 gauge catheters are used for therapy lasting fewer than 5 days. Adequate protection of IV site is required, especially with children. The catheter hub should be firmly secured at the puncture site preferably with transparent dressing to readily assess the IV site. Adhesive tape is used as needed to secure IV site without obscuring the puncture site.

2. *Answer:* B
   Rationale: An increase in pulse rate and blood pressure occur when there is an excessive strain on the circulatory system, such as a fluid volume overload. Increased pulse rate and decreased blood pressure occur with an excessive fluid volume loss. Options C and D are not applicable.

3. *Answer:* D
   Rationale: Approximately 75% to 80% of a full-term neonate's total body weight is water. Extracellular fluid (interstitial and intravascular) in an infant is much greater than that of an adult; this totals to 45% of an infant's body weight.

4. *Answer:* C
   Rationale: Neonates and infants have increased total body and extracellular water, which creates a larger volume of distribution. The larger volume requires administering a larger milligram per kilogram dose of water-soluble medication to neonates and infants.

5. *Answer:* B
   Rationale: The package insert or *PDR* will provide the safe dosage range for medications. The safe dose range for this medication is 25 to 50 mg/kg/day. The patient's weight should be converted to kilograms; divide 50 pounds by 2.2 kilograms, which gives you 23 kg. Calculate safe dose range by multiplying the child's weight and the safe dose range

which give you 575 to 1150 mg/day. The prescribed medication is 500 mg/day which is below the therapeutic benefits.

6. *Answer:* C
   Rationale: Conditions like gastritis can cause changes in gastric motility to increase. Gastric emptying time and gastroesophageal reflux can result in the regurgitation of orally administered drugs, producing irregular drug absorption.

7. *Answer:* A
   Rationale: Infants have a reduced amount of circulating albumin than adults. Albumin is responsible for binding acidic drugs, fatty acids, and bilirubin. There is a decrease affinity for protein binding during the neonatal period. These factors produce a larger volume of distribution and increased free drug concentration.

8. *Answer:* D
   Rationale: Intestinal peristalsis is rapid and unpredictable due to neuromuscular immaturity. Neonates and infants have irregular peristalsis, which can lead to enhanced absorption.

9. *Answer:* C
   Rationale: Body surface area is greatest in the infant and young child compared with older children and adults. Decreased thickness of the skin with increased skin surface hydration relative to body weight produces much greater percutaneous drug absorption.

10. *Answer:* D
    Rationale: A neonate liver is immature at birth and less effective for drug metabolism. In a neonate, medications may have a slow clearance rate and prolonged elimination half-life.

11. *Answer:* D
    Rationale: Pulling the pinna up and back straightens the ear canal in the child over 3 years of age. In children younger than 3 years of age, the pinna is gently pulled down and back to straighten the external ear canal.

12. *Answer:* C

Rationale: The package insert or *PDR* will provide the safe dosage range for medications. The safe dose range for this medication with a child's weight greater than 60 pounds: 600,000 to 1,200,000 Units daily. The prescribed dosage is 1,000,000 Units, which is within the range.

13. *Answer:* D
Rationale: EMLA, a topical anesthetic cream, must be applied at least 1 hour prior to a procedure to be effective. For maximum absorption, it should be covered after application. This also prevents the child from tasting it (which could anesthetize the gag reflex).

14. *Answer:* D
Rationale: Aspirin use and flu-like symptoms have been associated with Reye's syndrome. Aspirin or medication containing aspirin prolong bleeding/clotting time. Amoxicillin and cefaclor are antibiotics. Acetaminophen is a nonaspirin analgesic.

15. *Answer:* B
Rationale: Medication must be given on an empty stomach 1 hour before or 3 hours after meals; do not crush or chew tablets and do not give with fruit juice.

16. *Answer:* D
Rationale: Instilling eye drops in an infant can be difficult. The infant should be positioned in a supine position with the head supported due to the developmental age.

17 *Answer:* A
Rationale: The best strategy for increasing compliance includes prescribing drugs with once or twice daily administration schedules. Medications which have a pleasant taste or are affordable may not necessarily be beneficial for dosing schedules.

18. *Answer:* C
Rationale: Medications with narrow therapeutic windows are essential candidates for blood level monitoring. Among the many medications that require therapeutic drug monitoring are aminoglycosides, vancomycin, and antiepileptic drugs, to name a few.

19. *Answer:* C
Rationale: Even though several antibiotics can be used in the treatment of acute otitis media, amoxicillin remains the medication of choice for treating acute otitis media when the infecting organism is unknown.

20. *Answer:* C
Rationale: The treatment of choice for candidiasis is an antifungal, nystatin. Amoxicillin, erythromycin, and Omnicef are antibiotics and are not effective with candidiasis.

21. *Answer:* A
Rationale: Aggressive management to prevent serious complications requires immediate referral to an ophthalmologist and the use of systemic antibiotics is also required. Erythromycin is recommended for Chlamydia infections. Penicillin G is not available as a topical agent.

22. *Answer:* C
Rationale: Recommended regimen is 5% premethrin (Elimite) cream. Lindane should not be used in children younger than 24 months because children of this age have more permeable skin which may increase systemic absorption. Children 2 to 10 years of age use cautiously due to increase of toxicity. During pregnancy, there is an increased risk of CNS effect.

23. *Answer:* A
Rationale: Preferred IM injection sites for children under 4 years age of is the vastus lateralis or lateral aspect rectus femoris. Avoid posterior gluteal muscle in children under age 4 years. This muscle has not fully developed in children under 4 years of age.

24. *Answer:* D
Rationale: Recommended regimen for treatment of Chlamydia infection is azithromycin 1 g orally in a single dose. The Centers for Disease Control STD Guidelines recommends doxycycline as a 7-day treatment. Levofloxacin, a quinolone, is not recommended for use in 18-year-olds and younger. Clotrimazole is an antifungal.

25. *Answer:* C

Rationale: The Centers for Disease Control STD Guidelines recommends metronidazole 500 mg orally twice a day for 7 days as the treatment for bacterial vaginosis. Metronidazole gel is ordered as 0.75% for 5 days. Clindamycin ovules are prescribed for a course of 3 days. Clindamycin 300 mg is ordered for a course of 7 days.

BIBLIOGRAPHY

Baldwin, H.E., & Berson, D.S. (2005). *New perspectives in the management of acne, photodamage, and wound healing.* Cherry Hill, NJ: Elsevier.

Darmstadt, G.L., & Sidbury, R. (2004). The skin. In R.E. Behrman, R.M. Kliegman, & H.B. Jenson (Eds.). *Nelson textbook of pediatrics* (17th ed.). Philadelphia: Saunders.

Emslie, G.J. & Mayes, T.C. (2001). Mood disorders in children and adolescents: Psychopharmacological treatment. *Biological Psychiatry, 49*(12), 1082-1090.

McCormack, J., Brown, G., Levine, M., et al. (1996). *Drug therapy decision making guide.* Philadelphia: Saunders.

Parish, T.G. (2004). Inflammatory acne: Management in primary care. *Clin Rev, 14*(7), 40-45.

Reed, M.D., & Gal, P. (2004). Principles of drug therapy. In R.E. Behrman, R.M. Kliegman, & H.B. Jenson (Eds.). *Nelson textbook of pediatrics* (17th ed.). Philadelphia: Saunders.

Roberts, B.J., & Friedlander, S.F. (2005). Tinea capitis: A treatment update. *Pediatr Ann, 34*(3), 191-200.

Shields, B. (2003). Principles of newborn and infant drug therapy. In C. Kenner & J.W. Lott (Eds.). *Comprehensive neonatal nursing: A physiologic approach* (3rd ed.). Philadelphia: Saunders.

Silverman, M.A., & Bessman, E. (2005). Conjunctivitis. Retrieved November 30, 2005, from www.emedicine.com/EMERG/topic110.htm.

NOTES

55 Pain Management for Children

AMY K. FOY

Select the best answer for each of the following questions:

1. At what gestational age can a fetus perceive pain?
   A. 24 weeks.
   B. 28 weeks.
   C. 32 weeks.
   D. 16 weeks.

2. Acute pain elicits a stress response and affects multiple organ systems in the body. Common reactions include:
   A. Hypoglycemia, increased production of platelets, and decreased oxygen consumption.
   B. Increased gut motility, decreased cardiac output, and diuresis.
   C. Hypermetabolism, increased heart rate, increased blood pressure, and decreased tidal volume.
   D. Hyperventilation, decreased gastric acid secretion, decreased heart rate, and decreased platelet aggregation.

3. Which of the following demographic factors have been shown to influence assessment and management of pain?
   A. Sex, birth order, and age.
   B. Age, education level, and personal pain experience.
   C. Socioeconomic status, nutritional status, and sex.
   D. Degree of family support, race, and religion.

4. To avoid withdrawal syndrome, a child who has received opioids regularly for greater than 7 days should:

A. Begin ibuprofen and stop opioid.
B. Taper dose of opioid by decreasing dose amount by 50% each time.
C. Decrease daily dose by 10% each day or 20% every 2 to 3 days.
D. Continue same dose but lengthen intervals between administration by about 2 hours each day.

5. A 2-month-old is recommended to receive opiates at longer intervals than older infants because:
   A. Of increased risk of respiratory depression.
   B. The cytochrome P450 system is not fully developed at birth, resulting in prolonged elimination time.
   C. It may cause gastroesophageal reflux.
   D. Renal and liver metabolization does not mature until 4 months of age.

6. When assessing level of pain in a 3-year-old, you can expect:
   A. Restlessness, crying, and aggressive behavior.
   B. The child rating his/her pain less than 4 on a scale of 1 to 10.
   C. Denial, and pointing to a false area as the location of pain.
   D. A fairly good description of location, quality, and severity of pain.

7. Adolescents typically will not ask for pain medication because:
   A. They fear addiction.
   B. They do not want to appear weak.
   C. They do not want to appear to be drug-seeking.

D. Their pain is usually well-managed with over-the-counter medications like ibuprofen or acetaminophen.

8. Factors that influence perception and reporting of pain include ability to communicate, environmental factors, psychologic factors, cultural influences, and:
   A. Sleep deprivation.
   B. Fitness level.
   C. Nutritional status.
   D. Previous pain experience.

9. Traditional NSAIDs (i.e., ibuprofen, ASA, and ketorolac):
   A. Are used for management of moderate to severe pain.
   B. Inhibit the production of the COX-1 isoenzyme only.
   C. Are a less potent form of analgesia than acetaminophen.
   D. Inhibit production of central and peripheral prostaglandins.

10. Traditional NSAIDs should never be used in patients:
    A. Who are currently using opioids for pain management.
    B. With concomitant administration of other nephrotoxic agents.
    C. With a history of a metabolic disorder.
    D. With elevated liver enzymes.

11. Which pain mediation is indicated for mild to moderate pain, metabolized to morphine before it provides analgesia effects, and causes increased side effects in individuals sensitive to morphine?
    A. Codeine
    B. Tramadol
    C. Butorphanol
    D. Nalbuphine

12. Which medication is used for procedural pain management, is 80 times more potent than morphine, and the duration of action is less than 1 hour?
    A. Hydromorphone
    B. Oxycodone
    C. Meperidine
    D. Fentanyl

13. You are scheduling a 4-year-old with scoliosis for a full spine MRI to rule out tethered cord or lesion. Should you order the procedure with anesthesia, and if so, what medication do you order?
    A. No sedation needed. A 4-year-old should be able to lie still for 30 to 40 minutes without difficulty.
    B. Yes, chloral hydrate 500 mg orally 30 minutes before the procedure.
    C. Yes, Benadryl elixir 7.5 ml 30 minutes before the procedure.
    D. Yes, morphine 10 mg orally 1 hour before the procedure.

14. You are seeing a set of new parents at their newborn's 2-week checkup. They are anxious about pain associated with the immunizations scheduled for the 2-month visit. You counsel them by suggesting:
    A. ELA-Max to the infants lateral thighs 15 to 30 minutes before the appointment.
    B. A dose of Tylenol with codeine 30 minutes before appointment and you provide them with the prescription.
    C. Children's ibuprofen 1 teaspoon following the appointment.
    D. Ice directly to skin for 5 minutes prior to injection to numb the site.

15. You are a pediatric nurse practitioner working with a pediatric orthopedic surgeon. You are rounding one afternoon on the floor and one of your patients is preparing for discharge. He is a 14-year-old who is status postpatella realignment. He has been on a morphine PCA through the night. What is the drug of choice for pain management at home?
    A. Ibuprofen 800 mg orally every 4 hours as needed.
    B. Tylenol with codeine elixir 2 teaspoons orally every 4 to 6 hours as needed.
    C. Demerol 50 mg IM every 1 to 2 hours and instruct patient's caregiver on how to administer.
    D. Hydrocodone plus acetaminophen 5/325 mg orally every 4 to 6 hours as needed and recommend trying OTC ibuprofen 600 to 800 mg every 6 to 8 hours as needed a few days after discharge.

16. You are seeing an 8-year-old girl with varicella zoster. She is having moderate pain at the site of the lesions. In addition to prescribing acyclovir and Tylenol with codeine, you recommend:
   A. Applying hydrocortisone ointment to the lesions.
   B. Giving a stool softener for constipation caused by the Tylenol with codeine.
   C. Going to school as a means of distraction to get her mind off the pain.
   D. Benadryl elixir 12.5 mg/5 ml, 1 teaspoon at night to help her sleep.

17. An infant born at 28 weeks gestation is in the NICU and is showing signs of pain following a chest tube insertion. What is the pain medication of choice for neonates following painful procedures?
   A. IV fentanyl.
   B. IV meperidine.
   C. Tylenol with codeine elixir via nasogastric tube.
   D. IV morphine.

18. A 9-year-old with a seizure disorder is scheduled for a EEG. She is currently taking erythromycin for pertussis. Sedation medication of choice for this patient while undergoing the EEG would be:
   A. Valium.
   B. Pentobarbital.
   C. Ativan.
   D. Versed.

19. A 14-year-old with complex regional pain syndrome has severe right leg pain following a minor toe injury. Neuropathic pain is often treated with:
   A. Neurontin.
   B. Tylenol with codeine.
   C. Tramadol with acetaminophen.
   D. Valium.

20. You care for a competitive gymnast in your practice who has a connective tissue disorder causing ligamentous laxity. She frequently complains of back pain and other joint pain following a heavy practice session or meet. What are some nonpharmacologic suggestions you offer for pain management?
   A. Herbal tea.

   B. Art therapy.
   C. Music Therapy.
   D. Deep breathing, heat, and massage.

21. A 14-year-old comes in complaining of moderate to severe intermittent right lower quadrant abdominal pain. Her mother accompanies her and secretly tells you that she believes her daughter is "faking it because she wants attention." How do you assess her pain level?
   A. Obtain vital signs, ask her describe her pain using the Adolescent Pediatric Pain Tool (APPT), and offer support.
   B. Ask the girl if she is faking her pain and then conduct a clinical exam.
   C. Conduct a clinical exam and use the Children's Hospital of Eastern Ontario Pain Scale (CHEOPS) to determine severity of pain.
   D. Observation for 30 minutes to assess for facial grimacing, abdominal guarding, and crying.

22. You are volunteering at a local YMCA sports camp. An 11-year-old soccer player complains of aching pain below each knee while running. He states the pain is severe when his knees get hit by other players. After assessing him, you diagnose Osgood-Schlatter's disease and recommend:
   A. Ace wraps to each knee and Tylenol with codeine, 1 tablet every 4 hours for 3 days.
   B. Vioxx 25 mg each day for 3 weeks.
   C. Aspirin 650 mg every 4 hours for 24 hours.
   D. Naprosyn 250 mg every 12 hours for 3 weeks as well as rest and ice following heavy activity.

23. You have just diagnosed hand, foot, and mouth virus in a 19-month-old. You advise his mother to maintain hydration with cool fluids and popsicles and you recommend:
   A. Tylenol 15 mg/kg orally every 4 hours or 20 mg/kg rectally every 4 to 6 hours if unable to swallow the liquid medication.
   B. Lortab elixir 15 ml orally every 4 hours as needed.

C. Ibuprofen 20 mg/kg orally every 6 to 8 hours as needed.

D. Carbonated soda and salty foods.

24. You prefer using benzodiazepines when sedating pediatric patients for procedures. You must be sure the antagonist is available at all times. This drug is:

A. Naloxone.

B. Revex.

C. Ketamine.

D. Romazicon.

25. It is important for you as a pediatric nurse practitioner to identify whether a patient is suffering from nociceptive pain or neuropathic pain because this will determine the class of medication used for treatment as well as nonpharmacologic suggestions. You recognize that pain is nociceptive if it:

A. Is peripherally or centrally generated and reflects nervous system injury or impairment.

B. Is burning, tingling, knife-like or electric-feeling.

C. Requires adjunct therapy like anticonvulsants , tricyclic antidepressants, or local anesthetics.

D. Can be categorized into somatic or visceral pain.

NOTES

ANSWERS

1. *Answer:* A
   Rationale: Pathways for the transmission and perception of pain are developed at 24 weeks gestation.

2. *Answer:* C
   Rationale: Hypermetabolism, tachycardia, increased blood pressure, and decreased tidal volume are examples of multiple organ system responses to acute pain.

3. *Answer:* B
   Rationale: Research shows that demographic factors including age, education level, and personal pain experiences influence assessment and management of pain.

4. *Answer:* C
   Rationale: The recommended weaning plan to prevent to onset of withdrawal symptoms is to reduce the daily dose by 10% or 20% every 2 to 3 days.

5. *Answer:* B
   Rationale: Infants younger than 1 to 2 months of age may not need to receive opioids as often as older infants and children because the cytochrome P450 system is not fully developed at birth, thus resulting in prolonged elimination time.

6. *Answer:* A
   Rationale: These behaviors are age-appropriate indicators of pain in a 3-year-old.

7. *Answer:* B
   Rationale: Teenagers generally do not want to appear weak in front of family and friends.

8. *Answer:* D
   Rationale: Memories of pain and their circumstances and alterations in pain signal processing secondary to neurologic changes affect perception and reporting of pain.

9. *Answer:* D
   Rationale: NSAIDs function by inhibiting the production of prostaglandins both centrally and peripherally.

10. *Answer:* B
    Rationale: NSAIDs should never be used in patients with concomitant administration of nephrotoxic agents due to their associated risk for nephrotoxicity.

11. *Answer:* A
    Rationale: Codeine is indicated for mild to moderate pain, metabolized to morphine before it provides analgesia effects, and causes increased side effects in individuals sensitive to morphine.

12. *Answer:* D
    Rationale: Fentanyl is used for procedural pain management, is 80 times more potent than morphine, and the duration of action is less than 1 hour.

13. *Answer:* B
    Rationale: Chloral hydrate is used to produce immobility for nonpainful procedures. This is an appropriate dose for an average sized 4-year-old.

14. *Answer:* A
    Rationale: ELA-Max is a topical anesthetic which is safe to use in infants.

15. *Answer:* D
    Rationale: Hydrocodone and acetaminophen is a good transition drug from a morphine PCA as it provides similar analgesic effects.

16. *Answer:* B
    Rationale: All opioids decrease GI motility and cause constipation. It is recommended to start a stool softener or laxative at the same time opioid therapy is initiated.

17. *Answer:* D
    Rationale: Morphine is considered the gold standard because it has been the most widely studied in children. It is safe to use with neonates.

18. *Answer:* B
    Rationale: Benzodiazepine elimination can be affected by erythromycin due to the cytochrome P450 3a eAUenzymes. Pentobarbital is a barbiturate and is often used as

sedation for painless procedures (e.g., MRI, EEG).

19. *Answer:* A
Rationale: Anticonvulsants are often used for pain management of neuropathic pain.

20. *Answer:* D
Rationale: Examples of nonpharmacologic pain management include deep breathing, heat, and massage.

21. *Answer:* A
Rationale: These offer age-appropriate objective and subjective means of evaluating pain in addition to providing patient support. The CHEOPS is used to evaluate pain in children ages 1 to 7.

22. *Answer:* D
Rationale: Naprosyn is an excellent choice for mild to moderate musculoskeletal pain. This dose would be appropriate for an average-sized 11-year-old.

23. *Answer:* A
Rationale: Tylenol orally or rectally at this dose would be recommended for mild to moderate pain in a child. It is important to offer an alternate route of administration as hand, foot, and mouth virus can make it uncomfortable for a child to swallow.

24. *Answer:* D
Rationale: Flumazenil (Romazicon) is the medication indicated for the complete or partial reversal of benzodiazepine sedation.

25. *Answer:* D
Rationale: Nociceptive pain is normal pain transmission and can be categorized into somatic or visceral pain. Neuropathic pain is centrally and peripherally generated and reflects nervous system injury or impairment. Somatic is well-localized pain arising from the bone, muscles, tendons, joints, mucous membranes, skin, or connective tissue. Visceral pain is poorly localized pain arising from the visceral organs such as the lungs, pancreas, and GI tract.

BIBLIOGRAPHY

American Academy of Pain Medicine, American Pain Society, and American Society of Addiction Medicine. (AAPM, APS, & ASAM) (2001). *Definitions related to the use of opioids for the treatment of pain: A consensus document.* Retrieved July 25, 2005, from www.ampainsoc.org/advocacy/opioids2.htm.

American Academy of Pediatrics, & American Pain Society. (2001). The assessment and management of acute pain in infants, children, and adolescents. *Pediatrics, 108*(3), 793-797.

American Academy of Pediatrics, & Canadian Paediatric Society. (2000). Prevention and management of pain and stress in the neonate. *Pediatrics, 105*(2), 454-461.

American Pain Society. (1999). *Guideline for the management of acute and chronic pain in sickle cell disease.* Skokie, IL: Author.

American Pain Society. (2001). *Pediatric chronic pain: A position statement from the American Pain Society.* Retrieved July 25, 2005, from www.ampainsoc.org/advocacy/pediatric.htm.

American Pain Society. (2003). *Principles of analgesic use in the treatment of acute pain and cancer pain* (5th ed.). Skokie, IL: Author.

American Pain Society. (2005). *Pain control in the primary care setting.* Skokie, IL: Author.

Bauman, B.H., & McManus, J.G., Jr. (2005). Pediatric pain management in the emergency department. *Emerg Med Clin North Am, 23*(2), 393-414, ix.

Berry, P.H., Chapman, C.R., Covington, E.C., et al. (2001). Pain: Current understanding of assessment, management, and treatments. National Pharmaceutical Council, Inc. Retrieved July 25, 2005, from www.jcaho.org/news+room/health+care+issues/pain_mono_npc.pdf.

Beyer, J.E., Turner, S.B., Jones, L., et al. (2005). The alternate forms reliability of the Oucher pain scale. *Pain Manage Nurs, 6*(1), 10-17.

Cote, C.J., Karl, H.W., Notterman, D.A., et al. (2000). Adverse sedation events in pediatrics: Analysis of medications used for sedation. *Pediatrics, 106*(4), 633-644.

Di Maggio, T.J. (2002). Pediatric pain management. In B. St. Marie (Ed.). *Core curriculum for pain management nursing.* Philadelphia: Saunders.

Fitzgerald, M. (2000). Development of the peripheral and spinal pain system. *Pain Res Clin Manage, 10*, 9-21.

Franck, L.S., Greenberg, C.S., & Stevens, B. (2000). Pain assessment in infants and children. *Pediatr Clin North Am, 47*(3), 487-512.

Gerik, S.M. (2005). Pain management in children: Developmental considerations and mind-body therapies. *South Med J, 98*(3), 295-302.

Goldschneider, K.R., & Anand, K.S. (2003). Long-term consequences of pain in neonates. In N.L. Schecter, C.B. Berde, & M. Yaster (Eds.). *Pain in infants, children, and adolescents*. Baltimore: Lippincott Williams & Wilkins.

Golianu, B., Krane, E.J., Galloway, K.S., & Yaster, M. (2000). Pediatric acute pain management. *Pediatr Clin North Am, 47*(3), 559-587.

Joint Commission on Accreditation of Healthcare Organizations (JCAHO). (2000). *Pain assessment and management: An organizational approach*. Oakbrook Terrace, IL: Author.

Maunuksela, E., & Olkkola, K.T. (2003). Nonsteroidal anti-inflammatory drugs in pediatric pain management. In N.L. Schecter, C.B. Berde, & M. Yaster (Eds.). *Pain in infants, children, and adolescents*. Baltimore: Lippincott Williams & Wilkins.

McCaffery, M., & Pasero, C. (Eds.). (1999). *Pain: clinical manual* (2nd ed.). St Louis: Mosby.

McGrath, P.A., & Hillier, L.M. (2003). Modifying the psychologic factors that intensify children's pain and prolong disability. In N.L. Schecter, C.B. Berde, & M. Yaster (Eds.). *Pain in infants, children, and adolescents*. Baltimore: Lippincott Williams & Wilkins.

Mersky, H. (Ed.). (1986). Classification of chronic pain: Descriptions of chronic pain syndromes and definitions of pain terms. *Pain* (Suppl. 3, Pt II), S215-S221.

Pasero, C., Paice, J.A., & McCaffery, M. (1999). Basic mechanisms underlying the causes and effects of pain. In M. McCaffery, & C. Pasero (Eds.). *Pain: Clinical manual*. St. Louis: Mosby.

Rosenblum, R.K., & Fisher, P.G. (2001). A guide to children with acute and chronic headaches. *J Pediatr Health Care, 15*(5), 229-235.

Schecter, N.L. (2003). Management of pain problems in pediatric primary care. In N.L. Schecter, C.B. Berde, & M. Yaster, (Eds.). *Pain in infants, children, and adolescents*. Baltimore: Lippincott Williams & Wilkins.

Schecter, N.L., Berde, C.B. & Yaster, M. (Eds.) (2003). *Pain in infants, children, and adolescents*. Baltimore: Lippincott Williams & Wilkins.

Slater, J.A. (2003). Deciphering emotional aches and physical pains in children. *Pediatr Ann, 32*(6), 402-407.

Stanford, E.A., Chambers, C.T., & Craig, K.D. (2005). A normative analysis of the development of pain-related vocabulary in children. *Pain, 114*(1-2), 1-2, 278-284.

Sussman, E. (2005). Cancer pain management guidelines issued for children: Adult guidelines updated. *J Natl Cancer Inst, 97*(10), 711-712.

Tobias, J. (2000). Weak analgesics and NSAIDs in management of acute pain. *Pediatr Clin North Am, 47*(3), 527-543.

Van Hulle-Vincent, C. (2005). Nurses' knowledge, attitudes, and practices: Regarding children's pain. MCN: *Am J Matern Child Nurs, 30*(3), 177-183.

Walco, G.A., Burns, J.P., & Cassidy, R.C. (2003). The ethics of pain control in infants and children. In N.L. Schecter, C.B. Berde, & M. Yaster (Eds.). *Pain in infants, children, and adolescents*. Baltimore: Lippincott Williams & Wilkins.

Yaster, M., Kost-Byerly, S. & Maxwell, L.G. (2003). Opioid agonists and antagonists. In N.L. Schecter, C.B. Berde, & M. Yaster (Eds.). *Pain in infants, children, and adolescents*. Baltimore: Lippincott Williams & Wilkins.

56 Complementary and Alternative Therapy

RUEY JANE RYBURN

Select the best answer for each of the following questions:

1. Mrs. P. tells the pediatric nurse practitioner that she is giving Amy, her 4 year old daughter, one-half ounce daily of a phytonutrient liquid supplement from whole foods. This dosage is half the suggested adult dosage. Mrs. P. says she's been giving it to Amy for the last few months because she loves the taste. Your best response is:

A. "Oh, I agree. That must be fine for Amy, Mrs. P."

B. "Well, have you asked your pediatrician about this product, Mrs. P.?"

C. "Phytonutrients are regulated by the Food and Drug Administration as foods; the regulation is less stringent than the labeling for drugs. Could you bring in the bottle or give me the web site so I can check ingredients? I'm not comfortable giving approval for this product without seeing the contents and label."

D. "Amy likes the taste of this, you say? Well, since phytonutrients come from whole food sources, it is all right for Amy to continue taking it. However, I'd still like to check the product label for information. Could you please bring the bottle to the clinic for me to see what the package labeling indicates is in the product?"

2. The pediatric nurse practitioner does a readmission for Sam, a 10-year-old with metastatic brain cancer. During the intake assessment, the pediatric nurse practitioner asks the family whether they have utilized complementary and alternative medicine (CAM) during Sam's illness. The most appropriate way to ask is:

A. "Some of my other children's families have chosen to integrate therapies such as prayer, herbs, or massage to try to help their son or daughter. What, if any, options has your family chosen that are not mainstream Western medicine?"

B. "Because we need to know about all aspects of Sam's care, I'm wondering if there are any folk remedies or other unusual things you're doing that you haven't confessed to the doctor about to try and help your son?"

C. "I've heard that families are now choosing some strange therapies like waving hands in the air to help children with cancer. What are you folks doing?"

D. "Since your child has ADHD, asthma, cerebral palsy, cancer, JRA, or autism, I need to know what CAM therapies you are using for your child."

3. Sam's mother tells the pediatric nurse practitioner that she has been massaging lavender essential oil onto Sam's hands and feet at bedtime to help him relax, reduce his fears, and induce sleep. The pediatric nurse practitioner's best response is:

A. "I don't know about this use of lavender. I think it just smells good, but to help Sam relax or sleep sounds a little unusual."

B. "I think we'd better discuss with the physician your use of this oil, since

some oils applied directly to the skin cross the blood/brain barrier."
C. "Please discontinue the use of this oil, it will interfere with Sam's medical treatment."
D. "Lavender oil is known for having therapeutic properties indicated to help reduce Sam's symptoms. It must help for you to be able to comfort your son in this manner."

4. As the pediatric nurse practitioner during a well child exam, you note that Sherry, a 9-year-old, has a slightly raised, dry rash on her upper arms. In talking to the mother, you learn that Sherry is being raised as a vegan (no dairy, eggs, or meat). Your best reply to the mother is:
A. "How long has Sherry had this rash on her upper arms?"
B. "I would recommend that you start her on a fish oil supplement or other form of EFA such as flax or borage oil."
C. "I'd like to refer Sherry to our nutritionist immediately."
D. "I'm going to have my attending physician look at Sherry as soon as he can today because of this rash."

5. At your son's basketball game, another mother tells you, a pediatric nurse practitioner, that her children have received care from a naturopathic physician. They have only had homeopathic medications, never antibiotics. Your best response is:
A. "Wow, I wish I could say that about my son. He's had antibiotics several times for ear infections and strep throat. Are your children never sick?"
B. "I can't imagine any family able to keep their children well in this manner. Are you sure your naturopath hasn't prescribed antibiotics and you just didn't know?"
C. "I'm still learning about homeopathic medicines. When, how, and for what conditions do you use them for your son?"
D. "You know, if your children get strep throat or other untreated infections they may end up with permanent car-

diac or kidney problems. I'd be careful if I were you."

6. In discussion with several pediatricians and pediatric nurse practitioners at a national pediatric conference, you participate in a round table on CAM. Several of the participants complain that parents are being unrealistic when they use CAM on their children with special needs. Your most appropriate response is:
A. Surveys from many parts of the United States are finding from one-third to over one-half of parents are using CAM to assist their children.
B. There is not enough evidence to support the use of CAM for special needs children, while evidence to support Western medicine 'best practices' is well-supported.
C. Use of CAM is higher in well children than in children with chronic illness.
D. Acupuncture, chiropractic, and massage seem to be the safest and most used CAM therapies by parents for their children.

7. The variables most associated with CAM use in children are:
A. Parents of well children who use CAM therapies themselves.
B. Foreign-born parents of well children from religious families.
C. Foreign-born parents of children with chronic health issues.
D. Parents alienated from religion and Western medicine.

8. The Johnson family comes to the pediatric nurse practitioner for counseling regarding treatment for their 4-year-old son with leukemia. The family tells the pediatric nurse practitioner they are paying "out of pocket" for spiritual healing first before considering harsher chemotherapy and other "Western" medical practices. The most appropriate response by the pediatric nurse practitioner is:
A. "Has your child's pediatrician approved of your choice?"
B. "I can understand why you have made this choice, since chemotherapy has such harsh side effects."

C. "I urge you to see a psychologist or our chaplain to discuss this situation. I want to make sure you understand the untoward outcomes that will happen to your child for delaying medical treatment."

D. "I'm concerned about the costs you are incurring on this therapy not covered by insurance and with unknown therapeutic benefit."

9. Su, a 7-year-old Hmong (southeast Asian), is sent to the pediatric nurse practitioner school nurse because her teacher found symmetrical 5 cm circular welts on Su's back. The pediatric nurse practitioner's first action is to:

A. Call her back-up physician for suggestions on how to treat the welts.

B. Call Child Protective Services and request a social worker to make an immediate home visit to Su's family for obvious abuse.

C. Do nothing. This is a typical cultural practice of Hmong parents, and there is no outreach worker to talk to the parents anyway.

D. Ascertain from Su if she had been sick and who applied the Chinese medicine therapy of "coining" to her.

10. Three-year-old Sid was seen in clinic 5 times in 2 months for severe abdominal pain after his sister was born. Sid's mother then called the pediatric nurse practitioner to tell her that she'd started applying half-strength peppermint oil in a clockwise circular manner to Sid's abdomen with good results. The pediatric nurse practitioner replies:

A. "That's wonderful, there is some evidence that peppermint oil is effective for abdominal pain."

B. "I'm really concerned that you will cause Sid even greater problems in the long run even though the peppermint oil seems to be working now."

C. "I have no idea what you're talking about or why this would work, but keep it up."

D. "Even though the peppermint oil seems to be working, I'd recommend applying lavender oil instead since it seems to be so much gentler."

11. A pediatric nurse practitioner assigned to the neonatal intensive care unit (NICU) is contacted by parents wanting to massage their stable preterm infant. The pediatric nurse practitioner would best look for information to determine efficacy by choosing which of the following web sites?

A. Web site of University of Texas M.D. Anderson Cancer Center at www.mdanderson.org/departments/cimer.

B. Web site of American Association of Naturopathic Physicians at http://naturopathic.org.

C. Nonprofit corporation to combat health-related fraud at www.quackwatch.org.

D. Electronic database by NCCAM (National Center for Complementary and Alternative Medicine) and National Library of Medicine at www.nlm.nih.gov/nccam/camonpubmed.html.

12. A pediatric nurse practitioner intends to self-educate about CAM standards and therapies currently utilized by nurses in clinical practice. Her best web site to investigate is:

A. American Holistic Nurses Association at www.ahna.org.

B. Nurse-Healers Professional Associates International at www.therapeutic-touch.org.

C. The Center for Holistic Pediatric Education and Research (CHPR) at www.holistickids.org.

D. U.S. Pharmacopeia (USP) at www.usp.org.

13. John, a 16-year-old male, comes to clinic for his examination to clear him for football season. He has gained 40 pounds and "shows off" his muscles. When asked, John admits to taking pills from his friend to help him gain muscles. The pediatric nurse practitioner's initial intervention is to:

A. Send John for a blood test to determine if John has been taking anabolic steroids.

B. Call John's parents and ask if they are aware that their son is taking unprescribed pills to increase his weight for football season.

C. Call John's coach and ask if he is aware that some of his players are taking 'pills' to increase their weight and muscular development.
D. Inform John about the dangers of steroids including testicular atrophy, impotence, and breast enlargement.

14. Deana, a 16-month-old toddler, has developed diarrhea following a round of antibiotics for recurrent otitis media. Her mother calls clinic asking for help with the diarrhea. What complementary practice is documented safe and with some therapeutic efficacy for children?
A. Chamomile tea.
B. Powdered ginger.
C. Comfrey tea.
D. Lactobacillus.

15. According to the NCCAM (National Center for Complementary and Alternative Medicine), which therapy listed below is NOT categorized as a CAM therapy?
A. TCM or traditional Chinese medicine.
B. Therapeutic touch.
C. Massage.
D. Play therapy.

16. A parent of a 7-month-old baby returns for ear recheck with history of recurrent otitis media treated with frequent antibiotic therapy. The mother tells the pediatric nurse practitioner that she had tuning fork sound therapy applied to her baby's ears and energy field. The pediatric nurse practitioner notes that the ears are now clear. Her conclusion is:
A. She will suggest tuning fork sound therapy for recurrent otitis.
B. Tuning fork sound therapy should be researched for efficacy in recurrent otitis.
C. The improvement in the baby's ears was due to the most recent course of antibiotics, not sound therapy.
D. She is not responsible for knowing about unusual therapies with insufficient research to determine efficacy.

17. Parents of a 10-year-old boy come to see the pediatric nurse practitioner after their son fell off a rope swing at a friend's house. They ask about chiropractic therapy, since Tylenol and naproxen haven't helped his musculoskeletal pain and torqued posture. You tell them:
A. Acupuncture might be more helpful, since acupuncture meridians correspond to various body organs.
B. Aromatherapy might be work best, since oils applied to the areas of pain help reduce anxiety.
C. Ayurvedic treatment focused on energy and the mind and spirit might assist the boy.
D. Chiropractic spinal manipulation focused on righting body's structure to function seems worth trying.

18. Parents of a 10-month-old suffering from congenital heart disease tell the pediatric nurse practitioner that they are seeing an energy healer weekly to help their daughter maintain strength until her open-heart surgery in 2 months. The pediatric nurse practitioner's response is:
A. "I hope you are prepared to be responsible for any damage done by the healer to your baby."
B. "Please tell me about any changes you are noticing in your daughter's condition since seeing the healer."
C. "Have you shared with the cardiologist that you are exposing your daughter to an energy healer?"
D. "Acupuncture, herbs, or massage would be more helpful therapies than energy healing."

19. A health education teacher notes that two of her female students appear to have had significant weight loss over the course of the semester. She consults with the school pediatric nurse practitioner, and collectively the teacher and pediatric nurse practitioner decide to:
A. Counsel the girls individually to determine intake, supplements, and psychoemotional factors that might be responsible.
B. Send a note home to the parents suggesting that their daughters are either anorexic or bulimic.

C. Coteach a module on nutrition and supplements for wellness and health maintenance as a solution to this problem.

D. Suggest to the parents that they immediately take their daughters to their physicians for physicals to make sure they don't have parasites.

20. Parents of a 13-year-old male with cerebral palsy ask the pediatric nurse practitioner what he thinks about their son taking swimming lessons. The pediatric nurse practitioner responds:

A. "I can't see how swimming will help, since your son's lungs are compromised."

B. "What does your son's pulmonologist say?"

C. "I remember a recent study showed that swimming or aqua therapy was helpful for children with cerebral palsy."

D. "I would recommend that you research that question on the Internet."

21. The pediatric nurse practitioner is attempting to take a culturally sensitive, comprehensive history with a family recently moved to the United States from Indonesia. The most likely measure to elicit this goal is:

A. Hand the parents a printed health questionnaire to complete. Check for any blank answers when they return it to you.

B. Give the parents a questionnaire printed in their native language and expect that they will complete it correctly.

C. Determine the parents' ability to comprehend English before deciding whether to utilize a medical interpreter or language-sensitive questionnaire.

D. Conduct the interview slowly in English to help the parents acclimate to their new country.

22. The Smith family tells the pediatric nurse practitioner that they are utilizing herbs and essential oil to manage their 10-year-old child's chronic asthma in addition to traditional pharmaceutical inhalers and medications. The pediatric nurse practitioner's best response is:

A. "I think that is excellent that you are seeking other measures to help your son manage his asthma."

B. "Please list the herbs and oils and times and amounts of administration so that I can research if there are ways these may interfere negatively with his prescribed inhalers and medications."

C. "You need to stop all nonprescribed therapies now. They are likely to interfere with the medically prescribed therapy."

D. "I'm going to send you to the pharmacist at the clinic to have him discuss why using these other measures is not good, because they are interfering with your son's prescribed therapy."

23. The most appropriate sources for the pediatric nurse practitioner to access to determine effect of oils and herbs in interaction with pharmaceuticals include:

A. PDR (2001). *PDR for nutritional supplements*. Montvale, NJ: Medical Economics, Thomson Healthcare and http://nncam.nih.gov (National Institutes of Health, National Center for Complementary and Alternative Medicine).

B. www.quackwatch.org (Nonprofit corporation to combat health-related myths) and www.ncahf.org (National Council for Reliable Health Information).

C. www.usp.org (U.S. Pharmacopeia (USP) and http://ods.od.nih.gov (National Institutes of Health Office of Dietary Supplements).

D. www.mcp.edu/herbal (Longwood Herbal Task Force) and *PDR*. (2004). *PDR for Herbal Medicines* (3rd ed.). Montvale, NJ: Thomson PDR.

ANSWERS

1. *Answer:* C
   Rationale: Phytonutrients are regulated by the Food and Drug Administration as foods. Half of the adult dose may be too much for a 4-year-old even if the phytonutrient has 'safe' ingredients. The product should be checked for USP, GMP, or AHPA voluntary standards of purity and quality control by having the product brought in.

2. *Answer:* A
   Rationale: Asking the family gently about their use of complementary or integrative therapies is more likely to produce honest answers. Mentioning therapies as nonconventional or as not prescribed by the doctor can make a family feel judged or that their choices are disapproved by Western medicine—therefore, resulting in the family's greater reluctance to share this information. Labeling the child as falling into a disease category as a reason to ask about CAM practices is stigmatizing.

3. *Answer:* D
   Rationale: The pediatric nurse practitioner demonstrates an understanding of the therapeutic use of lavender essential oil. She supports the mother's attempts to help her son, and avoids making the mother feel defensive.

4. *Answer:* A
   Rationale: Although vegetarian diets can be deficient in essential fatty acids that can affect the skin, it is important to do a complete assessment of this skin condition before suggesting treatment. If the pediatric nurse practitioner determines the cause of this rash is related to her vegan diet, suggesting fish, flax, or borage oils because they are good sources of essential fatty acids may be appropriate.

5. *Answer:* C
   Rationale: Asking a mother experienced in the use of homeopathic medications and the care of a naturopath to tell the pediatric nurse practitioner about her wisdom is a practical way to learn more information about CAM. Comments or questions which sound demeaning or hostile stop the possibility of learning and have the potential to alienate the mother from both the pediatric nurse practitioner and the Western medical system.

6. *Answer:* A
   Rationale: Best practices in many of Western medicine's traditional therapies have not been studied with double-blinded randomized clinical trials as is true for CAM. Parents with special needs children according to several surveys from various regions of the United States are turning to CAM to assist their special needs children.

7. *Answer:* C
   Rationale: CAM use is highest among foreign-born parents who are religious, who use CAM themselves, and who have children with chronic health problems.

8. *Answer:* D
   Rationale: Costs for most CAM therapies are mostly not covered by insurance and the therapy may be without adequate research-based efficacy. The family has a right to choose their therapy, not the physician; the pediatric nurse practitioner's role is to express nonbias with the parents.

9. *Answer:* D
   Rationale: It is important for the pediatric nurse practitioner to be aware of usual cultural practices and must not assume a practice is either abusive or nonharmful without assessment. This is a situation within the pediatric nurse practitioner's domain to handle without physician oversight.

10. *Answer:* A
    Rationale: It is important for the pediatric nurse practitioner to have knowledge of the beginning evidence on effective therapies. It is unacceptable to claim ignorance or to suggest a parent may be harming a child with a CAM therapy without documentation supporting the conclusion. Lavender is not therapeutically indicated for abdominal pain; peppermint oil is.

11. *Answer:* D

Rationale: The NCCAM center of NIH maintains an excellent database covering published articles about CAM therapies. Quack Watch's purpose is directed toward disputing CAM therapies. The other two sites are not likely to have the information as one is more devoted to cancer therapies and the other a listing of naturopathic physicians.

12. *Answer:* A

Rationale: The American Holistic Nurses' Association is the organization setting standards of practice and endorsing complementary (holistic) therapeutic training programs in CAM therapies. The NCCAM center at NIH and The Center for Holistic Pediatric Education and Research offer mostly medicine-based therapies, but include nothing about standards of practice for nursing. Therapeutic Touch is one specific program offering CAM training but it does not offer overall information.

13. *Answer:* A

Rationale: Even though the weight gain and muscle "bulk" is suspicious, the pediatric nurse practitioner first needs to determine if John is taking an anabolic steroid before taking further action. The subsequent interventions may be needed, but are not the first step.

14. *Answer:* D

Rationale: Lactobacillus is safe for children and may help decrease duration and severity of diarrhea. The other three, ginger, comfrey, and chamomile are not indicated and/or deemed safe for young children.

15. *Answer:* D

Rationale: Play therapy is an approved psychologic intervention. The other three, therapeutic touch, massage, and traditional Chinese medicine are listed as CAM on the NCCAM web site.

16. *Answer:* B

Rationale: The pediatric nurse practitioner is responsible for learning about various CAM therapies. No conclusions can be drawn from a sample of one, but research of tuning fork sound therapy's efficacy for re-

current otitis media in infants is warranted due to its noninvasive nature compared to frequent antibiotics or ear tubes.

17. *Answer:* D

Rationale: Chiropractic treatment involves spinal manipulation and assists to realign the body righting structure and function. Acupuncture can ease pain, but the function of realigning energy meridians is not specific to the problem cited. Ayurvedic and aromatherapy applications are not indicated per the properties as listed.

18. *Answer:* B

Rationale: Exploring with the family any changes they see when energy is transmitted from the healer's hands to the baby's body to help restore balance is nonthreatening. The other responses indicate disapproval or ignorance about this modality of CAM therapy. It is important to not alienate families but to understand the CAM choices they make.

19. *Answer:* A

Rationale: Counseling the girls individually to try and determine the factors responsible for the weight loss is the most direct approach without being accusatory. Requesting the parents to take their daughters for a physical may or may not happen. Coteaching a health education module, while a worthwhile project, may not address the potential problem of the weight loss by the two students.

20. *Answer:* C

Rationale: A recent study does address the efficacy of aqua therapy for cerebral palsy. The pediatric nurse practitioner needs to address the parent's question. Suggesting that the parents do research on the Internet or talk to the pulmonologist is an avoidance of pediatric nurse practitioner role in this instance.

21. *Answer:* C

Rationale: Determining the parents' ability to speak English is essential before determining whether a medical interpreter is needed to either help conduct the interview or translate a printed interview. Proceeding with an interview in English without first determining the ability to comprehend English may prohibit a culturally sensitive history.

22. **Answer:** B

Rationale: Telling the parents that the herbs and oils are OK without research is irresponsible. Finding out the CAM herbs and oils being used and how so that the pediatric nurse practitioner can research possible adverse interactions are essential. The parents are likely to be alienated by being told to stop all CAM immediately, and the pharmacologist may not be trained to discuss herb and oil interactions.

23. **Answer:** D

Rationale: The sources with information about herbs are the most likely to be helpful. The other sources and sites are about dietary supplements or other health information.

BIBLIOGRAPHY

Allen, K.D. (2004). Using biofeedback to make childhood headaches less of a pain. *Pediatr Ann, 33*(4), 241-245.

American Academy of Family Physicians. (2003). Complementary practice. Retrieved on February 12, 2006, at www.aafp.org/x668.xml.

Committee on Children with Disabilities. (2001). American Academy of Pediatrics: Counseling families who choose complementary and alternative medicine for their child with chronic illness or disability. Committee on Children With Disabilities. *Pediatrics, 107*(3), 598-601.

American Holistic Nurses' Association (AHNA) Position Paper. (2004). AHNA: Position on the role of nurses in the practice of complementary and alternative therapies. Retrieved on February 11, 2006, at www.ahna.org/about/statments.html.

Anbar, R.D., & Hall, H.R. (2004). Childhood habit cough treated with self-hypnosis. *J Pediatr, 144*(2), 213-217.

Anderson, C., Lis-Balchin, M., & Kirk-Smith, M. (2000). Evaluation of massage with essential oils on childhood atopic eczema. *Phytother Res, 14*(6), 452-456.

Barnes, L., Risko, W., Nethersole, S., & Maypole, J. (2004). Integrating complementary and alternative medicine into pediatric training. *Pediatr Ann, 33*(4), 257-263.

Barrett, B.P., Brown, R.L., Locken, K., et al. (2002). Treatment of the common cold with unrefined echinacea. *Ann Intern Med, 137*(12), 939-946.

Bellas, A., Lafferty, W.E., Lind, B., & Tyree, P.T. (2005). Frequency, predictors, and expenditures for pediatric insurance claims for complementary and alternative medical professionals in Washington state. *Arch Pediatr Adolesc Med, 159*(4), 367-372.

Boyer, E.W., Kearney, S., Shannon, M.W., et al. (2002). Poisoning from a dietary supplement administered during hospitalization. *Pediatrics, 109*(3), E49.

Bronfort, G., Evans, R.L., Kubic, P., & Filkin, P. (2001). Chronic pediatric asthma and chiropractic spinal manipulation: A prospective clinical series and randomized clinical pilot study. *J Manipulative Physiol Ther, 24*(6), 369-377.

Bussing, R., Zima, B.T., Gary, F.A., & Garvan, C.W. (2002). Use of complementary and alternative medicine for symptoms of attention-deficit hyperactivity disorder. *Psychiatric Serv, 53*(9), 1096-1102.

CDC: Centers for Disease Control and Prevention. (2002). Hepatic toxicity possibly associated with kava-containing products—United States, Germany, and Switzerland, 1999-2002. (2002). *MMWR Morb Mortal Wkly Rep 51*(47), 1065-1067.

Cherkin, D.C., Deyo, R.A., Sherman, K.J., et al. (2002). Characteristics of visits to licensed acupuncturists, chiropractors, massage therapists, and naturopathic physicians. *J Am Board Fam Pract, 15*(6), 463-472.

Cohen, H.A., Varsano, I., Kahan, E., et al. (2004). Effectiveness of an herbal preparation containing echinacea, propolis, and vitamin C in preventing respiratory tract infections in children. A randomized, double-blind, placebo-controlled, multicenter study. *Arch Pediatr Adolesc Med, 158*(3), 217-221.

Dantas, F., & Rampes, H. (2000). Do homeopathic medicines provoke adverse effects? A systematic review. *Brit Homeopathic J, 89*(1), S35-S38.

Davis, M.P., & Darden P.M. (2003). Use of complementary and alternative medicine by children in the United States. *Arch Pediatr Adolesc Med, 157*(4), 393-396.

Doerr, L. (2001). Using homeopathy for treating childhood asthma: Understanding a family's choice. *J Pediatr Nurs, 16*(4), 269-276.

DSHEA: Dietary Supplement Health and Education Act of 1994. Public Law 103-417, 108 Statute 4325.

Eisenberg, D.M., Davis, R.B., Ettner, S.L., et al. (1998). Trends in alternative medicine use in the United States, 1990-1997: Results of a follow-up national survey. *JAMA, 280*(18), 1569-1575.

Ernst, E. (1999). Homeopathic prophylaxis of headaches and migraine? A systematic review. *J Pain Symptom Manage, 18*(5), 353-357.

Ernst, E., & Pittler, M.H. (2000). Efficacy of ginger for nausea and vomiting: A systematic review of randomised clinical trials. *Br J Anaesth, 84*(3), 367-71.

Ernst, E., Pittler, M., & Stevinson, C. (2002). Complementary/alternative medicine in dermatology: Evidence-assessed efficacy of two diseases and two treatments. *Am J Clin Dermatol, 3*(5), 341-348.

FDA: U.S. Food and Drug Administration (1995). Dietary supplement health and education act of 1994. Retrieved on February 12, 2005, at http://www.cfsan.fda.gov/~dms/dietsupp.html.

FDA: U.S. Food and Drug Administration. (2001). FDA warns consumers to discontinue use of botanical products that contain aristolochic acid. Consumer advisory, April 11, 2001. Retrieved June 24, 2005, from www.cfsan.fda.gov/~dms/addsbot.html.

FDA: U.S. Food and Drug Administration. (2004). Health effects of androstenedione. FDA white paper, March 11, 2004. Retrieved June 24, 2005, from www.fda.gov/oc/whitepapers/andro.html.

FDA: U.S. Food and Drug Administration. (2003). FDA warns consumers about use of "Litargirio"—Traditional remedy that contains dangerous levels of lead. FDA talk paper, T03-67. Retrieved June 24, 2005, from www.fda.gov/bbs/topics/ANSWERetS/2003/ANS01253.html.

Fetrow, C.W., & Avila, J.R. (2004). *Professional's handbook of complementary & alternative medicines.* Philadelphia: Lippincott Williams & Wilkins.

Field, T. (1999). Massage therapy: More than a laying on of hands. *Contemp Pediatr, 16*(5), 77-94.

Field, T. (1995). Massage therapy for infants and children. *J Dev Behav Pediatr, 16*(2), 105-111.

Francis, A.J., & Dempster, RJ. (2002). Effect of valerian, *Valeriana edulis,* on sleep difficulties in children with intellectual deficits: Randomised trial. *Phytomedicine, 9*(4), 273-279.

Gardiner, P., Dvorkin, L., & Kemper, K.J. (2004). Supplement use growing among children and adolescents. *Pediatr Ann, 33*(4), 227-232.

Grazzi, L., Andrasik, F., D'Amico, D., Leone, M., et al. (2001). Electromyographic biofeedback-assisted relaxation training in juvenile episodic tension-type headache: Clinical outcome at three-year follow-up. *Cephalalgia, 21*(8), 798-803.

Gross-Tsur, V., Lahad, A., & Shalev, R.S. (2003). Use of complementary medicine in children with attention deficit hyperactivity disorder and epilepsy. *Pediatr Neurol, 29*(1), 53-55.

Hrastinger, A., Dietz, B., Bauer, R., et al. (2005). Is there clinical evidence supporting the use of botanical dietary supplements in children? *J Pediatr, 146*(3), 311-317.

Hurvitz, E.A., Leonard, C., Ayyangar, R., & Nelson, V.S. (2003). Complementary and alternative medicine use in families of children with cerebral palsy. *Dev Med Child Neurol, 45*(6), 364-370.

Hypericum Depression Trial Study Group. (2002). Effect of *Hypericum perforatum* (St. John's wort) in major depressive disorder: A randomized controlled trial. *JAMA, 287*(14), 1807-1814.

Jacobs, J., Jonas, W.B., Jimenez-Perez, M., & Crothers, D. (2003). Homeopathy for childhood diarrhea: Combined results and meta-analysis from three randomized, controlled clinical trials. *Pediatr Infect Dis J, 22*(3), 229-234.

Jepson, R.G., Mihaljevic, L., & Craig, J. (2004). Cranberries for preventing urinary tract infections. *Cochrane Database Syst Rev,* (2):CD001321.

Kemp, A.S. (2003). Cost of illness of atopic dermatitis in children: A societal perspective. *PharmacoEconomics, 21*(2), 105-113.

Kemper, K.J. (2002). *The holistic pediatrician.* New York: Quill.

Kemper, K.J. (2001). Complementary and alternative medicine for children: Does it work? *Arch Dis Child, 84*(1), 6-9.

Kemper, K.J. (1998). "Something wicked this way comes"—herbs even witches should avoid. *Contemp Pediatr, 15*(6), 49-64.

Kemper, K.J. (1996). Seven herbs every paediatrician should know. *Contemp Pediatr, 13*(12), 79-91.

Kemper, K.J., & Gardiner, P. (2004). Herbal medicines. In R.E. Behrman, R.M. Kliegman, & H.B. Jenson (Eds.). *Nelson textbook of pediatrics* (17th ed.). Philadelphia: Saunders.

Kemper, K.J., & Lester, M.R. (1999). Alternative asthma therapies: An evidence-based review. *Contemp Pediatr, 16*(3), 162, 165, 167-168, 173, 177, 179-180, 186, 191-192, 195.

Kline, R.M., Kline, J.J., Di Palma, J., & Barbero, G.J. (2001). Enteric-coated, pH-dependent peppermint oil capsules for the treatment of irritable bowel syndrome in children. *J Pediatr, 138*(1), 125-128.

Krieger, D., & Krippner, S. (1993). *Accepting your power to heal: The personal practice of therapeutic touch.* Rochester, VT: Inner Traditions International, Limited.

Lanski, S.L., Greenwald, M., Perkins, A., & Simon, H.K. (2003). Herbal therapy use in a pediatric emergency department population: Expect the unexpected. *Pediatrics, 111*(5 Pt 1), 981-985.

Loman, D.G. (2003). The use of complementary and alternative health care practices among children. *J Pediatr Health Care, 17*(2), 58-63.

Magkos, F., Arvaniti, F., & Zampelas, A. (2003). Organic food: Nutritious food or food for thought? A review of the evidence. *International Journal of Food Sciences & Nutrition, 54*(5), 357-371.

McCrindle, B.W., Helden, E., & Conner, W.T. (1998). Garlic extract therapy in children with hypercholesterolemia. *Arch Pediatr Adolesc Med, 152*(11), 1089-1094.

McCurdy, E.A., Spangler, J.G., Wofford, M.M., et al. (2003). Religiosity is associated with the use of complementary medical therapies by pediatric oncology patients. *J Pediatr Hematol Oncol, 25*(2), 125-129.

Miller, S.K. (2004). Magnet therapy for pain control: An analysis of theory and research. *Adv Nurse Pract, 12*(5), 49-52.

Moyer, C.A., Rounds, J., & Hannum, J.W. (2004). A meta-analysis of massage therapy research. *Psychol Bull, 130*(1), 3-18.

NCCAM: National Center for Complementary and Alternative Medicine. (2002). What is complementary and alternative medicine? NCCAM Publication No. D156. Retrieved June 24, 2005, from http://nccam.nih.gov/health/whatiscam/#sup1.

NCCAM: National Center for Complementary and Alternative Medicine. (2003a). About chiropractic and its use in treating low-back pain. NCCAM Publication No. D196. Retrieved June 24, 2005, from http://nccam.nih.gov/health/chiropractic/index.htm.

NCCAM: National Center for Complementary and Alternative Medicine. (2003b). Questions and answers about homeopathy. NCCAM Publication No. D183. Retrieved June 24, 2005, from http://nccam.nih.gov/health/homeopathy/index.htm#37.

NCCAM: National Center for Complementary and Alternative Medicine. (2004). NCCAM consumer advisory on ephedra. Retrieved June 24, 2005, from http://nccam.nih.gov/health/alerts/ephedra/consumeradvisory.htm.

Ng, D.K., Pok-yu, M.S-p., Hong, S-h., et al. (2004). A double-blind, randomized, placebo-controlled trial of acupuncture for the treatment of childhood persistent allergic rhinitis. *Pediatrics, 114*(5), 1242-1247.

NIH: National Institutes of Health. (1997). Acupuncture. NIH Consensus Statement. *15*(5), 1-34. Retrieved June 24, 2005, from http://odp.od.nih.gov/consensus/cons/107/107_statement.htm.

Palm, L., Blennow, G., & Wetterberg, L. (1997). Long-term melatonin treatment in blind children and young adults with circadian sleep-wake disturbances. *Dev Med Child Neurol, 39*(5), 319-325.

PDR. (2001). *PDR for nutritional supplements.* Montvale, NJ: Medical Economics, Thomson Healthcare.

PDR. (2004). *PDR for herbal medicines* (3rd ed.). Montvale, NJ: Thomson PDR.

PDR. (2005). *PDR for nonprescription drugs and dietary supplements.* Montvale, NJ: Thomson PDR.

Perry, C.L., McGuire, M.T., Neumark-Sztainer, D., & Story, M. (2002). Adolescent vegetarians: How well do their dietary patterns meet the *Healthy People 2010* objectives? *Archives of Pediatrics & Adolescent Medicine, 156*(5), 431-437.

Pfaffenrath, V., Diener, H.C., Fischer, M., et al. (2002). The efficacy and safety of *Tanacetum parthenium* (feverfew) in migraine prophylaxis—A double-blind, multicentre, randomized placebo-controlled dose-response study. *Cephalalgia, 22*(7), 523-532.

Pitetti, R., Singh, S., Hornyak, D., et al. (2001). Complementary and alternative medicine use in children. *Pediatr Emerg Care, 17*(3), 165-169.

Portnoi, G., Chng, L.A., Karimi-Tabesh, L., et al. (2003). Prospective comparative study of the safety and effectiveness of ginger for the treatment of nausea and vomiting in pregnancy. *Am J Obstet Gynecol, 189*(5), 1374-1377.

Reznik, M., Ozuah, P.O., Fanco, K., et al. (2002). Use of complementary therapy by adolescents with asthma. *Arch Pediatr Adolesc Med, 156*(10), 1042-1044.

Sanders, H., Davis, M.F., Duncan, B., et al. (2003). Use of complementary and alternative medical therapies among children with special health care needs in southern Arizona. *Pediatrics, 111*(3), 584-587.

Sawni-Sikand, A., Schubiner, H., & Thomas, R.L. (2002). Use of complementary/alternative therapies among children in primary care pediatrics. *Ambul Pediatr, 2*(2), 99-103.

Scharff, L., & Kemper, K.J. (2003). For chronic pain, complementary and alternative medical approaches. *Contemp Pediatr, 20*(10), 117-118, 121-122, 130, 133, 137-138, 141.

Schlager, T.A., Anderson, S., Trudell, J., & Hendley, J.O. (1999). Effect of cranberry juice on bacteriuria in children with neurogenic bladder receiving intermittent catheterization. *J Pediatr, 135*(6), 698-702.

Sibinga, E., Ottoline, M.C., Duggan, A.K., & Wilson, M.H. (2004). Parent-pediatrician communication about complementary and alternative medicine use for children. *Clin Pediatr, 43*(4), 367-373.

Sinha, D., & Efron, D. (2005). Complementary and alternative medicine use in children with attention deficit hyperactivity disorder. *J Paediatr Child Health, 41*(1-2), 23-26.

Sparber, A. (2001). State boards of nursing and scope of practice of registered nurses performing complementary therapies. *Online J Iss Nurs, 6*(3), 1-10. Retrieved June 24, 2005, from www.nursingworld.org/ojin/topic15/tpc15_6.htm.

Stein, D. (1999). *Essential reiki: A complete guide to an ancient healing art*. Freedom, CA: The Crossing Press, Inc.

Stevinson, C., & Ernst, E. (2000). Valerian for insomnia: A systematic review of randomized clinical trials. *Sleep Medicine, 1*(2), 91-99.

Taylor, J.A., Weber, W., Standish, L., et al. (2003). Efficacy and safety of echinacea in treating upper respiratory tract infections in children: A randomized controlled trial. *JAMA, 290*(1), 2824-2830.

Tribal Connections. (2005). eHealth Information: Traditional healing. Retrieved June 24, 2005, from www.tribalconnections.org/ehealthinfo/trad_healing.html.

Van Niel, C.W., Feudtner, C., Garrison, M.M., & Christakis, D.A. (2002). Lactobacillus therapy for acute infectious diarrhea in children: A meta-analysis. *Pediatrics, 109*(4), 678-684.

Vogler, B.K., & Ernst, E. (1999). Aloe vera: A systematic review of its clinical effectiveness. *Brit J Gen Pract, 49*(447), 823-828.

Vogler, B.K., Pittler, M.H., & Ernst, E. (1998). Feverfew as a preventive treatment for migraine: A systematic review. *Cephalalgia, 18*(10), 704-708.

Wang, S.M., & Kain, Z.N. (2002). P6 acupoint injections are as effective as droperidol in controlling early postoperative nausea and vomiting in children. *Anesthesiology, 97*(2), 359-366.

Weydert, J.A., Ball, T.M., & Davis, M.F. (2003). Systematic review of treatments for recurrent abdominal pain. *Pediatrics, 111*(1), e1-e11.

WHCCAMP: White House Commission on Complementary and Alternative Medicine Policy. (2002). *White House Commission on Complementary and Alternative Medicine Policy: Final report*. Retrieved on June 24, 2005, at http://whccamp.hhs.gov/finalreport.html.

Winemiller, M.H., Billow, R.G., Laskowski, E.R., & Harmsen, W.S. (2003). Effect of magnetic vs. sham-magnetic insoles on plantar heel pain: A randomized controlled trial. *JAMA, 290*(11), 1474-1478.

Yuksek, M.S., Erdem, A.F., Atalay, C., & Demirel, A. (2003). Acupressure versus oxybutinin in the treatment of enuresis. *J Int Med Res, 31*(6), 552-526.

Zeltzer, L.K., Tsao, J.C.I., Stelling, C., et al. (2002). A phase I study on the feasibility and acceptability of an acupuncture/hypnosis intervention for chronic pediatric pain. *J Pain Symptom Manage, 24*(4), 437-446.

Zhdanova, I.V., Wurtman, R.J., & Wagstaff, J. (1999). Effects of a low dose of melatonin on sleep in children with Angelman syndrome. *J Pediatr Endocrinol Metab, 12*(1), 57-67.

CHAPTER

57 Nonpharmacologic Treatments and Pediatric Procedures

LINDA S. BLASEN

Select the best answer for each of the following questions:

1. Ross, a 4-year-old preschooler, is brought in by his mother for evaluation of eye pain. He was playing in the sandbox prior to the onset of the problem. You would apply ocular fluorescein staining to the eye surface to detect:
   A. Disruption of the corneal surface.
   B. Light sensitivity in the eye.
   C. Chalazion or hordeolum.
   D. Gonococcal conjunctivitis.

2. You find that Ross has a large grain of sand in his left eye, along with a localized corneal abrasion. Which is the appropriate sequence for attempting removal of ocular foreign body?
   A. Use an ocular burr; irrigate, and lift off with needle.
   B. Irrigate off, remove with moist cotton-tip applicator; use an ophthalmic burr.
   C. Irrigate off, remove with moist cotton-tip applicator, refer if unsuccessful with 2 to 3 attempts.
   D. Remove with moist cotton-tip applicator and refer at once.

3. Jaden, a 2-year-old male, is brought to your office for brown ear drainage. You discover a right external ear cerumen impaction. The tympanic membrane is obscured by the cerumen. The next step is:
   A. Irrigate with high-flow peroxide and reinspect the canal.
   B. Prescribe an otic antimicrobial as you cannot visualize the tympanic membrane.

   C. Prescribe an oral antimicrobial and refer to ENT at once.
   D. Use a plastic cerumen spoon to gently remove the plug and reinspect the canal.

4. Tonyette, a 3-year-old female, presents with a gumdrop in her left nostril. She put it there 2 hours ago at a birthday party. There is no epistaxis and she is relatively cooperative. How should the pediatric nurse practitioner proceed?
   A. Remove with a Yankauer suction device and give the gumdrop back to child.
   B. Provide local vasoconstriction and topical anesthetic then remove with a forceps or curette.
   C. Perform a Heimlich maneuver to dislodge the candy.
   D. Refer at once to ENT for conscious sedation and removal.

5. If a permanent tooth has been completely avulsed in the past 30 minutes, the pediatric nurse practitioner should clean the tooth and socket with sterile 0.9% sodium chloride and:
   A. Replace the tooth in the socket.
   B. Put the tooth in gauze and call a dentist.
   C. Call a dentist for instruction.
   D. Order a mandible CT to check the root structure.

6. Jess, age 4, fell against the edge of table. The right front tooth is pushed back and embedded into the soft tissue of the gum. Your best action is:

A. Try to pull it forward immediately.
B. Give an injection of lidocaine for comfort.
C. Refer to a dentist for evaluation.
D. Advise the parent it is unlikely the area will ever be normal.

7. You order home pulse oximetry monitoring for a 5-month-old patient with bradycardia. You educate the infant's parents about use of the device and advise them to avoid:
   A. Applying to an area of frequent movement for best tissue oxygenation.
   B. Using the probe on fingers or toes of patient.
   C. Applying in areas of good vascular supply.
   D. Shutting off the alarms on the device.

8. Evidenced-based information demonstrates that ventricular fibrillation or pulseless ventricular tachycardia responds best to early defibrillation. Which of the following statements regarding defibrillation is INACCURATE?
   A. Defibrillation is 90% effective if the initial shock is delivered within 4 minutes of cardiac arrest with CPR in progress.
   B. Defibrillation is 70% effective if the initial shock is delivered within 4 minutes of cardiac arrest without CPR in progress.
   C. Effectiveness of shocking in cardiac arrest decreases 10% each hour thereafter.
   D. Ventricular fibrillation occurs in 10% to 20% of pediatric cardiac arrests.

9. You are working in the pediatric emergency department when an 11-month-old infant is rushed through the door by his frantic parents. They report he was eating grapes and suddenly turned blue. He is not breathing but he is conscious. You act immediately by:
   A. Applying an external defibrillator and await cardiac arrest.
   B. Begin chest compressions at a rate of 100 per minute.
   C. Ordering a stat soft tissue neck film to identify the location of the foreign body.

D. Positioning the baby face down with his head lower than his torso over your forearm and deliver five midscapular back blows in rapid succession.

10. The action you selected in the previous question did not work. The infant is now unconscious. The pediatric nurse practitioner's next action is to:
    A. Position the infant on his back on a firm surface, open the airway with a tongue-jaw lift and use a finger-sweep to remove any visible objects.
    B. Position the infant prone and use successive combinations of five back blows until spontaneous respiration resumes.
    C. Prepare to intubate and hope the passage of the endotracheal tube will propel the foreign body down the esophagus.
    D. Obtain a Yankauer-type suction tip for direct suction to aid foreign body removal.

11. Damon is 10 years old and has an ileus postorthopedic surgery. He needs a nasogastric tube placed for decompression. The pediatric nurse practitioner should NOT include which of the following actions?
    A. Estimates length of tube by measuring from the earlobe to the xiphoid process and mark tube.
    B. Lubricates tube and passes through naris until the marked section reaches the edge of the nostril.
    C. Microwave the tube before tube placement but after measuring the tube for length.
    D. Verify placement by aspirating and checking the aspirate for a pH of 1.5 to 3.5.

12. Angel is 3 months old and needs a gastric tube placed for feeding supplementation. Which of the following actions is INCORRECT?
    A. Estimate tube length by measuring from the earlobe to the xiphoid process and marking the tube.
    B. Always place the tube through the naris of a young infant after lubrication.

C. Chill the tube in ice water to stiffen it prior to insertion.

D. Verify placement by aspirating and checking the aspirate for correct pH.

13. You need a urine specimen for protein and ketone testing from your patient. The most appropriate technique for collecting this specimen is:

A. Cleanse the periurethral area thoroughly and attach a collection bag in the noncontinent child or obtain the urine in a specimen container in the continent child.

B. Perform urethral catheterization regardless of age or continence for this specimen collection.

C. Send a disposable bedpan home with parent to use for attempting to catch urine for testing.

D. Perform a transabdominal percutaneous aspiration from the urinary bladder.

14. Two-year-old Joya has symptoms consistent with urinary tract infection. You know that urethral catheterization is indicated for collection of sterile urine specimens. Which of the following is an INCORRECT statement?

A. Contraindications included absolute neutropenia.

B. After the catheter has been placed and urine is returning, it is best to drain the specimen into an emesis basin.

C. The female patient should be supine and in a modified lithotomy-type position on the bed for catheterization.

D. The foreskin of the male patient should be retracted prior to cleaning if possible.

15. Kimberly, age 14, presents with a chief complaint of "lost tampon." You reassure her that the tampon has not moved out of the vaginal area and can be removed. All of the following are accurate EXCEPT:

A. This is not an unusual problem for an adolescent female.

B. The supine lithotomy position offers an opportunity for you to observe and remove the foreign body.

C. A stat gynecology consult is needed as the problem is likely to need surgical intervention.

D. The knee-chest position can be utilized for further removal efforts if initial attempt in the lithotomy position is unsuccessful.

16. Jaquee is 10 years old with a history of type 1 diabetes mellitus. She is premenarche. Her mother has noted an unpleasant odor in the child's genital area but cannot see anything except some whitish-grey clumps at the introitus. She is concerned and brings her in for an exam immediately. Which action is LEAST appropriate?

A. Obtain a thorough history including past GU complaints.

B. Attempt to identify if a potential foreign body may be in the vagina and the duration of insertion time.

C. Recall that a vaginal foreign body in a prepubertal child is always a sign of sexual abuse and notify authorities immediately.

D. Assist the child to a frog-leg position for inspection and begin a gentle initial exam examination.

17. Tommy presents with a 1 cm laceration of the right forearm. It occurred 3 days ago while playing outside. His father is concerned because the wound keeps opening. There is no sign of infection. The most appropriate action is to:

A. Irrigate with 300 ml after providing local anesthesia.

B. Clean the wound thoroughly and instruct Tommy's father regarding wound care and healing by secondary intention.

C. Suture the wound regardless of time frame since injury.

D. Cauterize wound margins in order to seal the epithelial cells.

18. The initial phase of wound healing consists of:

A. Neovascularization.

B. Epithelialization.

C. Remodeling.

D. Inflammation.

19. Major indications for suturing as an initial wound management technique include:
   A. Cosmetic appearance, hemostasis, and primary intention.
   B. Delayed closure of more than 24 hours.
   C. Heavily contaminated wounds worrisome for infection.
   D. Patient or parental preference for suturing.

20. In which body areas would the pediatric nurse practitioner NEVER infiltrate lidocaine with epinephrine for local anesthesia of a wound?
   A. Scalp, dorsal foot, calf.
   B. Forearm, forehead, wrist.
   C. Fingers, toes, penis.
   D. Thigh, buttock, upper arm.

21. Certain actions are essential prior to suturing a wound. Which of the following is MOST important action?
   A. A thorough neurovascular and functional assessment.
   B. Exsanguination of the extremity by compression.
   C. Evaluation of parental medication allergies.
   D. Consult a local surgeon for instructions.

22. In addition to assessing the wound, providing local anesthesia, and irrigating the wound well, it is important to AVOID:
   A. Repairing the wound symmetrically, placing sutures about .5 cm from the wound margin on either side.
   B. Placing the sutures as rapidly as possible.

C. Securing the child appropriately in a parent's arms or restraint.
   D. Discussing home care and wound observation with the parent.

23. Surgical skin glue preparations offer some advantage over suturing. On which of the following wounds might the pediatric nurse practitioner use a skin adhesive?
   A. A laceration over the right posterior elbow.
   B. A laceration more than 8 hours old.
   C. A simple straight laceration in a tension-free area.
   D. A laceration over the left prepatellar region.

24. Sprains and contusions represent common pediatric injuries. The mnemonic, "RICE," represents an effective way to create comfort and promote healing. The methods utilized by the RICE approach include:
   A. Warm moist heat, elevation, and rapid return to activity.
   B. Warm moist heat, elevation, and gradual return to activity.
   C. Rapid return to activity, ice, compression, and elevation.
   D. Rest, ice, compression, and elevation.

25. Subluxation of the radial head is colloquially referred to as "nursemaid's elbow." If there is no risk for fracture, which of the following reduction techniques is recommended?
   A. The supination-flexion maneuver.
   B. The flexion-supination maneuver.
   C. Use of finger traps with weight on humerus.
   D. The hypopronation and extension maneuver.

ANSWERS

1. *Answer:* A
   Rationale: Corneal foreign bodies and severe conjunctivitis can cause breakdown of the corneal surface, resulting in corneal abrasion. Fluorescein stain is taken up, or absorbed, in the area of disruption. It identifies the area and will also highlight a foreign body.

2. *Answer:* C
   Rationale: Attempts at removal of an ocular foreign body should progress from least invasive to most invasive.

3. *Answer:* D
   Rationale: If the tympanic membrane cannot be visualized, a perforation cannot be excluded. It is safest to attempt to remove enough wax to visualize the membrane before proceeding to irrigation.

4. *Answer:* B
   Rationale: With a cooperative child, there is a reasonable expectation of removal of a recently inserted nasal foreign body. Vasoconstriction will decrease the chance of epistaxis. Topical anesthetics increase comfort and increase patient cooperation.

5. *Answer:* A
   Rationale: If an avulsed permanent tooth and its socket are thoroughly cleansed and the tooth restored less than 90 minutes after the injury, there is a moderate possibility of successful reimplantation

6. *Answer:* C
   Rationale: An immediate dental referral is advised. The tooth may need realignment or other treatment.

7. *Answer:* A
   Rationale: Areas of high movement result in inaccurate measurement due to potential dislodging of the probe.

8. *Answer:* C

Rationale: Effectiveness of shocking decreases 10% each minute after the first 4 minutes.

9. *Answer:* D
   Rationale: The correct immediate action for a conscious choking infant under age 1 is to place the infant over your forearm with the head lower than the torso and deliver five back blows. Providing a list of safe finger-foods would be an appropriate teaching strategy after removing the obstruction.

10. *Answer:* A
    Rationale: The American Heart Association recommends that the unconscious choking infant be placed on his back on a firm surface, open his mouth by a tongue-jaw lift, and any visible foreign body be swept out with the fingers.

11. *Answer:* C
    Rationale: A nasogastric tube may require stiffening prior to placement, not heating. Microwave heating of any product of this nature may cause burning of the patient or product damage.

12. *Answer:* B
    Rationale: Infants under 6 months old who appear to be obligate nose breathers should have oral tube placement. The tube is measured differently.

13. *Answer:* A
    Rationale: Specimens obtained for testing purposes unrelated to evaluation of urinary tract infection do not need to be sterile.

14. *Answer:* B
    Rationale: All sterile urine specimen collection should drain from the catheter into a sterile container.

15. *Answer:* C
    Rationale: Surgery is not indicated. A "lost" tampon most often results when the strings ascend into the vagina and is usually simple to remove. In either case, sharing the information that her situation is not unusual

offers the adolescent reassurance at an awkward moment.

16. *Answer:* C

Rationale: You should consider the possibility of sexual abuse when a prepubescent adolescent has a vaginal foreign body. However, it is most prudent to include that concern as part of a wider differential diagnosis and then proceed with a detailed history and careful physical exam.

17. *Answer:* B

Rationale: It is inappropriate to suture the wound at this time. A high potential for infection exists as the wound is several days old.

18. *Answer:* D

Rationale: Inflammation constitutes the initial phase of wound healing. It begins immediately upon injury with triggering of the clotting cascade and initiation of the inflammatory response.

19. *Answer:* A

Rationale: Several reasons, including cosmetic appearance, hemostasis, and primary intention, support suturing as an initial wound management technique.

20. *Answer:* C

Rationale: Epinephrine causes significant vasoconstriction which precludes use in end-distal circulation, such as the fingers.

21. *Answer:* A

Rationale: This assessment should be performed as part of the initial assessment.

22. *Answer:* B

Rationale: Sutures must be placed carefully and symmetrically to avoid inversion or irregular approximation of wound edges.

23. *Answer:* C

Rationale: A wound with high tension, such as over the knee or elbow, will open under pressure if closed with skin adhesive. A dirty wound is best not repaired with adhesive.

24. *Answer:* D

Rationale: These measures treat inflammation and bleeding by cooling and elevation, promote venous return, and promote healing by providing a rest for the affected area.

25. *Answer:* A

Rationale: In this maneuver, the provider places his or her thumb over the patient's radial head with gentle pressure, fully supinates the arm, and then flexes the lower arm completely toward the upper arm. Most times, a click is felt. It helps to then stay out of child's sight, until a parent reports spontaneous use of affected arm. If there is any question of fracture, a radiograph should be obtained first.

BIBLIOGRAPHY

Adams, J. (2006). Genital complaints in prepubertal girls. Retrieved on May 27, 2006, from http://www.emedicine.com/ped/topic2894.htm.

American Heart Association (2005). BLS healthcare provider online renewal course. Retrieved July 19, 2005, from www.americanheart.org/presenter.jhtml?identifier=3019553.

Atkins, D.L., & Kenney, M.A. (2004). Automated external defibrillators: Safety and efficacy in children and adolescents. *Pediatr Clin North Am, 51*(5), 1443-1462.

Burns, C.E., Brady, M., Dunn, A., & Starr, N.B. (2000). *Pediatric primary care: A handbook for nurse practitioners.* Philadelphia: Saunders.

Colyar, M.R. & Ehrhardt, C. (2004). *Ambulatory care procedures for the nurse practitioner* (2nd ed.). Philadelphia: F.A. Davis.

Dermabond topical skin adhesives. (2006). Retrieved on June 28, 2006, from www.closuremed.com/products_professional.htm#dermabond.

Doud Galli, S.K., & Constantinides, M. (2004). Wound closure technique. Retrieved June 30, 2006, from www.emedicine.com/ent/topic35.htm.

Goepp, J.G., & Hostetler, M.A. (2001). *Procedures for primary care pediatricians.* St. Louis: Mosby.

Goodhue, C.J., & Brady, M.A. (2004). Respiratory disorders. In C.E. Burns, A.M. Dunn, M.A. Brady, et al. (Eds.). *Pediatric primary care* (3rd ed.). St. Louis: Saunders.

Marsden, J. (2002). Ophthalmic trauma in the emergency department. *Accident Emerg Nurs*, *10*(3), 136-142.

Nguyen, Q.A. (2005). Epistaxis. Retrieved on May 27, 2006, from http://www.emedicine.com/ent/topic701.htm.

Petersen-Smith, A.M. (2004). Ear disorders. In C.E. Burns, A.M. Dunn, M.A. Brady, et al. (Eds.). *Pediatric primary care* (3rd ed.). St. Louis: Saunders.

Schulze, S.L., Kerschner, J., & Beste, D. (2002). Pediatric external auditory canal foreign bodies: A review of 698 cases. *Otolaryngol Head Neck Surg*, *127*(1), 73-78.

Wall, E.J. (2000). Practical primary pediatric orthopedics. *Nurs Clin North Am*, *35*(1), 95.

NOTES

FUTURE EDUCATION AND PRACTICE ISSUES

58 Evolving Roles for Pediatric and Nurse Practitioners

KARI CRAWFORD AND STACEY TEICHER

Select the best answer for each of the following questions:

1. One of the best ways to promote the profession to lay people and medical professionals is to:
   A. Speak at schools of nursing.
   B. Introduce yourself as a pediatric nurse practitioner.
   C. Volunteer to take blood pressures at area health fairs.
   D. Wear a white lab coat to look professional.

2. Health care policies guide direction in health care and practice and support pediatric nurse practitioners as licensed and independent providers. One way to help promote continued autonomy is to:
   A. Be active in local health departments.
   B. Write articles for journals.
   C. Become active in the legislative process.
   D. Recruit new nurses to attend graduate school.

3. Across the country there are some restrictions to nurse practitioner practice that vary from state to state. One restriction present in many states is:
   A. Lack of full prescriptive authority.
   B. Inability to be recognized as nurse practitioners.
   C. No direct or indirect reimbursement.
   D. Inability to work in an acute care setting.

4. The Healthy Eating and Activity Together (H.E.A.T.) program, developed by members of NAPNAP, provides guidelines to prevent childhood obesity. This program is an example of how nurse practitioners can:
   A. Promote health through education.
   B. Write articles for journals.
   C. Advocate for families of children in the workplace.
   D. Affect change in legislation for nurse practitioner legal authority.

5. A Latino family has brought their 5-year-old into the emergency department for an asthma attack. The mother is quiet and sits in the corner of the room. Only the father answers the medical questions. The nurse caring for the patient is concerned by the mother's apparent lack of involvement. As a pediatric nurse practitioner you:
   A. Interrupt the procedures in the room, remove the mom from the room and see if she will answer questions.
   B. Assess the situation and inform the nurse that often in Latino cultures the husband is the head of the household
   C. You call social services when they are discharged to go to the home to investigate abuse.
   D. You reassure the nurse that nothing is wrong.

6. The role of the pediatric nurse practitioner has evolved over the past 30 years and many are working in nonprimary care settings such as:
   A. Private primary care physician offices.
   B. Well child clinics affiliated with university teaching hospitals.

C. Rural area clinics serving remote populations.

D. Specialty clinics like cardiology or oncology.

7. The limitations imposed on medical resident hours have opened up new opportunities for pediatric nurse practitioners in inpatient settings. The opportunity to work on inpatient teams provides patient continuity and:

A. Decreases job opportunities for pediatric nurse practitioners.

B. Offers cost-effective solutions to acute care facilities.

C. Increases bedside nursing in intensive care units.

D. Takes jobs away from physicians.

8. A new level of education, advocated by the American Colleges of Nursing, is geared to advance scientific knowledge in practice for the nurse practitioner is:

A. Doctor of Nursing Care (DNC).

B. Doctor of Nursing Science (DNS).

C. Doctor of Philosophy in Nursing (PhD).

D. Doctor of Nursing Practice (DNP).

9. One major advantage to joining national organizations such as the National Association of Pediatric Nurse Practitioners (NAPNAP) is:

A. Gain information about the location of conferences.

B. Ability to meet other types of health care providers.

C. Obtain professional education, advocacy, and support.

D. Identify other nurse practitioners in your local area.

10. One way to become involved in research projects is to:

A. Negotiate with your employer for time on the job set aside for research.

B. Ask other nurse practitioners what they do.

C. Ask the doctor in your practice to participate in his or her research projects.

D. Read research articles on your time off.

11. You are a pediatric nurse practitioner and you notice the physician in your practice has started treating otitis media with Zithromax instead of amoxicillin. You should:

A. Continue treating your otitis media patients with amoxicillin.

B. Start prescribing Zithromax for all otitis media infections.

C. Research the evidence to determine the most effective treatment.

D. Call the drug company and ask if Zithromax has been approved for treatment of otitis media in children.

12. What is one way pediatric nurse practitioners can eliminate barriers to reimbursement?

A. Educate yourself on state laws and requirements and keep abreast of new state regulations.

B. Participate in strikes and demonstrations.

C. Bill your services under the physician provider number.

D. Accept that pediatric nurse practitioners should not be reimbursed 100% of what the physicians are reimbursed.

13. You work for a physician who wants to bill your services under his provider number. You:

A. Agree since by doing so, the practice gets reimbursed at the physician rate for your services.

B. Call your state board of nursing and ask what the laws are regarding reimbursement.

C. Insist on using your own provider number for your services.

D. Ask other pediatric nurse practitioners what they are doing.

14. Changes in the curriculum in pediatric nurse practitioner programs are driven by:

A. Legislation.

B. The changing demands in the health care arena.

C. Physicians.

D. Public supply and demand.

15. The Doctor of Nursing Practice will allow advanced practice nurses the opportunity to have a degree comparable to:
   A. MD, DDS, PsyD.
   B. MBA, MBS.
   C. PPD, MD, DDP.
   D. PhD, MSN.

16. You are a pediatric nurse practitioner working in acute care at a large teaching hospital. You have been asked to provide an analysis of the nurse practitioner care in your department. The best way to do this is:

   A. Systematically collect data on pediatric nurse practitioner services and outcomes in the department.
   B. Ask patients and families how they rate the care from their pediatric nurse practitioner versus their physician.
   C. This is the job of the research team and refuse the assignment.
   D. Compare your patient volume to the physician's patient volume.

NOTES

_____

ANSWERS

1. *Answer:* B
Rationale: It is confusing in the health care arena for lay people to understand the various roles of the health care team. Introducing yourself as a pediatric nurse practitioner provides the opportunity to educate families on the role of pediatric nurse practitioners and the skills they bring to the health care team.

2. *Answer:* C
Rationale: Legislation moves forward only by active lobbying and organizations that make their message heard. If all pediatric nurse practitioners were active in legislation, Congress would face a very powerful team. This would help the profession move policy through faster and allow each individual to remain better informed.

3. *Answer:* A
Rationale: Across the country, practice patterns still vary which make it confusing for not only practicing pediatric nurse practitioners but the consumer as well. Several states still do not have prescriptive authority and many do not allow pediatric nurse practitioner to prescribe schedule II drugs.

4. *Answer:* A
Rationale: Nurse practitioners are well-known for their focus on prevention. Education of other health care members and the public are key components to this endeavor.

5. *Answer:* B
Rationale: In many cultures such as Asian, Islamic, and Latino, people view the male as head of household and the females are not to answer questions unless the male deems it appropriate. Pediatric nurse practitioners must be knowledgeable about the norm for their patients' cultures.

6. *Answer:* D
Rationale: With increasing demands for specialty services, more pediatric nurse practitioners are opting for positions in specialty clinics such as orthopedic, cardiology, and pulmonology.

7. *Answer:* B
Rationale: There are multiple changes in the acute care arena such as decreased resident work hours and increased number of patients. These changes have opened opportunities for pediatric nurse practitioners to provide care in acute settings such as pediatric inpatient units and intensive care units.

8. *Answer:* D
Rationale: Obtaining a terminal degree such as the DNP would allow pediatric nurse practitioners to have comparable educational credentials as other collaborating professions such as MD, PsyD, PharmD, or DDS.

9. *Answer:* C
Rationale: NAPNAP is an avenue to provide a voice to the pediatric nurse practitioners across the country to promote education, prevention, research, and advocacy.

10. *Answer:* A
Rationale: In a recent study conducted by NAPNAP, pediatric nurse practitioners said that they simply do not have time or feel that they have adequate time to conduct research. Negotiating on-the-job time to conduct research projects is one way to promote research in the clinical setting.

11. *Answer:* C
Rationale: Utilizing an evidenced-based approach to the treatment of disease in the pediatric setting is the best way to provide optimal care to children and their families. The pediatric nurse practitioner must be astute in his or her ability to use databases and libraries to seek out the best evidence available for patient health care.

12. *Answer:* A
Rationale: It is critical for nurse practitioners to fully understand reimbursement mechanisms and rules for the state where they practice. There are considerable penalties for incorrect billing and coding.

13. *Answer:* B
Rationale: Pediatric nurse practitioners must know the laws and regulations of their state regarding reimbursement and follow those laws accordingly.

14. *Answer:* B

Rationale: The ever-changing demands for health care services will often guide the direction for pediatric nurse practitioner curriculums. For example, to respond to the need for more inpatient focused pediatric nurse practitioners, many universities and colleges are creating acute care pediatric nurse practitioner programs.

15. *Answer:* A

Rationale: The DNP degree will be comparable to the Medical Doctor (MD), Doctor of Dentistry (DDS), Doctor of Physical Therapy (DPT), and Doctor of Psychology (PsyD).

16. *Answer:* A

Rationale: Collecting pediatric nurse practitioner services and outcome data will demonstrate the value and optimal health care services that they bring to the practice.

BIBLIOGRAPHY

American Association of Colleges of Nursing. (2004). AACN Position Statement on the Practice Doctorate in Nursing. Retrieved May 31, 2006, from www.aacn.nche.edu/DNP/pdf/DNP.pdf.

Bonnel, W.B., Starling, C.K., Wambach, K.A., & Tarnow, K. (2003). Blended roles: Preparing the advanced practice nurse educator/clinician with a web-based nurse educator certificate program. *J Prof Nurs, 19*(6), 347-353.

Burnweitt, C., Diana-Zerpa, J.A., Nahmad, N.H., et al. (2004). Nitrous oxide analgesia for minor pediatric surgical procedures: An effective alternative to conscious sedation. *J Pediatr Surg, 39*(3), 495-499.

Jackson, P.L., Kennedy, C., Sadler, L.S., et al. (2001). Professional practice of pediatric nurse practitioners: Implications for education and training of PNPs. *J Pediatr Health Care, 15*(6), 291-297.

Jackson, P.L., Kennedy, C., & Slaughter, R. (2003). Employment characteristics of recent PNPs. *J Pediatr Health Care, 17*(3), 133-139.

National Association for Pediatric Nurse Practitioners. (2006). Acute care NP's competencies. Retrieved on May 31, 2006, from http://www.napnap.org/index.cfm?page=10&sec=53.

Neiderhauser, V.P., & Kohr, L. (2005). Research endeavors among pediatric nurse practitioners (REAP) study. *J Pediatr Health Care, 19*(2), 80-89.

Pediatric Nursing Certification Board. (2006). PCNB acute care PNP certification exam. Retrieved on May 31, 2006, from http://www.pncb.org/ptistore/control/exams/ac/ac_news.

Sperhac, A.M., & Strodtbeck, F. (2001) Advanced practice in pediatric nursing: Blending roles. *Journal of Pediatric Nursing, 16*(2), 120-126.

Teicher, S., Crawford, K., Williams, B., Nelson, B., & Andrews, C. (2001). Emerging role of the pediatric nurse practitioner in acute care. *Pediatr Nurs, 27*(4), 387-390.

Wolfe, K.L. (2004). The role of the legal nurse consultant in risk management. *J Legal Nurse Consult, 15*(3), 13-14.

Wyatt, J. (2001). Continuing the discussion of advanced practice in acute care: Past and future. *Pediatr Nurs, 27*(4), 419-421.